Women's Mental Health

AF086745

Women's Mental Health

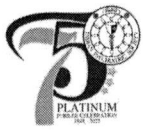

Indian Psychiatric Society Publication

Editors

Prabha S Chandra
MD FAMS FRCPsych FRCPE FRCOG (ad eundem)
Senior Professor
Department of Psychiatry
Dean, Behavioral Sciences
National Institute of
Mental Health and Neurosciences
Bengaluru, Karnataka, India
President
International Association of Women's Mental Health
Email: chandra@nimhans.ac.in

Aruna Yadiyal
MD
Professor
Department of Psychiatry
Father Muller Medical College and Hospital
Mangaluru, Karnataka, India
Email: aruna.g2779@gmail.com

Sai Krishna Tikka
DPM MD
Associate Professor
Department of Psychiatry
All India Institute of Medical Sciences
Bibinagar, Hyderabad, Telangana, India
Email: sai.psych@aiimsbibinagar.edu.in;
saikiatry@gmail.com

Debadatta Mohapatra
MD
Associate Professor
Department of Psychiatry
All India Institute of Medical Sciences
Bhubaneshwar, Odisha, India
Email: psych_debadatta@aiimsbhubaneswar.edu.in

Foreword
Florence Thibaut

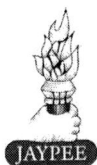

JAYPEE BROTHERS MEDICAL PUBLISHERS
The Health Sciences Publisher
New Delhi | London

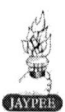 **Jaypee Brothers Medical Publishers (P) Ltd.**

Headquarters
Jaypee Brothers Medical Publishers (P) Ltd
EMCA House, 23/23-B
Ansari Road, Daryaganj
New Delhi 110 002, India
Landline: +91-11-23272143, +91-11-23272703
+91-11-23282021, +91-11-23245672
Email: jaypee@jaypeebrothers.com

Corporate Office
Jaypee Brothers Medical Publishers (P) Ltd
4838/24, Ansari Road, Daryaganj
New Delhi 110 002, India
Phone: +91-11-43574357
Fax: +91-11-43574314
Email: jaypee@jaypeebrothers.com

Overseas Office
JP Medical Ltd.
83, Victoria Street, London
SW1H 0HW (UK)
Phone: +44 20 3170 8910
Fax: +44 (0)20 3008 6180
Email: info@jpmedpub.com

Website: www.jaypeebrothers.com
Website: www.jaypeedigital.com

© 2024, Jaypee Brothers Medical Publishers and Indian Psychiatric Society

The views and opinions expressed in this book are solely those of the original contributor(s)/author(s) and do not necessarily represent those of editor(s) or publisher of the book.

All rights reserved. No part of this publication may be reproduced, stored or transmitted in any form or by any means, electronic, mechanical, photo copying, recording or otherwise, without the prior permission in writing of the publishers.

All brand names and product names used in this book are trade names, service marks, trademarks or registered trademarks of their respective owners. The publisher is not associated with any product or vendor mentioned in this book.

Medical knowledge and practice change constantly. This book is designed to provide accurate, authoritative information about the subject matter in question. However, readers are advised to check the most current information available on procedures included and check information from the manufacturer of each product to be administered, to verify the recommended dose, formula, method and duration of administration, adverse effects and contra indications. It is the responsibility of the practitioner to take all appropriate safety precautions. Neither the publisher nor the author(s)/editor(s) assume any liability for any injury and/or damage to persons or property arising from or related to use of material in this book.

This book is sold on the understanding that the publisher is not engaged in providing professional medical services. If such advice or services are required, the services of a competent medical professional should be sought.

Every effort has been made where necessary to contact holders of copyright to obtain permission to reproduce copyright material. If any have been inadvertently overlooked, the publisher will be pleased to make the necessary arrangements at the first opportunity.

Inquiries for bulk sales may be solicited at: jaypee@jaypeebrothers.com

Women's Mental Health

First Edition: **2025**

ISBN: 978-93-5696-722-9

Printed in India

Dedicated to

All the women who trusted us with their concerns, problems and feelings and from whom we learn daily.

Contributors

Abhilasha Das
MSc
PhD Scholar
Department of Clinical Psychology
National Institute of Mental Health
and Neurosciences
Bengaluru, Karnataka, India
Email: abhilashadas96@gmail.com

Adarsh Tripathi
MD
Professor
Department of Psychiatry
King Georges Medical University
Lucknow, Uttar Pradesh, India
Email: dradarshtripathi@gmail.com

Aishwariya Jha
MD
Senior Resident
Department of Psychiatry
National Institute of Mental Health
and Neurosciences
Bengaluru, Karnataka, India
Email: aishwariyajha0902@gmail.com

Amrit Pattojoshi
MD
Professor
Department of Psychiatry
Hi-Tech Medical College
Bhubaneshwar, Odisha, India
Email: dramritp@gmail.com

Anamika Das
MD
Assistant Professor of Psychiatry
IQ City Medical College
Durgapur, West Bengal, India
Email: dranamikadas.kgmu@gmail.com

Arthi R
MD
Consultant Psychiatrist
Schizophrenia Research Foundation
Chennai, Tamil Nadu, India
Email: aarthi@scarfindia.org

Aruna Yadiyal
MD
Professor
Department of Psychiatry
Father Muller Medical College
and Hospital
Mangaluru, Karnataka, India
Email: aruna.g2779@gmail.com

Arunashree B
MSc
PhD Scholar
Department of Clinical Psychology
National Institute of
Mental Health and Neurosciences
Bengaluru, Karnataka, India
Email: b.aruna2008@gmail.com

Ashlesha Bagadia
MRCPsych (UK) FRANZCP
Perinatal Psychiatrist and
Psychotherapist
The Green Oak Initiative
Bengaluru, Karnataka, India
Email: ashlesha.bagadia@gmail.com

Chandrima Naskar
MD
Senior Resident
Department of Psychiatry
All India Institute of Medical Sciences
Kalyani, West Bengal, India
Email: cnbondhu@gmail.com

Contributors

Debadatta Mohapatra
MD
Associate Professor
Department of Psychiatry
All India Institute of
Medical Sciences
Bhubaneshwar, Odisha, India
Email: psych_debadatta@
aiimsbhubaneswar.edu.in

Geetha Desai
MD PhD
Professor
Department of Psychiatry
National Institute of Mental Health
and Neurosciences
Bengaluru, Karnataka, India
Email: desaigeetha@gmail.com

Gunja Sengupta
MD
Post Doctoral Fellow in Women's
Mental Health
Department of Psychiatry
National Institute of Mental Health
and Neurosciences
Bengaluru, Karnataka, India
Email: gunja.s39@gmail.com

Imon Paul
DPM MD
Professor
Department of Psychiatry
IQ City Medical College
Durgapur, West Bengal, India
Email: dr.imonpaul@gmail.com

Karandeep Paul
MD
Consultant Psychiatrist
Department of Mental Health
and Behavioral Sciences
Artemis Hospitals
New Delhi, India
Email: karandeeppaul32@gmail.com

Lakshmi Vijayakumar
DPM PhD FRCP (Edin) FRCPsych(Hon)
Consultant Psychiatrist
Sneha Suicide Prevention Center and
Department of Psychiatry
Voluntary Health Services
Chennai, Tamil Nadu, India
Email: lakshmi@vijayakumars.com

Lavanya P Sharma
DPM MD PDF
Assistant Professor (Project)
Department of Psychiatry
National Institute of Mental Health
and Neurosciences
Bengaluru, Karnataka, India
Email: lava.sharma@gmail.com

Madhuri H Nanjundaswamy
MD PDF
Assistant Professor
Department of Psychiatry
National Institute of Mental Health
and Neurosciences
Bengaluru, Karnataka, India
Email: hnmadhuri@gmail.com

Mamta Sood
DPM MD
Professor, Department of Psychiatry
All India Institute of Medical Sciences
New Delhi, India
Email: soodmamta@gmail.com

Mangala Ramamurthi
MD
Consultant Psychiatrist
Schizophrenia Research Foundation
Chennai, Tamil Nadu, India
Email: mangala@scarfindia.org

Mohita Joshi
MD
Senior Resident
Department of Psychiatry
King Georges Medical University
Lucknow, Uttar Pradesh, India
Email: mohitajoshi123@gmail.com

Contributors

Nishant Goyal
DPM MD
Professor
Center for Child and Adolescent
Psychiatry and Center for
Cognitive Neurosciences
Central Institute of Psychiatry
Ranchi, Jharkhand, India
Email: psynishant@gmail.com

Prabha S Chandra
MD FAMS FRCPsych FRCPE FRCOG
(ad eundem)
Senior Professor
Department of Psychiatry
Dean, Behavioral Sciences
National Institute of
Mental Health and Neurosciences
Bengaluru, Karnataka, India
President
International Association of Women's
Mental Health
Email: chandra@nimhans.ac.in

Prerna Kukreti
MD
Professor
Department of Psychiatry
Lady Hardinge Medical College
New Delhi, India
Email: dr.prernakukreti@gmail.com

Ramachandran Padmavati
DPM MD
Consultant Psychiatrist and Director
Schizophrenia Research Foundation
Chennai, Tamil Nadu, India
Email: padmavati@scarfindia.org

Rashmi Arasappa
DPM MD
Associate Professor
Department of Psychiatry
National Institute of Mental Health
and Neurosciences
Bengaluru, Karnataka, India
Email: rashmia07@gmail.com

Rini Joseph
MD
Senior Resident
Department of Psychiatry
National Institute of Mental Health
and Neurosciences
Bengaluru, Karnataka, India
Email: rinijosephk5@gmail.com

Sai Chaitanya Reddy B
MD
Assistant Professor
Department of Psychiatry
National Institute of
Mental Health
and Neurosciences
Bengaluru, Karnataka, India
Email: chaitanyareddy557@gmail.com

Sai Krishna Tikka
DPM MD
Associate Professor
Department of Psychiatry
All India Institute of
Medical Sciences
Bibinagar, Hyderabad, Telangana, India
Email: sai.psych@aiimsbibinagar.edu.in;
saikiatry@gmail.com

Sai Spoorthy Mamidipalli
MD
Assistant Professor
Department of Psychiatry
All India Institute of
Medical Sciences
Bibinagar, Hyderabad, Telangana, India
Email: saispoorthy.m@gmail.com

Shalini Kumari
MD
Senior Resident
All India Institute of
Medical Sciences
Deoghar, Jharkhand, India
Email: sjshalini81@gmail.com

Contributors

Shivanee Kumari
MD
Senior Resident
Department of Psychiatry
National Institute of Mental Health
and Neurosciences
Bengaluru, Karnataka, India
Email: dr.shivaneekumari@gmail.com

Shobit Garg
DPM MD
Professor
Department of Psychiatry
Sri Guru Ram Rai Institute of
Medical and Health Sciences
Dehradun, Uttarakhand, India
Email: shobit.garg@gmail.com

Shree Mishra
MD
Associate Professor
Department of Psychiatry
All India Institute of
Medical Sciences
Bhubaneshwar, Odisha, India
Email: shreemishra09@gmail.com

Shyam Sundar Arumugham
MD
Professor
Department of Psychiatry
National Institute of
Mental Health
and Neurosciences
Bengaluru, Karnataka, India
Email: a.shyamsundar@gmail.com

Sonia Shenoy
MBBS MD PDF
Associate Professor
Department of Psychiatry
Kasturba Medical College
Udupi, Karnataka, India
Email: sonia.shenoy@manipal.edu

Sowmya Krishna
MD
Consultant Psychiatrist
Co-founder and Head of General
Psychiatric Services
The Green Oak Initiative
Bengaluru, Karnataka, India
Email: mindoverbodybengaluru@gmail.com

Srilakshmi Pingali
MD
Professor and Head
Department of Psychiatry
Government Medical College
Sangareddy, Telangana, India
Email: drpingali1@gmail.com

S Sireesha
MD
Professor and
Deputy Superintendent
Institute of Mental Health
Hyderabad, Telangana, India
Email: sireeshasvmc92@gmail.com

Sucharita Mandal
MD
Assistant Professor
Department of Psychiatry
All India Institute of
Medical Sciences
Kalyani, West Bengal, India
Email: drsucharitamandal08@gmail.com

Sundarnag Ganjekar
MD
Additional Professor
Department of Psychiatry
National Institute of
Mental Health
and Neurosciences
Bengaluru, Karnataka, India
Email: drbsnake@gmail.com

Sunita Simon Kurpad
MD
Professor
Department of Psychiatry
St John's Medical College and Hospital
Bengaluru, Karnataka, India
Email: simonsunita@gmail.com

Suresh Bada Math
MD PhD
Professor and Head of Forensic
Psychiatry Unit, Unit-5
Department of Psychiatry
National Institute of Mental Health
and Neurosciences
Bengaluru, Karnataka, India
Email: sureshbm@gmail.com

Tathagata Biswas
MD
Senior Resident
Department of Psychiatry
All India Institute of Medical Sciences
Bhubaneshwar, Odisha, India
Email: drtatz92@gmail.com

Upasna Gopalakrishna
MD PDF
Post-Doctoral Fellow in OCD
Department of Psychiatry
National Institute of Mental Health
and Neurosciences
Bengaluru, Karnataka, India
Email: upasna1511@live.com

Vasundhra Teotia
MD PDF
Post-Doctoral Fellow (Project)
Department of Psychiatry
National Institute of Mental Health
and Neurosciences
Bengaluru, Karnataka, India
Email: vasundhrat@gmail.com

Veena A Satyanarayana
MPhil PhD
Additional Professor
Department of Clinical, Psychology
National Institute of Mental Health
and Neurosciences
Bengaluru, Karnataka, India
Email: veenas@nimhans.ac.in

Venkata Lakshmi Narasimha
MD PDF DM
Assistant Professor
Department of Psychiatry
National Institute of Mental Health
and Neurosciences
Bengaluru, Karnataka, India
Email: narasimha.gvl.mbbs@gmail.com

Vikas Menon
MD DNB
Professor
Department of Psychiatry
Jawaharlal Institute of Postgraduate
Medical Education and Research
Puducherry, India
Email: drvmenon@gmail.com

Foreword

Sex-specific differences have been reported for various biological functions as well as in brain circuits, which result in differences in the prevalence, symptomatology, treatment responses and outcomes of neuropsychiatric disorders. As of 2021, 27 percent of females reported some type of mental illness in the past year compared to 18 percent of males. Women are more likely than men to be affected by internalizing disorders mainly depression and/or anxiety (but also eating disorders and borderline personality disorders); and have a higher risk of suicide attempts. In contrast, men have a higher prevalence of externalizing disorders (such as substance use disorders, antisocial personality disorders); neurodevelopmental disorders (e.g. psychotic disorders, learning disorders, ADHD); and a higher rate of completed suicide.

From a gender perspective, men and women are not equally exposed to psychosocial stressors, such as violence among other risk factors. Half of women who have mental health problems have also experienced physical and/or sexual abuse. Violence is known to impact physical, reproductive and mental health negatively.

It remains unclear to what extent sex and gender differences in mental health are due to biology or the consequences of behavioral and social factors. The association between biological sex and mental health in Europe is moderated by socioeconomic and family-related factors, which explain around 20% of the differences in mental health between women and men. Such factors are for example employment, education, housekeeping, looking after children and income (Otten et al. 2021).

Indeed, the integration of a gender-sensitive perspective in all aspects of mental health has become essential. Contemporary Issues in Women's Mental Health -a book for the practicing psychiatrist- edited by Professor Prabha Chandra is intended for training healthcare professionals and raising their awareness of the specificities of women's mental health. It perfectly integrates clinical descriptions of psychiatric disorders and their particularities in women, mental health in relation to reproduction, violence as a major contributing factor, sex- and gender-specific response to treatment, and finally it addresses the question of gender-sensitive mental health services.

Prabha Chandra is Senior Professor of Psychiatry and Dean of Behavioral Sciences, at the National Institute of Mental Health and Neurosciences in Bengaluru, India. She has been involved in the support of women facing various forms of gender-based violence. She has set up training programs in psychosocial issues and mental health care to support women facing gender-based violence. Her extensive experience in the field of women's health will provide readers with a very interesting insight into this major topic of interest.

Reference: Otten D, Tibubos AN, Schomerus G, Brähler E, Binder H, Kruse J, et al. Similarities and Differences of Mental Health in Women and Men: A Systematic Review of Findings in Three Large German Cohorts. Front. Public Health. 2021;9:553071. doi: 10.3389/fpubh.2021.553071

Florence Thibaut
University Paris Cité,
Department of Psychiatry and Addictive Disorders
University Hospital Cochin
Institute of Psychiatry and Neurosciences Paris, France
Chair of the Women's Mental Health
Section of the World Psychiatric Association and
Immediate Past President of the International Association of Women's Mental Health
Email: florence.thibaut@aphp.fr

Message

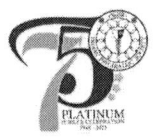 **Indian Psychiatric Society**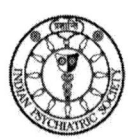

Scientifically speaking women are different, not only in terms of anatomy and physiology but also in terms of behavioral sciences and sociology. The bio-psycho-social construct of mind, mental health and mental illness underlines the importance of sex and gender issues in psychiatry rather more deeply. For any given diagnosis, women almost always express psychological distress differently. Management too needs gender sensitive approaches. In this context, the role of culture cannot be trivialized. So, there was a need for a book on Women's Mental Health from India to provide all relevant information and wisdom for students, researchers, and clinicians of the country.

It gives us satisfaction to remember that the Indian Psychiatric Society has had a Woman Specialty Section for more than 25 years which has become more proactive in organizing scientific programs in the last 10 years. We must admit that the idea of this book emerged during and due to the activities of this section.

We express our sincere thanks to all the editors and contributors for their commitment and hard work despite their own workload. It's a matter of pride that we have Prof Prabha S Chandra with us who is not only an experienced teacher but also a perinatal mental health researcher of international repute. She deserves appreciation to complete this exhaustive and arduous task within a year and we are all set to release this book in our Platinum Jubilee annual conference. We congratulate Dr Anil Kakunje and the team publication subcommittee for one more landmark publication. We must express our thanks to Jaypee Brothers Medical Publishers, especially, Ms Chetna Malhotra (Senior Director—Professional Publishing, Marketing and Business Development) and Pragati Singh (Development Editor) for timely and impressive production.

Vinay Kumar	**Laxmikant Rathi**	**Arabinda Brahma**
President	Vice President	Hon. General Secretary

Preface

We are delighted to write a preface for this compilation on all things related to women's mental health that is relevant to psychiatric practice in India and to other South Asian countries.

How do we make a book on women's mental health relevant to a psychiatry trainee or a practicing psychiatrist in India? This was the question we asked ourselves in the several editorial brainstorming exercises we held as we started conceptualizing the book.

Jostling for shelf space with many other books on mental health, we wanted this one to be something one could reach out to while conceptualizing the cultural aspects of mental health in a woman, addressing violence, using a life course approach or making a treatment plan or indeed in planning gender sensitive mental health.

After several animated and interesting conversations and much negotiation, we finalized on 22 chapters which we hope will cover the most relevant topics. We scanned the landscape of publications from India on all these areas and have chosen authors who we think will write with a passion for the subject and also discuss the latest evidence in a way that will pique the curiosity and interest of psychiatry trainees and practitioners.

In this volume, which was conceptualized as an 'Indian' book on women's mental health, we have tried to focus on cultural and social issues and review the relevant literature from India in addition to the latest evidence available globally.

The book is divided into four sections, each ably handled by a different editor.

Section 1 deals with psychiatric disorders disorders and focuses on clinical presentation, assessment and management of various mental health conditions among women. Having discussed the clinical disorders, we move into Section 2 to discuss the area of reproductive psychiatry. Here we have 3 chapters that focus on mental health aspects of gynecological conditions, the various reproductive life stages of women and the important area of perinatal psychiatry.

Section 3 dwells on important aspects of vulnerability, autonomy and power imbalances that affect women's mental health including gender-based violence that is indeed a harrowing indictment of our prevailing cultures, society and times. As adversities have the notoriety of leaving behind bio-psycho-social scars in the psyche of its victims, it is an expected fallout that women tend to have negative mental health consequences following these traumas. This section rightly explores these health outcomes in women who have faced gender-based violence and those in sexual minority groups. A chapter on the rights of women with mental health problems furthers our insights into legal provisions that protect the rights of women and offers recommendations on a rights-based approach to providing services. Finally, Section 4 has five chapters that look at more contemporary topics related to women's mental health. The themes are varied and offer guidance on how to view a woman's mental health from a gendered and cultural lens as well as an approach to developing gender sensitive mental health services. The chapter on measurement and assessment will be particularly useful for researchers who may be looking for tools related to women's mental health. There is a chapter on using neuromodulation among women and an important chapter on principles of psychopharmacology. We believe that both of these will offer the readers an insight into rational and evidence-based treatment methods that keep in mind women's biology, a factor which is usually sadly neglected.

We thank all the authors who have contributed their precious time with each chapter having several pearls of knowledge to offer. It is our endeavor with this book to shed light on the various dimensions of the mental health of women.

Margaret Atwood says "A word after a word after a word is power."

We hope that our readers will find what they want and through this book also want to read and learn more, that will then lead to better care of women with mental health concerns.

Prabha S Chandra
Aruna Yadiyal
Sai Krishna Tikka
Debadatta Mohapatra

Acknowledgments

The idea for this book emerged on a cold winter morning in Chandigarh where we were holding our 9th annual conference on women's mental health and perinatal psychiatry. After my keynote lecture on Priorities in Women's Mental Health and Perinatal Psychiatry, the President of the Indian Psychiatric Society, Dr Vinay Kumar with his usual enthusiasm approached me with the prospect of writing this book. His brief to me was that we should publish a book addressing different dimensions of women's mental health that would be relevant to Indian psychiatrists and specifically to trainees in India and South Asia. He also wanted the authors to be from premier institutions of India that have postgraduate psychiatry training and/or experts in the field. At that time, it indeed seemed a daunting task but with the help of my young and enthusiastic coeditors (all of whom are emerging leaders in the field) we have been able to fulfill our president's wish. A big thanks to him, to the Vice President, Dr Rathi, General Secretary, Dr Arabinda Brahma and other Office Bearers. We also want to thank the Chairperson of the Publication committee, Dr Anil Kakunje and other members of the publication committee of the Indian Psychiatric Society, for their support and encouragement. A special thanks to Dr Shubhangi Dere, Associate Professor of Psychiatry, MGM Medical College and Hospital, Navi Mumbai for the beautiful artwork on the cover.

Contents

SECTION 1: Clinical Issues

1. **Severe Psychiatric Illness in Women: Clinical Issues in Assessment and Management** 3
   Karandeep Paul, Mamta Sood

2. **Severe Psychiatric Illness in Women: Rehabilitation and Recovery** 16
   Ramachandran Padmavati, Mangala Ramamurthi, Arthi R

3. **Depressive and Anxiety Disorders** 33
   Srilakshmi Pingali, S Sireesha

4. **Obsessive-compulsive Related Disorders and Eating Disorders** 52
   Lavanya P Sharma, Vasundhra Teotia, Upasna Gopalakrishna, Shyam Sundar Arumugham

5. **Unraveling the Knots: Dissociation and Somatization in Women** 77
   Aishwariya Jha, Rashmi Arasappa, Geetha Desai

6. **Suicide and Self-harm in Women: A Gendered Approach** 108
   Aruna Yadiyal, Lakshmi Vijayakumar, Prabha S Chandra

7. **Substance Use and Externalizing Disorders in Women: The Indian Context** 123
   Venkata Lakshmi Narasimha, Shalini Kumari

8. **Sexual Problems and Management** 150
   Adarsh Tripathi, Mohita Joshi

9. **Psychiatric Disorders in Older Women** 176
   Debadatta Mohapatra, Tathagata Biswas, Shree Mishra

10. **Mood Swings and Mayhem: Personality Disorder in Women** 196
    Ashlesha Bagadia, Sowmya Krishna

SECTION 2: Reproductive Psychiatry

11. **Perinatal Psychiatry** 213
    Prerna Kukreti

12. **Gynecological Conditions and Mental Health** 249
    Sonia Shenoy

13. **Menarche, the Menstrual Cycle, and Menopause: Biological Cycles and Women's Mental Health** 268
   Imon Paul, Anamika Das

SECTION 3: Gender-based Violence and Vulnerable Groups

14. **Intimate Partner Violence: Impact on Mental Health and Evidence-based Interventions** 293
   Madhuri H Nanjundaswamy, Rini Joseph

15. **Rights of Women with Mental Illness** 316
   Shivanee Kumari, Sai Chaitanya Reddy B, Suresh Bada Math

16. **Mental Health Issues among Women in Sexual Minority Groups** 331
   Debadutta Mohapatra, Aruna Yadiyal, Amrit Pattojoshi

17. **Sexual Violence: Mental Health Consequences and Interventions** 348
   Arunashree B, Abhilasha Das, Veena A Satyanarayana

SECTION 4: Interventions and Services

18. **Cultural Formulation in Women's Mental Health** 365
   Sai Spoorthy Mamidipalli, Sucharita Mandal, Sai Krishna Tikka

19. **Gender-sensitive Mental Health Services and Ethical Issues in Care** 387
   Sunita Simon Kurpad

20. **Measurement and Assessment Tools for Women's Mental Health** 405
   Gunja Sengupta, Sundarnag Ganjekar

21. **Neuromodulation in Women** 443
   Nishant Goyal, Shobit Garg

22. **General Principles of Psychopharmacology in Women** 469
   Vikas Menon, Chandrima Naskar

Index 485

SECTION 1

Clinical Issues

- **Severe Psychiatric Illness in Women: Clinical Issues in Assessment and Management**
  Karandeep Paul, Mamta Sood

- **Severe Psychiatric Illness in Women: Rehabilitation and Recovery**
  Ramachandran Padmavati, Mangala Ramamurthi, Arthi R

- **Depressive and Anxiety Disorders**
  Srilakshmi Pingali, S Sireesha

- **Obsessive-compulsive Related Disorders and Eating Disorders**
  Lavanya P Sharma, Vasundhra Teotia, Upasna Gopalakrishna, Shyam Sundar Arumugham

- **Unraveling the Knots: Dissociation and Somatization in Women**
  Aishwariya Jha, Rashmi Arasappa, Geetha Desai

- **Suicide and Self-harm in Women: A Gendered Approach**
  Aruna Yadiyal, Lakshmi Vijayakumar, Prabha S Chandra

- **Substance Use and Externalizing Disorders in Women: The Indian Context**
  Venkata Lakshmi Narasimha, Shalini Kumari

- **Sexual Problems and Management**
  Adarsh Tripathi, Mohita Joshi

- **Psychiatric Disorders in Older Women**
  Debadatta Mohapatra, Tathagata Biswas, Shree Mishra

- **Mood Swings and Mayhem: Personality Disorder in Women**
  Ashlesha Bagadia, Sowmya Krishna

CHAPTER 1

Severe Psychiatric Illness in Women: Clinical Issues in Assessment and Management

Karandeep Paul, Mamta Sood

■ ABSTRACT

This chapter focuses on the distinctive clinical challenges in assessment and management among women with severe mental illness (SMI), with an emphasis on schizophrenia. It highlights how women's symptoms often differ from men's, influenced by hormonal factors and a higher prevalence of certain health conditions. It delves into the specific needs of women in terms of diagnosis, treatment, and the broader impact of SMI on their lives, including aspects like pregnancy, motherhood, and societal roles. The key points include the importance of a holistic approach to treatment, the role of caregivers, and the challenges posed by delayed diagnosis and stigma. Tailored interventions to address these unique challenges and support women's quality of life are also discussed.

Keywords: Schizophrenia, women's mental health, severe mental illness, pregnancy, childbirth

■ INTRODUCTION

Severe mental illnesses (SMIs) cause significant disability in the individuals and burden for families and society. Gender differences among SMI has long been known in terms of prevalence, clinical presentation, and factors influencing its course. Women with SMI may often have affective and paranoid symptoms, heightened anxiety, and fewer negative and cognitive symptoms.[1-3] Even at the time of initial presentation, women may often receive a preliminary diagnosis of a mood disorder. Women may frequently exhibit increased overt hostility, restlessness, sexual delusions, and emotional expression. Notably, there are certain differential diagnoses that are sometimes overlooked in women. These include conditions like thyroid disease, autoimmune disorders, corticosteroid treatment, and anorexia-related starvation. As these conditions are more prevalent in women, they must be thoroughly investigated.[4] Women may experience later onset of the illness, often during their late 20s to early 30s. This gender disparity is partly associated with neuromodulators, especially female sex hormones.[5] The "estrogen protection hypothesis" suggests that estrogen's impact on mood, cognition, and behavior may provide women with some advantages in managing schizophrenia.[6] Furthermore, in women, symptom severity tends to increase, relapses occur more frequently, and hospitalizations rise when sex hormone levels drop, such as during specific menstrual phases, postpartum, or following menopause.[7,8] Additionally, women are more likely to have a history of trauma, such as physical or sexual abuse, compared to men with the condition. Before diagnosis, women tend to exhibit better social functioning, but their social capabilities can decline more rapidly after diagnosis.[4] Although men with schizophrenia have a higher rate compared to women, but the suicide rate is higher in women with schizophrenia than in women without the condition. Women make more suicide attempts, but fewer are completed.[9,10] In the first 15 years following diagnosis, women tend to have a superior outcome, including lower rehospitalization rates. However, this advantage diminishes over time, and the long-term outcomes for women and men become roughly similar. Women with schizophrenia also tend to achieve better long-term outcomes, with higher remission rates and lower relapse rates. They are more likely to be employed, maintain social support, marry, and have children. Moreover, they enjoy a better quality of life, experience fewer negative symptoms, and endure less social and clinical disability. However, women with schizophrenia often face stigma- and gender-related discrimination, which negatively affects their treatment and recovery processes.[11-13]

In this chapter, we discuss clinical issues in assessment and management of women with SMI. For the purpose of this chapter, we will restrict ourselves to women with schizophrenia and related psychotic disorders will be covered under women with SMI.

APPROACHES TO ASSESSMENT AND MANAGEMENT OF WOMEN WITH SMI

The assessment and management of women with SMI are guided by certain pragmatic principles, which are mentioned as follows:
- Instead of introducing new interventions, the focus should be on utilizing existing recommendations and tailoring them to suit the specific needs of individuals and their caregivers within the local context.
- A biopsychosocial approach combined with keeping lens on both cross-sectional and longitudinal perspectives is helpful.
- There needs to be shifting of gaze beyond merely assessing symptoms and making diagnosis; there is need for emphasis on improving functioning and recovery.
- A collaborative, multidisciplinary approach is crucial. The management objectives encompass reducing the frequency, duration, and severity of symptoms, identifying and preventing relapses, and facilitating the patients' functioning within their sociocultural environment.

- This process of assessment and management is ongoing and dynamic, and it extends across multiple follow-up sessions.
- The involvement of caregivers is paramount; they are not only key resources but also active partners in the care process. Their collaboration is essential in planning and delivering interventions effectively.
- It is vital to acknowledge and integrate the distinct characteristics of the patient population like socioeconomic status, type of family, and area of residence.

Assessment and management of women with SMI pose several distinct challenges. Firstly, there is often a delay in making diagnosis in women compared to men, resulting in delayed treatment and poorer outcomes. This delay can stem from differences in symptom presentation and gender biases in healthcare. Secondly, women with SMI may exhibit atypical symptoms like mood swings, anxiety, and social withdrawal, leading to potential. Thirdly, these women are more likely to have co-occurring conditions like substance abuse, eating disorders, and post-traumatic stress disorder, complicating both diagnosis and treatment. Furthermore, stigma and discrimination, often due to gender and mental health status, can hinder their access to healthcare and suitable treatment. Trauma and victimization are additional concerns, impacting mental health and treatment engagement. Special reproductive health needs like contraception and pregnancy planning may be overlooked in routine mental health assessments. Lastly, cultural factors, including language barriers, cultural beliefs, and social norms, can affect how SMI is assessed and diagnosed in women from diverse backgrounds. Addressing these challenges is vital to ensuring effective care and support for women with SMI.[14-16]

The women patients with SMI may present to any of the settings ranging from community clinics or general hospitals or specialized clinics and hospitals. The levels of care vary as they transition from community (macro level) to specialized (micro level) care within the healthcare system. Various factors determine this transition, including the duration of illness, the number of episodes experienced, the response to treatment, the achievement of remission and functionality, and the frequency of hospitalization. These determinants collectively guide the decision to move from one level of care to another.

Level 1: Community/Primary Care Settings

In the context of community/primary care settings, crucial aspects of assessing and managing women patients with SMI are as follows:

While assessing, relevant sociodemographic and clinical information is collected. Duration of illness and whether it is the first episode, multiple episodes, or continuous occurrence is crucial information required to be collected. Identifying symptoms for diagnosis, assessing psychiatric and physical comorbidities, including body mass index (BMI) and substance use, is integral. A thorough risk assessment is conducted to gauge potential harm to oneself or others. The patient's level of functioning is evaluated, and insights into how the family perceives the illness and potential solutions are gained. Other pertinent issues, such as the distance traveled for treatment, need for hospitalization, and detailed workup requirements, are also considered. Psychometric evaluations are conducted when necessary.

The management strategies executed in these clinics encompasses several facets. Pharmacological treatment is initiated, while engagement with caregivers and psychoeducation occurs progressively through follow-up sessions. Patients and their caregivers receive information about the signs and symptoms of the illness and their broader impact on overall functioning. They are educated about the therapeutic effects and potential side effects of prescribed medications, with a focus on drug adherence. Reassurance is provided, and the significance of balanced nutrition, sufficient sleep, and mild-to-moderate exercise is emphasized. As acute symptoms subside, attention shifts to recognizing potential symptoms of relapse and implementing measures for relapse prevention. The importance of gradually resuming daily activities and functions, as psychopathological improvement becomes evident, is also highlighted. The scheduling of follow-up appointments is determined in collaboration with caregivers to ensure comprehensive care.

Level 2: General Hospitals/Secondary Care Settings

In these settings, a thorough and comprehensive evaluation and management approach is warranted under specific circumstances for schizophrenia patients. This applies when there are diagnostic complexities, instances of first episode psychoses or multi-episode psychoses with varying degrees of recovery and associated challenges, poor response to initial treatment in first episode psychoses, incomplete remission in cases of multi-episode psychoses, prolonged and continuous illness, and the need for extended engagement with healthcare services.

During this comprehensive assessment, various aspects are meticulously considered. This involves conducting detailed interviews to discern critical information, identifying underlying psychopathology, and documenting the repercussions of psychopathology on the individual's overall functioning. A comprehensive assessment of coexisting conditions, including physical, psychiatric, and substance-related concerns, is undertaken. The evaluation extends to medication adherence, probing reasons for noncompliance, and delving into psychosocial aspects. This includes assessing family and social dynamics as well as understanding how the family perceives the illness and copes with its challenges. In cases where appropriate, psychometric evaluations are conducted to further enhance understanding.

Subsequent to this in-depth assessment, a targeted course of action is initiated. This encompasses optimizing the dosage and duration of antipsychotic and other medications in alignment with established practice guidelines. Side effects stemming from medication are addressed, and if issues of nonadherence arise, the underlying reasons are explored and resolved. Lifestyle modifications, particularly weight reduction, are promoted. The management plan extends to addressing comorbid conditions. Additionally, considerations for interventions such as clozapine and depot antipsychotics are made as necessary.

Going beyond the scope of community-based interventions, a more comprehensive psychoeducational program is implemented over a series of follow-up visits. This program encompasses elements of supportive therapy, strategies for managing stressors, and collaborative problem-solving aimed at assisting caregivers in reestablishing disrupted social connections and work/school routines. Furthermore, the possibility of referral to specialized consultants, particularly those with expertise in psychology, is explored to provide targeted psychosocial interventions. The overarching objective is to deliver a thorough and tailored approach to the care of individuals navigating the challenges of schizophrenia.

Level 3: Special Services

At the level of focused care, often referred to as level 3 or micro level, special services are tailored for women grappling with SMIs who present intricate challenges. These services are designed specifically for patients who fall within the category of being difficult to treat or experiencing persistent psychopathology and dysfunction despite undergoing evidence-based treatment for a duration of 6 months.

The assessment process within these specialized services revolves around active engagement with both patients and their caregivers. This involves quantifying psychopathological manifestations across distinct domains, including positive, negative, mood, and cognitive symptoms. Quantification extends further to the evaluation of functioning and identification of deficits in various spheres: personal, biological, social, occupational, and recreational aspects. This quantification is often facilitated using tools such as the Visual Analog Scale (VAS). Additionally, there is a comprehensive reassessment of comorbidities spanning physical health, psychiatric well-being, and substance use. Delving into the factors underlying medication nonadherence is a critical facet of this evaluation.

The assessment process also includes a psychosocial dimension. Strengths and challenges faced by both caregivers/family and the patients themselves are thoroughly evaluated. Family burden is quantified, and detailed exploration of plans related to the patient's occupation or vocation is undertaken. Moreover, possibilities for engagement in occupational, recreational, or social activities within the patient's local environment, other areas, or nongovernmental organizations (NGOs) are explored.

The management approach adopted within these specialized clinics is grounded in a micromanagement principle. Each individual issue is meticulously addressed through targeted interventions, and the resultant changes are documented with precision in both quantitative and qualitative terms. Specific psychological interventions, such as cognitive behavioral therapy (CBT) for managing auditory hallucinations and cognitive remediation for addressing cognitive symptoms, are a vital part of the treatment strategy.

A dedicated social worker assumes a pivotal role in this context, offering essential services such as providing free medications for individuals holding below poverty line (BPL) status, offering vocational guidance, and potentially setting up reminders for follow-up appointments through phone calls on scheduled dates. The aim is to provide comprehensive care through a meticulous focus on each distinct aspect, ultimately leading to tangible enhancements in the well-being and overall functioning of patients contending with the complexities of SMIs, including schizophrenia.

SPECIAL CONSIDERATIONS
Drug Adverse Effects

Antipsychotic drugs can have varying effects on women. Both genders may experience sedation, which can impair scholastic abilities and driving skills. Women, particularly mothers, face additional challenges due to the need for alertness to their infants' needs. Women are more vulnerable to adverse effects due to sex-specific pharmacokinetics, resulting in higher concentrations of free drugs at target sites and subsequently more side effects compared to men. Estrogen hormones can enhance dopamine blockade, increasing the risk of side effects in women. The higher proportion of adipose tissue in women can lead to prolonged drug storage and higher drug concentrations. Additionally, women are more prone to immune reactions and drug–drug interactions due to comorbid illnesses. Prolongation of the QTc interval and hyperprolactinemia, with its associated health issues, affect women, especially older ones. Tolerability varies by gender, with more women reporting extrapyramidal and anticholinergic reactions, and more men experiencing sexual problems. A rare but serious side effect, agranulocytosis, is more frequent in women, necessitating careful monitoring, especially in those taking clozapine. Healthcare providers should be vigilant about these gender-related risks and tailor treatment plans to minimize side effects while maximizing treatment benefits.[4,17,18]

Suicide

Gender plays a significant role in suicide risk. Among individuals with this condition, men experience a decrease in suicide rates with age, while this trend does not hold for women. Over a two-decade longitudinal study, the suicide rate for men dropped from 10.5% in the first 2 years after hospital discharge to 0%, while women maintained a 6% rate that was more evenly distributed across the 20 years.[23] Schizophrenia and related psychotic disorders already increase suicide risk compared to the general population, with individuals being 13 times more vulnerable to suicide.[24] Nearly half of all patients with schizophrenia attempt suicide, and between 4 and 13% die by suicide. Men, especially within the first decade of diagnosis, face a higher mortality risk than women. However, the male to female suicide ratio is lower in SMI than in the general population, meaning that women with schizophrenia are at a comparatively greater risk of suicide compared to their counterparts in the general population than men with schizophrenia compared to healthy men. Women with schizophrenia and related psychotic disorders also contend with a higher risk of violent victimization, often due to domestic violence, with a prevalence of approximately 25% experiencing rape, possibly linked to the elevated occurrence of depressive symptoms among them. To prevent suicide, early identification of risk factors, including previous suicide attempts, depression, and substance abuse, is crucial, alongside providing suitable treatment and support. Treatment methods for schizophrenia, such as medication and psychotherapy, can effectively reduce suicide risk, and strong family and social support systems also play pivotal roles in prevention. Increasing awareness about suicide risk in schizophrenia and reducing mental health stigma can further encourage affected individuals to seek help and support when needed.[9,10,19]

Marriage

While considering marriage in women with SMI, there are several issues that are important. First, having schizophrenia and related disorders can lead to problems in getting married. Women with SMI have a harder time getting married or staying married compared to those without these conditions. This is because the effects of SMI can make it challenging to start or maintain a marriage.

In particular, women with SMI often face difficulties in their marital relationships, while men with the illness may struggle more with finding and keeping jobs. When women with schizophrenia do get married, they tend to experience more disability compared to their male counterparts with the same condition.[4]

One significant issue for women with SMI is the stigma they encounter, especially in the context of marriage, pregnancy, and childbirth. There are cultural beliefs and myths that can create barriers to getting married, and once married, these women may face challenges within their in-laws family due to these beliefs. This often leads women to hide their illness to avoid discrimination and stigma.[18]

The impact of SMI on women's marital experiences depends on various factors, including when the illness began (before or after marriage), the age at which they married, how long they've been married, and whether their husband and in-laws were aware of their condition when they got married. Access to mental health support and many other factors also play a role in shaping their experiences.[4]

In the Indian context, females typically marry at a young age, and most marriages are fairly equal in terms of gender roles. However, fewer males with schizophrenia tend to get married. Still, those who do often have stable marriages. In contrast, female patients, especially those without children, face a higher risk of marriage breakdown and separation. This is often related to the continuous or relapsing nature of their illness.

In marriages, men and women are usually assigned different roles, with women often expected to take on the primary role of a homemaker and child bearer. They often live with their husband's family for the rest of their lives after marriage and are culturally expected to have children early in their marriage.[4]

There is also a widespread belief that marriage can somehow cure mental illness, adding additional pressure to women with schizophrenia. Deciding whether or not to inform a potential husband and his family about their condition is a tough decision, as revealing it may lead to the withdrawal of a marriage proposal. Conversely, keeping the illness a secret and having it discovered later can result in a high risk of separation or divorce.[20]

Sexuality

Women with SMI encounter various difficulties when it comes to their sexuality. Having a mental illness does not mean that they lose interest in or engagement with sexual activities. However, there is limited information available about their sexuality, and the quality of their sexual experiences.[24]

They face multiple challenges related to their sexuality. They are at a higher risk of experiencing sexual coercion, violence, or engaging in prostitution, which also increases their vulnerability to human immunodeficiency virus (HIV) infection. They tend to have more sexual partners over their lifetime, are less likely to have a current partner, and often report lower satisfaction with their sex lives. Stigma and objectification linked to mental illness can undermine their autonomy and control over their sexual choices.[26]

Antipsychotic medications can affect their menstrual cycles, lower their desire for sex, and even cause galactorrhea (abnormal breast milk production).

Societal expectations based on gender can further diminish their sense of self and autonomy, making it harder for them to engage in safe sexual practices. Overall, women with schizophrenia spectrum disorders encounter many barriers to sexual satisfaction, often tied to their mental health condition and the discrimination they face because of it.

Due to difficulties in saying "no" to unwanted advances and social isolation, they are also more susceptible to sexual victimization. Some may turn to sex work due to poverty. Lack of contraception knowledge and access issues can lead to a higher rate of unwanted pregnancies among these women. They may not reliably use daily contraceptive pills, choosing methods like intrauterine devices, progesterone injections, or tubal ligation more suitable. Moreover, their lack of awareness about health risks and social isolation put them at greater risk of sexually transmitted infections (STIs).[10]

It is crucial for healthcare providers to create a safe and nonjudgmental space for women with schizophrenia to discuss their sexuality and related concerns, providing appropriate education, support, and treatment regarding contraception and STIs to ensure the best possible outcomes for these women.[21-23]

Pregnancy and Motherhood

Pregnancy and motherhood can be challenging for women with SMI. These women are more likely to have unplanned pregnancies because they may not have enough information about contraception. When pregnant, their schizophrenia symptoms can worsen, increasing the risk of relapse during the perinatal period. It is crucial for them to receive proper treatment during pregnancy and after childbirth. This often means adjusting their antipsychotic medication to minimize harm to the baby. Mothers with SMI need support to ensure safe and healthy motherhood, which involves following their treatment plan, knowing signs of relapse, and understanding legal issues related to mental health and custody.

These women also face an increased risk of problems during pregnancy and childbirth, such as premature birth and low birth weight. With the right treatment and support, these risks can be reduced. Mothers with SMI who consider breastfeeding should have a detailed discussion with their partner and healthcare provider about the pros and cons. In the first 6 weeks after giving birth, a higher dose of antipsychotic medication might be recommended to help manage symptoms during this vulnerable period. Home-based psychiatric services can be beneficial during this time since leaving the house can be challenging.[10]

Taking care of a child can be tough for women prone to psychosis, as they have a higher risk of losing custody. Children born to mothers with SMI also have a greater genetic risk for the condition and might show developmental delays.[24] Therefore, it is important to ensure these vulnerable children receive the support they need, as part of the overall treatment for psychosis in women. Mothers with schizophrenia may need ongoing support in their role as caregivers, and services like mother–infant units in hospitals are designed to address their unique needs.[5,24-26]

Stigma

Stigma poses a major hurdle for women diagnosed with schizophrenia and related psychotic disorders, influencing various aspects of their daily lives. It can be present at personal levels, where they might face negative attitudes from those around them like family, friends, or coworkers. This interpersonal stigma often leads to feelings of guilt, shame, and isolation, making it tough for these women to seek necessary help and resources. On a broader scale, structural stigma exists in policies and practices that restrict access to essential services, such as healthcare, housing, or job opportunities. For instance, they might face discrimination at their workplace or find it hard to get proper medical care. Additionally, intersectional stigma comes into play when these women belong to certain racial or ethnic groups, adding layers of discrimination and making resource access even harder. The families of these women, especially the female caregivers, can also be impacted by the stigma, experiencing feelings of depression and even greater stigma than their male counterparts.[4,27,28]

Addressing this issue demands a comprehensive strategy that encompasses raising public awareness, ensuring resource accessibility, and actively involving the women in their treatment plans. It is crucial to challenge prevailing negative perceptions and push for better policies that offer easier access to necessities. Advocacy at various levels, be it local, state, or national, is vital. It is equally important to forge supportive relationships with loved ones and communities who understand and empathize. Seeking timely mental health treatments can empower these women, helping them lead fulfilling lives despite the challenges. Worldwide efforts, like the World Health Organization's Dare to Care campaign and the World Psychiatric Association's global anti-stigma programs, are in place to tackle mental health stigma. To truly make a difference, education and awareness are key, as they can foster understanding and compassion for those living with mental health conditions.

Rehabilitation

Rehabilitating women with SMI has two main parts. First, there is clinical rehabilitation which helps manage their symptoms and reduces hospital visits. Second, there is disability support that helps them handle day-to-day tasks and improves their life skills based on their personal needs.[29]

For young, single women, families are a big help in the healing process. It is key to teach both the woman and her family about the illness. Also, they should be trained in essential skills, involving self-care, education, home maintenance, managing money, vocation, leisure, interpersonal and social skills, incorporate sex education and they should learn about reproductive health.

For married women, it is important to teach them about reproductive health, identify early if they are pregnant, and give them the right medication if they are pregnant or might become so. If they have just had a baby and need to stay in a hospital, it is good to let them spend time with their baby. Also, it is essential to help them become good parents, give advice on family planning, and help with any challenges they face while raising children.[8]

> **KEY POINTS**
> - *Delayed diagnosis:* Women with schizophrenia often experience delayed diagnosis with emotional and hormonal-influenced symptoms.
> - *Gender-specific treatment:* Treatment requires a holistic, gender-specific approach.
> - *Unique challenges:* They face higher suicide risk, trauma, and stigma.
> - *Positive long-term outcomes:* Generally positive long-term outcomes with stable social support.
> - *Focused rehabilitation:* Emphasis on life skills, reproductive health, and symptom management.

■ REFERENCES

1. Thomas N, Gurvich C, Hudaib AR, Gavrilidis E, Kulkarni J. Dissecting the syndrome of schizophrenia: Associations between symptomatology and hormone levels in women with schizophrenia. Psychiatry Res. 2019;280:112510.
2. Seeman MV. Men and women respond differently to antipsychotic drugs. Neuropharmacology. 2020;163:107631.
3. Seeman MV. Suicide among women with schizophrenia spectrum disorders. J Psychiatr Prac. 2009;15(3):235-42.
4. Thara R, Srinivasan TN. Outcome of marriage in schizophrenia. Soci Psychiatry Psychiatr Epidemiol. 1997;32:416-20.
5. Negash B, Asmamewu B, Alemu WG. Risky sexual behaviors of schizophrenic patients: a single center study in Ethiopia, 2018. BMC Res Notes. 2019;12:635.
6. Kaplan KJ, Harrow M, Clews K. The twenty-year trajectory of suicidal activity among post-hospital psychiatric men and women with mood disorders and schizophrenia. Arch Suicide Res. 2016;20(3):336-48.

7. Iversen TS, Steen NE, Dieset I, Hope S, Mørch R, Gardsjord ES, et al. Side effect burden of antipsychotic drugs in real life—Impact of gender and polypharmacy. Prog Neuropsychopharmacol Biol Psychiatry. 2018;82:263-71.
8. Hor K, Taylor M. Suicide and schizophrenia: a systematic review of rates and risk factors. J Psychopharmacol. 2010;24(4 Suppl):81-90.
9. Hanlon MC, Campbell LE, Single N, Coleman C, Morgan VA, Cotton SM, et al. Men and women with psychosis and the impact of illness-duration on sex-differences: The second Australian national survey of psychosis. Psychiatry Res. 2017;256:130-43.
10. González-Rodríguez A, Seeman MV. Pharmacotherapy for schizophrenia in postmenopausal women. Expert Opin Pharmacother. 2018;19(8):809-21.
11. González-Rodríguez A, Labad J, Seeman MV. Antipsychotic-induced hyperprolactinemia in aging populations: Prevalence, implications, prevention and management. Prog Neuropsychopharmacol Biol Psychiatry. 2020;101:109941.
12. Häfner H. From onset and prodromal stage to a life-long course of schizophrenia and its symptom dimensions: how sex, age, and other risk factors influence incidence and course of illness. Psychiatry J. 2019;2019:9804836.
13. Fernando P, Sommer IE, Hasan A. Do we need sex-oriented clinical practice guidelines for the treatment of schizophrenia? Curr Opin Psychiatry. 2020;33(3):192-9.
14. Dickerson FB. Women, aging, and schizophrenia. J Women Aging. 2007;19(1-2):49-61.
15. Abel KM, Drake R, Goldstein JM. Sex differences in schizophrenia. Int Rev Psychiatry. 2010;22(5):417-28.
16. Vigod SN, Kurdyak PA, Dennis CL, Gruneir A, Newman A, Seeman MV, et al. Maternal and newborn outcomes among women with schizophrenia: a retrospective population-based cohort study. BJOG: Int J Gynaecol Obstet. 2014;121(5):566-74.
17. Thorup A, Petersen L, Jeppesen P, Ohlenschlæger J, Christensen T, Krarup G, et al. Gender differences in young adults with first-episode schizophrenia spectrum disorders at baseline in the Danish OPUS study. J Nerv Ment Dis. 2007;195(5):396-405.
18. Thara R, Kamath S. Women and schizophrenia. Indian J Psychiatry. 2015;57(Suppl 2):S246.
19. Suparare L, Watson SJ, Binns R, Frayne J, Galbally M. Is intimate partner violence more common in pregnant women with severe mental illness? A retrospective study. Int J Soc Psychiatry. 2020;66(3):225-31.
20. Sood M, Krishnan V. Preventive psychiatry in clinical practice. Indian J Soc Psychiatry. 2017;33(2):79-85.
21. Sethuraman B, Rachana A, Kurian S. Knowledge, Attitude, and Practice Regarding Contraception among Women with Schizophrenia: An Observational Study from South India. Indian J Psychol Med. 2019;41(4):323-30.
22. Seeman MV. Gendering psychosis: the illness of Zelda Fitzgerald. Med Humanit. 2016;42(1):65-9.
23. Seeman MV. Women who suffer from schizophrenia: Critical issues. WJP. 2018;8(5):125-36.

24. Seeman MV. Women and Psychosis. Womens Health (Lond Engl). 2012;8(2):215-24.
25. Murthy GV, Janakiramaiah N, Gangadhar BN, Subbakrishna DK. Sex difference in age at onset of schizophrenia: discrepant findings from India. Acta Psychiatr Scand. 1998;97(5):321-5.
26. Miller LJ, Finnerty M. Family planning knowledge, attitudes and practices in women with schizophrenic spectrum disorders. J Psychosom Obstet Gynaecol. 1998;19(4):210-7.
27. Howard LM, Goss C, Leese M, Appleby L, Thornicroft G. The psychosocial outcome of pregnancy in women with psychotic disorders. Schizophr Res. 2004;71(1):49-60.
28. Hodgins S. Violent behaviour among people with schizophrenia: a framework for investigations of causes, and effective treatment, and prevention. Philos Trans R Soc Lond B Biol Sci. 2008;363(1503):2505-18.
29. Morin L, Franck N. Rehabilitation interventions to promote recovery from schizophrenia: a systematic review. Front Psychiatry. 2017;8:100.

CHAPTER 2

Severe Psychiatric Illness in Women: Rehabilitation and Recovery

Ramachandran Padmavati, Mangala Ramamurthi, Arthi R

ABSTRACT

This chapter provides some insights on gender-specific psychosocial intervention for women with serious mental illnesses (SMI). Literature review reveals the paucity of literature pertaining to women-centric approaches. However, the need for taking into account the needs of women in any psychosocial intervention is quite relevant. The impact of these gender-specific interventions needs more robust testing. The relevance of technology in the delivery of interventions also needs gender-specific interventions.

Keywords: Women centric approaches, psychosocial rehabilitation, severe mental illness

INTRODUCTION

Gender is an important element of mental health and mental illness. Women with a diagnosis of serious mental illnesses (SMI) are often doubly disadvantaged. Several gender-related structural factors like limited opportunities interpersonal violence, lack of social supports, poverty, and gender biases in mental health practice reduce accessibility to mental health services or keep the women living with SMI in psychiatric institutions. In contrast to conditions like depression or anxiety, the prevalence rates of schizophrenia and bipolar disorder do not show marked gender differences.[1,2]

Male and female gender vary with respect to age of onset, occurrence of psychotic symptoms, course and outcome of illness, and social functioning. Women with SMI demonstrate more affective symptoms, like depression, impulsivity, emotional instability, and sexual delusions as compared to men, who are at a greater risk of prominent negative symptoms.[3] Women with bipolar disorders present with a first episode of depression, higher frequency episodes of depression, "rapid cycling", and a higher comorbidity of hypothyroidism, migraine, and obesity.[4]

Although many studies, in developing countries have shown that female gender did better than men with respect to course and outcome of schizophrenia, recent studies have not demonstrated any gender difference.[5,6] There is a discrepancy between prevalence, access to and utilization of services, with more men accessing services than women. This is partially explained by the limited number of beds for women in the hospital settings. In a study of allotment of beds, only about a third of the beds were allocated for women.[7] The mental hospitals appear to provide services for men in distress.[7]

Despite the fact that rehabilitation in mental health within the framework of recovery, has been incorporated by many services across the world, in the context of gender, recovery and rehab need to viewed differently.

The implication of Anthony's[8] widely used definition of recovery is that it is an individualized process. There is mounting evidence that supports the value of psychosocial interventions to address mental ill-health, especially in low- and middle-income settings.[9,10] It has been observed that little attention has been paid to the special needs of women in psychosocial rehabilitation (PSR) programs. Social implications such as desertion by marital families, sexual abuse, infectious diseases, and homelessness contribute to the difficulties of rehabilitation of women.[11] In addition to the family hierarchy and the consequent limitations in decision-making about their own lives, women face other forms of woman-specific discrimination, limits to healthcare access, education, and economic independence, and restrictive role delineation as carers of others in the family.[12]

There is a need for PSR services that are gender-sensitive for women with SMI. This chapter details rehabilitation programs of the mentally ill women in India in various contexts, drawing from published reports and personal contributions from service providers. We discuss the meaning of recovery in the global and Indian contexts and why women require special rehabilitation services. Psychopharmacological management of women with schizophrenia can be exceptionally challenging with several biological factors that play significant roles on the prescription practice. This chapter, however, does not include a discussion on the subject.

■ NEEDS FOR WOMEN WITH SMI—INTEGRAL TO RECOVERY

Needs assessment forms the foundation of rehabilitation programs, individually tailored to promote recovery in keeping with the implication of a multimodal approach to recovery.[13] Several meta-analyses have emphasized on "the need to address the complex health, social, and economic needs of those diagnosed with a chronic and highly disabling illness such as schizophrenia."[14] Assessment of needs of persons with SMI has been reported by several studies in outpatient and inpatient setup.[15-18] Specific to women, the common needs expressed across these studies included welfare benefits, money, company and/or intimate relationships, and more financial incentives for working in day care, along with variety in food and grooming items.[19] Community outreach programs, was a felt need expressed by persons with SMI admitted in a tertiary hospital, especially in areas where limited psychiatric services are available.[20]

Several studies have explored the facilitators and barriers for women with SMI needing PSR.[18] Medication adherence, having a work experience, support from family and coworkers, and financial gain from employment were noted to be facilitators. Lack of motivation, medication side effects, lack of proof of identity, stigma from the community, social exclusion, lack of empowerment, and a male-dominated mindset were the key barriers.[21]

Rehabilitation programs need to keep in mind the felt needs of caregivers as well. Several studies have reported on the needs of the families. Family caregivers expressed needs for improvement in hygiene, employment for patients,[15,22] admission for patients to hospitals and help for caregivers for outpatients,[23] and social skills[24] help with changing attitudes for other family members[16,17] vocational training and psychosocial modification.[22] Help in procuring welfare benefits and dealing with psychological distress were the other needs reported by families.[25] A community sample of caregivers also wanted skills training for the patients and jobs.[26] In a study using focused group discussion methodology, caregivers of inpatients with persons with SMI wanted support in managing behavioral problems and social and vocational problems of patients, their own personal health, education about schizophrenia, and managing marital and sexual problems of patients.[18] None of these studies were specific to women.

The context of needs assessments is integral to recovery. It is important that rehabilitation strategies are linked to the needs of patients and their families, in general and specifically for women. In a study conducted on 100 patients and 80 caregivers, 88% of the sample reported that absence of symptoms was an indicator of recovery. Being independent and getting to professional life was perceived as recovery by more than three quarters of the sample in the same study. In this study, women reported that stopping medications was the indicator for recovery.[27] A comprehensive case management would include psychoeducation, social skills training, peer support systems in addition to cognitive remediation, skills training or vocational rehabilitation.[28] Systematic analysis of effective techniques of psychosocial interventions revealed that cognitive remediation, social skills training, psychoeducation, and cognitive therapy (CT) are recommended techniques to promote recovery.[29]

Most reported literature that report general psychosocial interventions are nongender-specific. In a situational analysis of psychosocial interventions programs provided in existing services in two study sites in India and Pakistan, a collaborative and integrated approach when delivering mental health care to patients with psychosis was noted.[30] This approach was noted to be crucial to the long-term and comprehensive management of persons with severe mental health conditions.[31]

PSYCHOSOCIAL INTERVENTIONS DELIVERED TO WOMEN WITH SMI

A large majority of the population of persons with SMI live with their families. However, it has been noted that the ratio of access to treatment between men and women is 3:1.[11] This reiterates the need for psychosocial interventions be delivered at the outpatient setting specific to meet the needs of women.

Cognitive Interventions for Psychosocial Interventions

Cognitive deficits play a major role in impairments on functioning in persons with SMI. The association between deficits in cognition and day-to-day functioning in psychosis has good evidence.[32,33] Both genders with schizophrenia performed poorly when compared to normal controls, in a study of cognitive deficits. The same study also showed that among persons with schizophrenia, men had more serious cognitive deficits than women, in immediate and delayed memory, but not in language, visuospatial, and attention indices.[34] A 12-week, group CT intervention that focused on compensatory strategies and habit learning, Twamley and others[35] proposed that cognitive interventions emphasizing habit learning are likely to result in long-term changes in ability to function independently in the community. In India, Gopal et al.[36] have culturally adapted and tested the feasibility of the English version of the compensatory cognitive training (CCT) manual to suit Indian culture. It remains to be seen if this intervention will be useful for activities of daily living (ADL), especially for women with SMI.

Activities of Daily Living

Activities of daily living comprise tasks such as grooming, clothing nutrition, eating, and exercise, and more complex activities for independent living, such as managing finances and medication. Interventions delivered in a community-driven program.[37,38] by lay community workers.[39] or by trained staff[40] appeared to improve patient functioning in the domains of personal care, interpersonal activities, communication, and work. The studies showed that with intervention, improvement in scores of disability and/or functioning were the same or better in women as compared to men. There is little research on gender-specific interventions.

Domestic Chores—A Felt Need

Domestic chores form an integral part of most of the women in Indian setting. Planning for a meal, buying the ingredients, financial management, time management alongside donning multiple hats at home can be quite challenging. In a study with 31 participants (both men and women) who trained for an hour every day for 5 days, the researchers reported that the mental well-being of the participants improved after 2 and 4 weeks.[41] In this study, more females chose to participate. The researchers opined that a nonjudgmental atmosphere in a day care center, peer learning, and appreciation were important factors for the success of the program.

Further, this program could easily be replicated in resource-scarce settings as it did not require mental health professionals to participate.

At the Schizophrenia Research Foundation (SCARF), a Household Management Efficiency Unit (HOME Unit) has been initiated wherein training for domestic chores would be provided for 4 weeks (5 days per week and 3 hours per day). Vocational skills training for financial sustenance (self-employed or to be employed) and work behavior training (training of soft skills like punctuality, regularity, grooming, working in a team, how to handle success, criticism, stress management) would be dealt with. This program is currently work in progress.

Employment

Work and employment are viewed as important for social inclusion in the community or society.[42,43] Persons with SMI want to work and earn a living. Being employed, in addition to economic gains, also improves self-reliance, self-confidence, being respected by others and facilitates community integration.[44] There are several interventions that have proved to improve employment outcomes for persons with SMI.

Better outcomes of being employed have been reported for with schizophrenia in low- and middle-income country (LMIC). This has been explained on the basis of supportive family, workplace colleagues who are helpful, less stressful, and an informal work opportunities, work timings flexibility, and the lack of high disability pension that acts as a disincentive to work that is given in high-income countries.[45] In addition to the various psychosocial challenges they face, women with SMI have limited access to gainful employment. From a gender perspective, other researchers have stressed on the need for inclusive care centers focusing in skills training for chronic mentally ill women that could facilitate employment opportunities.[10]

In a psychosocial service initiative to improve supportive employment, the Roses Café was initiated as a supportive employment program. It aimed to empower both inpatients and daycare patients in catering skills. Over two-thirds of the persons employed in this activity were women. This program demonstrated that it is possible to empower persons with mental illnesses to live a life of dignity if provided opportunities for a livelihood.[46]

Studies show that opportunities for employment appear to be better in the rural areas for women with mental illnesses as they can be involved in agricultural work, cattle rearing, and related jobs. Jobs are also made available for women through the MNREGA scheme (Mahatma Gandhi National Rural Employment Guarantee Act) which assures 100 days of paid work for one member of the family per year. Flexibility at work and support of family and others at workplace makes it easier for women to sustain in them. Other associated jobs in the agrarian industry like bamboo basket weaving, making broomsticks, thatched leaves, cow dung cakes, and vermicompost can be done from the comfort of their homes.[47] Another study in rural Karnataka highlights the systemic and personal barriers of rural women in finding jobs and sustaining in them which includes stigma and lack of access to benefits and means.[21] Self-help groups (SHGs) are another resource for many women in rural areas. Many treated women with SMI are seen to be part of regular SHGs. Women with severe mental illnesses are incorporated in "special" disability (other than mental illness) SHG.[48]

On background of increasing evidence that being employed reduces chances of relapse and also reduce stigma discrimination significantly, there is a great need to move beyond the routine thinking around employment and financial inclusion of people with SMIs. The THRIVE (Therapeutic interventions, Habit and routine, Relational-social, Individual differences, Values and beliefs, and Emotional factors) model, developed by Parivarthan an nongovernmental organization (NGO) in Maharashtra, is based on an adaptation of the social ecological model. While this is not gender-specific, it offers a good opportunity to women with SMI.

Peer Support

Recent literature has focused on the role of peer support as an established intervention for a person who has lived with mental illness. In India, the first effort at involving persons with lived experience was the peer support program as part of the quality rights program in Gujarat.[49] A survey of patients with psychoses, their families and mental health clinicians to understand the feasibility and acceptance of peer support volunteers led interventions, in a tertiary care setting, showed that majority of the participants accepted peer support interventions. Women caregivers in this study reinforced the need for peer support for their relatives especially for day-to-day living.[50]

Rehabilitation of Women in an Inpatient Setting

Reviews about inadequacies in mental health care for women have been voiced by a number of researchers[10] care providers[4] users and activists.[42] In UK, a strategy document that provided guidelines to organizations on planning and delivery of mental health services for women[51,52] included the need for access to services exclusively for women–group and social activities; single-sex lounges, sleeping, toilet and bathing facilities. Service evaluation reported that most projects provided dedicated spaces for women, female service users had a female case manager. However, the uptake of women-only groups and activities was limited. This report recommended a focus on working together with female service users to identify and set up programs that appeal to women service users was critical to worthwhile engagement.[51]

In a study conducted at a private medical college hospital, inpatients with schizophrenia were provided interventions for 4 weeks on a self-care module. There was improvement on post scores, with both men and women showing improvement.[53] It remains to be seen whether group interventions for cognitive deficits as recommended by Twamley et al.[35] and Gopal et al.[36] is feasible in a residential care setting.

Admissions to residential care can happen due to various reasons other than crisis management. A third of persons with chronic conditions require long-term care.[46] Admissions provide opportunities to develop emotional, personal, cognitive, social, intellectual, and occupational skills needed to live in the community with minimal professional support toward an feasible recovery.[54]

The few published studies on PSR in a residential setting from India report that as assessed at the time of the first intake of the inpatient referrals, vocational rehabilitation is the most common need for planning psychosocial interventions.[55] A study from another half-way home reports that interventions that include individuals and families are effective.[56] There are no details of the methods of interventions in these reports. When a woman is admitted for residential care, families expect the woman to be able to handle household responsibilities independently when they return home. These include doing the laundry, cooking, and cleaning chores. It is important that these activities get incorporated into the routine of the inpatient facility.[56]

Rehabilitation at a Residential Facility Run by an NGO

Experience at Bavishya Bhavan, the residential facility for women, run by the SCARF, India, indicates that improvement in personal care and hygiene is very often a felt need. Women with difficulty in attending to brushing and bathing may have to be trained to do so and supervised regularly to ensure that the task is done. Menstrual hygiene, including education about use of sanitary napkins, safe disposal, keeping clean, and proper washing of soiled clothes are areas that need address. Women are encouraged to keep their rooms clean or participate in cleaning a small area of the facility under supervision. They are engaged in simple tasks like peeling skins of vegetables, separating greens from stems, or cutting vegetables under supervision. Training in making meal plans, in execution of cooking recipes by breaking them into smaller steps, allowing them to cook small portions of simple recipes under supervision or engaging them in fireless cooking, helps to make them more functional when they return to their homes. To meet the need for vocational rehabilitation,[48] a vocational training center within the inpatient premises will help in the rehabilitation process. Activities like sewing, embroidery, tailoring, and craft activities, can be made available besides opportunities for leisure activities like drawing, coloring, and music. Following a structured schedule, for a significant amount of time in a residential facility till it becomes an easy routine for the person, helps them to step back into their roles in the outside world with ease. Unpublished qualitative feedback from the staff (nurses, psychiatric social workers, and occupational therapists) indicates that these interventions can be systematically delivered in a residential care setup.

Residential centers are places where peer support comes to play in a significant way in our experience. Women develop close friendships with other residents which can be exploited to benefit all, but may need some supervision and guidance. The instinctive caregiving tendencies of women can be put to good use in helping those in distress or need and they can become an ally in taking care of difficult, dysfunctional patients.

With reduced life expectancy for persons with SMI attributed to physical health conditions,[57] researchers have recommended to role of physical activity in different forms.[58-60] Although gender-specific literature is limited, it is important to include adequate physical activities like yoga, dance, and walking to improve their mobility, control weight gain, and feel better. At SCARF, emphasis is laid on graded physical activity that includes yoga and walking. Personal and staff narratives report the value of this practice. This however, needs to be examined in a systematic manner.

Where families are available, it is important to engage in dialogs with the patient and caregivers and make a clear post-discharge plan. It is important to keep the family informed about progress happening in their ward while in the facility and encourage them to visit the patient regularly. Getting into their roles at home can become difficult if the period of stay in a structured environment is prolonged.

All efforts in rehabilitation in a residential facility is incomplete without ensuring continuity of care in the community. This is important to sustain the improvement gained in the residential facility.

Women who stay for longer periods in a rehabilitation facility with no imminent exit plans have a different set of needs besides those mentioned above. They need to be engaged adequately to maintain or improve their functionality to prevent deterioration. Providing avenues to express themselves through activities and responsibilities improves self-esteem and mental wellness in these women. Celebrating important festivals, national days, birthdays, and specific days on the mental health calendar and allowing them to entertain themselves by showcasing their skills, preparing special food, and dressing up well help in improving the mood and general sense of well-being among residents. Incentivizing some of the tasks in cash or kind infuses lots of enthusiasm and pride in what they do.

While television and newspapers do help them to stay in touch with the outside world, it is important that they are allowed to go out as often as possible in groups or alone, accompanied by someone if needed, for specific needs or for recreation. This allows them to have a sense of freedom and belonging to the world outside.

ROLE OF NURSING CARE IN AN INPATIENT SETTING

Nurses play a major role in the inpatient setting. In any psychiatric setting, it is the nurse who spends maximum time interacting with the patients, for a better understanding of their background and problems. However, there is limited literature on nurses and nursing care in a psychiatric in patient facility from India. In a study of nurses who completed a self-report questionnaire to assess knowledge and perceptions toward mental illness, it was observed that the respondents noted adequate knowledge on mental illness among nurses. However, the responses also reflected negative attitudes, implying stigma toward mental illness.[61]

GROUP INTERVENTIONS

Psychosocial groups have been recommended as relevant intervention in communities. In a scoping review of group interventions in south east Asia, this intervention was recommended as effective to promote and increase awareness of mental health in communities[9] and in mental health centers.[18] At SCARF group activities including games, reading, and listening, conversations are used as methods to improve communication skills and social interactions.

Does it Matter How and Where It is Offered?

One study highlighted that brief outpatient-based across-the-table psychosocial interventions were as effective as structured facility-based interventions, highlighting that setting did not matter as long as the techniques were feasible and pragmatic. A retrospective chart analysis of the PSR techniques showed that including "regular telephonic interventions to face-to face PSR sessions" were as advantageous as "only face-to-face interventions", for those patients who could not attend for interventions in person. Thus, technology can be used to deliver psychosocial interventions.[62]

IMPROVING ACCESS TO WELFARE BENEFITS AS PART OF PSYCHOSOCIAL INTERVENTIONS

Community-based interventions play an important role to reintegrate persons with lived experiences of mental illnesses into the society. It has been demonstrated repeatedly that it is cost-effective to include mental healthcare in community-based rehabilitation (CBR) programs. It allows for equal opportunities and full participation for persons with all disabilities to access their resources.[63] Analysis of data from a SCARF led TElepsychiatry program in Pudukkottai (STEP) in the rural communities of Tamil Nadu, which showed that a range of PSR activities were provided to persons with SMI and their family members. These included enabling securing disability and welfare benefits, help with getting jobs, obtaining loans from banks to start small businesses, help with mental health crisis situations including admissions. This data demonstrated that it was feasible to integrate psychosocial interventions in community-based programs for persons with SMI.[48] Both reports were not gender-specific.

PREGNANCY, LACTATION, AND PARENTING IN WOMEN WITH SEVERE MENTAL DISORDERS

Women with SMI get married and have children.[64] However, negative sequelae of pregnancy and the subsequent postpartum period have also been noted.[65] Women with schizophrenia and related disorders were noted to be younger, had more relapses, had less family support, were more likely to be single, and had a higher prevalence of smoking and substance misuse during pregnancy compared with women with affective illnesses. This suggests that women with severe mental disorders need more support to optimize both psychiatric and obstetric adverse outcomes. Psychosocial interventions that meet the special needs of mothers with schizophrenia and their children are limited.[66] A higher rate of unplanned and unwanted pregnancies has been noted in women with schizophrenia and related disorders.[41] There indicates a dire need for psychosocial interventions to support these women to make decisions about birth control as well as care during pregnancy. Medication during pregnancy and the postpartum periods are of special concern and need to be addressed.[67] Mother and baby units (MBUs) in inpatient mental health service for women experiencing acute severe postpartum psychiatric difficulties to be admitted with their babies has been a significant development. The first MBU in India was started in 2009 at NIMHANS (National Institute of Mental Health and Neurosciences), Bengaluru, as a five-bedded unit.[65] Bonding interventions and maintenance or restitution of lactation were an important part of care in an MBU. Chandra et al.[68] emphasized on the need for assessments and interventions to provide care for the mother and infant dyad that included both clinical management, infant health, and handling of mother–infant interactions. This study demonstrated that clinical outcomes for the mother with SMI were significantly good as was the relationship between the mother and the infant dyad. More such units are now being established across in the country in both private and government institutions.

Parenting is a rewarding experience for women with severe mental illness, giving hope and satisfaction. Studies have shown that parents are more hopeful than nonparents and hope plays a big role in the individual's recovery process.[69] However parenting can pose a huge challenge to the woman placing high demands on her, affecting parenting methods and impacting the children too. They end up as single parents with provider role added on the parenting role. They are afraid to express their concerns about their challenges as they run a risk of losing the custody of the children. Stigma and societal attitudes also affect the parents and the children.[70]

■ OTHER INTERVENTIONS

The challenges like difficulty in access to services, shortage of mental health professionals, poor mental health awareness, religious beliefs, stigma and poverty contribute to significant mental morbidity, and stress on the need for innovations in care services.[48] While they are not always women-specific, some of them have been useful in the rehabilitation of women with SMI. We have highlighted some of them in this section.

Women Self-help Groups

Providing interventions like psychoeducation, peer support, and referral, with women from SHGs has a positive impact on their mental health. A study showed that women felt relaxed and were comfortable in sharing their problems with peers, experienced reduced emotional distress and physical symptoms, and slept better.[48]

Collaborative Community-based Interventions

It has been shown that CBR delivered using community health workers alongside mental health specialists is feasible and effective in improving clinical and social outcomes of persons with schizophrenia.[38] The COPSI (Care for People with Schizophrenia in India) study provides rigorous evidence about effectiveness of use of supervised community health workers, most of them being women in service delivery in resource-depleted places. This research demonstrated the feasibility and acceptability of community-based intervention which showed a positive impact on reducing disability for a majority of people with psychotic disorders in low-resource settings.[39] However, women-centric evidence needs to be generated.

Family-centric Rehabilitation for Women

The Indian family system values interdependence and mutual concern as key elements and play a vital role in recovery of persons with SMI.[10] Caregiver burden and its impact on their quality of life expressed as physical, emotional, and financial difficulties has been recognized across several studies.[71,72] To address this, a model that included whole families as target for intervention was conceptualized. This study[71] showed that the process facilitates families to reach optimal level of functioning. There is, however, limited research addressing women specifically.

Namma Area (Our Space)

As an experiment at SCARF, a hangout space for persons with lived experiences of mental illnesses was conceived to improve socialization, independence, and reduce apathy and avolition. This facility, underway at SCARF premises twice a week for 4 hours each day, with an average 8–10 men and women is currently being evaluated. The place is owned by the members who use it and activities are planned by them which includes games, music, watching movies, group discussions on themes chosen by them. This also includes group outings accompanied by staff from SCARF. Anecdotal reports from service users and families show that this service has benefitted the mental wellness of the persons using it and has improved communication and social interactions and interest to work in a group.

Homelessness

Circumstances leading to homelessness among women with chronic mental illness is not satisfactorily represented in research and at policy levels. Homeless women are "invisible", and when women with mental illness have wandered for a period, the family seldom take them back home.[73] Homeless mentally ill women are at high risk of exploitation, sexual and physical abuse, unwanted pregnancies or infectious diseases like human immunodeficiency virus (HIV) besides loss of dignity.[74] The need for better shelter homes for homeless women with mental illness has been stressed upon by several studies.[74] A study done on women in a shelter home showed that many women had insight about their illness, its impact on their functioning and need for medication. But reintegration with families remains a challenge as families lack awareness, experience stigma and fear the possibility of relapse which can create problems for the whole family.[73] This underlines the importance of regular psychoeducation for the families and sensitizing local communities about mental illnesses to facilitate reintegration.

Several state-run and NGO-operated institutions are actively involved in rehabilitating homeless women and reintegrating them with families and in the community.[74] These include state-run institutions such as the Hospital for Mental Health (Ahmedabad) and the *Institute for Health and Behavioural Sciences* (Delhi) and nongovernmental agencies, such as *Ashadeep* (Guwahati), *Iswar Sankalp* (Kolkata), *Koshish* (Mumbai), *Banyan* (Chennai), and *Parivartan* (Maharashtra) are actively involved in rehabilitating homeless women and reintegrating them with families and in the community.[74] It would be worthwhile to collate these different experiences to help create a knowledge base to develop socially relevant policy and robust evidence-based practices.

> **KEY POINTS**
> - Addressing several and complex health, social, and economic needs of those diagnosed with SMI are integral to recovery.
> - Nurses play a major role in the inpatient rehabilitation.
> - Psychosocial interventions delivered to women with SMI include cognitive Interventions, peer support, group interventions, etc.
> - Improving access to welfare benefits is an important part of psychosocial interventions.
> - Collaborative community-based interventions and family-centric rehabilitation for women is also very important.

■ REFERENCES

1. Thara R, Patel V. Role of non-governmental organizations in mental health in India. Indian J Psychiatry. 2010;52(7):S389-95.
2. Seedat S, Scott KM, Angermeyer MC, Berglund P, Bromet EJ, Brugha TS, et al. Cross-National Associations Between Gender and Mental Disorders in the World Health Organization World Mental Health Surveys. Arch Gen Psychiatry. 2009;66(7):785-95.
3. Mendrek A, Mancini-Marïe A. Sex/gender differences in the brain and cognition in schizophrenia. Neurosci Biobehav Rev. 2016;67:57-78.
4. Pillai M, Munoli RN, Praharaj SK, Bhat SM. Gender Differences in Clinical Characteristics and Comorbidities in Bipolar Disorder: a Study from South India. Psychiatr Q. 2021;92(2):693-702.
5. Rangaswamy T. Twenty-five years of schizophrenia: The Madras longitudinal study. Indian J Psychiatry. 2012;54(2):134-7.
6. Mayston R, Kebede D, Fekadu A, Medhin G, Hanlon C, Alem A, et al. The effect of gender on the long-term course and outcome of schizophrenia in rural Ethiopia: a population-based cohort. Soc Psychiatry Psychiatr Epidemiol. 2020;55(12):1581-91.
7. Davar B. Mental Health of Indian Women: A Feminist Agenda. New Delhi: Sage Publications, 1999. Sci Technol Soc. 2000;5(2):263.
8. Anthony WA. Recovery from mental illness: The guiding vision of the mental health service system in the 1990s. Psychosoc Rehabil J. 1993;16(4):11-23.
9. Mathias K, Jain S, Fraser R, Davis M, Kimijima-Dennemeyer R, Pillai P, et al. Improving mental ill-health with psycho-social group interventions in South Asia–A scoping review using a realist lens. PLOS Glob Public Health. 2023;3(8):e0001736.
10. Thara R, Kamath S. Women and schizophrenia. Indian J Psychiatry. 2015;57(Suppl 2):S246-51.
11. Malhotra S, Shah R. Women and mental health in India: An overview. Indian J Psychiatry. 2015;57:S205-11.
12. Tirupati S, Ramachandran P. Schizophrenia, recovery and the individual-cultural considerations. Australas Psychiatry. 2020;28(2):190-2.
13. Slade M, Leese M, Taylor R, Thornicroft G. The association between needs and quality of life in an epidemiologically representative sample of people with psychosis. Acta Psychiatr Scand. 1999;100(2):149-57.

14. Solmi M, Croatto G, Piva G, Rosson S, Fusar-Poli P, Rubio JM, et al. Efficacy and acceptability of psychosocial interventions in schizophrenia: systematic overview and quality appraisal of the meta-analytic evidence. Mol Psychiatry. 2023;28(1):354-68.
15. Nagaswami V, Valecha V, Thara R, Rajkumar S, Menon MS. Rehabilitation needs of schizophrenic patients—a preliminary report. Indian J Psychiatry. 1985;27(3):213-20.
16. Pillai R, Sahu K, Mathew V, Sahu S, Chandran P, Ram D. Rehabilitation Needs of Persons with Major Mental Illness in India. Int J Psychosoc Rehabil. 2010;14:95-104.
17. Pavithra SR, Niveditha S, Dharitri R. Rehabilitation Needs of Persons with Schizophrenia and their Families. Artha J Soc Sci. 2013;12(2):33-46.
18. Jagannathan A, Thirthalli J, Hamza A, Hariprasad VR, Nagendra HR, Gangadhar BN. A Qualitative Study On the Needs of Caregivers of Inpatients With Schizophrenia in India. Int J Soc Psychiatry. 2011;57(2):180-94.
19. Waghmare A, Sherine L, Sivakumar T, Kumar CN, Thirthalli J. Rehabilitation Needs of Chronic Female Inpatients Attending Day-care in a Tertiary Care Psychiatric Hospital. Indian J Psychol Med. 2016;38(1):36-41.
20. Chadda RK, Pradhan SC, Bapna JS, Singhal R, Singh TB. Chronic psychiatric patients: an assessment of treatment and rehabilitation-related needs. Int J Rehabil Res. 2000;23(1):55-8.
21. Meera J, Sivakumar T, Shanivaram RK, Kumar D, Chandra PS. (2023). Facilitators and Barriers Faced by Women With Severe Mental Illness in Gaining Employment—a Qualitative Study From Rural India. [online] Available from: https://www.researchsquare.com/article/rs-2663405/v1 [Last accessed December, 2023].
22. Shihabuddeen I, Bilagi S, Krishnamurthy K, Chandran M. Rehabilitation needs and disability in persons with schizophrenia and the needs of the care givers. Delhi Psychiatry J. 2012;(15):118-21.
23. Gandotra S, Paul SE, Daniel M, Kumar K, Raj HA, Sujeetha B. A Preliminary Study of Rehabilitation Needs of In-patients and Out-patients with Schizophrenia. Indian J Psychiatry. 2004;46(3):244-55.
24. Singh TB, Kaloiya GS, Kumar S, Chadda RK. Rehabilitation need assessment of severely mentally ill and effect of intervention. Delhi Psychiatry J. 2010;13:109-16.
25. Kulhara P, Avasthi A, Grover S, Sharan P, Sharma P, Malhotra S, et al. Needs of Indian schizophrenia patients: an exploratory study from India. Soc Psychiatry Psychiatr Epidemiol. 2010;45(8):809-18.
26. Shivakumar P, SK M, Ramaprasad D. Prafulla S, Murthy SK, Ramaprasad D. Family Burden and Rehabilitation Need of beneficiaries of a Rural Mental Health Camp in a Southern state of India. Int J Psychosoc Rehabil. 2010;15:5-12.
27. Gopal S, Mohan G, John S, Raghavan V. What constitutes recovery in schizophrenia? Client and caregiver perspectives from South India. Int J Soc Psychiatry. 2020;66(2):118-23.
28. Yildiz M. Psychosocial Rehabilitation Interventions in the Treatment of Schizophrenia and Bipolar Disorder. Noro Psikiyatri Arsivi. 2021;58(Suppl 1):S77-82.
29. Morin L, Franck N. Rehabilitation Interventions to Promote Recovery from Schizophrenia: A Systematic Review. Front Psychiatry. 2017;8:100.

30. Bird VJ, Davis S, Jawed A, Qureshi O, Ramachandran P, Shahab A, et al. Implementing psychosocial interventions within low and middle-income countries to improve community-based care for people with psychosis-A situation analysis. Front Psychiatry. 2022;13:807259.
31. Khenti A, Fréel S, Trainor R, Mohamoud S, Diaz P, Suh E, et al. Developing a holistic policy and intervention framework for global mental health. Health Policy Plan. 2016;31(1):37-45.
32. Twamley EW, Jeste DV, Bellack AS. A review of cognitive training in schizophrenia. Schizophr Bull. 2003;29(2):359-82.
33. Green MF, Kern RS, Braff DL, Mintz J. Neurocognitive Deficits and Functional Outcome in Schizophrenia: Are We Measuring the "Right Stuff"? Schizophr Bull. 2000; 26(1):119-36.
34. Han M, Huang XF, Chen DC, Xiu MH, Hui L, Liu H, et al. Gender differences in cognitive function of patients with chronic schizophrenia. Prog Neuropsychopharmacol Biol Psychiatry. 2012; 39(2):358-63.
35. Twamley EW, Savla GN, Zurhellen CH, Heaton RK, Jeste DV. Development and Pilot Testing of a Novel Compensatory Cognitive Training Intervention for People with Psychosis. Am J Psychiatr Rehabil. 2008;11(2):144-63.
36. Gopal S, Balasubramanian S, Venkatraman L, Akshaya A, Pavithra R, Padmavati R, et al. Compensatory Cognitive Training—Cultural Adaptation to Persons with Schizophrenia in India. J Psychosoc Rehabil Ment Health. 2022;9(1):21-32.
37. Balaji M, Chatterjee S, Koschorke M, Rangaswamy T, Chavan A, Dabholkar H, et al. The development of a lay health worker delivered collaborative community based intervention for people with schizophrenia in India. BMC Health Serv Res. 2012;12(1):42.
38. Chatterjee S, Naik S, John S, Dabholkar H, Balaji M, Koschorke M, et al. Effectiveness of a community-based intervention for people with schizophrenia and their caregivers in India (COPSI): a randomised controlled trial. Lancet. 2014;383(9926):1385-94.
39. Chatterjee S, Pillai A, Jain S, Cohen A, Patel V. Outcomes of people with psychotic disorders in a community-based rehabilitation programme in rural India. Br J Psychiatry. 2009;195(5):433-9.
40. Ravindren R, Jose K. Psychosocial rehabilitation, disability, and quality of life in patients with schizophrenia residing in long-stay homes. Indian J Soc Psychiatry. 2021;37(4):446.
41. Ambika S, Radhakrishnan G, Sivakumar T, Shamala A. Effectiveness of Domestic Skills Training on Well-Being Among the Persons with Mental Illness Attending Psychiatric Rehabilitation Service. J Psychosoc Rehabil Ment Health. 2020;7(3):295-9.
42. Waghorn G, Lloyd C. The employment of people with mental illness. Aust E-J Adv Ment Health. 2005;4(2):129-71.
43. Yang LH, Phillips MR, Li X, Yu G, Zhang J, Shi Q, et al. Employment outcome for people with schizophrenia in rural v. urban China: population-based study. Br J Psychiatry J Ment Sci. 2013;203(3):272-9.
44. Drake RE, Wallach MA. Employment is a critical mental health intervention. Epidemiol Psychiatr Sci. 2020;29:e178.

45. Isaac M, Chand P, Murthy P. Schizophrenia outcome measures in the wider international community. Br J Psychiatry. 2007;191(S50):s71-7.
46. Gandhi S, Jayaraman S, Sivakumar T, John AP, Joseph A, Prathyusha PV. Can employment in a café change Clientele Attitude towards the staff when they are Persons with Mental Illness? Int J Soc Psychiatry. 2022;68(3):541-7.
47. Sivakumar T, Thirthalli J. Employment of Persons with Severe Mental Illness in Low and Middle-Income Countries: Need for Regionally Relevant Models. J Psychosoc Rehabil Ment Health. 2023;10(3):271-5.
48. Rao K, John S, Kulandesu A, Karthick S, Senthilkumar S, Gunaselvi T, et al. Psychosocial Rehabilitation of Persons with Severe Mental Disorders in Rural South India: Learnings from Step Project. J Psychosoc Rehabil Ment Health. 2022;9(3):335-43.
49. Sheth S, Mehta R, Chauhan A. Humanizing mental health care-Experiences of Peer Support in two different settings in Gujarat after WHO Quality Rights Project. IJMSCR. 2019;2:71-80.
50. Sims S, Hepsipa Omega Juliet S, Joseph J, Gopal S, Raghavan V, Venkatraman L, et al. Acceptability of Peer Support for People With Schizophrenia in Chennai, India: A Cross Sectional Study Amongst People With Lived Experience, Caregivers, and Mental Health Professionals. Front Psychiatry. 2022;13:797427.
51. Taylor TL, Dorer G, Bradfield S, Killaspy H. Meeting the Needs of Women in Mental Health Rehabilitation Services. Br J Occup Ther. 2010;73(10):477-80.
52. Department of Health. (2002). Women's Mental Health: Into the Mainstream. Strategic Development in Women's Mental Health Care. [online] Available from: http://data.parliament.uk/DepositedPapers/Files/DEP2009-0974/DEP2009-0974.pdf [Last accessed December, 2023].
53. Kalavalli, Kanniammal, Malarvizhi. Effectiveness of Practicing Self-Care Module on Activities of Daily Living (ADL) among Patients with Schizophrenia in a Selected Hospital. Int J Res Pharm Sci. 2021;12(1).
54. Manjunatha N, Agarwal PP, Shashidhara HN, Palakode M, Raj EA, Kapanee ARM, et al. First 2 Years of Experience of "Residential Care" at "Sakalawara Rehabilitation Services," National Institute of Mental Health and Neurosciences, Bengaluru, India. Indian J Psychol Med. 2017;39(6):750-5.
55. Desai G, Narasimha A, Harihara SN, Dashrath MS, Bhola P, Berigai PN, et al. A Study on First Intake Assessments of In-patient Referrals to Psychiatric Rehabilitation Services. Indian J Psychol Med. 2014;36(3):236-8.
56. Chowdur R, Dharitri R, Kalyanasundaram S, Suryanarayana Rao N. Efficacy of psychosocial rehabilitation program: The RFS experience. Indian J Psychiatry. 2011;53(1):45.
57. Laursen TM, Munk-Olsen T, Vestergaard M. Life expectancy and cardiovascular mortality in persons with schizophrenia. Curr Opin Psychiatry. 2012;25(2):83-8.
58. Firth J, Carney R, Pownall M, French P, Elliott R, Cotter J, et al. Challenges in implementing an exercise intervention within residential psychiatric care: a mixed methods study. Ment Health Phys Act. 2017;12:141-6.
59. Cherubal AG, Suhavana B, Padmavati R, Raghavan V. Physical activity and mental health in India: A narrative review. Int J Soc Psychiatry. 2019;65(7-8):656-67.
60. Kodama S. Cardiorespiratory Fitness as a Quantitative Predictor of All-Cause Mortality and Cardiovascular Events in Healthy Men and Women: A Meta-analysis. JAMA. 2009;301(19):2024.

61. Gandhi S, Poreddi V, Govindan R, G J, Anjanappa S, Sahu M, et al. Knowledge and perceptions of Indian primary care nurses towards mental illness. Investig Educ En Enferm. 2019;37(1):e7.
62. Juliet SHO, Joseph J, Sims S, Annamalai K, Venkatraman L, Raghavan V, et al. Does Telephone Based Intervention Combined with Face to Face Contact Improve Socio-Occupational Functioning of Persons with Schizophrenia? A Retrospective Chart Review. J Psychosoc Rehabil Ment Health. 2022;9(1):99-105.
63. Janardana N, Naidu DM. Inclusion of people with mental illness in community based rehabilitation: Need of the day. Int J Psychosoc Rehabil. 2012;16(1):117-24.
64. Aggarwal S, Grover S, Chakrabarti S. A comparative study evaluating the marital and sexual functioning in patients with schizophrenia and depressive disorders. Asian J Psychiatry. 2019;39:128-34.
65. Taylor CL, Stewart R, Ogden J, Broadbent M, Pasupathy D, Howard LM. The characteristics and health needs of pregnant women with schizophrenia compared with bipolar disorder and affective psychoses. BMC Psychiatry. 2015;15(1):88.
66. Gearing RE, Alonzo D, Marinelli C. Maternal schizophrenia: psychosocial treatment for mothers and their children. Clin Schizophr Relat Psychoses. 2012;6(1):27-33.
67. Babu GN, Desai G, Chandra PS. Antipsychotics in pregnancy and lactation. Indian J Psychiatry. 2015;57(Suppl 2):S303-307.
68. Chandra P, Desai G, Reddy D, Thippeswamy H, Saraf G. The establishment of a mother-baby inpatient psychiatry unit in India: Adaptation of a Western model to meet local cultural and resource needs. Indian J Psychiatry. 2015;57(3):290.
69. Bonfils KA, Adams EL, Firmin RL, White LM, Salyers MP. Parenthood and severe mental illness: relationships with recovery. Psychiatr Rehabil J. 2014;37(3):186-93.
70. Thara R, Srinivasan TN. How stigmatising is schizophrenia in India? Int J Soc Psychiatry. 2000;46(2):135-41.
71. Stanley S, Balakrishnan S, Ilangovan S. Psychological distress, perceived burden and quality of life in caregivers of persons with schizophrenia. J Ment Health. 2017;26(2):134-41.
72. Raj E, Shiri S, Jangam K. Subjective burden, psychological distress, and perceived social support among caregivers of persons with schizophrenia. Indian J Soc Psychiatry. 2016;32(1):42.
73. Nagawanshi A. Do shelter homes recover mental health? A case study on women with mental illness in rural community. J Surv Fish Sci. 2023;10-1(S):3787-91.
74. Narasimhan L, Kishore Kumar KV, Regeer B, Gopikumar V. Homelessness and women living with mental health issues: lessons from the banyan's experience in Chennai, Tamil Nadu. In: Anand M (Ed). Gender and Mental Health. Singapore: Springer Singapore; 2020. pp. 173-91.

Depressive and Anxiety Disorders

Srilakshmi Pingali, S Sireesha

■ ABSTRACT

The biological and psychosocial challenges women face throughout out their lifetime make them vulnerable to mood and anxiety disorders. This chapter intends to discuss the depressive and anxiety disorders in general in females with a special focus on the episodes that are unique to women such premenstrual dysphoric disorder, perinatal and post-menopausal depression. To begin with we discuss epidemiology and then subsequently discuss diagnostic indicators, risk factors and special considerations such as suicide, inflammatory hypothesis, assessment tools and management, for both depressive and anxiety disorders separately.

Keywords: Perinatal depression and anxiety disorders, premenstrual dysphoric disorder, postmenopausal depression, stress and inflammation

■ INTRODUCTION

Depressive and anxiety disorders are more common in women and the difference in genders becomes prominent after puberty. The hormonal fluctuations and the unique psychosocial challenges women face throughout their reproductive age starting from menarche to menopause and beyond increase vulnerability to these disorders. The influence of the reproductive hormones on the central nervous system (CNS) and the mediating role of the process of inflammation are proposed to be responsible for these disorders. Moreover, exposure to psychotropics used in pregnancy and lactation to fetus and infant and the risk-benefit ratio for the use of psychotropics during pregnancy and lactation are challenges in the treatment of women with depressive and anxiety disorders.

■ DEPRESSIVE DISORDERS IN WOMEN

Mood disorders are syndromes consisting of a cluster of signs and symptoms, sustained over a period of weeks to months, that represent a marked departure from a person's habitual functioning, in which pathological moods and related vegetative and psychomotor disturbances dominate the clinical picture. Depression is the most common mood disorder in women.[1]

Epidemiology

Depression is more common in women of reproductive age and present with more internalizing symptoms, while men present with more externalizing symptoms. Women are both biologically and psychosocially vulnerable. The fluctuations in gonadal hormones throughout their reproductive life span are implicated as one of the factors. This concept is further strengthened by the fact that the rates of depression are equal in both sexes before puberty and after age 65. The stressors faced by women are also unique, contributing to their vulnerability.

In India, it is estimated that nearly one third of patients seeking help from healthcare facilities could have symptoms related to depression. The National Mental Health Survey of India,[2] which is a multisite population-based cross-sectional study across 12 states, has shown that the weighted prevalence of depression for both current and lifetime to be 2.7% and 5.2%, respectively. The survey also showed that lifetime prevalence was more in females (5.72%) when compared with males (4.75%). The lifetime prevalence was also higher among urban population, lower income groups, lower levels of education, and those recently divorced or widowed. Prevalence of current depression in females was 23% more likely than males. The treatment gap was 80% in women.

It has been postulated that this increased prevalence in women is associated with female-specific reproductive events such as perimenstrual changes, pregnancy, postpartum period, and menopause.[3]

Diagnostic Criteria

International Classification of Diseases 11[4]

The International Classification of Diseases (ICD) describes depressive disorders in the BlockL2-6A7. The disorders included in this category include single-episode depressive disorder, recurrent depressive disorder, dysthymic disorder, mixed depressive and anxiety disorders. Premenstrual dysphoric disorder (PMDD) is coded under *GA34.41*, postpartum depression is coded under mental or behavioral disorders associated with pregnancy, childbirth, and the puerperium, with/without psychotic symptoms *(6E20/21)*.

Depressive disorders are characterized by depressive mood (e.g., sad, irritable, and empty) or loss of pleasure, accompanied by other cognitive, behavioral, or neurovegetative symptoms such as difficulty concentrating, feelings of worthlessness, excessive or inappropriate guilt, hopelessness, recurrent thoughts of death or suicide, changes in appetite or sleep, psychomotor agitation or retardation, and reduced energy or fatigue that significantly affect the individual's ability to function. The symptoms should last at least 2 weeks and occur daily.

The depressive episode has been classified further as mild, moderate, and severe depending on intensity of symptoms and effect on functioning. According to course of the episode, the specifier of partial or full remission is added. For example, single-episode depressive disorder, currently in partial remission means a prior diagnosis of a depressive disorder has been met, but currently the full definitional requirements are not met, though some significant mood symptoms remain.

Other specifiers include prominent anxiety symptoms in mood episodes, panic attacks in mood episodes, persistent depressive episodes, and melancholic depressive episodes.

Difference between International Classification of Diseases 10 and 11[5]

Features of ICD-11 contrasting to the ICD-10 are:
- Expansion of criteria for quality of mood as sad, irritable, or empty
- Exclusion of reduced energy or fatigue from essential criteria
- Inclusion of suicidal thoughts and psychotic symptoms from moderate depressive episode onward
- Severity is classified according to degree of functional impairment rather than a count of symptoms
- Symptomatic and course qualifiers for mood episodes

Risk Factors[6,7]

Risk factors for depression can be both psychosocial and biological.

Psychosocial Factors

The psychosocial factors that put the female at a disadvantage and hence vulnerable to depression are given in **Table 1**.

TABLE 1: Psychosocial factors for depression in women.

Partner and family factors	- Excessive partner alcohol use - Sexual and physical violence by the husband - Widowed or separated - Low autonomy in decision-making - Low levels of support from one's family - Relationship difficulties
Stressful life events	- Childbirth and maternal roles - Caring and nurturing the old and sick of the family - Lesser opportunities of education and employment - Societal expectations such as birth of a girl child when a boy is desired

Biological Factors

The increased vulnerability to depression during major events of the reproductive life span such as puberty, premenstrual period, and postpartum and perimenopausal period show a role of reproductive hormones, especially estrogen. Estrogen has a protective effect on the pathology that underlies depression and decreases in estrogen may increase the risk for depression.

The low rate of depression in men may be accounted for by the fact that in the male brain testosterone is converted into estrogen by endogenous aromatase. Since testosterone does not cycle in men as estrogen does in women, there may be a more consistent protection in men.[8]

How Depression Differs between Men and Women?

- Depression is not only more in women but is also more persistent.
- Women tend to have more symptoms and higher symptom severity and report more subjective distress.
- Melancholic features are more common in women.
- Women are more likely to have a comorbid anxiety disorder and men a comorbid substance abuse disorder.
- There are no sex differences in antidepressant response.
- The subgenual anterior cingulate cortex (sgACC) which has elevated metabolic activity in depression is higher in women.
- Reduced expression of somatostatin (SST), a marker for inhibitory gamma-aminobutyric acid (GABA) neurons implicated in the network of mood regulation [sgACC amygdala and dorsolateral prefrontal cortex (DLPFC) is more marked in females.

Depression and Suicide[9-11]

Indian women have twice the suicide death rate compared with the global average for women. Presence of mood disorder increases the risk of suicide. About 15% of patients with depression die by suicide.

Risk Factors of Suicide

- *History:* Study on inpatients admitted for major depressive disorders in India showed severity of depression and history of suicidal attempts predicted the presence and severity of current suicidal ideation.
- *Clinical features:* Hopelessness, worthlessness, inappropriate guilt, thoughts of death, or suicidal ideation.
- *Comorbidities:* Substance use disorders, anxiety disorders, disabling medical illness.
- *Personality traits:* Impulsivity, aggression, pessimism, and few reasons for living.

- *Attachment:* Insecure attachment with affective dysregulation.
- *Family history of suicide:* Familial aggregation of suicide may be attributed to genetic vulnerability to major psychiatric disorders, genetic nature of impulsive–aggressive personality traits, and in some cases copycat mechanisms.
- *Stressful life events:* As predisposing or precipitating factors.

Neurobiology of Depression

Genetics, personality traits, and epigenetic modifications due to stress are all implicated in depression.

Genetics

Heritability of depression is around 37%. Among the various genes associated with the increased risk of depression, the allele that codes for the promoter region of serotonin transporter is best studied. It moderates the association between stressful life events and depression.

Personality Traits

Traits such as harm avoidance and low levels of novelty seeking are also partially heritable and increase the vulnerability to depression.

Epigenetic Modification

Where acute stress can act as both precipitating and perpetuating factors in depression, prolonged stress may bring about epigenetic changes affecting brain structure, one such being reduced volume of hippocampus in patients of depression, increasing the vulnerability to depression. Maltreatment in the form of physical, verbal, or sexual abuse and parental neglect in childhood increase the risk of depression by two- to threefold. Similarly, major life events involving interpersonal loss coupled with social rejection are the most common precipitants of depression, with up to 44% of depressive episodes being preceded by such stress.

Stress, Inflammation, and Depression[12]

Inflammation probably links stress to depression. This is further supported by the fact that other illnesses that have inflammation as underlying mechanism such as obesity, diabetes, cardiovascular diseases, and rheumatoid arthritis co-occur with depression.

Stress is associated with elevated inflammatory activity. These effects are apparent for both early life stress and adulthood life stress and they have been demonstrated at the protein level (i.e., proinflammatory cytokines), intracellular signaling level (i.e., transcription factors), and genome-wide expression level (i.e., gene programs and transcriptional skewing). The inflammation in turn can cause sad mood, anhedonia, fatigue, and social withdrawal.

The increased proinflammatory cytokines in the brain activate both the sympathetic nervous system and the hypothalamic–pituitary axis. Animal models' cytokines were found to modulate various neurotransmitters in the brain such as serotonin, dopamine, etc., leading to decreases in daytime activity, decreased interest in feeding, grooming, socializing, and mating, and hedonic behaviors. These behaviors have been collectively called sickness behaviors and it has been hypothesized that similar mechanisms occur in humans to cause symptoms of depression.

Sex Chromosomes, Steroids, and Inflammation[13]

- Sex chromosomes are intricately involved in the development and organization of the immune system. The X chromosome contains more immune-related genes than any other chromosome. Some genes residing on the X chromosome are resistant to inactivation, resulting in a double dose of the gene product for females.
- Sex steroids including estrogens, progesterone, and androgens—all influence immune cell population. Progesterone is anti-inflammatory, while estrogen in low concentration is proinflammatory and at high concentration anti-inflammatory. Androgens are generally immunosuppressive.
- Receptors for estrogen and progesterone are present in areas of brain involved with emotion and cognition, such as amygdala and hippocampus. They also affect receptors that modulate GABA, serotonin, dopamine, and N-methyl-D-aspartate (NMDA). Estrogen fluctuations across the menstrual cycle alter mood and neural responses to psychosocial stress.

Gut Microbiome and Inflammation[14]

Alteration of the gut microbiota or dysbiosis and the consequent alteration of intestinal permeability lead to the production and spread into the bloodstream of a potent proinflammatory endotoxin, lipopolysaccharide (LPS). This small molecule has an important influence on the modulation of the CNS, increasing the activity of areas such as amygdala. It also leads to activation of inflammatory and immune response.

Assessment

History

A diagnosis of depression is done by a thorough history from multiple sources, including family and past records. History should also include substance use, history of similar or manic symptoms, or other medical illnesses in order to rule out comorbidities and to differentiate depression due to substance use, due to medical condition, or a depressive episode in bipolar disorder.

Physical Examination

General physical and systemic examination including examination for thyroid swelling and any nutritional deficiencies

Assessment Tools

Tools for screening, assessment of the severity, and the changeover time with treatment can be used.
- *Across lifespan:*
  - Becks depression inventory—for use between ages 13 and 80 years; self-report scale; 21 items
  - Hamilton depression rating scale—rater administered; scored on 17 items
  - Montgomery-Åsberg depression rating scale—administered above age 18; sensitive to change over time; 10 items
- *Scale for PMDD:*
  - Premenstrual symptom screening tool—allows rating of symptom severity; 19 items
  - Daily record of severity of symptoms—34 items scale
- *Scale for perimenopausal depression:*
  - Meno D—self/clinician rated; 12 items
- *Scale for peripartum depression:*
  - Edinburgh postnatal depression scale—used in pregnancy and postpartum; 10 items
  - Postpartum depression rating scale

Investigations

- Complete hemogram, liver and kidney function tests, blood sugar, and lipid levels
- Neuroimaging in late-onset depression or with neurological signs

By the end of all assessments, the following objectives should be met:[15]
- Assessment of need
- Development of a treatment plan
- Physical health problems to be considered
- Coexisting mental health problems to be considered
- Review reasons for relapse, noncompliance, and admission in the past
- Previous treatment history to be considered
- Risk to self and others to be assessed and the setting of treatment as outpatient or hospitalization of patient to be considered

Management

Indications for Inpatient Treatment
- Risk of harm to self or others
- Severe side effects
- Diagnostic clarification
- Unmanageable in outpatient setup
- Management of other medical or psychiatric comorbidities requiring inpatient care

The management of depression depends on the stage of illness, severity of illness, past response, comorbidities, and risk of harm to self and others

Acute Phase[16]
- *Psychotherapy:* In patients with mild-to-moderate depression, psychotherapy is considered as an initial treatment. Psychotherapy is also used in case of significant psychosocial stressors, intrapsychic conflict, and interpersonal difficulties. Some of the therapies are cognitive behavior therapy, interpersonal therapy, marital therapy, etc.
- *Antidepressants:* Antidepressant medication may be used as initial treatment modality for patients with mild, moderate, or severe major depressive disorder. The choice of antidepressants depends on past response, side effect profile, patient preference, and comorbidities among others.
- *Electroconvulsive therapy (ECT):*[17]

Indications of ECT in a patient of depression include the following:
- Poor oral intake
- High suicidal risk
- High level of distress requiring rapid symptom remission
- Psychotic features
- Melancholic features
- Peripartum depression
- Treatment resistance
- With severe mixed affective features

Continuation Phase
The continuation phase lasts for a period of 16–24 weeks at the same dose of the drugs that helped in acute phase.

Maintenance Phase
Maintenance treatment has to be considered due to risk of recurrence, which happens in 50–85% of cases. The duration of treatment is decided based on

previous treatment history and number of previous depressive episodes. Patients with three or more relapses need to be given long-term treatment. When the decision is made to discontinue maintenance pharmacotherapy, it is best to taper the medication over the course of at least several weeks to few months.

ANXIETY DISORDERS IN WOMEN

Anxiety disorders are characterized by anxious apprehension or fear in response to a perceived threat. Core features of anxiety disorders include subjective anxiety or fear, physiologic reactivity, and avoidance behavior followed by functional impairment.

While fear represents a reaction to perceived imminent threat in the present, anxiety is more about perceived anticipated threat. A key differentiating feature among the various anxiety and fear-related disorders is disorder-specific foci of apprehension.[4]

Epidemiology[18]

An estimated 4.05% of the global population has an anxiety disorder, translating to 301 million people. Women are 1.66 times more likely to be affected by anxiety disorders than men in India, which is around 2.57% as per the national mental health survey done in 2016. Specific phobias are the most common anxiety disorders.

The age of onset for anxiety disorders differs among the disorders. Separation anxiety disorder and specific phobia start during childhood (7 years), followed by social anxiety (13 years), agoraphobia without panic attacks (20 years), and panic disorder (24 years). Generalized anxiety disorder (GAD) starts later in life. Anxiety disorders tend to run a chronic course, with symptoms fluctuating in severity.[19]

Diagnostic Criteria

International Classification of Diseases 11[4]

The ICD-11 classifies anxiety or fear-related disorders in BlockL1-6B0. It includes GAD, panic disorder, agoraphobia, specific phobia, social anxiety disorder (SAD), selective anxiety disorder, and selective mutism.
- *GAD:* Marked symptoms of anxiety that persist for at least several months, for more days than not, manifested by either general apprehension (i.e., "free-floating anxiety") or excessive worry focused on multiple everyday events, most often concerning family, health, finances, and school or work, together with additional symptoms such as muscular tension or motor restlessness, sympathetic autonomic overactivity, subjective experience of nervousness, difficulty maintaining concentration, irritability, or sleep disturbance.

- *Panic disorder:* Recurrent unexpected panic attacks that are not restricted to particular stimuli or situations. Panic attacks are discrete episodes of intense fear or apprehension, accompanied by the rapid and concurrent onset of several characteristic symptoms (e.g., palpitations or increased heart rate, sweating, trembling, shortness of breath, chest pain, dizziness or lightheadedness, chills, hot flushes, and fear of imminent death). There is persistent concern about the recurrence or significance of panic attacks or behaviors intended to avoid their recurrence
- *Agoraphobia:* Marked and excessive fear or anxiety that occurs in response to multiple situations where escape might be difficult or help might not be available, such as using public transportation, being in crowds, and being outside the home alone. The individual is consistently anxious about these situations due to a fear of specific negative outcomes.
- *Specific phobia:* It is characterized by a marked and excessive fear or anxiety that consistently occurs when exposed to one or more specific objects or situations and that is out of proportion to actual danger.
- *SAD:* Marked and excessive fear or anxiety that consistently occurs in one or more social situations such as social interactions, being observed, or performing in front of others (e.g., giving a speech). Fear of being negatively evaluated by others. Such situations are avoided or endured with difficulty.
- *Separation anxiety disorder:* Marked and excessive fear or anxiety about separation from specific attachment figures. In children, separation anxiety focuses on caregivers, parents, or other family members. In adults, it is a romantic partner or children, thoughts of harm or untoward events befalling the attachment figure, reluctance to go to school or work, recurrent excessive distress upon separation, reluctance or refusal to sleep away from the attachment figure, and recurrent nightmares about separation.
- *Selective mutism:* Consistent selectivity in speaking (for example, speaks at home but not at school), not confined to first month in school and not due to lack of knowledge of the spoken language.

Differences between International Classification of Diseases 10 and 11[20]

- In ICD-10, anxiety disorders are classified under neurotic, stress-related, and somatoform disorders, whereas in ICD-11 included under anxiety and fear-related disorders.
- Emphasizes the wide range of possible emotional responses which may include shame, anger, or disgust.
- Agoraphobia is a separate diagnostic entity with a panic attack specifier.

- The definition has been elaborated to several scenarios where escape may be hard or where help may not be obtainable.
- Social phobia has been renamed as SAD.
- Duration for GAD is now several months.

Risk Factors[21,22]

Psychosocial Factors

- *Female gender:* Females were 1.66 times more affected than men. Hypothesized—to be due to poor social support, differential access to care, and an increased tendency of worrying.
- Age group of 40–59 years
- *Urban metro dwellers:* Due to reasons of overcrowding, poor social support, social isolation, migration, and poor quality of life.

Biological Factors

- The difference between men and women starts around puberty with worry cognitions affecting day-to-day activities increasing in girls around puberty.
- Anxiety disorders among women often precipitate at times of hormonal fluctuations including puberty, premenstrual period, pregnancy, postpartum, and menopausal transition. For instance, first attack of panic disorder occurs perinatally in 3–11% of women and panic disorder may start or worsen during menopause. Women with history of GAD was more likely to recur perinatally.

Biopsychosocial Model of Anxiety[23-26]

A combination of biological, psychological, and social factors influences the sex differences and course of anxiety disorders over female lifespan.

Girls experience multiple forms of abuse, including sexual abuse, household dysfunction, and neglect at a higher rate than boys. Women are physiologically more reactive to stressors and exhibit a ruminative coping style and often seek support from others in times of stress. Women exhibit greater anxiety sensitivity than men as defined by catastrophic interpretations of bodily sensations such as heart pounding or dizziness. All women experience hormonal fluctuations at different phases of their life, but not all women develop anxiety disorders. Thus, it is not just hormone levels that determine vulnerability but their interactions with brain.

At puberty, ovarian hormones fluctuate and at the same time, brain remodeling occurs in areas implicated in anxiety disorders such as amygdala. This remodeling may program the brain's responsivity to trophic and steroid hormones, persisting into adulthood. Altered interactions between

Allopregnanolone (Allo) and GABA A receptors across menstrual cycle may contribute to anxiety and affective disorders. Allo is a potent positive allosteric modulator of the GABA A receptor with anxiolytic, anesthetic, and sedative properties.

Assessment

The plan of assessment follows the same as for depression; however, certain conditions such as substance-induced anxiety disorders, hypoglycemia, hypo/hyperthyroidism, cardiac disorders, chronic respiratory disease, vitamin B deficiency, and inner ear conditions can present with anxiety symptoms and hence need to be focused on.

Scales for Assessment of Anxiety Disorders

- GAD:
  - GAD-7 scale—a screening instrument with sensitivity of 89% and a specificity of 82%; scores above 10 indicate need for further evaluation
- Agoraphobia:
  - The severity measure for agoraphobia—adult is a 10-item measure that assesses the severity of symptoms of agoraphobia in individuals above age 18; administered following a diagnosis of agoraphobia
- Panic disorder:
  - The panic disorder severity scale (PDSS)—self-report scale that measures the severity of panic attacks and panic disorder symptoms. It is appropriate for use with adolescents (13+) and adults; 7 items scale
- Specific phobia:
  - Specific phobia questionnaire—screening tool for assessing fear of a broad range of phobic stimuli and the extent to which fear interferes with daily life
- Separation anxiety disorder:
  - The adult separation anxiety symptom questionnaire (ASA-27) self-report measure of adult separation anxiety (ASA)
- Social phobia:
  - Social phobia inventory (SPIN)-17 item; self-rated
- Selective mutism:
  - The Frankfurt Scale of Selective Mutism—detects selective mutism and its severity from the perspective of parents of children between the ages of 3 and 18 years; 10 items

Management

The treatment includes psychotherapy, pharmacotherapy, or a combination. The choice of treatment depends on stage of illness, severity of illness, past response, comorbidities, and risk of harm to self and others.

Psychotherapy

Cognitive behavioral therapy has the highest level of evidence for treatment of anxiety disorders among other psychotherapies. If avoidance of feared situations is a relevant factor, exposure techniques should be included in the treatment schedule.

Treatment resistant anxiety: Before considering a patient to be treatment unresponsive, the points to considered are whether the diagnosis was correct, whether the adherence was sufficient, and was the drug prescribed for adequate dose and duration. If after treatment, at what is considered an adequate dose for 4-6 weeks, a patient shows no response, the medication should be changed to another selective serotonin reuptake inhibitor (SSRI) or a selective norepinephrine reuptake inhibitor (SNRI).

Pharmacotherapy[27]

First-line drugs are the SSRIs and serotonin–norepinephrine reuptake inhibitors. When developing a treatment plan, efficacy, adverse effects, interactions, costs, and the preference of the patient should be considered. Anxiolytic effect of these antidepressants has a latency of 2-4 weeks. Starting doses in the lower part of the therapeutic range is recommended. Drug treatment should be continued for 12 months or more after remission has occurred. When the decision to taper has been made; the dose should be slowly tapered off over a period of 2 weeks at treatment termination.

MOOD AND ANXIETY DISORDERS SPECIFIC TO WOMEN AND RELATED ISSUES

Premenstrual Dysphoric Disorder[28]

Premenstrual dysphoric disorder includes a constellation of mood, behavioral, and physical changes that occur in a cyclic pattern prior to menstruation and then wane off after the menstrual period in women of reproductive age. Duration of symptoms vary from a few days to 2 weeks and intensify 2-6 days before and resolve completely after 1 week following the onset of menses. It occurs in about 3-8% and causes significant distress and functional impairment.

It is coded as a separate disorder in ICD-11 in diseases of the genitourinary system and cross-listed in the subgrouping of depressive disorders due to the prominence of mood symptomatology.

The symptoms include:
- Mood symptoms (depressed mood and irritability)
- Somatic symptoms (lethargy, joint pain and overeating)
- Cognitive symptoms (concentration difficulties and forgetfulness)

Premenstrual dysphoric disorder often has a comorbid anxiety disorder such as GAD (40%), panic disorder (25%), and SAD (20%). Women with anxiety disorders may also develop premenstrual exacerbation of symptoms.

Etiology
- PMDD is in part attributable to luteal phase abnormalities in serotonergic activity.
- A suboptimal luteal phase GABA A receptor sensitivity to Allo is proposed as a mechanism for PMDD pathogenesis.
- Deficiencies of certain vitamins and minerals including vitamin B, vitamin D, calcium, and magnesium may play a role.

Management
- *SSRIs* are effective in intermittent dosing as they enhance the formation of neuroactive steroids, Allo, especially for irritability, affect lability, and mood swings, while having a weaker effect on depressed mood and somatic symptoms.
- *Combined hormonal contraceptive (CHC) pills*, especially 20 µg ethinyl estradiol/3 mg drospirenone in a 24/4 extended cycle regimen has been shown to significantly improve the emotional and physical symptoms of PMDD. Drospirenone can counteract estrogen-induced stimulation of the renin–angiotensin–aldosterone system that can lead to sodium and water retention and symptoms such as breast tenderness and edema.
- *Copper intrauterine devices (IUDs)* are recommended for those not seeking hormonal contraceptives.
- *Gonadotropin hormone-releasing hormone (GnRH) agonists:* In resistant cases, artificially induced menopause with medical (GnRH agonists) or surgical (oophorectomy) menopause usually eliminates symptoms.

Postpartum Depression

A syndrome associated with pregnancy or commencing within 6 weeks of delivery involving significant mental and behavioral features such as mood lability, sadness, dysphoria, emotional confusion, and tearfulness. Though 4-6 weeks have been cited as variable by different classificatory systems, the first year after delivery continues to be a high-risk period for depression.

Risk Factors
- History of depression
- Past psychiatric conditions such as bipolar disorder, obsessive-compulsive disorder, eating disorder, and schizophrenia increase the chances of postpartum depression.

Management

The challenge of treating depression during pregnancy is manifold. The risk of untreated depression versus exposure of fetus to psychotropics.

Effect of Untreated Depression in Pregnancy[29]

- *In mother*: Risk of inadequate maternal weight gain, substance abuse, and preeclampsia.
- *In fetus*: Risk of preterm birth, low birth weight, fetal distress, increased risk of cesarean birth, increased risk of neonatal intensive care unit (NICU) admission.

Use of Antidepressants in Perinatal Period[30,31]

Pregnancy

Decisions about psychiatric medication use during and after pregnancy should be ideally made before conception. In euthymic women with a history of major depression, the planned, voluntary withdrawal of antidepressant medication prior to conception is associated with a fivefold increase in the risk of relapse during pregnancy. Certain things to remember in these scenarios are that a longer duration of illness and a larger number of past depressive episodes each predict an increased risk of relapse and about half of the relapses occur during the first trimester. In general, psychotherapy is recommended for mild-to-moderate depression.[32-34] and antidepressants should be reserved for moderate-to-severe depression. Before starting an antidepressant, an individualized risk–benefit assessment should be done, including:
- Psychiatric history
- Response to prior or ongoing antidepressants
- Mental health outcomes following prior attempts to discontinue the medication
- Woman's treatment preference.

Most guidelines have shown a preference to sertraline. Paroxetine is not preferred due to its reported cardiac effects on fetus. However, switching treatment in ongoing, stable patient is discouraged. The use of a single medication at a higher dosage is preferred over multiple medications and those with fewer metabolites, higher protein binding, and fewer interactions with other medications are also preferred. SSRIs and tricyclic antidepressants (TCAs) had some evidence for effectiveness in anxiety disorders in perinatal period. If women are not willing for medications, cognitive behavioral therapy (CBT) may be a good alternative for women with panic disorder and phobia.

Effects of Antidepressants in Pregnancy

- The concern about using antidepressants in pregnancy is whether they cause pregnancy complications such as miscarriages or preterm deliveries and congenital anomalies in the developing fetus or cause long-term neurodevelopmental problems.
- Studies have not shown any causal relations between use of SSRIs and its dose with miscarriage. It is likely due to other factors including the pathophysiology of mood disorders and substance abuse.
- The increased cardiac risk in developing fetus was found to be largely due to secondary factors associated with underlying depression.
- However, SSRIs were found to be associated with preterm birth and neonatal complications, such as a risk for lower Apgar scores and admission to the neonatal intensive care unit and may persist 30 days postdelivery.
- An elevated risk of intellectual disability in children born to women who used antidepressant medication during pregnancy is likely attributable to illness related and not to the antidepressant medication itself.

Lactation[35]

In mild-to-moderate depression, psychotherapy is the first line of treatment and antidepressant medications are recommended for moderate-to-severe depression. Maternal lactation status should not delay treatment. During pregnancy, an individualized risk–benefit analysis, mother's clinical history and response to treatment, the risks of untreated depression, the risks and benefits of breastfeeding, the benefits of treatment, the known and unknown risks of the medication to the infant, and the mother's wishes are taken into consideration. Sertraline has lower levels in human milk and infant serum is often a first choice. If there has been response to a particular antidepressant in the past, it should be considered as a first-line treatment if there are no contraindications.

Perimenopausal Depression[36,37]

The pooled prevalence of depression in perimenopausal and postmenopausal women in India was found to be 42.47%. Risk for depressive symptoms increases with the beginning of the menopausal transition and stays elevated through early postmenopause and decreases 5–10 years after menopause. Perimenopausal depression presents with classic depressive symptoms in combination with menopause symptoms such as vasomotor symptoms and sleep disturbance and the various psychosocial challenges midlife brings with it. During the perimenopausal period, these normally cyclic hormonal fluctuations become increasingly erratic followed by progressively longer periods of estrogen withdrawal. It has been postulated that changes in these hormonally mediated neuromodulatory effects may heighten the risk for mood disorders in women with sensitivity-to-normal hormonal fluctuations.

Risk Factors

Along with other risk factors for depression, negative attitudes toward aging and menopause and menopausal symptoms such as hot flashes and poor sleep are independently associated with depression.

Management[38]

Antidepressants and psychotherapy are the frontline treatments for perimenopausal depression. Estrogen therapy due to its side effects such as increased risk for breast cancer and thromboembolism is not approved to treat perimenopausal depression, but when used to treat vasomotor symptoms, it has shown to improve mood symptoms when given closer to menopause.

> **KEY POINTS**
> - While treating the depressive and anxiety disorders in women, the psychosocial stressors specific to women should be taken in to utmost consideration.
> - Also the hormonal fluctuations throughout the reproductive cycle influence the course as well as treatment of depressive and anxiety disorders.
> - In pregnant women with depressive and anxiety disorders the risk to the growing fetus, from both the illness per se and the pharmacological agents should be considered.
> - Management protocols keeping the special unmet needs of women in mind should be developed.

■ REFERENCES

1. Sadock BJ, Ruiz P, Sadock VA (Eds). Kaplan and Sadock's Comprehensive Textbook of Psychiatry, 10th edition. USA: Lippincott Williams and Wilkins; 2017. pp. 4997.
2. Gururaj G, Varghese M, Benegal V, Rao GN, Pathak K; NMHS collaborators group. National Mental Health Survey of India, 2015-16. Bengaluru: NIMHANS; 2016.
3. Kessler RC, Berglund P, Demler O, Jin R, Koretz D, Merikangas KR, et al. The epidemiology of major depressive disorder: results from the National Comorbidity Survey Replication (NCS-R). JAMA. 2003;289:3095-105.
4. International Classification of Diseases, Eleventh Revision (ICD-11); World Health Organization (WHO). (2019/2021). ICD-11 for Mortality and Morbidity Statistics (ICD-11 MMS). [online] Available from https://icd.who.int/browse11 [Last accessed December, 2023].
5. Gaebel W, Stricker J, Kerst A. Changes from ICD-10 to ICD-11 and future directions in psychiatric classification. Dialogues Clin Neurosci. 2020;22(1):7-15.

6. Malhotra S, Shah R. Women and mental health in India: An overview. Indian J Psychiatry. 2015;57(Suppl 2):S205-11.
7. Poongothai S, Pradeepa R, Ganesan A, Mohan V. Prevalence of Depression in a Large Urban South Indian Population—The Chennai Urban Rural Epidemiology Study (Cures—70). PLoS One. 2009;4(9):e7185.
8. Albert PR. Why is depression more prevalent in women? J Psychiatry Neurosci. 2015;40(4):219-21.
9. Dandona R, George S, Kumar GA. Sociodemographic characteristics of women who died by suicide in India from 2014 to 2020: findings from surveillance data. Lancet Public Health. 2023;8(5):e347-55.
10. Lalthankimi R, Nagarajan P, Menon V, Olickal JJ. Predictors of Suicidal Ideation and Attempt among Patients with Major Depressive Disorder at a Tertiary Care Hospital, Puducherry. J Neurosci Rural Pract. 2021;12(1):122-8.
11. Belsiyal CX, Rentala S, Das A. Frequency of suicide ideation and attempts and its correlates among inpatients with depressive disorders at a tertiary care center in North India. J Family Med Prim Care. 2022;11:2537-44.
12. Slavich GM, Irwin MR. From stress to inflammation and major depressive disorder: a social signal transduction theory of depression. Psychol Bull. 2014;140(3):774-815.
13. Rainville JR, Hodes GE. Inflaming sex differences in mood disorders. Neuropsychopharmacology. 2019;44(1):184-99.
14. Mangiola F, Ianiro G, Franceschi F, Fagiuoli S, Gasbarrini G, Gasbarrini A. Gut microbiota in autism and mood disorders. World J Gastroenterol. 2016;22(1):361-8.
15. National Institute for Health and Care Excellence (NICE). Depression in adults: treatment and management. London: NICE; 2022.
16. Gautam S, Jain A, Gautam M, Vahia VN, Grover S. Clinical Practice Guidelines for the Management of Depression. Indian J Psychiatry. 2017;59(Suppl 1):S34-50.
17. Thirthalli J, Sinha P, Sreeraj VS. Clinical Practice Guidelines for the Use of Electroconvulsive Therapy. Indian J Psychiatry. 2023;65(2):258-69.
18. Javaid SF, Hashim IJ, Hashim MJ, Stip E, Samad MA, Ahbabi AA. Epidemiology of anxiety disorders: global burden and sociodemographic associations. Middle East Curr Psychiatry. 2023;30:44.
19. Manjunatha N, Jayasankar P, Suhas S, Rao GN, Gopalkrishna G, Varghese M, et al.; NMHS National Collaborators Group. Prevalence and its correlates of anxiety disorders from India's National Mental Health Survey 2016. Indian J Psychiatry. 2022;64(2):138-42.
20. El Khoury JR, Baroud EA, Khoury BA. The revision of the categories of mood, anxiety and stress-related disorders in the ICD-11: a perspective from the Arab region. Middle East Curr Psychiatry. 2020;27:7.
21. Bandelow B, Michaelis S, Wedekind D. Treatment of anxiety disorders. Dialogues Clin Neurosci. 2017;19(2):93-107.
22. Claudia P, Andrea C, Chiara C, Stefano L, Giuseppe M, Vincenzo DL, et al. Panic disorder in menopause. a case control study. Mauritas. 2004:48:147-54.
23. Gorey KM, Leslie DR. The prevalence of child sexual abuse: integrative review adjustment for potential response and measurement biases. Child Abuse Negle. 1997;21:391-8.

24. Mich LC, Mc Laughlin KA, Shepherd K, Nolen-Hoeksema S. Rumination as a mechanism linking stressful life events to symptoms of depression and anxiety: longitudinal evidence in early adolescents and adults. J Abnorm Psychol. 2013;122:339-52.
25. Nillni YI, Toufexis DJ, Rohan KJ. Anxiety sensitivity, the menstrual cycle and panic disorder: epidemiology and treatment. Curr Psychiatry Rep. 2015;17:87.
26. Alarcon G, Cservenka A, Rudolph MD, Fair DA, Nagel BJ. Developmental sex differences in resting functional connectivity of amygdala subregions. Neuroimage. 2015;115:235-44.
27. Gautam S, Jain A, Gautam M, Vahia VN, Gautam A. Clinical Practice Guidelines for the Management of Generalised Anxiety Disorder (GAD) and Panic Disorder (PD). Indian J Psychiatry. 2017;59(Suppl 1):S67-73.
28. Hantsoo L, Epperson CN. Premenstrual Dysphoric Disorder: Epidemiology and Treatment. Curr Psychiatry Rep. 2015;17(11):87.
29. Andersen JT, Andersen NL, Horwitz H, Poulsen HE, Jimenez-Solem E. Exposure to selective serotonin reuptake inhibitors in early pregnancy and the risk of miscarriage. Obstet Gynecol. 2014;124(4):655-61.
30. Betcher HK, Wisner KL. Psychotropic Treatment During Pregnancy: Research Synthesis and Clinical Care Principles. J Womens Health. 2020;29(3):310-8.
31. Viktorin A, Uher R, Kolevzon A, Reichenberg A, Levine SZ, Sandin S. Association of Antidepressant Medication Use During Pregnancy With Intellectual Disability in Offspring. JAMA Psychiatry. 2017;74(10):1031-8.
32. Molenaar NM, Kamperman AM, Boyce P, Bergink V. Guidelines on treatment of perinatal depression with antidepressants: An international review. Aust N Z J Psychiatry. 2018;52(4):320-7.
33. Kittel-Schneider S, Felice E, Buhagiar R, Lambregtse-van den Berg M, Wilson CA, Banjac Baljak V, et al. Treatment of Peripartum Depression with Antidepressants and Other Psychotropic Medications: A Synthesis of Clinical Practice Guidelines in Europe. Int J Environ Res Public Health. 2022;19(4):1973.
34. Marchesi C, Osola P, Amerio A, Daniel BD, Tonna M, De Panfilis C. Clinical management of perinatal anxiety disorders: a systematic review. J Affect Disord. 2016;190:543-50.
35. Carrie Armstrong. ACOG Guidelines on Psychiatric Medication Use During Pregnancy and Lactation. Am Fam Physician. 2008;78(6):772-8.
36. Yadav V, Jain A, Dabar D, Goel AD, Sood A, Joshi A, et al. A meta-analysis on the prevalence of depression in perimenopausal and postmenopausal women in India. Asian J Psychiatr. 2021;57:102581.
37. Bromberger JT, Matthews KA, Schott LL, Brockwell S, Avis NE, Kravitz HM, et al. Depressive symptoms during the menopausal transition: The Study of Women's Health Across the Nation (SWAN). J Affect Disord. 2007;103(1-3):267-72.
38. Maki PM, Kornstein SG, Joffe H, Bromberger JT, Freeman EW, Athappilly G, et al. Guidelines for the Evaluation and Treatment of Perimenopausal Depression: Summary and Recommendations. J Womens Health (Larchmt). 2019;28(2):117-34.

CHAPTER 4

Obsessive-compulsive Related Disorders and Eating Disorders

Lavanya P Sharma, Vasundhra Teotia, Upasna Gopalakrishna, Shyam Sundar Arumugham

ABSTRACT

The objective of this chapter is to provide an overview of obsessive-compulsive disorder (OCD), body dysmorphic disorder (BDD), body-focused repetitive behavior disorders (BFRBs), and eating disorders (ED) through the lens of gender, specifically women's mental health. These disorders are characterized by intense preoccupation and/or pathological compulsive "habits". They have an onset in adolescence/early adulthood and often run a chronic course. They are often underdiagnosed due to the associated guilt and shame. Some of these conditions, especially eating disorders are predominantly seen in females. Puberty, perinatal period, and menopause influence the clinical presentation and treatment of these conditions. We discuss the influence of sociocultural, neurobiological, and experiential aspects of gender on the pathogenesis, epidemiology, clinical manifestation, and treatment of obsessive-compulsive related disorders and eating disorders.

Keywords: Obsessive compulsive disorder, body dysmorphic disorder, body focused repetitive behavior disorders, eating disorders

INTRODUCTION

Obsessive-compulsive disorder (OCD) and related disorders are grouped under a separate category in the current classificatory systems. These obsessive-compulsive spectrum disorders (OCSDs) include OCD, body dysmorphic disorder (BDD), and body-focused repetitive behavior (BFRBs) disorders. In addition to the shared heritability and comorbidity patterns, these disorders are characterized by the presence of underlying compulsivity.[1] Compulsivity may be defined as a tendency to perform repetitive behaviors in a stereotypical or habitual pattern, which does not align with an individual's overall goal.[2,3] The OCSDs are characterized by a shift in balance away from goal-directed control toward pathological habitual response patterns. The psychopathology of eating disorders can also be described using the transdiagnostic rubric of compulsivity or maladaptive habit.[4]

Sex and gender play important roles in the manifestation of OCSD. Sex implies the biological characteristics assigned at birth, while gender is a psychosocial phenomenon moderated by environmental factors and can

CHAPTER 4: Obsessive-compulsive Related Disorders and Eating Disorders

fluctuate throughout life.[4] There is a female predilection for BFRBs, while in OCD, rates tend to be evenly represented in clinical samples, with slightly more female preponderance in community samples.[5] Gender and life stage may also influence the clinical presentation and comorbidity, coping styles, pathways to care, and help-seeking in these disorders. In addition to the unique lived experiences of womanhood and their impact on the course and outcome of these disorders, the neurobiological effects of puberty, the menstrual cycle, pregnancy, postpartum, lactation as well as the menopausal period influence the pathogenesis, course, choice of and response to treatment.

Understanding the role of gender in the pathophysiology of eating disorders relies on not just sex-dependent neurobiological underpinnings but also a deeper understanding of current gender roles and body ideals, integrated with an individual's lived experience and engagement with the prevalent socio-cultural discourse.[6] Feminist literature understands gender as a social construct that attaches specific expectations and meanings to people's bodies. It further draws on gendered "dualism", which implies that women are more often "objectified" through the lens of their bodies and may consider bodily self-control as a means of achieving agency.[7] The relative suppression of one's needs as a part of the traditional gender role, being in a position of disempowerment, bodily valuation, objectification, and discrimination are important factors to consider when understanding eating disorder (ED) through the lens of gender.[8,9]

This chapter discusses the influence of sociological, neurobiological, and experiential aspects of gender/sex on the pathogenesis, clinical manifestation, and treatment of OCSDs and eating disorders.

■ OBSESSIVE-COMPULSIVE DISORDER IN WOMEN

Epidemiology

Obsessive-compulsive disorder (OCD) is a heterogeneous neuropsychiatric condition with a lifetime prevalence of 1–3% with women having a 1.6-fold higher likelihood of illness.[10] The onset in women has bimodal peaks-one in late adolescence/adulthood and one in late adulthood. The first onset occurs later in women (20–24 years) compared to men (13–15 years).[11,12] Consequently, there is a male preponderance in pediatric OCD samples. Men are likely to show higher dysfunction, possibly due to the earlier age-at-onset. Women with OCD are more likely to be married.[13] Comorbid depression and suicidality are higher in women.[13] OCD impacts the sexual functioning of women irrespective of the medication being taken or the symptom dimension. Women with OCD often report experiencing more sexual disgust, less sexual desire, sexual arousal, and satisfying orgasms than women without OCD.[14]

Phenomenology

Cluster analytical studies show that females have a higher preponderance of contamination obsessions and cleaning/washing compulsions.[15] Studies on a large Indian cohort ($n = 545$) corroborated this finding. Excessive cleaning may be perceived as culturally acceptable, which may explain their late presentation to clinics for treatment.[13] Men tend to experience more sexual and aggressive obsessions.[13]

Etiology

Cortico-striato-thalamo-cortical (CSTC) circuits involving the cognitive, affective, sensorimotor, and motivational circuit abnormalities are well studied in OCD.[16] Evidence for the involvement of serotonergic, dopaminergic, and glutamatergic neurotransmitter systems comes from pharmacotherapy and animal studies.[16] Regarding neuropsychological tasks, one study found that women with OCD perform worse on verbal memory tasks. There are no gender differences in response inhibition task performance among patients with OCD.[17] Structural and functional imaging changes in the orbitofrontal cortex (OFC) and anterior cingulate cortex (ACC) are found in patients with OCD; however, there is no evidence to suggest gender differences. Gender differences in genetic studies indicate a higher frequency of homozygosity for the low activity allele of the monoamine oxidase A gene in females with OCD, whereas males have the high activity allele.[18] Similarly, another study found a higher prevalence of the 5HT 2A promoter polymorphism allele in women with OCD.[19]

Evaluation and Treatment

A thorough evaluation of the obsessions and neutralizing behaviors, including physical and mental compulsions, avoidance, safety behaviors, and proxy compulsions, should be done. An assessment of family accommodation also helps in planning therapy. The Yale-Brown Obsessive Compulsive Scale (YBOCS)[20] checklist and severity scores help comprehensively assess symptoms. Item 11 of the YBOCS assesses for insight, essential while planning therapy or prognosticating. Dimensional YBOCS[21] and Family Accommodation Scale (FAS)[22] can also be applied to get a complete idea of the severity of each dimension (if the patient has multiple principal dimensions) and the maintaining factors, respectively.

First-line treatment for OCD includes high-dose serotonin reuptake inhibitors (SSRIs) and cognitive behavior therapy (CBT) involving exposure response prevention (ERP). Augmentation agents such as antipsychotics (risperidone, aripiprazole, and haloperidol), 5HT3 antagonists, memantine, and lamotrigine can be used when there is a partial response to an SRI. There is preliminary evidence for noninvasive brain stimulation techniques such as repetitive transcranial magnetic stimulation (rTMS) and transcranial direct current stimulation (tDCS). Ablative surgeries or deep brain stimulation (DBS) can be considered in severe, chronic, and treatment-refractory OCD.[23]

RELATION OF OBSESSIVE-COMPULSIVE DISORDER WITH REPRODUCTIVE CYCLE EVENTS AND THE INFLUENCE OF HORMONES

Exacerbations (21.6–49.2%) or new onset of OCD symptoms (25%) have been noted to occur during different phases of the reproductive lifecycle. A multicenter retrospective study found that OCD may have an onset (start within 12 months) following reproductive life events—menarche (13%), pregnancy (5.1%), postpartum (4.7%), and at menopause (3.7%), suggesting a potential relationship to hormonal fluctuations.[24] OCD worsening during the premenstrual period was seen in 37.6% of women, and exacerbations during pregnancy, postpartum, and menopause were seen in 33, 46.6, and 32.7 of women, respectively. If a woman has an exacerbation during her first pregnancy or first postpartum period, it is associated with a risk of exacerbation in the subsequent pregnancy or postpartum period as well.[24] Factors predictive of OC symptoms exacerbations are depression during pregnancy,[25] contaminations/symmetry obsessions with washing/arranging compulsions,[25] and premenstrual worsening of symptoms.[26] Premenstrual worsening of symptoms is associated with comorbid social anxiety, and these patients also score higher on suicidality and sexual and religious obsessions.[27]

Furthermore, polycystic ovarian syndrome (PCOS) is also significantly associated with an increased risk of a diagnosis of OCD,[28] which supports the hormonal fluctuation hypothesis. Fluctuating estrogen, progesterone, and oxytocin levels can play a role in reducing serotonin and increasing dopamine and glutamate, which can worsen OCD symptoms.[29] Estradiol can increase serotonin synthesis, reduce its breakdown, modulate the serotonin transporter (SERT) and receptors, and increase the expression of genes coding for synapse molecules in serotonin neurons.[29] Further supporting the estrogen hypothesis, mood, and OCD symptoms tend to fluctuate in OCD patients taking oral contraceptive (OC) pills.[30,31] Short-term administration of estrogen inhibits monoamino oxidase-A (MAO-A) activity, leading to a decrease in serotonin breakdown at the synapse. This explains the worsening of OC symptoms before the onset of menstruation, as estrogen levels suddenly drop around the 22nd day in a 28-day cycle. At the same time, chronic administration of estrogen can set in negative feedback loops when there are increased serotonin levels, leading to the activation of the MAO-A enzyme, possibly explaining the fluctuations noted with women taking OC pills.[29] Postdelivery, there is a 1,000-fold drop in estrogen levels. This period is associated with a higher risk of OCD symptoms.[32] Weaker ventral striatum-generated reward prediction errors mediated by dopaminergic activity can increase the propensity for habits/compulsivity.[33] Estrogen influences the release (increases release in caudate, putamen, and nucleus accumbens) and uptake (reducing uptake in nucleus accumbens) of dopamine and striatal D2 receptor affinity (shifting it to low affinity from high affinity), providing indirect evidence for its role in OCD.[27] Estrogen can also increase glutamate levels in the hippocampus and hypothalamus. It can also have neuroprotective effects against glutamate toxicity.[29]

There are relatively fewer studies evaluating the role of progesterone. Progesterone increases serotonin signaling and can modulate dopamine release, especially when primed with estrogen.[29] The levels of progesterone during the luteal phase of the menstrual cycle can increase checking symptoms by modulating response/error monitoring.[34] This study also demonstrated that error-related negativity signals fluctuate during the follicular and luteal phase of the menstrual cycle and could play a role in OCD symptoms.[34] Elevated levels of oxytocin are found in patients with OCD.[35] Increased levels during delivery or breastfeeding may contribute to worsening of OCD in vulnerable women in the postpartum period.

OBSESSIVE COMPULSION DISORDER IN THE PERINATAL PERIOD

It is crucial to recognize and treat perinatal OCD earlier, as it can have adverse maternal and neonatal outcomes. Gestational hypertension, gestational diabetes,[36] preeclampsia, premature rupture of membranes, venous thromboembolism, and instrumental/cesarean deliveries are more common in pregnant women with OCD than those without OCD.[37] Women with OCD can also have worse neonatal outcomes in the form of lower birth weight,[38] preterm birth,[38] fetal neuroinflammation,[39] low APGAR scores at 5 minutes,[40] and neonatal respiratory distress.[40]

Postpartum women often present with intrusive, violent, infant-related harm thoughts, which could be accidental or intentional harm to the infant.[41] These are common in new mothers, but sleep deprivation (due to nocturnal child care, breastfeeding),[42] negative mood, and fatigue can contribute to developing OCD.[41] Women with infant-related harm obsessions may be embarrassed to reveal such symptoms due to their social unacceptability and often remain undiagnosed. Discussion of such symptoms during a routine postnatal visit in a nonjudgmental manner may help in early detection. They may even be misdiagnosed as postpartum psychosis, which can also present with thoughts of infant-related harm. Here, the differentiating features of OCD include ego dystonicity, the presence of insight, the distressing nature of the thoughts, avoidance of the infant, and neutralizing behavior. Women with infant-related harm obsessions may engage in either washing (excessively cleaning anything that could come in contact with the baby) or checking compulsions (repeatedly checking if something terrible has happened to the baby), and severe OCD can lead to complete avoidance of the baby, hampering the mother-infant bonding and attachment.[43]

MANAGEMENT OF PERINATAL OBSESSIVE COMPULSION DISORDER

Consensus recommendations about assessing and treating perinatal OCD are summarized in **Table 1**. For new-onset OCD, CBT/ERP should be considered as the first line.[23] In terms of pharmacotherapy, SSRIs can be used for perinatal OCD.[23] Clomipramine can be used in postpartum OCD. Paroxetine is associated with an increased risk of cardiac septal defects (1.5-2%). Hence, it is best avoided during pregnancy.[23] SSRIs late in pregnancy can increase the risk of persistent pulmonary hypertension. Although rare, first-trimester use of SSRIs is associated with anencephaly, omphalocele, and craniosynostosis. Neonates should be monitored for serotonin toxicity and discontinuation symptoms. Relative infant dose of sertraline, fluvoxamine, and paroxetine is lower in breastfed infants and higher with fluoxetine.[45] Low doses of quetiapine may be beneficial in those with associated sleep deprivation.[42]

POSTMENOPAUSAL OBSESSIVE COMPULSION DISORDER

There is a dearth of research on perimenopausal OCD. The prevalence of OCD in menopausal women is around 7.1%.[47] Preexisting OCD may worsen (29.4%) or improve (23.5%) during the perimenopausal period. Geriatric OCD is also represented by a higher female prevalence.[48] Common obsessions noted during the postmenopausal period are contamination and symmetry obsessions with washing and checking compulsions. Comorbidity was seen in 63.2% of women, with GAD being the most common comorbidity. In general, there are lower rates of treatment with CBT in the older population.[48] Treatment options would be the same as in the younger population with attention paid to medical comorbidities, interactions with other medications, and higher risks of hyponatremia with SSRIs.

BODY DYSMORPHIC DISORDER IN WOMEN

Epidemiology

Body dysmorphic disorder has a point prevalence of 1.6-2.9%, is often missed, and is more common in women (60%) than men (40%).[49] The prevalence is higher in specific populations such as dermatology clinics (9.2-11.3%), cosmetic dentistry (5.2%), rhinoplasty (20.1%), general cosmetic

TABLE 1: Assessment and treatment of perinatal obsessive compulsion disorder (OCD).[44]

Step	Components
Screening	• Expectant mothers with a history of mood, anxiety or OCD symptoms should be routinely screened for perinatal OCD • Screening tools developed for perinatal OCD: Perinatal obsessive-compulsive scale (POCS),[46] Y-BOCS can be administered to ascertain the severity of OCD[18]
Assessment	• Describe nature of assessments, maintain confidentiality and obtain informed consent for assessments. Embarrassment/child safeguarding due to disclosure can lead to refusal of consent • Mental health professionals (MHPs) should assess for taboo thoughts, such as sexual or aggressive thoughts with harm to infant • Assess for compulsions, especially excessive cleaning, checking, reassurance seeking, avoidance of the infant, and mental compulsions like praying • Assess the duration, frequency, distress, resistance of thoughts and compulsions, insight, impairment of biological or occupational functioning • Assess for onset before pregnancy if any, course, worsening during premenstrual period, worsening during pregnancy • Assessment of impact on infant, caregiver behavior, safety of mother and the fetus/infant • Assess for comorbid psychiatric illnesses and suicidality
Differential diagnosis	• Determine whether the obsessions are ego-syntonic (in keeping with the patient's beliefs) or ego-dystonic (inconsistent with the beliefs, senseless, and intrusive) • Differentiate fears that are senseless (e.g., contaminating the baby by changing nappy), from depressive ruminations that are characteristically pessimistic views of oneself and the world (e.g., "I'm an inadequate mother") and delusions, which are false fixed firm beliefs (e.g., "My enemies are coming to take my baby") • Differentiate avoidance from social withdrawal and amotivation associated with depression and schizophrenia respectively
Treatment	• For subclinical symptoms, provide psychoeducation about perinatal OCD, including treatment options should it develop, and how to access treatment • For syndromal OCD, provide information to the patient about pharmacotherapy, psychotherapy, and somatic treatments like repetitive transcranial magnetic stimulation, transcranial direct current stimulation, efficacy of each option and side effects along with risks during pregnancy and breastfeeding, risk of not taking treatment, mother's preferences regarding infant feeding, and take a collaborative decision with the patient

Contd...

Contd...

Step	Components
	- CBT with ERP should be offered as first line, and the infant can safely be involved in exposures
- In case of comorbid psychiatric illness or psychosocial issues, multidisciplinary approach should be considered
- Where warranted (suicidal risk, concerns about mother-infant relationship) an admission to a mother baby unit should be considered to provide intensive care
- Review treatment plan in case of inadequate response to pharmacotherapy or CBT
- Review the patient regularly for at least 12 months posttreatment completion
Psychoeducation	- Psychoeducating expectant mothers about perinatal mental illnesses and OCD
- Normalizing intrusive thoughts of infant related harm
- Onset or worsening in the perinatal period, reasons for onset (role transition, lack of sleep, and stress), course, and availability of treatment
- Common themes/content of intrusions and common compulsions, and those unique to perinatal period
- Ego-dystonic nature of thoughts and that yielding compulsions are counterproductive
Partners and families	- Ask the mother whom she is comfortable involving them in the treatment.
- Psychoeducate the partner and immediate family about perinatal OCD, nature and goals of treatment, and how to support the mother experiencing perinatal OCD.
- Address family accommodation, which can maintain the symptoms.

(CBT: cognitive behavior therapy; ERP: exposure response prevention; OCD: obsessive compulsion disorder)

surgery (13.2%), and women predominate in all settings except dermatology and cosmetic settings.[50] BDD onset tends to occur before the age of 18 years, more commonly in the adolescence between 12 and 13 years.[49] The course is chronic; BDD has the highest association with suicidal ideation (81%) and lifetime suicidal attempts (58%). Suicidality positively correlates with the severity of BDD.[51]

Phenomenology

Body dysmorphic disorder is characterized by extreme preoccupations about one's appearance or perceived defects that are not or only mildly discernible to others.[52] These are associated with repetitive behaviors such as mirror gazing, camouflaging, excessive grooming, skin picking, reassurance seeking, compulsively taking selfies, information seeking for cosmetic surgeries, and excessive shopping for cosmetic products; and mental acts like comparing one's appearance with others.[52] Appearance-related concerns commonly involve skin, hair, and nose. Girls or women are preoccupied with more body areas than men, including breasts, hips, legs, excessive body hair,[53] and female external genitalia/labia.[54] Girls or women with BDD are more likely to engage in mirror gazing, camouflaging, skin picking, and changing outfits.[53] Women with BDD also have poorer insight and frequently present with comorbid depression, whereas substance use disorder is commoner in men.[55,56] It is also seen that girls are less functionally impaired than men.[53]

Muscle dysmorphia is an understudied concept in women. It is the preoccupation with being insufficiently muscular or lean accompanied by excessive workouts, steroid use, and strict diets. In women, gender role stress due to physical appearance, aerobic exercise, and sociocultural factors may predict muscle dysmorphia, whereas in men, gender role stress related to physical capability may predict muscle dysmorphophobia.[57]

Etiology

Between 5.8 and 6.4% of first-degree relatives of patients with BDD can have BDD.[58] The heritability of BDD ranges from 37 to 49% and is higher in women.[59] A single-photon emission computed tomography (SPECT) study suggests changes in temporoparietooccipital regions.[60] There are also biases in visual processing, leading to a focus on the minute details rather than the bigger picture.[61] Sex-specific differences in genetics and neuroimaging in BDD need to be studied. Oxytocin, a hormone important for social cognition, is found to be increased in BDD patients and is correlated with symptom severity.[62] Interestingly, increased oxytocin levels are also seen in patients with OCD. It is unclear whether the increased oxytocin contributes to psychopathology or is a compensatory mechanism for other deficits.

Environmental factors, including adverse childhood experiences (ACEs) such as bullying [$r = 0.282$, 95% CI (0.206, 0.354)] and teasing [$r = 0.423$, 95% CI (0.360, 0.482)] have low to moderate association with BDD symptomatology and gender moderated the association between the ACEs and BDD symptomatology.[63] Internet and social media use also affect body satisfaction. Women (12–29 years) spending 11–20 hours online were more likely to be dissatisfied with their body image.[64] The increase in social network use (Instagram, TikTok, Facebook, and Twitter) during the COVID-19 pandemic lockdown and following appearance-focused accounts on Instagram, is associated with a rise in body dissatisfaction, drive for thinness, and low self-esteem, especially in younger women.[65] Viewing appearance-focused comments on Instagram can have negative implications on body image.[66] Body image concerns can also involve the genitalia. Major motivators for gynecological surgeries like labiaplasty are psychological reasons/low self-esteem (39.4%), sexual reasons like self-consciousness during intimacy or fear of being negatively evaluated by the partner during sexual intercourse (46.5%), and aesthetic reasons (52.1%).[67] These are influenced by how the mass media and pornographic content portray the "perfect" female body type.[68]

Evaluation

Patients often hesitate to reveal body image concerns because of the fear of being judged, shamed, embarrassed, or due to the belief that cosmetic surgeries would help. BDD can be confused with an eating disorder (concerns about body weight), social anxiety disorder (social anxiety in BDD is due to appearance-related concerns), psychosis (due to poor insight or bizarre appearance if attempts at camouflaging are excessive), skin picking disorder, trichotillomania (in case hair pulling is accompanied by preoccupation about excessive body hair patient should be diagnosed with BDD), and gender dysphoria.[69] BDD-YBOCS is a 12-item clinician-rated scale that can be used to assess the severity of BDD and capture the changes over the course of treatment.[70] Other scales that can be used include body dysmorphic disorder examination (BDDE),[71] and the psychiatric status rating scale for body dysmorphic disorder (BDD-PSR).[72] Gender differences are found in rating scales as well, with BDDE showing higher scores in females, whereas BDD-PSR shows higher scores in males.[72]

Treatment

Cognitive behavior therapy is recommended as the first line of treatment with components consisting of psychoeducation, cognitive restructuring, exposures usually to social situations, behavioral experiments, response prevention of excessive behaviors such as mirror checking, mirror retraining, relapse prevention, and motivational interviewing during therapy due to poorer insight.[69] Other individualized components, such as habit reversal training, can be included for skin-picking or hair-pulling behaviors secondary to BDD are present. The newer therapist-assisted internet-based CBT or BDD-NET is gaining popularity, which can be provided to patients who are hesitant to access treatment due to shame and stigma.[73]

Clomipramine and SSRIs in high doses are the recommended pharmacotherapy for BDD. SSRIs have been found to be helpful irrespective of the level of insight, while there is no evidence for the efficacy of antipsychotic monotherapy, even in delusional BDD.[74,75] The duration of a trial with a serotonin reuptake inhibitor (SRI) should be 12–16 weeks. It is to be noted that medication discontinuation is strongly associated with relapse.[76] Although data is limited, atypical antipsychotics, N-acetyl cysteine, and buspirone can be added for augmentation in case of a partial response.[69] For severe symptoms, a combination treatment of CBT with SRI is recommended.[77]

Women with BDD often undergo cosmetic treatments such as rhinoplasty. Such cosmetic treatments do not improve BDD symptoms and sometimes may worsen them.[78] Given that BDD is more prevalent in women seeking breast reconstruction than the general population,[79] and labiaplasties, it is important to keep cosmetic surgeons and gynecologists[54] well informed about BDD.

REPRODUCTIVE ASPECTS OF BODY DYSMORPHIC DISORDER

The onset of BDD in women is often seen around the time of menarche (12–13 years), and there may be worsening during the premenstrual period, especially in women who have PMDD.[69] Sexual intimacy can be affected by BDD and lead to lower pregnancy rates.[69] BDD may also be observed during the perinatal period. A study from the US found that 14.9% of women experience marked BDD symptoms in the third trimester of pregnancy and 11.8% during the postpartum period.[80] Unlike OCD, the phenomenology of symptoms during the perinatal period is not well studied. In a systematic review of qualitative studies of body image experiences during the perinatal period, themes such as limiting weight gain during pregnancy and returning to prepregnancy weight, body image concerns about the breast and stomach had emerged.[81] Those with syndromal BDD during the perinatal period might require treatment in the form of CBT and/or SSRI. Medications can be advised considering the severity, comorbidity, and previous treatment history.

BODY FOCUSED REPETITIVE BEHAVIORS

Body focused repetitive behaviors are a collection of repetitive and destructive behaviors targeted toward the body. They include a variety of behaviors such as skin picking, hair pulling, lip biting, and nail-biting, the most recognized of which are trichotillomania (TTM) and skin picking disorder (SPD). Due to shared features with OCD in terms of phenomenology, neurobiology, family history, etc., these disorders have been grouped under OCRD in the ICD-11.[82]

Epidemiology

Large epidemiological studies for BFRBs are lacking. Studies have generally found prevalence rates ranging from 0.5 to 2% for TTM and 2–4% for SPD in community samples.[83] Although there is some inconsistency, women account for the majority of those with TTM and SPD.[84,85] It is hypothesized that women are overrepresented in clinical populations because they are more likely to face the negative social consequences of hair loss or scarred skin. In contrast, men may find it easier to camouflage their hair loss.[86]

The onset of TTM is usually during adolescence with women having an earlier onset than men (14.8 years as opposed to 19 years in one large study).[86] TTM generally has a chronic course with waxing and waning symptoms. A putative subtype of TTM has been characterized with onset in childhood (sometimes termed "Baby Trich"), which appears to have an equal sex ratio, run a more benign course, and is thought to have neurodevelopmental origins.[87]

Etiology

The etiology of BFRBs remains unknown and is likely to result from the interaction of genetic and environmental influences. A few studies have suggested that BFRBs are highly heritable, with heritability estimates ranging from 32 to 78% for TTM.[88] A study from the UK Twin registry found that genetic factors accounted for 40% of the variance in skin picking.[89] Neurobiological studies are limited and lacking in consistent findings, have small sample sizes, and are conducted mostly in women. Abnormalities have been found in neuroimaging studies, such as excessive gray matter density in the striatum, amygdala, and medial frontal cortices in TTM.[90] Similarly, diffusion tensor imaging studies in both TTM and SPD found decreased functional integrity of white matter tracts of the sensorimotor and response inhibition circuits, which may be involved in habit generation and suppression.[83]

Psychological theories of BFRBs suggest that individuals with BFRBs have a deficit in emotional regulation, leading to BFRBs as a way of coping with negative affect.[91] Several studies have found an association with traumatic experiences, often just preceding the onset of BFRBs.[92,93] BFRBs lead to a sense of unattractiveness and disgust with their bodies, which leads to a cycle where the individual increases their pulling/picking behavior to cope with their sense of shame.[94]

Clinical Features

In both disorders, individuals experience a recurrent urge to pull their hair or pick their skin. Picking or pulling behavior is often preceded by a sense of mounting tension and followed by a sense of relief or gratification. Individuals develop negative consequences such as areas of scarring or hair loss, which causes distress and leads to multiple attempts to stop the behavior. This behavior can be wholly conscious and "focused" or unconscious and "automatic". After pulling or picking, individuals may engage in rituals such as chewing their hair or lining it up. Triggers for hair pulling include negative affective states such as anxiety or boredom and sensory triggers such as areas of uneven skin or coarse hair. Women are more likely than men to pull hair from the scalp alone, whereas men are more likely to pull from multiple sites such as beard and eyebrows.[95] A study comparing skin picking in men and women showed similar impairment and distress. However, women had lower family loading and were more likely to pick from scalp, back, and breasts.[85] Patients can also ask others to pull their hair or feel the urge to pull the hair of others. This TTM by proxy was reported by 37% of patients in one study.[96] An Indian case study reported a patient with trichotillomania who stopped pulling her hair after treatment but started pulling that of her child.[97]

Much has been written about the secretiveness of BFRBs and the strong sense of shame and guilt felt by individuals with BFRBs.[98,99] Individuals go to great lengths to conceal the evidence of their BFRB. This might involve avoidance of certain clothing, avoidance of social activities, and physical intimacy. Many patients keep their hair pulling a secret from loved ones.[96] BFRBs are often perceived as bad habits, leading to delays in treatment seeking.[100,101] Due to the relative rarity of the disorders, patients may find support on social media platforms like YouTube and online forums, where they exchange advice and encouragement.[102]

Treatment

Treatment leads to symptom reduction and improved psychosocial functioning.[83] Psychotherapy with habit reversal therapy (HRT) and CBT is the mainstay of treatment. It involves techniques such as self-awareness of pulling/picking behaviors and using competing responses, coping strategies, and relaxation exercises. There are no Food and Drug Administration (FDA)-approved drugs for BFRBs. There is evidence for the efficacy of NAC (1200–3000 mg/day), memantine (10–20 mg), and olanzapine (up to 20 mg).[103-106] The evidence for SRIs is equivocal. Case reports exist of successful treatment with naltrexone and antipsychotics.[107]

■ EATING DISORDERS

Eating disorders (ED), such as anorexia nervosa (AN), bulimia nervosa (BN), and binge eating disorder (BED) can be highly disabling and even potentially lethal. DSM-5 and ICD-11 recognize AN, BN, BED, avoidant restrictive food intake disorder (ARFID), Pica, and Rumination Disorder as feeding and eating disorders.[108] For a long time, eating disorders were seen as affecting women and girls exclusively. Several explanations have been put forth to explain the unique vulnerability of women to eating disorders, from feminist theories to sociocultural ones.

Epidemiology

A meta-analysis of 15 studies found that the estimated lifetime prevalence of any ED was 1.01%, and those of AN, BN, and BED were 0.21, 0.81, and 2.22%, respectively.[109]

More than 90% of EDs occur in women. AN and BN typically have their onset in adolescence and are more common in the upper class of industrialized Western nations. AN is commonly associated with comorbid depression, OCD, and other anxiety disorders. BN is frequently associated with depression and high impulsivity.[110]

Eating disorders were once considered "culture bound" to Western societies and relatively rare in non-Western cultures. With globalization, the prevalence of EDs is rising in non-Western countries. It has been observed that individuals with restrictive eating in non-Western countries do not report a fear of fatness that is considered pathognomonic of AN. Some authors have suggested that the increased prevalence in the West might be due to the biased diagnostic criteria, which reflect symptoms commonly seen in the West, whereas individuals with restrictive eating in non-Western countries are more likely to be categorized as ED, not otherwise specified.[111,112]

There is a lack of epidemiological studies on ED in India. A few studies have assessed disordered eating primarily among Indian college students and found rates ranging from 4 to 29%.[113] A survey conducted among psychiatrists in an urban area found that two-thirds reported seeing at least one case of ED, suggesting that ED is not uncommon in India.[114] AN is higher in certain professions where appearance and weight are emphasized, such as dancers and athletes. A study done among Kathak dancers found greater body dissatisfaction and disordered eating attitudes compared to controls.[115]

Etiology

Feminist perspectives suggest that EDs are a kind of rebellion against the demands imposed by patriarchy.[116] A woman's value in society is measured by her appearance, and thinness is idealized as beautiful. Cultural explanations have been suggested, pointing to the differential emphasis on appearance placed by different societies. In non-Western countries such as Fiji, studies have shown the rise in body dissatisfaction and disordered eating associated with the spread of Western culture through TV and social media.[112] Genetic studies have implicated genes involved in serotonin receptors and transporter.[117] Studies have implicated personality traits such as perfectionism associated with AN and impulsivity with BN.[110]

Eating Disorder in Puberty

Puberty is a time of increased risk for developing EDs. Girls become more aware of their bodies and society's expectations, and body dissatisfaction grows.

In addition, levels of reproductive hormones such as estrogen and progesterone increase during puberty. Estrogen is an important modulator of transcription of genes involved in neurotransmitter production and transmission, secretion of neurotrophic factors like BDNF, etc. It is hypothesized that estrogen may be involved in activating some of the genes involved in developing EDs.[118,119]

Eating Disorder during the Menstrual Cycle

Estrogen inhibits appetite. Studies have also shown variations in appetite associated with estrogen concentrations in the menstrual cycle, with binge eating being inversely proportional to estrogen concentration. Both binge eating and bulimic symptoms are raised in the luteal phase compared to the follicular and ovulatory phases. AN is associated with reduced concentrations of both estrogen and progesterone, which is a consequence of starvation and leading to amenorrhea.[119] Amenorrhea is not found to be a good indicator of disease severity or a reflection of psychological symptoms. Currently, it is understood to be a consequence of nutritional status. Hence, it is no longer considered an essential diagnostic criterion for AN.[120]

Eating Disorder in Perinatal Period

Women with ED are at an increased risk of infertility. A systematic review examining ED in women seeking infertility treatment found that anorexia nervosa or bulimia nervosa was reported by up to 2% and 10.3% of women, respectively. In comparison, a history of anorexia nervosa or bulimia nervosa was reported by up to 8.5% and 3.3% of women, respectively.[121] However, it is important not to dismiss the risk of pregnancy in AN, as irregular menstruation can occur even in severe AN, and ovulation can occur in the absence of menstruation. Amenorrhea might lead to inadequate use of contraception and increased risk of unplanned pregnancies.[121,122]

Studies show that 1 in 20 pregnant women may have some form of disordered eating. Pregnancy has been shown to be associated with increased binge eating and dissatisfaction with weight and appearance.[122] ED has a variable course during pregnancy, with some studies showing improvement during pregnancy and increased risk for relapse in the postpartum period.[122,123]

Pregnancy in women with AN is considered high risk. It is ideally recommended that intervention for AN occurs before conception. A systematic review of obstetric complications in women with AN found an increased risk of anemia, cesarean section, intrauterine growth restriction, preterm birth, small-for-gestational-age birth, and low birth weight. The rates of GDM and PPH were lower in women with AN. In BN, increased risk of hyperemesis, babies with microcephaly, induced abortions, and small for gestational age have been reported.[122] It is important to differentiate between hyperemesis gravidarum and purging in AN and BN. In addition to routine obstetric care, psychiatric intervention and active nutritional rehabilitation would be required.[124]

Eating Disorder in Older Women

There is growing recognition that disordered eating can also occur in older women. One study found a 12-month prevalence of eating disorders of 3.6% among middle-aged women.[125] ED in midlife may be associated with medical comorbidities. Women in the perimenopausal age group have a slightly higher risk, leading some authors to consider perimenopausal eating disorders as separate entities. Binge eating is more common than food restriction in this age group. The perimenopausal period is known to have fluctuations in estrogen, which might play a role in influencing appetite.[126]

Eating Disorder in Minority Groups

Although the transgender population is under-represented in ED research, some literature suggests that gender and sociocultural body image norms may uniquely influence the manifestation of body image issues and ED. A proposed explanatory model for ED in minority groups is the minority stress model. This refers to the health disparities in the lived experience of individuals from stigmatized groups, including sexual and gender minorities. Exposure to higher stress levels and stigma and victimization experiences may put individuals at higher risk of ED.[127] Transgender people often experience intense levels of body dissatisfaction, which may increase their vulnerability to disordered eating.[128,129]

In particular, gender-nonconforming adults assigned female at birth may have higher lifetime ED risk.[130] It is known that hormone therapy as a part of gender-affirming treatment may alleviate bodily dissatisfaction and reduce disordered eating behaviors.[128] It is thus important to assess for gender dysphoria in vulnerable individuals who may first present with disordered eating.

Treatment

Psychotherapy, including enhanced CBT (CBT-E), family therapy, and interpersonal therapy (IPT), is the treatment of choice for AN and BN. CBT-E, a modification of CBT for eating disorders, focuses on the cognitive behavioral factors associated with the development and maintenance of eating disorders. Medications are used to manage co-occurring conditions such as depression and anxiety. SSRIs are ineffective in improving core symptoms of anorexia nervosa but have shown some benefit in BN. Limited evidence exists for atypical antipsychotics like olanzapine and quetiapine in improving weight gain. Exogenous administration of reproductive hormones has been studied with little evidence and no effect on bone density. Despite advancements, AN remains notoriously difficult to treat and is associated with the highest mortality rate of any mental disorder. It would require a skilled multidisciplinary management of the psychopathology, nutrition, and physical consequences of malnutrition. The level of care may be decided based on the severity of symptoms and dysfunction.

> **KEY POINTS**
> - Gender and sex can have an ongoing impact on the course and presentation of obsessive-compulsive related disorders (OCRD) and eating disorders (EDs) and must be approached with sensitivity during clinical evaluation.
> - Hormonal and reproductive cycles can influence clinical presentation and management.
> - They are often underreported due to the associated guilt and shame and hence a detailed empathetic evaluation may facilitate early diagnosis.

Disclosures: None.
Conflicts of interest: None.

REFERENCES

1. Reddy YCJ, Simpson HB, Stein DJ. Obsessive-compulsive and Related Disorders in International Classification of Diseases-11 and Its Relation to International Classification of Diseases-10 and Diagnostic and Statistical Manual of Mental Disorders-5. Indian J Soc Psychiatry. 2018;34:S34.
2. Luigjes J, Lorenzetti V, de Haan S, Youssef GJ, Murawski C, Sjoerds Z, et al. Defining Compulsive Behavior. Neuropsychol Rev. 2019;29:4-13.
3. Fineberg NA, Chamberlain SR, Goudriaan AE, Stein DJ, Vanderschuren LJ, Gillan CM, et al. New developments in human neurocognition: clinical, genetic, and brain imaging correlates of impulsivity and compulsivity. CNS Spectr. 2014;19(1):69-89.
4. Tannenbaum C, Greaves L, Graham ID. Why sex and gender matter in implementation research. BMC Med Res Methodol. 2016;16:145.
5. Lochner C, Stein DJ. Gender in obsessive-compulsive disorder and obsessive-compulsive spectrum disorders. Arch Womens Ment Health. 2001;4:19-26.
6. Springmann ML, Svaldi J, Kiegelmann M. Theoretical and Methodological Considerations for Research on Eating Disorders and Gender. Front Psychol. 2020;11.
7. MacSween M, Macsween M. Anorexic Bodies: A Feminist and Sociological Perspective on Anorexia Nervosa. United Kingdom: Routledge, Taylor and Francis Group; 2013.
8. Piran N. Journeys of Embodiment at the Intersection of Body and Culture: The Developmental Theory of Embodiment. United States: Academic Press; 2017.
9. Kwee J, Macbride H. Embodiment and Eating Disorders: Theory, Research, Prevention and Treatment. United Kingdom: Routledge, Taylor and Francis Group; 2018.

10. Fawcett EJ, Power H, Fawcett JM. Women Are at Greater Risk of OCD Than Men: A Meta-Analytic Review of OCD Prevalence Worldwide. J Clin Psychiatry. 2020;81(4):19r13085.
11. Rasmussen SA, Eisen JL. Epidemiology of obsessive-compulsive disorder. J Clin Psychiatry. 1990;51(Suppl):10-4.
12. Nestadt G. Obsessive-compulsive disorder issues pertinent to women. Women's health (London, England). 2008;4(4):311-3.
13. Cherian AV, Narayanaswamy JC, Viswanath B, Guru N, George CM, Bada Math S, et al. Gender differences in obsessive-compulsive disorder: findings from a large Indian sample. Asian J Psychiatry. 2014;9:17-21.
14. Vulink NC, Denys D, Bus L, Westenberg HG. Sexual pleasure in women with obsessive-compulsive disorder? J Affect Disord. 2006;91(1):19-25.
15. Koumantanou L, Kasvikis Y, Giaglis G, Skapinakis, Mavreas V. Differentiation of 2 Obsessive-Compulsive Disorder Subgroups with Regard to Demographic and Phenomenological Characteristics Combining Multiple Correspondence and Latent Class Analysis. Psychopathology. 2021;54(6):315-24.
16. Stein DJ, Costa DLC, Lochner C, Miguel EC, Reddy YCJ, Shavitt RG, et al. Obsessive-compulsive disorder. Nat Rev Dis Primers. 2019;5(1):52.
17. Hallion LS, Sockol LE, Wilhelm S. Obsessive-Compulsive Disorder. In: Stein D, Vythilingum B (eds). Anxiety Disorders and Gender. United States: Springer, Cham; 2015.
18. Lochner C, Hemmings SM, Kinnear CJ, Moolman-Smook JC, Corfield VA, Knowles JA, et al. Corrigendum to 'gender in obsessive-compulsive disorder: clinical and genetic findings'. Eur Neuropsychopharmacol. 2004;14:105-13. Updated: Eur Neuropsychopharmacol: J Eur Coll Neuropsychopharmacol. 2004;14(5):437–45.
19. Enoch MA, Greenberg BD, Murphy DL, Goldman D. Sexually dimorphic relationship of a 5-HT2A promoter polymorphism with obsessive-compulsive disorder. Biol Psychiatry. 2001;49(4):385-8.
20. Goodman WK, Price LH, Rasmussen SA, Mazure C, Fleischmann RL, Hill CL, et al. The Yale-Brown Obsessive Compulsive Scale: I. Development, use, and reliability. Arch Gen Psychiatry. 1989;46(11):1006-11.
21. Rosario-Campos MC, Miguel EC, Quatrano S, Chacon P, Ferrao Y, Findley D, et al. The Dimensional Yale-Brown Obsessive-Compulsive Scale (DY-BOCS): an instrument for assessing obsessive-compulsive symptom dimensions. Mol Psychiatry. 2006;11(5):495-504.
22. Wu MS, Pinto A, Horng B, Phares V, McGuire JF, Dedrick RF, et al. Psychometric properties of the Family Accommodation Scale for Obsessive–Compulsive Disorder—Patient Version (FAS-PV). Psychol Assess. 2016;28(3):251-62.
23. Janardhan Reddy YC, Sundar AS, Narayanaswamy JC, Math SB. Clinical practice guidelines for Obsessive-Compulsive Disorder. Indian J Psychiatry. 2017;59(Suppl 1):S74-90.
24. Guglielmi V, Vulink NC, Denys D, Wang Y, Samuels JF, Nestadt G. Obsessive-compulsive disorder and female reproductive cycle events: results from the OCD and reproduction collaborative study. Depress Anxiety. 2014;31(12):979-87.
25. Uguz F, Kaya V, Gezginc K, Kayhan F, Cicek E. Clinical correlates of worsening in obsessive-compulsive symptoms during pregnancy. General Hospital Psychiatry. 2011;33(2):197-9.

26. Forray A, Focseneanu M, Pittman B, McDougle CJ, Epperson CN. Onset and exacerbation of obsessive-compulsive disorder in pregnancy and the postpartum period. J Clin Psychiatry. 2010;71(8):1061-8.
27. Moreira L, Bins H, Toressan R, Ferro C, Harttmann T, Petribú K, et al. An exploratory dimensional approach to premenstrual manifestation of obsessive-compulsive disorder symptoms: a multicentre study. J Psychosomatic Res. 2012;74(4):313-9.
28. Brutocao C, Zaiem F, Alsawas M, Morrow AS, Murad MH, Javed A. Psychiatric disorders in women with polycystic ovary syndrome: a systematic review and meta-analysis. Endocrine. 2018;62(2):318-25.
29. Karpinski M, Mattina GF, Steiner M. Effect of Gonadal Hormones on Neurotransmitters Implicated in the Pathophysiology of Obsessive-Compulsive Disorder: A Critical Review. Neuroendocrinology. 2017;105(1):1-16.
30. Labad J, Menchón JM, Alonso P, Segalàs C, Jiménez S, Vallejo J. Oral contraceptive pill use and changes in obsessive-compulsive symptoms. J Psychosomatic Res. 2006;60(6):647-8.
31. Vulink NC, Denys D, Bus L, Westenberg HG. Female hormones affect symptom severity in obsessive-compulsive disorder. Int Clin Psychopharmacol. 2006;21(3):171-5.
32. Sacher J, Wilson AA, Houle S, Rusjan P, Hassan S, Bloomfield PM, et al. Elevated brain monoamine oxidase A binding in the early postpartum period. Arch Gen Psychiatry. 2010;67(5):468-74.
33. Balleine BW, O'Doherty JP. Human and rodent homologies in action control: corticostriatal determinants of goal-directed and habitual action. Neuropsychopharmacology : Am Coll Neuropsychopharmacol. 2010;35(1):48-69.
34. Mulligan EM, Hajcak G, Klawohn J, Nelson B, Meyer A. Effects of menstrual cycle phase on associations between the error-related negativity and checking symptoms in women. Psychoneuroendocrinology. 2019;103:233-40.
35. Marazziti D, Baroni S, Giannaccini G, Catena-Dell'Osso M, Piccinni A, Massimetti G, et al. Plasma Oxytocin Levels in Untreated Adult Obsessive-Compulsive Disorder Patients. Neuropsychobiology. 2015;72(2):74-80.
36. Holingue C, Samuels J, Guglielmi V, Ingram W, Nestadt G, Nestadt PS. Peripartum complications associated with obsessive compulsive disorder exacerbation during pregnancy. J Obsess Compuls Disord. 2021;29:100641.
37. Nasiri K, Czuzoj-Shulman N, Abenhaim HA. Association between obsessive-compulsive disorder and obstetrical and neonatal outcomes in the USA: a population-based cohort study. Arch Women Ment Health. 2021;24(6):971-8.
38. Uguz F, Yuksel G, Karsidag C, Guncu H, Konak M. Birth weight and gestational age in newborns exposed to maternal obsessive-compulsive disorder. Psychiatry Res. 2015;226(1):396-8.
39. Uguz F, Onder Sonmez E, Sahingoz M, Gokmen Z, Basaran M, Gezginc K, et al. Neuroinflammation in the fetus exposed to maternal obsessive-compulsive disorder during pregnancy: a comparative study on cord blood tumor necrosis factor-alpha levels. Comprehen Psychiatry. 2014;55(4):861-5.
40. Fernández de la Cruz L, Joseph KS, Wen Q, Stephansson O, Mataix-Cols D, Razaz N. Pregnancy, Delivery, and Neonatal Outcomes Associated With Maternal

Obsessive-Compulsive Disorder: Two Cohort Studies in Sweden and British Columbia, Canada. JAMA Network Open. 2023;6(6):e2318212.
41. Fairbrother N, Thordarson DS, Challacombe FL, Sakaluk JK. Correlates and Predictors of New Mothers' Responses to Postpartum Thoughts of Accidental and Intentional Harm and Obsessive Compulsive Symptoms. Behav Cogn Psychotherapy. 2018;46(4):437-53.
42. Sharma V. Role of sleep deprivation in the causation of postpartum obsessive-compulsive disorder. Med Hypotheses. 2019;122:58-61.
43. Hudepohl N, MacLean JV, Osborne LM. Perinatal Obsessive-Compulsive Disorder: Epidemiology, Phenomenology, Etiology, and Treatment. Curr Psychiatry Reports. 2022;24(4):229-37.
44. Mulcahy M, Long C, Morrow T, Galbally M, Rees C, Anderson R. Consensus recommendations for the assessment and treatment of perinatal obsessive-compulsive disorder (OCD): A Delphi study. Arch Women Ment Health. 2023;26(3):389-99.
45. Abel KM, Taylor D, Duncan D, McConnell H, Kerwin R. The Maudsley Prescribing Guidelines in Psychiatry. United States: John Wiley & Sons, Ltd.; 1999.
46. Lord C, Rieder A, Hall GB, Soares CN, Steiner M. Piloting the perinatal obsessive-compulsive scale (POCS): development and validation. J Anxiety Disorders. 2011;25(8):1079-84.
47. Uguz F, Sahingoz M, Gezginc K, Karatayli R. Obsessive-compulsive disorder in postmenopausal women: prevalence, clinical features, and comorbidity. Australian New Zealand J Psychiatry. 2010;44(2):183-7.
48. Dell'Osso B, Benatti B, Rodriguez CI, Arici C, Palazzo C, Altamura AC, et al. Obsessive-compulsive disorder in the elderly: A report from the International College of Obsessive-Compulsive Spectrum Disorders (ICOCS). Eur Psychiatry: J Assoc Eur Psychiatr. 2017;45:36-40.
49. Bjornsson AS, Didie ER, Grant JE, Menard W, Stalker E, Phillips KA. Age at onset and clinical correlates in body dysmorphic disorder. Comprehen Psychiatry. 2013;54(7):893-903.
50. Veale D, Gledhill LJ, Christodoulou P, Hodsoll J. Body dysmorphic disorder in different settings: A systematic review and estimated weighted prevalence. Body Image. 2016;18:168-86.
51. Phillips KA. Suicidality and aggressive behavior in body dysmorphic disorder. In: Phillips KA (ed). Body dysmorphic disorder: Advances in research and clinical practice. New York, NY: Oxford University Press; 2017. pp. 155-72.
52. American Psychiatric Association. Diagnostic and statistical manual of mental disorders: DSM-5. Washington (DC): American Psychiatric Publishing; 2013.
53. Gazzarrini D, Perugi G. Gender and body dysmorphic disorder. In: Phillips KA (ed). Body dysmorphic disorder: Advances in research and clinical practice. New York, NY: Oxford University Press; 2017. pp. 187-94.
54. Dworakowski O, Drüge M, Schlunegger M, Watzke B. Body dysmorphic disorder of female genitalia: a qualitative study of Swiss obstetrician-gynecologists' experiences and practices. Arch Gynecol Obstet. 2022;305(2):379-87.
55. Phillips KA, Kelly MM. Body Dysmorphic Disorder: Clinical Overview and Relationship to Obsessive-Compulsive Disorder. Focus (American Psychiatric Publishing). 2021;19(4):413-9.

56. Malcolm A, Pikoos TD, Castle DJ, Rossell SL. An update on gender differences in major symptom phenomenology among adults with body dysmorphic disorder. Psychiatry Res. 2021;295:113619.
57. Tucker R, Watkins PL, Cardinal BJ. Muscle dysmorphia, gender role stress, and sociocultural influences: an exploratory study. Res Quart Exer Sport. 2011;82(2):310-9.
58. Phillips KA, Menard W, Fay C, Weisberg R. Demographic characteristics, phenomenology, comorbidity, and family history in 200 individuals with body dysmorphic disorder. Psychosomatics. 2005;46(4):317-25.
59. Enander J, Ivanov VZ, Mataix-Cols D, Kuja-Halkola R, Ljótsson B, Lundström S, et al. Prevalence and heritability of body dysmorphic symptoms in adolescents and young adults: a population-based nationwide twin study. Psychol Med. 2018;48:2740-7.
60. Carey P, Seedat S, Warwick J, van Heerden B, Stein DJ. SPECT imaging of body dysmorphic disorder. J NeuroPsychiatry Clin Neurosci. 2004;16(3):357-9.
61. Feusner JD, Townsend J, Bystritsky A, Bookheimer S. Visual information processing of faces in body dysmorphic disorder. Arch Gen Psychiatry. 2007;64(12):1417-25.
62. Fang A, Jacoby RJ, Beatty C, Germine L, Plessow F, Wilhelm S, et al. Serum oxytocin levels are elevated in body dysmorphic disorder and related to severity of psychopathology. Psychoneuroendocrinology. 2020;113:104541.
63. Longobardi C, Badenes-Ribera L, Fabris MA. Adverse childhood experiences and body dysmorphic symptoms: A meta-analysis. Body Image. 2022;40:267-84.
64. Carter A, Forrest JI, Kaida A. Association Between Internet Use and Body Dissatisfaction Among Young Females: Cross-Sectional Analysis of the Canadian Community Health Survey. J Med Internet Res. 2017;19(2):e39.
65. Vall-Roqué H, Andrés A, Saldaña C. The impact of COVID-19 lockdown on social network sites use, body image disturbances and self-esteem among adolescent and young women. Prog Neuropsychopharmacol Biol Psychiatry. 2021;110:110293.
66. Tiggemann M, Barbato I. 'You look great!': The effect of viewing appearance-related Instagram comments on women's body image. Body Image. 2018;27:61-6.
67. Dogan O, Yassa M. Major Motivators and Sociodemographic Features of Women Undergoing Labiaplasty. Aesthetic Surg J. 2019;39(12):NP517-NP527.
68. Müllerová J, Weiss P. Plastic surgery in gynaecology: Factors affecting women's decision to undergo labiaplasty. Mind the risk of body dysmorphic disorder: a review. J Women Aging. 2020;32(3):241-58.
69. Phillips KA, Susser LC. Body Dysmorphic Disorder in Women. Psychiatric Clin North Am. 2023;46(3):505-25.
70. Phillips KA, Hollander E, Rasmussen SA, Aronowitz BR, DeCaria C, Goodman WK. A severity rating scale for body dysmorphic disorder: development, reliability, and validity of a modified version of the Yale-Brown Obsessive Compulsive Scale. Psychopharmacol Bulletin. 1997;33(1):17-22.
71. Rosen JC, Reiter J. Development of the body dysmorphic disorder examination. Behav Res Ther. 1996;34(9):755-66.
72. Phillips KA, Menard W, Fay C, Weisberg R. Gender similarities and differences in 200 individuals with body dysmorphic disorder. Compr Psychiatry. 2006b;47(2):77-87.

73. Lundström L, Flygare O, Ivanova E, Mataix-Cols D, Enander J, Pascal D, et al. Effectiveness of Internet-based cognitive-behavioural therapy for obsessive-compulsive disorder (OCD-NET) and body dysmorphic disorder (BDD-NET) in the Swedish public health system using the RE-AIM implementation framework. Internet Interventions. 2023;31:100608.
74. Phillips KA, Hollander E. Treating body dysmorphic disorder with medication: evidence, misconceptions, and a suggested approach. Body Image. 2008;5(1):13-27.
75. Phillips KA, McElroy SL, Keck PE Jr, Hudson JI, Pope HG Jr. A comparison of delusional and nondelusional body dysmorphic disorder in 100 cases. Psychopharmacol Bull. 1994;30(2):179-86.
76. Phillips KA, Keshaviah A, Dougherty DD, Stout RL, Menard W, Wilhelm S. Pharmacotherapy Relapse Prevention in Body Dysmorphic Disorder: A Double-Blind, Placebo-Controlled Trial. Am J Psychiatry. 2016;173(9):887-95.
77. NICE. Obsessive-compulsive disorder and body dysmorphic disorder: treatment. National Inst Heal Care Excell. 2005.
78. Phillips KA, Grant J, Siniscalchi J, Albertini RS. Surgical and nonpsychiatric medical treatment of patients with body dysmorphic disorder. Psychosomatics. 2001;42(6):504-10.
79. Metcalfe DB, Duggal CS, Gabriel A, Nahabedian MY, Carlson GW, Losken A. Prevalence of Body Dysmorphic Disorder Among Patients Seeking Breast Reconstruction. Aesthetic Surg J. 2014;34(5):733-7.
80. Miller ML, Roche AI, Lemon E, O'Hara MW. Obsessive-compulsive and related disorder symptoms in the perinatal period: prevalence and associations with postpartum functioning. Arch Women Ment Health. 2022;25(4):771-80.
81. Watson B, Fuller-Tyszkiewicz M, Broadbent J, Skouteris H. The meaning of body image experiences during the perinatal period: A systematic review of the qualitative literature. Body Image. 2015;14:102-13.
82. Stein DJ, Kogan CS, Atmaca M, Fineberg NA, Fontenelle LF, Grant JE, et al. The classification of Obsessive-Compulsive and Related Disorders in the ICD-11. J Affect Disord. 2016;190:663-74.
83. Grant JE, Chamberlain SR. Trichotillomania and Skin-Picking Disorder: Different Kinds of OCD. FOCUS. 2015;13(2):184-9.
84. Grant JE, Christenson GA. Examination of Gender in Pathologic Grooming Behaviors. Psychiatr Q. 2007;78(4):259-67.
85. Grant JE, Chamberlain SR. Skin picking disorder: Does a person's sex matter? Ann Clin Psychiatry Off J Am Acad Clin Psychiatr. 2022;34(1):15-20.
86. Grant JE, Dougherty DD, Chamberlain SR. Prevalence, gender correlates, and co-morbidity of trichotillomania. Psychiatry Res. 2020;288:112948.
87. Snorrason I, Ricketts EJ, Stein AT, Thamrin H, Lee SJ, Goldberg H, et al. Sex Differences in Age at Onset and Presentation of Trichotillomania and Trichobezoar: A 120-Year Systematic Review of Cases. Child Psychiatry Hum Dev. 2022;53(1):165-71.
88. Monzani B, Rijsdijk F, Harris J, Mataix-Cols D. The structure of genetic and environmental risk factors for dimensional representations of DSM-5 obsessive-compulsive spectrum disorders. JAMA Psychiatry. 2014;71(2):182-9.
89. Monzani B, Rijsdijk F, Cherkas L, Harris J, Keuthen N, Mataix-Cols D. Prevalence and heritability of skin picking in an adult community sample: a twin study.

Am J Med Genet Part B Neuropsychiatr Genet Off Publ Int Soc Psychiatr Genet. 2012;159B(5):605-10.
90. Chamberlain S, Menzies L, Fineberg N, Del Campo N, Suckling J, Craig K, et al. Grey matter abnormalities in trichotillomania: Morphometric magnetic resonance imaging study. Br J Psychiatry. 2008;193(3):216-21.
91. Roberts S, O'Connor K, Bélanger C. Emotion regulation and other psychological models for body-focused repetitive behaviors. Clin Psychol Rev. 2013;33(6):745-62.
92. Houghton DC, Mathew AS, Twohig MP, Saunders SM, Franklin ME, Compton SN, et al. Trauma and trichotillomania: A tenuous relationship. J Obsessive-Compuls Relat Disord. 2016;11:91-5.
93. Özten E, Hızlı Sayar G, Kağan G, Işık S, Karamustafalıoğlu O, Eryilmaz G. The relationship of psychological trauma with trichotillomania and skin picking. Neuropsychiatr Dis Treat. 2015;11:1203-10.
94. Weingarden H, Renshaw KD. Shame in the obsessive compulsive related disorders: A conceptual review. J Affect Disord. 2015;171:74-84.
95. Grant JE, Redden SA, Leppink EW, Chamberlain SR, Curley EE, Tung ES, et al. Sex differences in trichotillomania. Ann Clin Psychiatry Off J Am Acad Clin Psychiatr. 2016;28(2):118-24.
96. Falkenstein MJ, Haaga DAF. Symptom accommodation, trichotillomania-by-proxy, and interpersonal functioning in trichotillomania (hair-pulling disorder). Compr Psychiatry. 2016;65:88-97.
97. De Sousa A. Trichotillomania by Proxy. Int J Trichology. 2015;7(1):24-5.
98. Anderson S, Clarke V. Disgust, shame and the psychosocial impact of skin picking: Evidence from an online support forum. J Health Psychol. 2019;24(13):1773-84.
99. Stemberger RM, Thomas AM, Mansueto CS, Carter JG. Personal toll of trichotillomania: behavioral and interpersonal sequelae. J Anxiety Disord. 2000;14(1):97-104.
100. Soriano JL, O'Sullivan RL, Baer L, Phillips KA, McNally RJ, Jenike MA. Trichotillomania and self-esteem: a survey of 62 female hair pullers. J Clin Psychiatry. 1996;57(2):77-82.
101. Woods DW, Flessner CA, Franklin ME, Keuthen NJ, Goodwin RD, Stein DJ, et al. The Trichotillomania Impact Project (TIP): Exploring Phenomenology, Functional Impairment, and Treatment Utilization. J Clin Psychiatry. 2006;67(12):21754.
102. Ghate R, Hossain R, Lewis SP, Richter MA, Sinyor M. Characterizing the content, messaging, and tone of trichotillomania on YouTube: A content analysis. J Psychiatr Res. 2022;151:150-6.
103. Grant JE, Chesivoir E, Valle S, Ehsan D, Chamberlain SR. Double-Blind Placebo-Controlled Study of Memantine in Trichotillomania and Skin-Picking Disorder. Am J Psychiatry. 2023;180(5):348-56.
104. Grant JE, Odlaug BL, Kim SW. N-acetylcysteine, a glutamate modulator, in the treatment of trichotillomania: a double-blind, placebo-controlled study. Arch Gen Psychiatry. 2009;66(7):756-63.
105. Grant JE, Chamberlain SR, Redden SA, Leppink EW, Odlaug BL, Kim SW. N-Acetylcysteine in the Treatment of Excoriation Disorder: A Randomized Clinical Trial. JAMA Psychiatry. 2016;73(5):490-6.

106. Van Ameringen M, Mancini C, Patterson B, Bennett M, Oakman J. A randomized, double-blind, placebo-controlled trial of olanzapine in the treatment of trichotillomania. J Clin Psychiatry. 2010;71(10):1336-43.
107. França K, Kumar A, Castillo D, Jafferany M, Hyczy da Costa Neto M, Damevska K, et al. Trichotillomania (hair pulling disorder): Clinical characteristics, psychosocial aspects, treatment approaches, and ethical considerations. Dermatol Ther. 2019;32(4):e12622.
108. Claudino AM, Pike KM, Hay P, Keeley JW, Evans SC, Rebello TJ, et al. The classification of feeding and eating disorders in the ICD-11: results of a field study comparing proposed ICD-11 guidelines with existing ICD-10 guidelines. BMC Med. 2019;17(1):93.
109. Qian J, Hu Q, Wan Y, Li T, Wu M, Ren Z, et al. Prevalence of eating disorders in the general population: a systematic review. Shanghai Arch Psychiatry. 2013;25(4):212-23.
110. Mitchell AM, Bulik CM. Eating Disorders and Women's Health: An Update. J Midwifery Womens Health. 2006;51(3):193-201.
111. Sharan P, Sundar AS. Eating disorders in women. Indian J Psychiatry [Internet]. 2015;57(Suppl 2):S286-S295.
112. Keel PK, Klump KL. Are eating disorders culture-bound syndromes? Implications for conceptualizing their etiology. Psychol Bull. 2003;129(5):747-69.
113. Vaidyanathan S, Kuppili PP, Menon V. Eating Disorders: An Overview of Indian Research. Indian J Psychol Med. 2019;41(4):311-7.
114. Chandra PS, Abbas S, Palmer R. Are eating disorders a significant clinical issue in urban India? A survey among psychiatrists in Bangalore. Int J Eat Disord. 2012;45(3):443-6.
115. Kulshreshtha M, Babu N, Goel NJ, Chandel S. Disordered eating attitudes and body shape concerns among North Indian Kathak dancers. Int J Eating Disor. 2021;54(2):148-54. https://doi.org/10.1002/eat.23425.
116. Ahlin T. What keeps Maya from eating? A case study of disordered eating from North India. Transcult Psychiatry. 2018;55(4):551-71.
117. Baker JH, Schaumberg K, Munn-Chernoff MA. Genetics of Anorexia Nervosa. Curr Psychiatry Rep. 2017;19(11):84.
118. Klump KL. Puberty as a Critical Risk Period for Eating Disorders: A Review of Human and Animal Studies. Horm Behav. 2013;64(2):399-410.
119. Baker JH, Girdler SS, Bulik CM. The role of reproductive hormones in the development and maintenance of eating disorders. Expert Rev Obstet Gynecol. 2012;7(6):573-83.
120. Attia E, Roberto CA. Should amenorrhea be a diagnostic criterion for anorexia nervosa? Int J Eat Disord. 2009;42(7):581-9.
121. Hecht LM, Hadwiger A, Patel S, Hecht BR, Loree A, Ahmedani BK, et al. Disordered eating and eating disorders among women seeking fertility treatment: A systematic review. Arch Women Ment Health. 2022;25(1):21-32.
122. Martínez-Olcina M, Rubio-Arias JA, Reche-García C, Leyva-Vela B, Hernández-García M, Hernández-Morante JJ, et al. Eating Disorders in Pregnant and Breastfeeding Women: A Systematic Review. Medicina (Mex). 2020;56(7):352.
123. Ward VB. Eating disorders in pregnancy. BMJ. 2008;336(7635):93-6.
124. Pan JR, Li TY, Tucker D, Chen KY. Pregnancy outcomes in women with active anorexia nervosa: a systematic review. J Eat Disord. 2022;10:25.

125. Micali N, Martini MG, Thomas JJ, Eddy KT, Kothari R, Russell E, et al. Lifetime and 12-month prevalence of eating disorders amongst women in mid-life: a population-based study of diagnoses and risk factors. BMC Med. 2017;15:12.
126. Baker JH, Runfola CD. Eating disorders in midlife women: a perimenopausal eating disorder? Maturitas. 2016;85:112-6.
127. Breton É, Juster RP, Booij L. Gender and sex in eating disorders: a narrative review of the current state of knowledge, research gaps, and recommendations. Brain Behav. 2023;13(4):e2871.
128. Jones BA, Haycraft E, Bouman WP, Brewin N, Claes L, Arcelus J. Risk Factors for Eating Disorder Psychopathology within the Treatment Seeking Transgender Population: The Role of Cross-Sex Hormone Treatment. Eur Eating Disord Rev: J Eating Disord Associat. 2018;26(2):120-8.
129. Watson RJ, Veale JF, Saewyc EM. Disordered eating behaviors among transgender youth: Probability profiles from risk and protective factors. Int J Eat Disord. 2017;50(5):515-22.
130. Diemer EW, White Hughto JM, Gordon AR, Guss C, Austin SB, Reisner SL. Beyond the Binary: Differences in Eating Disorder Prevalence by Gender Identity in a Transgender Sample. Transgender Health. 2018;3(1):17-23.

CHAPTER 5

Unraveling the Knots: Dissociation and Somatization in Women

Aishwariya Jha, Rashmi Arasappa, Geetha Desai

▮ ABSTRACT

Women who suffer from dissociation and somatization constitute a large percentage of outpatient consultations and inpatient hospitalizations, they incur significant healthcare costs and have higher rates of absenteeism, disability, mood and anxiety disorders, poorer quality of life, unsatisfying healthcare contact, and increased use of prescription medication. Although these conditions are not limited to women as was historically popularized, they evidently occur more often in women. Our growing understanding of the etiology and presentation of these two, sometimes intertwined conditions, is reflected in our current classificatory systems and treatment approaches. This chapter provides an overview of the history, nosology, clinical presentation, course, outcomes, challenges, assessment, and treatment of "Dissociation and Somatization".

Keywords: Dissociative disorders, conversion disorders, somatization disorders

▮ INTRODUCTION

In Greco-Roman literature and the Hippocratic corpus, "Hysterika" was derived from the root Greek and Latin "Hysterikos" and "Hystera" respectively for uterus, the organ most condemned for the suffocation, palpitations, and convulsions that women at the time suffered from.[1] It was believed that the uterus rendered dry from a lack of fluids or pregnancy would wander to various sites in the body which would explain its protean manifestations. Today, we understand that these incorrect and gendered connotations are barely based in clinical reality, but at the time, this was a prevalent belief and laid the foundation for treatments like ovarian compression, sexual intercourse, massages, and chemical treatments to coax the wandering womb back to its place.[2,3] For centuries, such symptoms were marked off as maladies confined to women. Before the 17th century, the other theories included demonic possession, punishment for sins, and witchcraft due to which many women were subjected to cruelty. Physicians and the lay public alike were repulsed by the condition and to this day, the term "hysterical" serves a negative connotation in common parlance.

In the 19th century, the permeable boundaries between psychism and brain sciences allowed physicians and scientists to speculate on another organ that may be operating in hysteria—the brain. Several revered greats such as Charcot, Janet, Babinski, Tourette, and Freud studied "Hysteria".[1] Charcot famously demonstrated theatrical hysterical expressions to his fascinated students.[4] Sigmund Freud, a student of Charcot, too believed that the origins of these symptoms resided in the psyche and introduced the concept of conversion. According to Freud, suppressed impulses manifest as bodily or behavioral manifestations.[5] The notion that hysterical manifestations stemmed from a disordered brain was further expanded on and described in both men and women by Thomas Willis and Thomas Sydenham.[6,7]

Throughout history, the origins of the malady continued to dumbfound physicians. More questions arose as time passed by: What do we call it, how do we classify it, and more importantly—what can we do about it?

Women who suffer from dissociation and somatization constitute a large percentage of outpatient consultations, they incur significant healthcare costs, have higher rates of absenteeism, have higher rates of disability, comorbid mood disorders, and anxiety disorders, poorer quality of life, increased subjective suffering, unsatisfying healthcare contact, increased use of prescription medication, more requirement of pain control and are at a greater risk of abuse and misuse of substances and medication.[8-13]

This chapter is on "Dissociation and Somatization" as we know them today. However, these two conditions inter alia originated from the initial descriptions of "Hysteria". Thus, the nosology, presentation, evaluation, and management will be discussed in tandem. Although there are several synonymous and confusing terms in the literature, the terms "dissociation" and "somatization" will be used when referring to the now known dissociative disorders and bodily distress/somatic symptom disorders, respectively.

NOSOLOGICAL EVOLUTION OF DISSOCIATION AND SOMATIZATION

Table 1 describes the evolution of the nosology of dissociation and somatization in the two classificatory systems: the International Classification of Diseases (ICD) and the Diagnostic Statistical Manual of Mental Disorders (DSM).

In the ICD-11, the "bodily distress" disorder subsumes all somatoform disorders and neurasthenia, thus simplifying the entity.[22] The fundamental revision, however, is the abolition of the need for the somatic complaint to be medically unexplained. The revised classification defines the condition based on a feature that is *present*—the distress, rather than what is *absent*—the physical or medical basis for the complaint.[23]

The most recent revisions of both the ICD and the DSM have highlighted that a single symptom causing significant distress is adequate for a diagnosis—which is a valid argument considering that even significant pain can be

TABLE 1: Evolution of Dissociation and Somatization in the International Classification of Diseases (ICD) and the Diagnostic Statistical Manual of Mental Disorders (DSM).

5th Century BC	*Hippocrates first coined Hysteria: "the moving uterus"*	
1940s–1960s	DSM-I and II included a diagnosis of hysteria/hysterical neurosis[14]	The ICD-6 mentioned psychoneuroses with somatic symptoms and psychoneuroses without anxiety which included hysteria. This was later modified to psychoneuroses with somatic symptoms affecting other systems in ICD-7. The term hysteria was retained in ICD-8[15,16]
1970s–1980s	• DSM-III removed hysterical neurosis and instead added the St Louis criteria for Briquet syndrome (14 of 37 possible symptoms). The DSM-III included conversion disorder, psychogenic pain disorder, hypochondriasis, and atypical somatoform disorders • The DSM-III R included somatoform pain disorder[17]	• ICD-9: The term "hysteria" was retained • ICD-10: The term "somatoform disorder" was introduced. Dissociative and conversion disorders were grouped under a different category[18] • Dissociative disorders included dissociative amnesia, fugue, stupor, conversion disorders with motor symptoms/deficits, seizures, sensory symptoms/deficits, dissociative identity disorder, and other mixed and unspecified conditions
1994–2000	In DSM-IV and DSM-IV-TR, somatization disorder needed only 8 out of the 32 symptoms. The name of somatoform pain disorder was changed to pain disorder[19]	
2013–2019	• The DSM-5 saw the emergence of somatic symptoms and related disorders (SSD), a diagnosis that required one or more physical symptoms that caused distress or significant disruption of daily life. The requirement that the symptoms are medically unexplained has not been included in SSD criteria	• ICD-11 in 2019 introduced the term "bodily distress disorder" which criteria is one or more symptoms that attract excessive attention and the ensuing distress cannot be alleviated by reassurance, examination, or investigations • Hypochondriasis, which was long believed to be a related condition, was moved to the obsessive-compulsive and related disorders group

Contd...

Contd...

5ᵗʰ Century BC	Hippocrates first coined Hysteria: "the moving uterus"	
	• There is no requirement that the symptom(s) must be associated with psychological conflicts or stressors. The criteria require a duration of 6 months with a "persistent" specifier if the symptoms are for >6 months. A specifier for the severity of SSD as mild, moderate, or severe based on the number of symptoms present has been added[20]	• Chronic pain has been moved out and is an entity of its own. It includes cancer, neuropathic, visceral, musculoskeletal, headache, and orofacial pain • The ICD-11 dissociative disorders group includes dissociative neurological symptom disorder, dissociative identity disorder, and dissociative amnesia. The term "conversion" has been removed entirely and the two broad categories under dissociation have multiple specifiers for the type of symptom presentation • There are two separate diagnoses for trance disorder and possession disorder. Depersonalization and derealization have been moved to the dissociative disorders grouping[21]

excessively bothersome, comparable to or perhaps more so, than multiple such somatic symptoms.

However, the evolution of these conditions is not limited to the field of "Psychiatry and Mental Health". The terms "Functional symptoms", "Medically unexplained symptoms", "Persistent physical symptoms", "Psychosomatic disorders", "Functional somatic symptoms", "Multiple somatic symptoms", "Somatothymic symptoms", "Health worry", and "Idiopathic symptoms" among others have been used as diagnostic labels across the clinical practice. This terminological divide could be partly due to the physician's perception of the mind and body as two separate entities, reflecting the historical divide between what is "organic" and what is "functional".

UNDERSTANDING DISSOCIATION AND SOMATIZATION

After Janet developed the modern approaches to dissociative disorders,[24] and Freud and Breuer described their case studies on "hysteria",[25] the notion that such symptoms were harvested from trauma became evident. In the often-cited case of Anna O, for example, the unconscious intrapsychic conflicts that gave rise to the symptoms of hysteria were treated with cathartic talk therapy.[26]

CHAPTER 5: Unraveling the Knots: Dissociation and Somatization in Women

Therefore, dissociative symptoms and somatization symptoms involve both externally visible experiences and intrapsychic genealogy. Locating symptom origins in the mind or the psyche tends to ascribe responsibility to the patient. There is significant moral blame since psychological issues are perceived to be reversible and under volitional control. Therefore, such explanations elicit less empathy from family, peers, employers, and physicians alike. On the contrary, illness that is attributable to physical causes is often viewed as uncontrollable and evokes more concern from the onlooker.

Thus, an individual with such complaints may often initially seek medical attention for physical symptoms.[27] Moreover, the individual rarely has insight into the link between the psychological distress and the physical symptoms. The psychological issues are then unidentified and undertreated or untreated.

Both dissociation and somatization are unconscious physical expressions of emotional distress. The etiology of dissociation and somatization may involve a complex interplay of factors that may not be immediately evident. Some of these may include:

- Negative life experiences and trauma, adverse childhood experiences and emotional neglect, ongoing stress, or recent stressful events[28-34]
- Personality factors such as neuroticism, negative affectivity, and impaired normalizing attributions[35,36]
- Social learning and gain seeking
- Comorbid psychiatric illnesses[37]
- Biologically derived vulnerabilities, epigenetics, trauma-related neurobiological responses[38-42]
- Cultural factors and acculturation stress[11,43-45]

The interactions of these factors may lead to:

> - A heightened awareness of bodily sensations and physical symptoms → Somatization
> - An altered state of consciousness in a state of intolerable emotions → Dissociation

These processes are not limited to the "invisible mind", but also have a neurobiological basis. In somatization, a cognitive phenomenon called somatosensory amplification has been proposed by Barsky, 1992[46] which translates to a heightened focus on one's own body and bodily complaints. Another neurobiological process known as "central sensitization" has been used to explain a sensitive and hyperresponsive neural network[47-49] such that these patients perceive an innocuous stimulus to be noxious due to central augmentation of pain signals.[47] Neuroimaging techniques have demonstrated differences in pituitary, hippocampal, and amygdalae volumes.[50,51] The insula, which is implicated in pain processing,[52] threat detection,[53] and emotional regulation[54] has been implicated in the central sensitization process[55,56] along with the anterior cingulate cortex,[57,58] which processes emotions,[59,60] attention[61] and pain,[62] and the striatum which is critical in salience detection.[63] Pain catastrophizing is also correlated with the neural circuitry between the anterior cingulate cortex and the prefrontal cortex.[64] Somatic symptoms have also been correlated with hypothalamic pituitary axis dysfunction[65] and inflammatory and oxidative stress pathways.[66]

Research on dissociative amnesia has reported autobiographical retrieval deficits and dysfunction in the frontal executive systems.[67] Research on depersonalization proposes a cortico-limbic disconnection model.[68] Increased activity in the dorsolateral prefrontal cortices via the anterior cingulate cortex leads to a decrease in the activity of the amygdala which is integral to the responsivity to stressful and fear-inducing stimuli.[69-71] Dissociation as a phenomenon in posttraumatic stress disorder (PTSD) has been linked to an increase in self-control and arousal modulation, i.e., an increase in the prefrontal activity and decreased activation in the amygdala and insula.[72] The re-experiencing phenomenon in PTSD is associated with a reversal of this neural mechanism. Patients who suffer from dissociative motor symptoms have been shown to have differences in the amygdala, dorsolateral prefrontal, temporal cortices, thalamus, insula, and primary motor cortices when compared to healthy controls.[56] These neural areas are involved in motor activity (planning and selection) and autonomic arousal.

Dissociation and somatization as phenomena may be viewed on a spectrum of physical manifestations of underlying emotional distress, rather than truly separate entities. The spectrum approach is based on the evidence that these two disorders often share etiologies, vulnerabilities, behaviors, and symptomatology.[31,73-75] This would serve two purposes—one, that we would not confine our understanding of either to the "disorders" described in nosology and thus address them in the whole scope of other psychiatric and systemic illnesses, and the other, that we would understand these manifestations on a vertical level, and modify our approach to help our patients better.

■ DISSOCIATIVE DISORDERS

A Ms M, a 25-year-old single woman, presented to the emergency with jerky movements of the hands and legs, apparent unawareness of her surroundings, and sporadic vocalization and aggressive behavior. Upon evaluation, there were no focal deficits, and no past history of epilepsy, and the MRI brain and electroencephalogram (EEG) were normal. There was a history of similar episodes in the preceding week wherein she would also speak in a strange voice, laugh, cry, scream, throw items, bang her head against the wall, and throttle her neck. Upon further exploration, she revealed that her elder brother who had reportedly sexually harassed her in childhood had recently lost his job and had to move back in with her family.

CHAPTER 5: Unraveling the Knots: Dissociation and Somatization in Women

Dissociative symptoms and experiences range from minor lapses in memory and attention and daydream-like state to the more debilitating symptoms of dissociative identity disorder (DID), depersonalization/derealization disorder (DDD), and dissociative amnesia. The disorder is diagnosed when there is evidence of significant disturbances in the integration of consciousness, emotions, memory, motor processes, perceptual experiences, bodily representation, and identity.[76] Approximately a fifth of outpatients in psychiatric settings report clinically significant dissociative symptoms.[77] Dissociative disorders evidently worsen the quality of life, lead to recurrent hospitalizations, and are associated with higher rates of suicide and disability.[78,79]

The lifetime prevalence of DDD in the United States is 1–3%.[80,81] A recent systematic review on the prevalence of DDD reported that the prevalence rates in the general population ranged from 0 to 1.9%, 5–20% in outpatients, and 17.5–41% in inpatients, 1.8–5.9% in addictive disorders, 3.3–20.2% in anxiety disorders, 16.3% in patients with schizophrenia, 17% in borderline personality disorder, 50% in depression, and 25–54% in patients who experiences abuse.[82]

A study from a tertiary neuropsychiatry center in South India reported a prevalence of 1.5–15 per 1,000 outpatients and 1.5–11.6 per 1,000 inpatients.[83] In this study, the highest percentage of patients were diagnosed with dissociative motor disorders and convulsions, and a female preponderance was reported across all subtypes of dissociative disorders except dissociative fugue.[83]

Estimates of the prevalence of DID and dissociative amnesia vary widely across literature. The prevalence in the general population is approximately 1–2% with higher rates in inpatient settings (1–9.6%).[84,85]

Although this section speaks of dissociative "disorders", dissociation as a *phenomenon* or symptom can occur in women who suffer from various other conditions. There is a significant clinical overlap with more than half of such patients also meeting diagnostic criteria for borderline personality disorder,[86,87] and nearly three-fourths of BPD patients reporting dissociative symptoms.[88] Moreover, patients with dissociative disorders often meet the criteria for depression, PTSD, panic disorder, obsessive-compulsive disorders (OCD), social anxiety, and somatization disorder.[37,85] The most common comorbidity overall appears to be mood disorders and these patients often report childhood abuse.[37] Different ways in which dissociation may present are described in **Table 2**.

Assessment, Course, and Outcome of Dissociative Disorders

The assessment of dissociative disorders is usually through a clinical history and mental status examination.[93] Clinicians may also adopt tools

TABLE 2: Presentation and differentials in dissociative disorders.

S. No.	Dissociative disorder	Clinical presentation	Differential diagnoses
1	Dissociative neurological symptom disorder	The presence of motor, sensory, and cognitive symptoms that involuntarily interrupt normal behavior and cannot be explained by diseases of the nervous system. These symptoms may include visual/auditory disturbances, dizziness, other sensory perceptions, nonepileptic seizures, speech disturbances, weakness, gait abnormalities, movement disorder symptoms, or impaired cognitive performance[21]	Corresponding neurological condition. Requires a detailed history, neurological examination, EEG, neuroimaging, and blood investigations as needed
2	Dissociative amnesia	• The inability to recall pertinent personal information usually has a stressful or traumatic aspect and is to an extent that cannot be explained by forgetfulness. Usually, it has a clear onset, and can be either an abrupt amnesia of personal events or more commonly, a deletion from conscious memories.[67] • If the individual has fugue, the essential symptom is that one travels away from their usual place of residence suddenly and is unable to recall events of their past life. A fugue usually occurs after unbearable life circumstances[21,89]	• Dementia • Delirium • Korsakoff psychosis • Stroke • Postoperative amnesia • CNS infections • Epilepsy • Transient global amnesia • Electroconvulsive therapy associated with amnesia • Toxin and substance-related disorders

Contd...

Contd...

S. No.	Dissociative disorder	Clinical presentation	Differential diagnoses
3	Trance and possession disorders	• Trance is a temporary alteration of the present state of consciousness which is either demonstrable by a loss of sense of personal identity, narrowing of awareness of the environment, or a drastic reduction in movements, postures, and speech which may be stereotyped and perceived as outside of one's control[21] • Possession is a state wherein the individual believes that a foreign entity, a spirit/power/deity, or another person has taken over the body and mind. Thus, the individual takes on a new identity with partial or complete amnesia for the events that occurred when possessed[21]	• Epilepsy • Head injury • Postconcussion • CNS infections or space-occupying lesions • Neurodegenerative conditions
4	Dissociative identity disorder	The presence of two or more identities/alter-egos or personalities within an individual that alternatively takes over the person's consciousness and behaviors. As a result, there are large gaps in memory. These symptoms may be accompanied by feelings of detachment from self, symptoms of passive influence, and depersonalization[21,90,91]	• PTSD • Schizophrenia • Malingering • Borderline personality disorder

Contd...

Contd...

S. No.	Dissociative disorder	Clinical presentation	Differential diagnoses
5	Depersonalization and derealization disorder	A subjective sense of estrangement from oneself or one's reality. It can be described as a transient dream-like state that is outside of one's control. Such patients may be unable to fully explain what they are feeling at the time these events occur. An emotional numbing and sense of detachment may be described. Objects may be perceived as farther away and with reduced depth perception. Auditory percept may be muffled, distorted, and unclear. Other perceptions such as vividness of color may also appear to reduce[21,92]	• Epilepsy • Borderline personality disorder • Panic attacks and anxiety disorders • Depression • Schizophrenia • Brain tumors • Postconcussion • Metabolic abnormalities • Vertigo, Meniere's disease • Head injury • Substance-induced states

(CNS: central nervous system; EEG: electroencephalogram; PTSD: posttraumatic stress disorder) such as the dissociative experiences scale (DES) which is a 28-item self-report questionnaire[94] or the structured clinical interview for DSM-IV dissociative disorders–revised (SCID-D-R).[95] A culturally sensitive approach to assessment with the exploration of the patient and caretaker's experiences and explanatory models is especially pertinent in trance and possession disorders.

The usual onset is adolescence or adulthood, and the condition may persist lifelong with exacerbations at times of acute stress or high levels of sensory input.[82,96] Most dissociative disorders follow an episodic or relapsing-remitting course and the outcomes are positive when the patient is safely removed from the overwhelming situation and when timely intervened.[92] However, in many cases, somatic/sensory symptoms may persist for several years in the presence of chronic stress. The resolution of symptoms may take a variable amount of time contingent on whether the traumatic or overwhelming situation has improved and the patient's coping skills and personality traits. Such conditions are likely to persist if there is continued exposure to interpersonal abuse and there is a high risk of self-harm and suicide.[97]

In the case of trance and possession disorders, patients are likely to make first contact with traditional folk healers, and shamans and resort to magico-religious practices and exorcism. Outcomes can be positive for 95% of individuals if the stressful factor underlying psychiatric illness or cause of psychological distress is appropriately addressed.[98]

Treatment of Dissociative Disorders

The first step is to ensure the patient's safety, manage acute distress, and educate. The subsequent steps would be to focus on the integration of traumatic memories and subsequent resolution. This process can be facilitated with timely pharmacotherapy and psychotherapy.[99,100]

Brand et al. have suggested a phasic approach to the treatment of dissociative disorders:[101,102]

- Safety and symptom stabilization
- Traumatic memory recovery and processing
- Reintegration

Pharmacological strategies usually include antidepressants and anxiolytics such as benzodiazepines and prazosin or clonidine for hyperarousal. Paroxetine and naloxone have been studied in randomized controlled trials for depersonalization symptoms and dissociation symptoms in patients with PTSD and borderline personality disorder.[103]

Psychotherapy for dissociation would include the following:
- *Developing a therapeutic alliance:* Studies have shown that the development of a therapeutic alliance is critical in determining the outcomes of patients with dissociative disorders.[104]
- An initial phase focused on gathering a deeper understanding about the client's experiences, coping mechanisms and relationships would help to engage the client and develop tailor-made interventions.[105]
- Uncovering core conflicts in a safe and trusting environment.
- Processing uncovered material and engaging the client in a mind-body formulation.
- Interventions aimed at developing adaptive coping skills and enhancing self-esteem would decrease the frequency of "escape" events in dissociative disorders.[106]
- Grounding skills, improving sensory awareness, and raising distress tolerance can aid in improving the client's initial sense of control over symptoms.[107]
- *Skill building:* Mindfulness,[108] problem solving, emotional regulation, and improving communication.[107]
- Practicing these skills in therapy with simulations.
- Family psychoeducation.
- Environmental modification, if feasible.

Psychodynamic psychotherapy is often utilized for memory recovery and processing of complex emotions. Supportive psychotherapy and cognitive behavioral psychotherapy that focuses on increasing stress tolerance and reducing avoidance behaviors may also be employed to help aid the recovery of such patients. Above all, a nonjudgmental and flexible approach to evaluation and treatment is decisive in the management of these disorders. Secondary gain in such disorders may be discussed with the family members as a means to decrease the intensity and frequency of dissociative motor episodes, among others.

Dissociation in Women

The epidemiologically apparent dominance of dissociative phenomena in women[109,110] may reflect the higher prevalence of adverse childhood events,[111] psychosocial stressors[112] such as domestic violence,[113] and increased help-seeking in women.[114] Moreover, women may be subject to oppression and victimization as a result of, but not limited to, patriarchal norms established in society. Therefore, calling dissociation merely a defense mechanism in women could be reductionistic, it may rather be a representation of how silenced women's bodies speak when their minds cannot.

CHAPTER 5: Unraveling the Knots: Dissociation and Somatization in Women

Women who suffer from dissociation may be younger than men and may have higher rates of derealization and depersonalization.[115] Studies have also shown that women with dissociative convulsions endorse more number of dissociative symptoms.[116] Soon after a traumatic event, women may be more likely to suffer from peritraumatic dissociation and subsequently PTSD.[117,118] In response to stress, women may have more emotion- and avoidance-focused coping styles, and women are, thus, more prone to psychological dissociation compared to men.[119-121] Moreover, sensitized hypothalamic pituitary adrenal axis systems, oxytocin-mediated responses, and the effect of sex hormones may also hold specific relevance to how women cope with stressful situations.[122] Dissociative experiences may be linked to ego dysfunction and studies have found that dissociative experiences in women may be associated with abnormal eating and eating disorders.[123,124]

Studies on dissociation in India have also reported a female preponderance in dissociation symptoms.[83,125,126] Moreover, socioeconomic status and family-related precipitants to dissociation may be important in Indian settings.[126] The predominant presentation in India appears to be motor symptoms especially "pseudo-seizures" (or dissociative convulsions).[126]

While assessing women with dissociation it may be important to:
- Ensure privacy and safety during the interview.
- Accumulate corroborative information from witnesses and close caregivers.
- Appropriately evaluate for differential diagnoses with investigations and liaison as necessary.
- Approach labels sensitively and establish a transparent therapeutic relationship.

The establishment of a psychological link may be met with resistance and confusion since most women have partial to no recollection of dissociative episodes. Even if the experience is reported, openness to treatments aimed at psychiatric causes may be hampered by stigma. A psychiatric label may imply to their families that the symptom expressions are under volitional control. Women suffering from dissociative motor or sensory symptoms may be justifiably anxious that the symptoms are being caused by something more sinister. In certain clinical scenarios involving possession episodes, these women may embody powerful female deities who are given importance, worshipped, and offered gifts. Therefore, a culturally sensitive approach is important when assessing and treating (or when culturally accepted, not treating) such episodes. Since the underlying stress and nuances of the patient's life dynamics may not be apparent in the initial interviews, these women may benefit from longitudinal assessments and treatment.

SOMATIZATION DISORDERS

> Ms. A is a 38-year-old office worker who has consulted her general physician for the third time in 2 months about abdominal pain and bloating, which are both worse after meals and have been present for several months. Similar symptoms occurred a year ago for around four months but then disappeared for some months. Her routine blood tests (including antibodies for celiac disease and lactose intolerance) are normal. She has stopped going out for meals with friends because of her symptoms. She also experiences dizziness (without vertigo), fatigue, and difficulty concentrating. She has been unable to go to work for the last 3 weeks because of her symptoms. She has occasional migraines and more frequent milder tension-type headaches, which occur 2 or 3 days per week at work. Nevertheless, she manages to continue bringing up her young family with her husband, who works as an engineer in a factory currently under threat of closure. Her husband usually has a drink in the evenings but on some evenings, he drinks heavily and gets loud and verbally abusive.

Clinical Presentation

These disorders are characterized by the presence of distressing bodily symptoms that urge the individual to divert attention toward them. This attention may be excessive in its intensity, duration, level of distress, or all of the above.

Earlier, the term somatization precluded the diagnosis of anything "medically explainable". However, today, it has evolved to mean that even *if* there is another health condition that may cause or exacerbate the presenting symptoms, the level of distress that accompanies it is clearly in excess and is causing significant dysfunction. Moreover, such distress is persistent on most days for several months and is not alleviated by extensive clinical and laboratory evaluation. They are generally accompanied by worries about the symptoms themselves, bodily sensations, and overall health resulting in multiple visits to medical specialists.

There may be one primary and several secondary symptoms, only one symptom, or several equally distressing symptoms that along with the distress and preoccupation hamper at least some impact on one or many aspects of the individual's functioning. According to the ICD-11, the entity bodily distress disorder excludes all obsessive-compulsive related disorders, movement disorders including tic disorder and Tourette's syndrome, postviral fatigue and chronic fatigue, sexual pain and sexual dysfunction disorders, and myalgic encephalomyelitis.[21]

Studies in India have also explored "female dhat" syndrome as a somatic expression of distress. A study in rural India reported that 87% of women attending a gynecology outpatient clinic attributed bodily weakness to the loss of vaginal fluid. The same study has also reported that other somatic symptoms such as backache and abdominal pain were linked to vaginal discharge.[127]

Vaginal discharge was also believed to be responsible for decrease in stamina, thin physique, and sleep disturbances by respondents.[128] About 38% of women with Dhat syndrome have a psychiatric comorbidity and 68% report higher levels of perceived stress.[129]

Challenges in Somatization Disorders

There have been numerous challenges in the nosology and clinical delineation of somatization disorders due to the lack of consistent terminology and several overlapping entities. There have been disparities among physicians on the labels we assign somatic symptoms. One medical specialty may extend attention to specific symptom characteristics that relate to the organ system they most deal with, for example, Rome Diagnostic Criteria for Functional Gastrointestinal disorders.[130] However, in such an approach, multiple other systems and the root cause of the condition may be overlooked. On the other hand, psychiatric classificatory systems have historically overlooked the pattern of the symptoms and the characteristics of these symptoms and may have instead paid more attention to the number of symptoms, the presence of psychological criteria, or the amount of healthcare visits.

Clinicians may also face a dilemma in the risks of under-investigating a diagnosis that may be missed versus the risks of over-investigating an individual whose primary concern is psychological.[131] For example, in conditions like multiple sclerosis, nonspecific bodily symptoms like pain and fatigue may very well predate the more obvious neurological signs and symptoms that lead to its diagnosis. The confirmation of the presence or absence of an "organic" condition sometimes requires longitudinal evaluation and patience from both ends of the table. Therefore, the presence or absence of conclusive objective proof should not lead to ignorance of the body or the mind. In the presence of comorbid abnormal illness behaviors, discouraging repeated investigations and unnecessary treatments becomes critical to the management of both abnormal behaviors and somatization.[132]

The development and utilization of objective measures that can capture subjective experiences such as pain and emotional distress have been challenging. There are several scales for the assessment of somatic symptoms such as the Swartz somatization index,[133] the Patient Health Questionnaire-15,[134] the scale for assessment of somatic symptoms,[135] and the Somatic Symptom Scale-8[136] among others. However, in clinical practice, these scales are seldom utilized and their utility in prognostication and treatment may not have been fully explored.[137]

The poor response to treatment and the resistance from the patient to treatments aimed at psychological conditions leads to frustration. There is a difference of opinion between the physician and the patient about the patient's health. Patients are largely unaware of the link between the psychological distress and the bodily symptoms. Therefore, there is obvious resistance to receiving psychiatric care when the physical symptoms are in plain sight and what the patient wants most help with. This can lead to poor rapport, frequent changes in provider and overall morbidity, and decreased quality of life.

Communication with the patient and the family about the diagnosis and their barriers to the acceptance of such a condition is a significant challenge. There is a risk of miscommunication that one carries while communicating to the patient's family about the "nonexistence" of a medically attributable cause to their patient's distress when none is found. It may perpetuate the cycle of neglect and invalidation that the patient has faced earlier which may worsen the clinical condition.[131]

Lastly, the idioms of distress and explanatory models vary in different sociocultural settings.[138-142] Each individual may have their own expression of distress and explanations for their current symptoms borne out of their socioeconomic, educational, cultural, familial, societal, and politico-religious background. In a country as culturally diverse as India, if the medical practitioner is not aware of or sensitive to such variations, there may be risks of overpathologizing or under-recognition of medical and psychiatric conditions.

Prevalence of Somatization and How it Affects Women

The epidemiology of such disorders has been historically challenging to ascertain due to the nosological overlaps and varied clinical presentations as has been highlighted above. It is estimated that somatization disorders have a prevalence of 16.1% in primary care settings in the Netherlands,[143] a lifetime prevalence of 12.9%,[144] and an annual prevalence of 6.3%[145] in hospital settings in Germany. Further, inpatient settings have reported a prevalence as high as 18.4%.[146]

Somatoform disorders have been reported more often in women.[147-150] One study from a neuropsychiatric center in India reported a prevalence of 10.84 per 1,000 population with nearly double the prevalence in women compared to men.[151]

The high rates of somatization in women may reflect the higher prevalence of chronic pain disorders, self-reported psychological distress, anxiety, and depression in this population.[147,152-155] Women have been shown to report more numerous, more frequent, and more chronic symptoms.[156-158] This can also partly be explained by a difference in reporting style[159,160] and more healthcare-seeking in women.

The increased prevalence in women has been attributed in part to the gender-based differences in perception and modulation of painful stimuli, including the central processing of pain, the autonomic arousal in response to pain, pain-related memory, and the pain-regulation systems.[159,161-165] Nociception may also be determined by the hormonal cycle in women such that women may experience more sensitivity to pain in the luteal phase of their menstrual cycle.[166,167] The relationship between sex hormones and pain-related neurotransmitter activity has also been studied.[168]

Chronic pain, particularly pain in the pelvis region, has been linked to physical abuse, including sexual abuse in childhood.[169-175] The literature estimates that childhood sexual abuse is 12–17% in girls, almost double that reported for boys,[176] although the reasons for this variation may be many. Since sexual abuse is reported more in girls in the available literature, it could explain, in part, the increase in the prevalence of somatization in women. Women may be subject to more interpersonal violence, intimate partner violence, and domestic violence around the world[177-180] including India.[113] Oppression, victimization, and violence may also explain the increased prevalence of somatization in women.[181]

Another interesting theory on gender-based pain and somatization differences is about social roles and the socialization process. Growing up, in most societies, boys are taught to be less expressive about pain and illness, thus paving the way for men to seldom admit weakness and distress in adulthood.[162] Conversely, it may be more acceptable to express distress as a female. Women have also been shown to be ready to consult health services for medical problems, seek help for interpersonal problems, and on average have more physician visits annually.[182-184]

Lastly, there appears to be a gender bias in research and clinical practice when it comes to somatization which may account partly for this prevalence in women.[185-187] Studies have found that there may be physician-specific gender bias in the diagnosis of somatization.[188] Such biases have potential implications for the physician-patient relationship and the patient's outcomes.

However, despite these biases, there is overwhelming evidence as demonstrated above that the phenomenon does seem to be more common in women overall. This conclusion should neither in any way mean that only women suffer nor that women over-report their distress. It simply cautions the reader and sensitizes the physician to the factors that exist when caring for a woman with somatization.

Assessment of Somatization Disorders

A comprehensive assessment should include:
- The description and pattern of somatic symptoms, their frequency, duration, intensity, number, and the systems involved. Similar to the clinical evaluation of any medical symptom, a thorough history of the

- onset, duration, severity, aggravating, and relieving factors followed by a systematic clinical examination is necessary.
- The subjective descriptions of such symptoms in the local dialect and relevant to the sociocultural setting are also integral to such descriptions. The beliefs and explanations that surround such symptoms should also be elicited. The assessment should include the subjective distress and bio-socio-occupational dysfunction as a result of such distress.
- A psychiatric screening for comorbid or past mental illnesses and a review of past medical and treatment history.
- Psychosocial factors related to somatic symptoms, genetic vulnerabilities, early life events, recent or chronic stress, coping styles, lifestyle, personality factors, support systems, and cultural factors. It would be relevant to address sexual abuse in any patient suffering from somatization.[189]
- The assessment may also include strategic relevant investigations and liaison with other specialists. Limiting the number of tests and specialist referrals may also be part of the treatment and thus this step can seem counterintuitive in some situations.

A comprehensive assessment of all somatic symptoms for both men and women would aid in reducing the overpsychologizing rare medical syndromes and overmedicalizing psychological distress. Both can coexist and can occur in both genders.

Treatment of Somatization Disorders

Nonpharmacological interventions appear to be the first-line treatment for somatization disorders.[190] A thorough history and clinical examination serve as important starting points in making the patient feel heard and validated. Establishing a therapeutic alliance and providing a validating environment is the crux upon which any treatment can be planned. An honest and transparent discussion about the symptoms can be attempted once the assessment is completed. However, such conversations can be challenging for the practitioner and frustrating for the patient.

A doctor's common response to a somatizing patient may imply that their illness is "not real" or "all in their head" which would provoke the patient and cause doctor-patient conflict. Moreover, it may be a physician's belief that a patient should, in a sense, listen to reason and reassurance but patients with somatization do not often fit this paradigm.

The following are examples of approaches that can be employed to aid in engagement in treatment:
- *Self-disclosure and re-focus:* "The tests and evaluation do not really give us an answer as to why you are suffering from back pain—and I do not have all the answers either. But, your pain is certainly there and because of it, you are quite upset. Do you think we can talk about that for a bit?"

Acknowledging uncertainty about the cause of symptoms and steering the conversation to their distress may help to initiate treatment.

- *Psychological link:* "*I can understand your pain is quite severe. I would like to help with that. May I offer a theory that may not be restricted to a condition in your back? The mind is connected to the body and helps it do several things throughout the day. We have some evidence to believe that if the mind is stressed, that can affect the body as well.*"

  The dualism of the mind and body is engrained in the minds of most patients (and physicians). Helping the patient understand the link and gently moving the discussion toward the possible psychological etiology is an important stepping stone in treatment.

- *Partnering while not denying the reality of the physical symptom:* "*I can see that your pain has been troubling you for several years now. I believe the pain is very much there, even if nothing is showing up on the tests. Because of it, you are constantly worried about sitting in a position for too long, you have left your desk job and you cannot sleep very well anymore. The secondary problems that have arisen due to the pain are very real too, can we work on those for now till we find a solution to the pain?*"

  The somatic symptom is indeed very real and very distressing to the patient. Addressing sleep, depressive symptoms, worries, and other psychological problems around the somatic symptom may help to relieve some distress and also demonstrate the link in real-time. During interviews and therapy sessions, the conversation from the patient's end may be largely focused on the physical symptom(s). Shifting the focus to the functionality, output, routines, and biological activities may help to provide a passageway into other aspects of their lives. This approach can also help to reset the treatment goals to improve their overall functioning and quality of life rather than finding a singular solution to the somatic symptom.

The nonpharmacological treatments for somatization disorder include psychoeducation, cognitive behavioral therapy,[191-193] reattribution therapy,[194] problem-solving therapy, biofeedback, supportive psychotherapy, mindfulness-based approaches,[195,196] acceptance and commitment therapy, relaxation therapy and guided imagery.[197] Other therapeutic approaches used are family therapy and short-term psychodynamic psychotherapy.[198,199] During therapy, early identification of dependence, management of crises, decisions on settings of therapy (inpatient versus outpatient), and termination can be especially challenging. Following a predetermined schedule for sessions and follow-ups may be vital to treatment. An important but overlooked aspect of nonpharmacological treatment is communication with the caregivers about the nature of the illness the concept of secondary gains and how to reduce or eliminate them.[200]

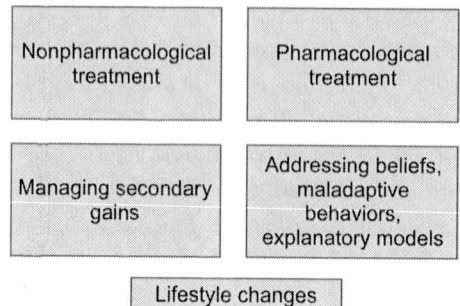

Fig. 1: Treatment of somatization disorders.

Usual pharmacological strategies are aimed at the treatment of comorbid depression, anxiety, or sleep disturbances. This population is especially vulnerable to the misuse and abuse of pain medication[201] and thus, the clinician should be wary of the benefits and risks of pain management. Neuromodulation especially transmagnetic stimulation (TMS) is an option for select candidates in the management of chronic pain.[202] **Figure 1** describes a practical model for management.

> **KEY POINTS**
> - *Women suffering from dissociation and somatization disorders need to be heard.* Their physical symptoms are likely manifestations of intrapsychic pain and conflict.
> - *Nonpharmacological treatments are the first line.* Providing a nonjudgmental and safe space to discuss their physical and psychological complaints is vital in building a therapeutic relationship.
> - *Flexibility is key in all aspects of care.* The physician may have to keep an open mind about differentials, revisit diagnoses, partner with other specialists, collaborate with the patient and their caregivers, and be open to alternative strategies in therapy or pharmacological treatments.
> - *Treatment is long-term.* Patients with dissociation and somatization may require long-term interventions and follow-ups. The relapsing-remitting and unpredictable course may be challenging to the practitioner and distressing to the patient.

REFERENCES

1. Tasca C, Rapetti M, Carta MG, Fadda B. Women And Hysteria In The History Of Mental Health. Clin Pract Epidemiol Ment Health CP EMH. 2012;8:110-9.
2. Wolfsohn jm. The treatment of hysteria: successful results of a rapid re-education method. JAMA. 1918;71(25):2057-62. [online] Available from https://jamanetwork.com/journals/jama/article-abstract/219872 [Last accessed December, 2023].
3. Komagamine T, Kokubun N, Hirata K. Battey's operation as a treatment for hysteria: a review of a series of cases in the nineteenth century. Hist Psychiatry. 2020;31(1):55-66.
4. Waraich M, Shah S. The life and work of Jean-Martin Charcot (1825–1893): 'The Napoleon of Neuroses.' J Intensive Care Soc. 2018;19(1):48-9.

5. Michael MT. On the scientific prospects for Freud's theory of hysteria. Neuropsychoanalysis. 2018;20(2):87-98.
6. Pearce JMS. Sydenham on Hysteria. Eur Neurol. 2016;76(3-4):175-81.
7. Eadie MJ. A pathology of the animal spirits—the clinical neurology of Thomas Willis (1621–1675) Part I—Background, and disorders of intrinsically normal animal spirits. J Clin Neurosci. 2003;10(1):14-29.
8. Hoedeman R, Blankenstein AH, Krol B, Koopmans PC, Groothoff JW. The contribution of high levels of somatic symptom severity to sickness absence duration, disability and discharge. J Occup Rehabil. 2010;20(2):264-73.
9. Barsky AJ, Orav EJ, Bates DW. Somatization Increases Medical Utilization and Costs Independent of Psychiatric and Medical Comorbidity. Arch Gen Psychiatry. 2005;62(8):903-10.
10. Löwe B, Spitzer RL, Williams JBW, Mussell M, Schellberg D, Kroenke K. Depression, anxiety and somatization in primary care: syndrome overlap and functional impairment. Gen Hosp Psychiatry. 2008;30(3):191-9.
11. Kirmayer LJ, Robbins JM, Dworkind M, Yaffe MJ. Somatization and the recognition of depression and anxiety in primary care. Am J Psychiatry. 1993;150(5):734-41.
12. Černis E, Evans R, Ehlers A, Freeman D. Dissociation in relation to other mental health conditions: an exploration using network analysis. J Psychiatr Res. 2021;136:460-7.
13. Badura AS, Reiter RC, Altmaier EM, Rhomberg A, Elas D. Dissociation, Somatization, Substance Abuse, and Coping in Women With Chronic Pelvic Pain. Obstet Gynecol. 1997;90(3):405-10.
14. US Army. (2023). DSM-1 Full PDF [Internet]. 1952 [cited 2023 Aug 20]. [online] Available from http://archive.org/details/dsm-1 [Last accessed December, 2023].
15. World Health Organization. (2023). Manual of the international statistical classification of diseases, injuries, and causes of death: sixth revision of the International lists of diseases and causes of death, adopted 1948 [Internet]. World Health Organization; 1948 [cited 2023 Aug 20]. [online] Available from https://apps.who.int/iris/handle/10665/42893 [Last accessed December, 2023].
16. World Health Organization. (2023). Manual of the international statistical classification of diseases, injuries, and causes of death: based on the recommendations of the seventh revision Conference, 1955, and adopted by the ninth World Health Assembly under the WHO Nomenclature Regulations [Internet]. World Health Organization; 1957 [cited 2023 Aug 20]. [online] Available from https://apps.who.int/iris/handle/10665/42900 [Last accessed December, 2023].
17. Volkmar FR. DSM-III. In: Volkmar FR (Ed). Encyclopedia of Autism Spectrum Disorders [Internet]. New York, NY: Springer; 2013. pp. 999-1001.
18. ICD. (2022). ICD-10 Version:2010 [Internet]. [cited 2022 Jun 12]. [online] Available from https://icd.who.int/browse10/2010/en#/ [Last accessed December, 2023].
19. Wiley Online Library. (2023). Diagnostic and Statistical Manual of Mental Disorders (DSM-IV-TR) - Segal - Major Reference Works - Wiley Online Library [Internet]. [cited 2023 Aug 20]. [online] Available from https://onlinelibrary.wiley.com/doi/abs/10.1002/9780470479216.corpsy0271 [Last accessed December, 2023].
20. Diagnostic and statistical manual of mental disorders: DSM-5™, 5th edition. Arlington, VA, US: American Psychiatric Publishing, Inc.; 2013. p. xliv, 947.

21. ICD. (2022). ICD-11 [Internet]. [cited 2022 Jun 12]. [online] Available from https://icd.who.int/en [Last accessed December, 2023].
22. Reed GM, First MB, Kogan CS, Hyman SE, Gureje O, Gaebel W, et al. Innovations and changes in the ICD-11 classification of mental, behavioural and neurodevelopmental disorders. World Psychiatry. 2019;18(1):3-19.
23. Basavarajappa C, Dahale AB, Desai G. Evolution of bodily distress disorders. Curr Opin Psychiatry. 2020;33(5):447-50.
24. Hart O, Horst R. The dissociation theory of Pierre Janet. J Trauma Stress. 1989;2:397-412.
25. Freud S, Breuer J. Studies in hysteria. London, United Kingdom: Penguin; 2004.
26. Forrester J. The true story of Anna O. Soc Res. 1986;53:327-47.
27. Lipowski ZJ. Review of Consultation Psychiatry and Psychosomatic Medicine: II. Clinical Aspects. Psychosom Med. 1967;29(3):201.
28. Dalenberg CJ, Brand BL, Gleaves DH, Dorahy MJ, Loewenstein RJ, Cardeña E, et al. Evaluation of the evidence for the trauma and fantasy models of dissociation. Psychol Bull. 2012;138(3):550-88.
29. Schimmenti A, Caretti V. Linking the overwhelming with the unbearable: Developmental trauma, dissociation, and the disconnected self. Psychoanal Psychol. 2016;33(1):106-28.
30. Farina B, Liotti G. Does a traumatic-dissociative dimension exists? A review of dissociative processes and symptoms in developmental trauma spectrum disorders. Clin Neuropsychiatry. 2013;10:11-8.
31. van der Kolk BA, Pelcovitz D, Roth S, Mandel FS, McFarlane A, Herman JL. Dissociation, somatization, and affect dysregulation: the complexity of adaptation of trauma. Am J Psychiatry. 1996;153(7 Suppl):83-93.
32. Granot M, Yovell Y, Somer E, Beny A, Sadger R, Uliel-Mirkin R, et al. Trauma, attachment style, and somatization: a study of women with dyspareunia and women survivors of sexual abuse. BMC Womens Health. 2018;18(1):29.
33. Moran JK, Jesuthasan J, Schalinski I, Kurmeyer C, Oertelt-Prigione S, Abels I, et al. Traumatic Life Events and Association With Depression, Anxiety, and Somatization Symptoms in Female Refugees. JAMA Netw Open. 2023;6(7):e2324511.
34. Simeon D, Guralnik O, Schmeidler J, Sirof B, Knutelska M. The role of childhood interpersonal trauma in depersonalization disorder. Am J Psychiatry. 2001;158(7):1027-33.
35. Hollifield M, Tuttle L, Paine S, Kellner R. Hypochondriasis and somatization related to personality and attitudes toward self. Psychosomatics. 1999;40(5):387-95.
36. Russo J, Katon W, Sullivan M, Clark M, Buchwald D. Severity of somatization and its relationship to psychiatric disorders and personality. Psychosomatics. 1994;35(6):546-56.
37. Ellason JW, Ross CA, Fuchs DL. Lifetime axis I and II comorbidity and childhood trauma history in dissociative identity disorder. Psychiatry. 1996;59(3):255-66.
38. Koh KB, Choi EH, Lee YJ, Han M. Serotonin-related gene pathways associated with undifferentiated somatoform disorder. Psychiatry Res. 2011;189(2):246-50.
39. Guze SB. Genetics of Briquet's syndrome and somatization disorder. A review of family, adoption, and twin studies. Ann Clin Psychiatry Off J Am Acad Clin Psychiatr. 1993;5(4):225-30.

40. Klengel T, Heck A, Pfister H, Brückl T, Hennings JM, Menke A, et al. Somatization in major depression – clinical features and genetic associations. Acta Psychiatr Scand. 2011;124(4):317-28.
41. Şar V, Dorahy MJ, Krüger C. Revisiting the etiological aspects of dissociative identity disorder: a biopsychosocial perspective. Psychol Res Behav Manag. 2017;10:137-46.
42. Jang KL, Paris J, Zweig-Frank H, Livesley WJ. Twin study of dissociative experience. J Nerv Ment Dis. 1998;186(6):345-51.
43. Barbati A, Geraci A, Niro F, Pezzi L, Sarchiapone M. Do Migration and Acculturation Impact Somatization? A Scoping Review. Int J Environ Res Public Health. 2022;19(23):16011.
44. Bhavsar V, Ventriglio A, Bhugra D. Dissociative trance and spirit possession: Challenges for cultures in transition. Psychiatry Clin Neurosci. 2016;70(12):551-9.
45. Krüger C. Culture, trauma and dissociation: A broadening perspective for our field. J Trauma Dissociation Off J Int Soc Study Dissociation ISSD. 2020;21(1):1-13.
46. Barsky AJ. Amplification, somatization, and the somatoform disorders. Psychosomatics. 1992;33(1):28-34.
47. Bourke JH, Langford RM, White PD. The common link between functional somatic syndromes may be central sensitisation. J Psychosom Res. 2015;78(3):228-36.
48. Nijs J, Meeus M, Van Oosterwijck J, Ickmans K, Moorkens G, Hans G, et al. In the mind or in the brain? Scientific evidence for central sensitisation in chronic fatigue syndrome. Eur J Clin Invest. 2012;42(2):203-12.
49. Phillips K, Clauw DJ. Central pain mechanisms in chronic pain states—maybe it is all in their head. Best Pract Res Clin Rheumatol. 2011;25(2):141-54.
50. Yildirim H, Atmaca M, Sirlier B, Kayali A. Pituitary Volumes Are Reduced in Patients with Somatization Disorder. Psychiatry Investig. 2012;9(3):278-82.
51. Atmaca M, Sirlier B, Yildirim H, Kayali A. Hippocampus and amygdalar volumes in patients with somatization disorder. Prog Neuropsychopharmacol Biol Psychiatry. 2011;35(7):1699-703.
52. Peyron R, Frot M, Schneider F, Garcia-Larrea L, Mertens P, Barral FG, et al. Role of operculoinsular cortices in human pain processing: converging evidence from PET, fMRI, dipole modeling, and intracerebral recordings of evoked potentials. NeuroImage. 2002;17(3):1336-46.
53. Critchley HD, Mathias CJ, Dolan RJ. Fear conditioning in humans: the influence of awareness and autonomic arousal on functional neuroanatomy. Neuron. 2002;33(4):653-63.
54. Gray MA, Harrison NA, Wiens S, Critchley HD. Modulation of Emotional Appraisal by False Physiological Feedback during fMRI. PLoS One. 2007;2(6):e546.
55. Perez DL, Barsky AJ, Vago DR, Baslet G, Silbersweig DA. A neural circuit framework for somatosensory amplification in somatoform disorders. J Neuropsychiatry Clin Neurosci. 2015;27(1):e40-50.
56. Boeckle M, Schrimpf M, Liegl G, Pieh C. Neural correlates of somatoform disorders from a meta-analytic perspective on neuroimaging studies. NeuroImage Clin. 2016;11:606-13.
57. Egloff N, Sabbioni MEE, Salathé C, Wiest R, Juengling FD. Nondermatomal somatosensory deficits in patients with chronic pain disorder: clinical findings and hypometabolic pattern in FDG-PET. Pain. 2009;145(1-2):252-8.

58. Valet M, Gündel H, Sprenger T, Sorg C, Mühlau M, Zimmer C, et al. Patients with pain disorder show gray-matter loss in pain-processing structures: a voxel-based morphometric study. Psychosom Med. 2009;71(1):49-56.
59. Kawamoto T, Onoda K, Nakashima K, Nittono H, Yamaguchi S, Ura M. Is dorsal anterior cingulate cortex activation in response to social exclusion due to expectancy violation? An fMRI study. Front Evol Neurosci. 2012;4:11.
60. Killgore WDS, Yurgelun-Todd DA. Unconscious processing of facial affect in children and adolescents. Soc Neurosci. 2007;2(1):28-47.
61. Nebel K, Wiese H, Stude P, de Greiff A, Diener HC, Keidel M. On the neural basis of focused and divided attention. Brain Res Cogn Brain Res. 2005;25(3):760-76.
62. Büchel C, Bornhövd K, Quante M, Glauche V, Bromm B, Weiller C. Dissociable Neural Responses Related to Pain Intensity, Stimulus Intensity, and Stimulus Awareness within the Anterior Cingulate Cortex: A Parametric Single-Trial Laser Functional Magnetic Resonance Imaging Study. J Neurosci. 2002;22(3):970-6.
63. Itti L, Koch C. Computational modelling of visual attention. Nat Rev Neurosci. 2001;2(3):194-203.
64. Seminowicz DA, Davis KD. Cortical responses to pain in healthy individuals depends on pain catastrophizing. Pain. 2006;120(3):297-306.
65. Rief W, Shaw R, Fichter MM. Elevated levels of psychophysiological arousal and cortisol in patients with somatization syndrome. Psychosom Med. 1998;60(2):198-203.
66. Maes M. Inflammatory and oxidative and nitrosative stress pathways underpinning chronic fatigue, somatization and psychosomatic symptoms. Curr Opin Psychiatry. 2009;22(1):75-83.
67. Staniloiu A, Markowitsch HJ. Dissociative amnesia. Lancet Psychiatry. 2014;1(3):226-41.
68. Sierra M, Berrios GE. Depersonalization: neurobiological perspectives. Biol Psychiatry. 1998;44(9):898-908.
69. Phillips ML, Medford N, Senior C, Bullmore ET, Suckling J, Brammer MJ, et al. Depersonalization disorder: thinking without feeling. Psychiatry Res. 2001;108(3):145-60.
70. Sierra M, Senior C, Dalton J, McDonough M, Bond A, Phillips ML, et al. Autonomic response in depersonalization disorder. Arch Gen Psychiatry. 2002;59(9):833-8.
71. Davis M, Whalen PJ. The amygdala: vigilance and emotion. Mol Psychiatry. 2001;6(1):13-34.
72. Lanius RA, Vermetten E, Loewenstein RJ, Brand B, Schmahl C, Bremner JD, et al. Emotion Modulation in PTSD: Clinical and Neurobiological Evidence for a Dissociative Subtype. Am J Psychiatry. 2010;167(6):640-7.
73. Irpati AS, Avasthi A, Sharan P. Study of stress and vulnerability in patients with somatoform and dissociative disorders in a psychiatric clinic in North India. Psychiatry Clin Neurosci. 2006;60(5):570-4.
74. Espirito-Santo H, Pio-Abreu JL. Psychiatric symptoms and dissociation in conversion, somatization and dissociative disorders. Aust N Z J Psychiatry. 2009;43(3):270-6.
75. Atlas JA, Wolfson MA, Lipschitz DS. Dissociation and somatization in adolescent inpatients with and without history of abuse. Psychol Rep. 1995;76(3 Pt 2):1101-2.
76. American Psychiatric Association, American Psychiatric Association. Diagnostic and statistical manual of mental disorders: DSM-5. 5th ed. Washington, DC: American Psychiatric Association; 2013. p. 947.

77. Yanartas O, Ozmen H, Çıtak S, Zincir S, Sunbul E, Kara H. Childhood Traumatic Experiences and Trauma Related Psychiatric Comorbidities in Dissociative Disorders. Bull Clin Psychopharmacol. 2015;25:381-9.
78. Polizzi CP, Aksen DE, Lynn SJ. Quality of life, emotion regulation, and dissociation: Evaluating unique relations in an undergraduate sample and probable PTSD subsample. Psychol Trauma Theory Res Pract Policy. 2022;14(1):107-15.
79. Langeland W, Jepsen EKK, Brand BL, Kleven L, Loewenstein RJ, Putnam FW, et al. The economic burden of dissociative disorders: a qualitative systematic review of empirical studies. Psychol Trauma Theory Res Pract Policy. 2020;12(7):730-8.
80. Aderibigbe YA, Bloch RM, Walker WR. Prevalence of depersonalization and derealization experiences in a rural population. Soc Psychiatry Psychiatr Epidemiol. 2001;36(2):63-9.
81. Ross CA. Epidemiology of multiple personality disorder and dissociation. Psychiatr Clin North Am. 1991;14(3):503-17.
82. Yang J, Millman LSM, David AS, Hunter ECM. The Prevalence of Depersonalization-Derealization Disorder: A Systematic Review. J Trauma Dissociation Off J Int Soc Study Dissociation ISSD. 2023;24(1):8-41.
83. Chaturvedi SK, Desai G, Shaligram D. Dissociative Disorders in a Psychiatric Institute in India: A Selected Review and Patterns Over a Decade. Int J Soc Psychiatry. 2010;56(5):533-9.
84. Chiu CD, Meg Tseng MC, Chien YL, Liao SC, Liu CM, Yeh YY, et al. Dissociative disorders in acute psychiatric inpatients in Taiwan. Psychiatry Res. 2017;250:285-90.
85. Lynn SJ, Maxwell R, Merckelbach H, Lilienfeld SO, Kloet D van H van der, Miskovic V. Dissociation and its disorders: Competing models, future directions, and a way forward. Clin Psychol Rev. 2019;73:101755.
86. Coons PM, Bowman ES, Milstein V. Multiple personality disorder. A clinical investigation of 50 cases. J Nerv Ment Dis. 1988;176(9):519-27.
87. Horevitz RP, Braun BG. Are multiple personalities borderline? An analysis of 33 cases. Psychiatr Clin North Am. 1984;7(1):69-87.
88. Sar V. The scope of dissociative disorders: an international perspective. Psychiatr Clin North Am. 2006;29(1):227-44, xi.
89. Loewenstein RJ. Dissociative Amnesia and Dissociative Fugue. In: Michelson LK, Ray WJ (Eds). Handbook of Dissociation: Theoretical, Empirical, and Clinical Perspectives [Internet]. Boston, MA: Springer US; 1996. pp. 307-36.
90. Kluft RP. Diagnosing Dissociative Identity Disorder: Understanding and assessing manifestations can help clinicians identify and treat patients more effectively. Psychiatr Ann. 2005;35(8):633-43.
91. Kluft RP. Dissociative Identity Disorder. In: Michelson LK, Ray WJ (Eds). Handbook of Dissociation: Theoretical, Empirical, and Clinical Perspectives [Internet]. Boston, MA: Springer US; 1996. pp. 337-66.
92. Roberts LW, Hoop JG, Heinrich TW. Clinical Psychiatry Essentials. Philadelphia, Pennsylvania: Lippincott Williams & Wilkins; 2010.
93. Loewenstein RJ. An office mental status examination for complex chronic dissociative symptoms and multiple personality disorder. Psychiatr Clin North Am. 1991;14(3):567-604.
94. Bernstein EM, Putnam FW. Development, reliability, and validity of a dissociation scale. J Nerv Ment Dis. 1986;174(12):727-35.

95. Steinberg M. Depersonalization: Systematic Assessment. In: Fink G (Ed). Encyclopedia of Stress (Second Edition) [Internet]. New York: Academic Press; 2007. pp. 736-40.
96. Simeon D. Depersonalization disorder. In: Dell PF, O'Neil JA (Eds). Dissociation and the dissociative disorders: DSM-V and beyond. New York, NY, US: Routledge/Taylor & Francis Group; 2009. pp. 435-44.
97. Ford JD, Gómez JM. The relationship of psychological trauma and dissociative and posttraumatic stress disorders to nonsuicidal self-injury and suicidality: a review. J Trauma Dissociation Off J Int Soc Study Dissociation ISSD. 2015;16(3):232-71.
98. During EH, Elahi FM, Taieb O, Moro MR, Baubet T. A Critical Review of Dissociative Trance and Possession Disorders: Etiological, Diagnostic, Therapeutic, and Nosological Issues. Can J Psychiatry. 2011;56(4):235-42.
99. Putnam FW. Diagnosis and Treatment of Multiple Personality Disorder. New York: Guilford Press; 1989. p. 376.
100. Loewenstein R. Psychopharmacologic Treatments for Dissociative Identity Disorder. Psychiatr Ann. 2005;35:666.
101. Brand BL, Loewenstein RJ, Spiegel D. Dispelling Myths About Dissociative Identity Disorder Treatment: An Empirically Based Approach. Psychiatry Interpers Biol Process. 2014;77(2):169-89.
102. Loewenstein RJ. DID 101: A Hands-on Clinical Guide to the Stabilization Phase of Dissociative Identity Disorder Treatment. Psychiatr Clin North Am. 2006;29(1):305-32.
103. Sutar R, Sahu S. Pharmacotherapy for dissociative disorders: a systematic review. Psychiatry Res. 2019;281:112529.
104. Cronin E, Brand BL, Mattanah JF. The impact of the therapeutic alliance on treatment outcome in patients with dissociative disorders. Eur J Psychotraumatology. 2014;5.
105. Sahota PBK, D'Mello RJ, Shanbhag V, Nanjundaswamy MH, Ganjekar S, Kashyap H, et al. Finding One's Voice: Psychotherapy for Dissociative Motor Disorders in the Indian Context. J Contemp Psychother. 2022;52(3):249-55.
106. Nicholson TR, Aybek S, Craig T, Harris T, Wojcik W, David AS, et al. Life events and escape in conversion disorder. Psychol Med. 2016;46(12):2617-26.
107. Subramanyam AA, Somaiya M, Shankar S, Nasirabadi M, Shah HR, Paul I, et al. Psychological Interventions for Dissociative disorders. Indian J Psychiatry. 2020;62(Suppl 2):S280-9.
108. Zerubavel N, Messman-Moore TL. Staying Present: Incorporating Mindfulness into Therapy for Dissociation. Mindfulness. 2015;6(2):303-14.
109. Coons PM. The dissociative disorders. Rarely considered and underdiagnosed. Psychiatr Clin North Am. 1998;21(3):637-48.
110. Ross CA. History, Phenomenology, and Epidemiology of Dissociation. In: Michelson LK, Ray WJ (Eds). Handbook of Dissociation [Internet]. Boston, MA: Springer US; 1996. pp. 3-24.
111. Trickett PK, Putnam FW. Impact of Child Sexual Abuse on Females: Toward a Developmental, Psychobiological Integration. Psychol Sci. 1993;4(2):81-7.
112. Najavits LM, Sonn J, Walsh M, Weiss RD. Domestic violence in women with PTSD and substance abuse. Addict Behav. 2004;29(4):707-15.

113. Kalokhe A, Del Rio C, Dunkle K, Stephenson R, Metheny N, Paranjape A, et al. Domestic violence against women in India: a systematic review of a decade of quantitative studies. Glob Public Health. 2017;12(4):498-513.
114. Tedstone Doherty D, Kartalova-O'Doherty Y. Gender and self-reported mental health problems: predictors of help-seeking from a general practitioner. Br J Health Psychol. 2010;15(Pt 1):213-28.
115. Spitzer C, Klauer T, Grabe HJ, Lucht M, Stieglitz RD, Schneider W, et al. Gender Differences in Dissociation: A Dimensional Approach. Psychopathology. 2003;36(2):65-70.
116. Myers L, Trobliger R, Bortnik K, Lancman M. Are there gender differences in those diagnosed with psychogenic nonepileptic seizures? Epilepsy Behav. 2018;78:161-5.
117. Grieger TA, Fullerton CS, Ursano RJ. Posttraumatic stress disorder, alcohol use, and perceived safety after the terrorist attack on the pentagon. Psychiatr Serv Wash DC. 2003;54(10):1380-2.
118. Bryant RA. Early predictors of posttraumatic stress disorder. Biol Psychiatry. 2003;53(9):789-95.
119. Lipschitz DS, Grilo CM, Fehon D, McGlashan TM, Southwick SM. Gender differences in the associations between posttraumatic stress symptoms and problematic substance use in psychiatric inpatient adolescents. J Nerv Ment Dis. 2000;188(6):349-56.
120. Langeland W, Brink W, Draijer N. (2005). Gender and the relationship between childhood trauma dissociation and alcohol dependence. [cited 2023 Aug 27]. [online] Available from https://www.semanticscholar.org/paper/Gender-and-the-relationship-between-childhood-and-Langeland-Brink/fd6a44ab45a1ca55394a68bc45b0e8022dc0dd88 [Last accessed December, 2023].
121. Ouimette P, Brown PJ. Trauma and substance abuse: Causes, consequences, and treatment of comorbid disorders. Washington, DC, US: American Psychological Association; 2003. p. xiii, 315..
122. Olff M, Langeland W, Draijer N, Gersons BPR. Gender differences in posttraumatic stress disorder. Psychol Bull. 2007;133(2):183-204.
123. Valdiserri S, Kihlstrom JF. Abnormal eating and dissociative experiences. Int J Eat Disord. 1995;17(4):373-80.
124. Meyer C, Waller G. Dissociation and eating psychopathology: gender differences in a nonclinical population. Int J Eat Disord. 1998;23(2):217-21.
125. Reddi VSK, Salian HH, Muliyala KP, Chandra PS. Profile and outcome of dissociative disorders presenting as psychiatric emergencies to a tertiary hospital setting in India. Asian J Psychiatry. 2019;44:187-8.
126. Deka K, Chaudhury PK, Bora K, Kalita P. A study of clinical correlates and socio-demographic profile in conversion disorder. Indian J Psychiatry. 2007;49(3):205.
127. Mehra A, Kathirvel S, Gainder S, Avasthi A, Grover S. Female Dhat syndrome in primary care setting. Ind Psychiatry J. 2021;30(2):278-84.
128. Grover S, Avasthi A, Gupta S, Hazari N, Malhotra N. Do female patients with nonpathological vaginal discharge need the same evaluation as for Dhat syndrome in males? Indian J Psychiatry. 2016;58(1):61-9.
129. Joshi S, Tripathi A, Agarwal S, Singh N, Gupta B, Nischal A, et al. Phenomenology, disability and sexual functioning in female Dhat syndrome: a study of tertiary care gynaecology outpatients. Gen Psychiatry. 2022;35(5):e100863.

130. Lacy BE, Patel NK. Rome Criteria and a Diagnostic Approach to Irritable Bowel Syndrome. J Clin Med. 2017;6(11):99.
131. Desai G, Chaturvedi SK. Ethical dilemmas of medically unexplained symptoms [Internet]. Indian J Med Ethics. 2016;1(2):129
132. Chaturvedi SK, Desai G, Shaligram D. Somatoform disorders, somatization and abnormal illness behaviour. Int Rev Psychiatry Abingdon Engl. 2006;18(1):75-80.
133. Swartz M, Hughes D, George L, Blazer D, Landerman R, Bucholz K. Developing a screening index for community studies of somatization disorder. J Psychiatr Res. 1986;20(4):335-43.
134. Kroenke K, Spitzer RL, Williams JBW. The PHQ-15: validity of a new measure for evaluating the severity of somatic symptoms. Psychosom Med. 2002;64(2):258-66.
135. Desai G, Chaturvedi SK, Dahale A, Marimuthu P. On Somatic Symptoms Measurement: The Scale for Assessment of Somatic Symptoms Revisited. Indian J Psychol Med. 2015;37(1):17-9.
136. Gierk B, Kohlmann S, Kroenke K, Spangenberg L, Zenger M, Brähler E, et al. The somatic symptom scale-8 (SSS-8): a brief measure of somatic symptom burden. JAMA Intern Med. 2014;174(3):399-407.
137. Chaturvedi SK, Desai G. Measurement and assessment of somatic symptoms. Int Rev Psychiatry. 2013;25(1):31-40.
138. Keyes CLM, Ryff CD. Somatization and mental health: A comparative study of the idiom of distress hypothesis. Soc Sci Med. 2003;57(10):1833-45.
139. Parsons CDF, Wakeley P. Idioms of distress: Somatic responses to distress in everyday life. Cult Med Psychiatry. 1991;15(1):111-32.
140. Saint Arnault D, Kim O. Is There an Asian Idiom of Distress?: Somatic Symptoms in Female Japanese and Korean Students. Arch Psychiatr Nurs. 2008;22(1):27-38.
141. So JK. Somatization as cultural idiom of distress: rethinking mind and body in a multicultural society. Couns Psychol Q. 2008;21(2):167-74.
142. Nichter M. Idioms of Distress Revisited. Cult Med Psychiatry. 2010;34(2):401-16.
143. de Waal MWM, Arnold IA, Eekhof JAH, van Hemert AM. Somatoform disorders in general practice: prevalence, functional impairment and comorbidity with anxiety and depressive disorders. Br J Psychiatry J Ment Sci. 2004;184:470-6.
144. Meyer C, Rumpf HJ, Hapke U, Dilling H, John U. Lifetime prevalence of mental disorders in general adult population. Results of TACOS study. Nervenarzt. 2000;71(7):535-42.
145. Wittchen HU, Nelson CB, Lachner G. Prevalence of mental disorders and psychosocial impairments in adolescents and young adults. Psychol Med. 1998;28(1):109-26.
146. Pieh C, Lahmann C, Heymann FV, Tritt K, Loew T, Busch V, et al. Prevalence and comorbidity of somatoform disorder in psychosomatic inpatients: a multicentre study. Z Psychosom Med Psychother. 2011;57(3):244-50.
147. Mirza I, Jenkins R. Risk factors, prevalence, and treatment of anxiety and depressive disorders in Pakistan: systematic review. BMJ. 2004;328(7443):794.
148. Koch H, van Bokhoven MA, ter Riet G, van der Weijden T, Dinant GJ, Bindels PJE. Demographic characteristics and quality of life of patients with unexplained complaints: a descriptive study in general practice. Qual Life Res Int J Qual Life Asp Treat Care Rehabil. 2007;16(9):1483-9.
149. Barsky AJ, Peekna HM, Borus JF. Somatic Symptom Reporting in Women and Men. J Gen Intern Med. 2001;16(4):266-75.

150. Seeman MV. Gender and Psychopathology. United States: American Psychiatric Publishing, Inc.; 1995. p. 424.
151. Desai G, Chaturvedi SK. Gender and somatoform disorders: Do subtypes of somatoform disorders differ? Asian J Psychiatry. 2013;6(6):609-10.
152. Golding JM, Smith GR, Kashner TM. Does somatization disorder occur in men? Clinical characteristics of women and men with multiple unexplained somatic symptoms. Arch Gen Psychiatry. 1991;48(3):231-5.
153. Linzer M, Spitzer R, Kroenke K, Williams JB, Hahn S, Brody D, et al. Gender, quality of life, and mental disorders in primary care: results from the PRIME-MD 1000 study. Am J Med. 1996;101(5):526-33.
154. Lynn R, Martin T. Gender differences in extraversion, neuroticism, and psychoticism in 37 nations. J Soc Psychol. 1997;137(3):369-73.
155. Jorm AF. Sex differences in neuroticism: a quantitative synthesis of published research. Aust N Z J Psychiatry. 1987;21(4):501-6.
156. Kroenke K, Spitzer RL. Gender differences in the reporting of physical and somatoform symptoms. Psychosom Med. 1998;60(2):150-5.
157. Piccinelli M, Simon G. Gender and cross-cultural differences in somatic symptoms associated with emotional distress. An international study in primary care. Psychol Med [Internet]. 1997;27(2):433-44.
158. Unruh AM. Gender variations in clinical pain experience. Pain. 1996;65(2-3):123-67.
159. Fillingim RB, Maixner W. Gender differences in the responses to noxious stimuli. Pain Forum. 1995;4(4):209-21.
160. Kroenke K, Mangelsdorff AD. Common symptoms in ambulatory care: incidence, evaluation, therapy, and outcome. Am J Med. 1989;86(3):262-6.
161. Derbyshire SWG. Sources of variation in assessing male and female responses to pain. New Ideas Psychol. 1997;15(1):83-95.
162. Verbrugge LM. Sex differences in complaints and diagnoses. J Behav Med. 1980;3(4):327-55.
163. Lieban RW. Gender and symptom sensitivity: report on a Philippine study. Am J Orthopsychiatry. 1985;55(3):446-50.
164. Warner CD. Somatic awareness and coronary artery disease in women with chest pain. Heart Lung J Crit Care. 1995;24(6):436-43.
165. Jamison RN, Sbrocco T, Parris WCV. The influence of physical and psychosocial factors on accuracy of memory for pain in chronic pain patients. Pain. 1989;37(3):289-94.
166. Fillingim RB, Maixner W, Girdler SS, Light KC, Harris MB, Sheps DS, et al. Ischemic but not thermal pain sensitivity varies across the menstrual cycle. Psychosom Med. 1997;59(5):512-20.
167. Pfleeger M, Straneva PA, Fillingim RB, Maixner W, Girdler SS. Menstrual cycle, blood pressure and ischemic pain sensitivity in women: a preliminary investigation. Int J Psychophysiol Off J Int Organ Psychophysiol. 1997;27(2):161-6.
168. Berkley KJ. Sex differences in pain. Behav Brain Sci. 1997;20(3):371-80; discussion 435-513.
169. McCauley J, Kern DE, Kolodner K, Dill L, Schroeder AF, DeChant HK, et al. Clinical characteristics of women with a history of childhood abuse: unhealed wounds. JAMA. 1997;277(17):1362-8.

170. Craig TK, Boardman AP, Mills K, Daly-Jones O, Drake H. The South London Somatisation Study. I: Longitudinal course and the influence of early life experiences. Br J Psychiatry J Ment Sci. 1993;163:579-88.
171. Briere J, Runtz M. Symptomatology associated with childhood sexual victimization in a nonclinical adult sample. Child Abuse Negl. 1988;12(1):51-9.
172. Cunningham J, Pearce T, Pearce P. Childhood Sexual Abuse and Medical Complaints in Adult Women. J Interpers Violence. 1988;3(2):131-44.
173. Laws A. Does a History of Sexual Abuse in Childhood Play a Role in Women's Medical Problems? A Review. J Womens Health. 1993;2(2):165-72.
174. Leserman J, Drossman DA. Sexual and physical abuse history and medical practice. Gen Hosp Psychiatry. 1995;17(2):71-4.
175. Reiter RC, Shakerin LR, Gambone JC, Milburn AK. Correlation between sexual abuse and somatization in women with somatic and nonsomatic chronic pelvic pain. Am J Obstet Gynecol. 1991;165(1):104-9.
176. Gorey KM, Leslie DR. The prevalence of child sexual abuse: integrative review adjustment for potential response and measurement biases. Child Abuse Negl. 1997;21(4):391-8.
177. McCauley J, Kern DE, Kolodner K, Dill L, Schroeder AF, DeChant HK, et al. The "battering syndrome": prevalence and clinical characteristics of domestic violence in primary care internal medicine practices. Ann Intern Med. 1995;123(10):737-46.
178. Naumann P, Langford D, Torres S, Campbell J, Glass N. Women battering in primary care practice. Fam Pract. 1999;16(4):343-52.
179. Elliott BA, Johnson MM. Domestic violence in a primary care setting. Patterns and prevalence. Arch Fam Med. 1995;4(2):113-9.
180. Haywood YC, Haile-Mariam T. Violence against women. Emerg Med Clin North Am. 1999;17(3):603-15, vi.
181. Koss MP, Heslet L. Somatic consequences of violence against women. Arch Fam Med. 1992;1(1):53-9.
182. Verbrugge LM. Gender and health: an update on hypotheses and evidence. J Health Soc Behav. 1985;26(3):156-82.
183. Mustard CA, Kaufert P, Kozyrskyj A, Mayer T. Sex differences in the use of health care services. N Engl J Med. 1998;338(23):1678-83.
184. Hoeper EW, Nycz GR, Regier DA, Goldberg ID, Jacobson A, Hankin J. Diagnosis of mental disorder in adults and increased use of health services in four outpatient settings. Am J Psychiatry. 1980;137(2):207-10.
185. Verbrugge LM, Wingard DL. Sex differentials in health and mortality. Women Health. 1987;12(2):103-45.
186. Wenger NK, Speroff L, Packard B. Cardiovascular health and disease in women. N Engl J Med. 1993;329(4):247-56.
187. Levine FM, Lee De Simone L. The effects of experimenter gender on pain report in male and female subjects. Pain. 1991;44(1):69-72.
188. Claréus B, Renström EA. Physicians' gender bias in the diagnostic assessment of medically unexplained symptoms and its effect on patient-physician relations. Scand J Psychol. 2019;60(4):338-47.
189. Paras ML, Murad MH, Chen LP, Goranson EN, Sattler AL, Colbenson KM, et al. Sexual abuse and lifetime diagnosis of somatic disorders: a systematic review and meta-analysis. JAMA. 2009;302(5):550-61.

190. van Dessel N, den Boeft M, van der Wouden JC, Kleinstäuber M, Leone SS, Terluin B, et al. Non-pharmacological interventions for somatoform disorders and medically unexplained physical symptoms (MUPS) in adults. Cochrane Database Syst Rev. 2014;(11):CD011142.
191. Liu J, Gill NS, Teodorczuk A, Li Z jiang, Sun J. The efficacy of cognitive behavioural therapy in somatoform disorders and medically unexplained physical symptoms: a meta-analysis of randomized controlled trials. J Affect Disord. 2019;245:98-112.
192. Menon V, Rajan TM, Kuppili PP, Sarkar S. Cognitive Behavior Therapy for Medically Unexplained Symptoms: A Systematic Review and Meta-analysis of Published Controlled Trials. Indian J Psychol Med. 2017;39(4):399-406.
193. Looper KJ, Kirmayer LJ. Behavioral medicine approaches to somatoform disorders. J Consult Clin Psychol. 2002;70(3):810-27.
194. Goldberg D, Gask L, O'Dowd T. The treatment of somatization: teaching techniques of reattribution. J Psychosom Res. 1989;33(6):689-95.
195. Lakhan SE, Schofield KL, Sampson M. Mindfulness-Based Therapies in the Treatment of Somatization Disorders: A Systematic Review and Meta-Analysis. PLoS One. 2013;8(8):e71834.
196. Fjorback LO, Arendt M, Ornbøl E, Walach H, Rehfeld E, Schröder A, et al. Mindfulness therapy for somatization disorder and functional somatic syndromes: randomized trial with one-year follow-up. J Psychosom Res. 2013;74(1):31-40.
197. Palsson OS, van Tilburg M. Hypnosis and Guided Imagery Treatment for Gastrointestinal Disorders: Experience With Scripted Protocols Developed at the University of North Carolina. Am J Clin Hypn. 2015;58(1):5-21.
198. Kleinstäuber M, Witthöft M, Hiller W. Efficacy of short-term psychotherapy for multiple medically unexplained physical symptoms: a meta-analysis. Clin Psychol Rev. 2011;31(1):146-60.
199. Abbass A, Kisely S, Kroenke K. Short-term psychodynamic psychotherapy for somatic disorders. Systematic review and meta-analysis of clinical trials. Psychother Psychosom. 2009;78(5):265-74.
200. Agarwal V, Nischal A, Praharaj SK, Menon V, Kar SK. Clinical Practice Guideline: Psychotherapies for Somatoform Disorders. Indian J Psychiatry. 2020;62(Suppl 2):S263-71.
201. Lee SJ, Koussa M, Gelberg L, Heinzerling K, Young SD. Somatization, mental health and pain catastrophizing factors associated with risk of opioid misuse among patients with chronic non-cancer pain. J Subst Use. 2020;25(4):357-62.
202. Oriuwa C, Mollica A, Feinstein A, Giacobbe P, Lipsman N, Perez DL, et al. Neuromodulation for the treatment of functional neurological disorder and somatic symptom disorder: a systematic review. J Neurol Neurosurg Psychiatry. 2022;93(3):280-90.

Suicide and Self-harm in Women: A Gendered Approach

Aruna Yadiyal, Lakshmi Vijayakumar, Prabha S Chandra

■ ABSTRACT

Suicide and self-harm though are major health issues worldwide, the burden of both behaviors is more in low- and middle-income countries with India accounting for the largest proportion of self-harm episodes and suicidal deaths globally. Although rates of suicide are higher in males, self-harm is more common in females, and hence suicidal behaviors, which include self-harm and suicides, among Indian women, are higher and continues to be twice the global rate. This chapter sheds light on suicidal behaviors in women and also discusses the confluence of diverse, yet significant factors involved. Along with description of general preventive approaches with universal, selected and indicated strategies, a discussion on a focused interventional framework, which can be both gender sensitive and region specific is envisaged, which will hopefully and effectively protect women at risk from suicidal behaviors across all cultures.

Keywords: Suicide, self-harm, women, gendered approach

■ INTRODUCTION

Suicide and self-harm, though are behaviors that are intensely individualistic and experiential, often indicative of underlying psychological pain, are also issues of major health and societal concern. Societal, cultural, and economic factors affect the statistics of suicide and self-harm as shown by global estimates. Also, most epidemiological studies from diverse nations and cultures show distinct differences in suicidal behavior, across gender and life span, independent of methodological issues. With majority of the suicides occurring in low- and middle-income countries, it comes as no surprise that India has the ignominy of having the highest number of suicide deaths in the world, with suicide being the leading cause of death in the 15–39 years age group. India also accounts for the largest proportion (30%) of global self-harm episodes, though self-harm surveillance systems and data worldwide are few and complex to compare and conclude.[1,2] Gender also appeared quite frequently as a pertinent associated factor for suicidal behaviors worldwide, with India's contribution to global suicide deaths increasing much more among its female population in comparison with their male counterparts in the last three decades. Suicidal deaths rose from 27.3% in 1990 to 36.5%

in 2019 among women and girls and from 16.7% in 1990 to 20.9% in 2019 among men and boys in the Indian subcontinent. This makes the suicide rate among Indian girls and women to be twice the global rate also.[3] Though the global age-standardized suicide rate for males (13.7 per 100,000) was higher by 1.8 times than that of females (7.5 per 100,000) in most countries,[4] the prevalence of suicide attempts were two to three times higher than suicides which was clearly more in women everywhere. This gender paradox was found reversed in few countries like China, Bangladesh, Lesotho, Morocco, and Myanmar, according to recent most estimates by the WHO. For young women aged 15–29 years, suicide was found to be the second leading cause of death, globally. The South-East Asia region had a much higher female age-standardized suicide rate of 11.5 per 100,000 versus the 7.5 per 100,000 rate of the global female average. Women in the low- and middle-income countries had the highest suicide rate of 9.1 per 100,000, when compared across other income groups too. All these data point reasonably to the fact that suicidal behaviors in women are a significant problem, unique enough to warrant a separate focus and discussion.[5,6]

■ EPIDEMIOLOGY

Suicide is said to be the leading cause of death in age group of 15–34 years with some country and gender-specific exceptions. It was clearly found to be higher in women and girls aged 15–29 years in India. Although male suicide deaths outnumber female suicide deaths globally, in several countries like India and China, this sex ratio is much narrower or is even reversed in certain areas. Suicide rates for females in low- and middle-income countries appear to be the highest in younger age groups rather than increasing with age, which appears to be the trend elsewhere globally.[2,7] The Global Burden of Disease (GBD) Study for India reported suicidal rates with substantial sex differences with age standardized suicidal rates to be 12.1 per 100,000 population in women and 15.6 per 100,000 population for men. But, these national-level estimates mask a 15-times variation for women versus a 7-times variation for men at individual state levels in India. However, in the younger age group of 15–39 years, 52.6% of all deaths were from suicide among women, whereas it was 47.4% among men.[3,8]

Though the exact number of self-harm episodes is unknown, owing to few self-harm surveillance systems worldwide and particularly in low- and middle-income countries, comparing self-harm data across countries and understanding international patterns, even with the limitations is found to be useful. The Global Burden of Disease Study estimates point out to approximately 20 self-harm episodes for each suicide death every year. The age-standardized incidence rate of self-harm is 62.5 per 100,000 with higher rates in women (74.0 per 100,000) than men (51.0 per 100,000). Though India accounts for the largest proportion of global self-harm episodes (30%), these incidences appeared to be the highest in the northern hemisphere with lowest rates in Africa, Latin America, and the Caribbean group. In Indian population older than 18 years of age, it was estimated that 5.1% had some level of suicidality in 2015-16 with the ratio of suicidality in men to women reported at 0.68.[2,3,9,10]

■ METHODS OF SUICIDAL BEHAVIOR AND GENDER

Exact knowledge of the various methods used for suicide and self-harm across countries, though is limited, research information about the same is important for devising strategies for suicide prevention, especially if it highlights variations across age, gender and cultures. Firearms, hanging or suffocation, poisoning and overdose, jumps, cuts, and burning have been the methods for suicidal behavior listed commonly in studies across the world. A 2008 bulletin by the WHO has highlighted regional differences clearly. According to this report, poisoning by pesticide was common in many Asian countries and in Latin America whereas poisoning by drugs was common in both Nordic countries and the United Kingdom. Hanging was the preferred method of suicide in eastern Europe, as was firearm suicide in the United States and jumping from a high place in cities and urban societies such as Hong Kong Special Administrative Region, China. This analysis showed that pesticide suicide and firearm suicide replaced traditional methods like hanging in many countries.[11] More recent national estimates from India, however, reports hanging as the most common method of death by suicide, followed by pesticide ingestion, overdose of medicines, and self-immolation, the last especially being more common in females.[12] Suicide by burning oneself is deemed to be both a private and a cultural act and varies greatly in acceptability and meanings attributed to such acts, across cultures. Self-immolation has been documented in suicidal research from several countries like Iran, Iraq, Afghanistan, Tajikistan, Uzbekistan, India, Sri Lanka, and Africa where majority of the victims were women. Suicidal self-burning was also seen in countries like China, Vietnam, and parts of Eastern Europe which highlighted the gender and cultural variations in the presentations of suicidal behaviors across countries. Self-immolation in women was mostly seen as a protest against the institutionally–enabled social injustices and persecution from proximal sources, like their family and community, while in case of men, it was scripted as a protest against distal oppressors, authorities, institutions, or situations with social explanations getting all the attention.[13] Some Indian studies have shed light on the gender-related differences in the methods of suicidal behaviors, wherein, the most common methods in both genders were poison consumption and drug overdose with majority of the attempters being young and of female gender. Though females outnumbered males in deliberate self-harm behaviors, the gender-specific rates were found to be considerably low when compared to developed countries with the gender disparity appearing to be slowly reducing in India. Males from urban background and single unmarried females had higher odds of attempting suicide by poison consumption and females from urban background had higher odds of attempting self-harm by drug overdose. Most of the attempts were of low intentionality, low lethality, and high impulsivity and were precipitated by a psychosocial stressor. Suicide attempt in an intoxicated state was significantly higher in males when compared to females. Though gender differences among attempters appeared less pronounced in the Indian setting compared to the worldwide literature, more studies are clearly needed to draw meaningful inferences from it. Nevertheless, studies on suicidality with a gendered lens may point to some important differences between male and female self-harm attempters which may further have implications for specific preventive work in the area.[14]

FACTORS IN SUICIDAL BEHAVIOR OF WOMEN

Gender factors: As gender is one of the most frequently replicated predictors of suicide, understanding the gender differences in suicidal behavior, and not just suicide, will hopefully lead us also to consider current suicide prevention strategies with a gendered lens. Several studies have pointed toward differences in suicidality between men and women. While completed suicides are more in men in most countries, women attempt to take their life two to three times more than men, though this attempt to completed suicide rates ratio tends to fall as both genders move to age more.[15] Unlike in men, where older age has a higher risk for suicide, in women it is younger age that appears to confer a higher risk. More differences seem to appear in suicidal behavior in women across cultures and nations, unlike in males, where findings are more stable and similar cross culturally. Differences in cognitive styles related to suicidal behavior also have been described with women tending to have overthinking, inclusive thinking, considering feelings of others, and being more ready to seek and get help. Men appear to think less, have a more decided attitude, are more planned or action oriented, and often refuse help. Women tend to have higher rates of suicidal thinking and nonfatal suicidal behavior in addition to higher suicidal attempts. Suicidal methods chosen differ with women tending to choose less lethal or less violent methods. Poisoning appears to be the most common method and in case women use a gun, they seldom shoot themselves on the face.[16] Also, women have been shown to have different and unique risk and protective factors when compared to men. For example, pregnancy and parenthood appeared to be protective, and postpartum psychiatric disorders, abortions, infertility, death of children proved to be risk factors unique to female gender.

Marriage, found to be a protective factor for men, was not always so for women, and varied across cultures. Forced marriage, early marriage, marriage to an older man and intimate partner violence were found to be risk factors arising out of marriage for women, predominantly so in developing countries. Depression, which was one of the most prominent risk factors for suicide, also differs in its manifestation and course across gender. Also, comorbid psychiatric illnesses such as anxiety disorders, eating disorders, body dysmorphic disorder, and physical illnesses were more burdensome in females rather than males. Though 70% of antidepressants use is noted in women, attempted suicides and suicidal behavior are more subjected to under reporting in many countries, especially non-Western societies due to stigma associated with suicidality among women.[17-20]

Sociocultural factors: Diverse cultural patterns with gender-specific undertones seem to add varying dimensions in the unfolding saga of female suicidality, which impact each gender differently. Understanding these patterns may help us devise interventions, that acknowledge the interface between gender and culture.

The cultural milieu of mankind has so far been hostile to the female gender, which is evident, by the negative impact it has on female suicidal behavior. Suicide rates among women diverge among countries, wherein rates are the highest in older age groups (>75 years) in Europe, Russia, Korea, and China, in the age group of 45-54 years in the USA and a much younger age group in South Asia. The method of suicide also varied across cultures, with women in Western countries using over the counter or prescribed medications in overdose, followed by use of firearms. Asian women have been found to use more lethal methods, often without more intent, but rather due to easy accessibility and availability such as consuming pesticides. Self-immolation is also chosen by a sizeable number of women in developing countries because of prevailing sociocultural norms and higher acceptability. Marriage, seen as a sociocultural construct, also varies across cultures and genders in its impact on suicidal behavior. Marriage tends to be less protective for females than males across cultures, and even turns into a risk factor for suicidal behavior in younger women in developing countries in South Asia. This seems to be because of the life and marital circumstances, rather than marriage itself, which increases their vulnerability toward suicidal behavior. The most common circumstances include forced and early marriages, dowry issues, young motherhood, low social status, economic dependency, and domestic violence. Intimate partner violence and domestic violence are associated with suicidal risk and behavior in females worldwide, more strikingly so in developing countries of Asia and Middle East, as it is partially condoned and accepted as a sociocultural norm in these communities. Studies revealed staggering figures where, 48% of women in Brazil, 61% in Egypt, 64% in India,

11% in Indonesia, and 28% in Philippines showed a significant correlation between spousal violence and suicidal behavior.[21-23] Recently published systematic reviews have shown strong association between cultural practices like female genital mutilation and adverse mental health outcomes including increased risk of suicidal behavior in women.[21] Substance use disorders independently increase risk of suicidal behavior, more so in men and elderly populations. But, with increasing substance use disorders in females, globally, and with its association with violence and risk-taking behavior, substance use disorders in both genders need to be considered as a significant risk factor in female suicidal behavior across cultures.[22,23]

Childhood adversities such as physical, emotional, and sexual abuse and violence are also associated with suicidal behavior in women. Consistent risk factors which weighed heavily toward female suicidality included intimate partner violence, nonpartner physical violence, childhood sexual abuse, being widowed, divorced or separated, and history of partner violence in mother, according to a WHO multi-country study.[22] Sporadic risk factors were also found in some western countries in migrant and minority communities. More common risk factors predominant in western cultures were being widowed, divorced, being single, death of partner, death of child, and occasionally abortion and infertility. Pregnancy and childbirth, considered as protective factors, may not be applicable uniformly across all countries. In high income countries, suicide is one of the important causes of maternal mortality during pregnancy and related events like abortion and miscarriage, highlighting the cultural variance of suicidal behavior in females.[24,25] Contrary to research findings from developing countries, reports from developed countries like Australia suggest psychiatric illness in young mothers as one of the leading causes of maternal mortality, with most suicides by violent means.[25] WHO, in its report, in 2017, highlighted the fact that low- and middle-income countries account for 78% of world's death by suicide and studies in these cultures pointed toward family conflict, emotional distress, poverty, and illness to be major risk factors for suicidal behavior in women of these cultures.[26,27] Various studies done in war zones and conflict areas such as Pakistan, Afghanistan, Jordan, and Thai-Burma borders have shown that women in these contexts become refugees and are victims of endless traumas including physical and sexual violence, abduction, forced prostitution, and forced sale of their children. A range of trauma-related psychological aftermath including suicidal behavior has been noted in these women.[28] The sociocultural milieu of India, though unique, has not been kind toward the female gender, where patriarchy is the main flavor on any day. Culturally, colored-risk factors in Indian women include stifling patriarchy, archaic stances on sexuality, marriage and female autonomy, sexual and emotional victimization of women, problematic spousal substance abuse, domestic violence, poor physical health, and economic impoverishment. Some cultural factors which were found to be protective in Indian women were support from extended family systems, religiosity, resilience, good coping skills, and scriptural wisdom in the face of continuing adversities.[29,30] With Islam being the fastest growing religion in the world, the higher rates of suicide among young Middle Eastern Muslim females also warrant special attention. Though their religion forbids suicide, there is cultural discrimination between sexes, with high illiteracy and socio-economic impoverishment among women. Many women suffer from mental health disorders, the most common being depression, with no access to mental health services. Marriage is more of a risk factor, again, with domestic violence, arranged or forced marriage with much older males, overall oppression in marriage, polygamy practices and secondary designated role in marriage and society as subfactors. The rights of the men are forced upon at the cost of liberty of women leading to irrational traditions like honor killing. Restrictions about clothes and movement are also enforced upon women. Infertility, childlessness, abortions, and lack of control over one's birthing rights or bodily issues are unique and culturally biased risk factors pushing these women, especially the young ones, toward suicidal behavior.[31]

Suicidal studies in women from China highlight the fact that cultural, social, and economic deprivation and abuse, as well as violence in the context of family and community, are potent suicidal risk factors for women, especially in communities where there is no culturally acceptable option for women to escape the deprivation, abuse, and violence, except via suicide. Further, studies of suicidal women in China, India, and a range of Muslim-majority countries may capture the experiences of thwarted individuation (a frustrated desire for individuality and independence) and may be at the center of a general theory of women's suicidality versus that of similar studies in United States, where popular theories of perceived burdensomeness (feeling that one is a burden to others) and thwarted belongingness (a frustrated desire for closer ties with others) are considered to be universal experiences in the path to suicidality. A study using United Nations data shows that women's suicide rates were lower in countries with more egalitarian gender norms, with strong human development capabilities, hence shifting the focus of suicide prevention strategies in women toward eliminating culturally embedded gender discrimination.[32]

The interactions of these gender and sociocultural factors with mental health antecedents and consequences among women explain the significant roles these factors play in the unfolding of the suicidal behaviors in females, further advocating the need for more culture-sensitive and gender-specific interventions **(Fig. 1)**.

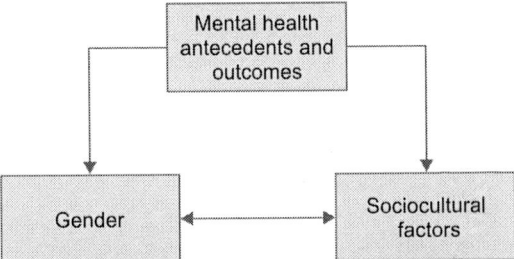

Fig. 1: The interactive pattern between sociocultural factors, gender, and mental health antecedents and outcomes in women.

> **BOX 1:** Specific protective factors for suicidality in women.
> - Healthy reproductive health outcomes: Pregnancy, motherhood (planned and wanted)
> - Accomplishments in vocational and social spheres
> - Children when very young and dependent
> - Supportive and positive relationships in family and society
> - Obligations, precommitments toward family
> - Adequate regulation of emotions
> - Good social/verbal skills
> - Sufficient satisfaction/Gratification in life
> - Proactive problem-solving skills/coping with stress abilities
> - More acceptance toward health seeking and treatment
> - Psychological responsiveness and readiness for psychological interventions
> - Less lethality of means of suicide
> - Intractability in reality-testing
> - Resilience secondary to religiosity or spirituality

Risk and Protective factors: Suicide prevention strategies to be appropriate, effective, and relevant to women need to consider risk factors and protective factors specific to women and aim to mitigate risk factors and bolster protective factors, which might vary across cultures and nations[20-22,32-34] **(Boxes 1 and 2).**

Suicide prevention interventions: Suicide prevention strategies need to take into account the magnitude of suicide and suicidality and the scope of preventable deaths between them. Though these interventions are limited in developing countries, various preventive approaches, along the lines of universal, selective, and indicated interventions have been in implementation among developed ones. Universal interventions target whole populations and work toward reducing risk factors across populations. Selective interventions target subgroups of people, with risk factors, but with no suicidal behavior as yet. Indicated interventions attend exclusively to people who already have exhibited some suicidal behavior such as plans, attempts, or to survivors of suicide.[35]

> **BOX 2:** Specific risk factors for suicidality in women.
>
> - *Comorbid mental illnesses:* Depression, anxiety, personality disorders, etc.
> - Psychiatric disorders in postpartum period
> - Reproductive difficulties like infertility, IVF treatments
> - *Stressors in perinatal period:* Abortion, miscarriages, and malnutrition
> - *Stressors in family members:* Death/disability in children, early spousal death
> - Violence by spouse, partner, and family members
> - Caregiving responsibilities and associated stress
> - *Childhood history of abuse:* Physical/emotional/sexual
> - Disturbances in body image
> - Invasive surgeries like mastectomy and hysterectomy
> - Marriage with postmarriage living and sociocultural contexts
> - Spousal use of substances, especially alcohol
> - Pregnancy/Motherhood, when unwanted and unexpected
> - Stressors, stigma, restrictions associated with menstrual cycles
> - Dependency status in sociocultural sphere
> - Missed and limited opportunities in vocational, educational areas
> - Pressure on personal issues/agency by society and family
> - Increased sensitivity toward criticism and emotional issues
> - Sexual discrimination/harassment/everyday sexism
> - *Media reporting of suicides:* Inappropriate, inaccurate, and sensitization
> - Laws which criminalize suicide (in some countries)

But, these interventions, though effective, are gender-neutral and hence cannot be applied universally across all regions and cultures and fail to focus on vulnerable specific groups such as women. Some studies which have included a social, judicial, and context perspective have rightly pointed out that the vast majority of existing suicide prevention programs targeting women's suicidality are still individual-based and psychocentric.[36] So, it would serve us well to innovate ways to modify these interventions to become more region-specific, culture-sensitive, and gender-focused. Existing scant evidence indicates that for suicide prevention interventions to be specifically effective for females, it needs to be multipronged, addressing social, economic, political factors, and structural inequalities within these factors.[37]

Gender specific interventions for suicide prevention: Suicide prevention strategies along the lines of universal, selective, and indicated interventions can be tweaked and refined to be more women-centric, so that they become useful for a sizable proportion of victims of suicidal behavior across cultures.

Universal interventions here could include investing in robust public awareness campaigns advocating for gender equality among masses, programs to empower women through educational and economic opportunities, creating women peer support groups, pressing for laws to protect women's rights, laws against female feticide and female genital mutilation, bolstering existing laws on marital rape, domestic violence, birthing rights and work place benefits, focusing on reducing menace of spousal drinking problems, advocating for compulsory and universal education of girls, abolition of dowry system and child marriages, striving for better representation of women in policy and decision making forums, making access to mental healthcare more easy to women, or supporting NGOs working in area of women welfare.[38] As women are significant victims of postdisaster situations, disaster intervention programs should work toward gender equity too. Development of support network around women and their care as a family unit would make disaster response strategies more empowering and sensitive toward women needs.[39] Given the significance of social, economic, and legal discrimination in women's suicidality, context- and social-justice perspectives need to be incorporated in initiatives aiming at preventing women's suicidality too.[37] Women empowerment programs which aim for socioeconomic freedom for women effectively help in suicide prevention, given the close links between female suicidality and sociocultural factors. Laws in certain countries (including India) that perpetuate certain risk factors against women, such as those pertaining to marital rape and intimate partner violence, needs to be changed. Bebbington et al., back in 2009 itself, showed in their study that lifetime risk of suicide attempts would reduce by almost 28% in women if sexual abuse could somehow be eliminated. A study from India noted a changing profile in suicidal methods in women, wherein suicides by hanging and insecticide consumption showed an increasing trend between 2014 and 2021. Decreased self-immolation rates during the same period might be because of the welfare initiative to provide clean cooking fuel to households during that period. Since reducing access to means comes under the umbrella of universal interventions, a ban on lethal pesticides here might help lower insecticide poisoning suicide rates. However, all these universal interventions, hence, must be multipronged and nested into existing platforms of social, educational, and health services, for wider reach and better impact.[40,41]

Selective interventions could be strengthening screening and referral services to mental health service for women in peripartum conditions, integrating mental health into routine antenatal healthcare and developing a chain of mother-baby care units as part of psychiatry in patient services across tertiary care centers. This should also include gender-specific school mental health programs for addressing mental health needs of adolescent girls, reproductive health programs for both genders, gender sensitization programs across all work sectors, establishment of internal complaint committee and grievance cells for women in all workplaces, advocating for maternity leaves and benefits in all higher educational and occupational organizations, and strengthening of responses to domestic and sexual violence through better managed shelters, one-stop centers, and women mental health services specifically across the country.[39,42] By sensitizing health sector workers toward violence against women, they can be made to respond appropriately, which may subsequently reduce the health burden associated with violence and suicidal behavior in women.[24] A multi-level program aiming at effective detoxification, followed by rehabilitation and recovery programs in wards specially earmarked for women, would be a very desired gender-specific approach for women with suicidal behavior and comorbid substance use disorders.

Indicated interventions could include assertive follow-ups and treatment of perinatal women with psychiatric morbidity through accessible psychiatric services, including liaison consultations, which can address suicide in these indicated cases. Along with this routine perinatal check-ups, psychosocial screening programs with clear referral protocols, and treatment of significant psychiatric morbidity during perinatal period could be chosen indicated strategies here. Clinicians should be made aware of the need for continuity of care between primary, mental health and maternity care, so that suicides become more preventable in this vulnerable group.[24,43] Indicated interventions could adopt a more empathetic approach, exploring the cultural, social, and clinical risk factors in each context, providing continuity of care and outreach through women personnel, and work toward teaching effective coping skills in order to build resilience and to avert suicidal thoughts and behavior in the face of continuing adversities in the future[38,40,41] **(Fig. 2)**.

Though these interventions are largely touted as being women-centric, the overall goal would be to bring in a much desired and deserved change in the sociocultural scene of the society as a whole, which should then ideally involve the male counterparts as well. Especially in many South Asian and Middle Eastern countries this would include involving men to decrease patriarchy and change traditional masculine roles and power equations.[6]

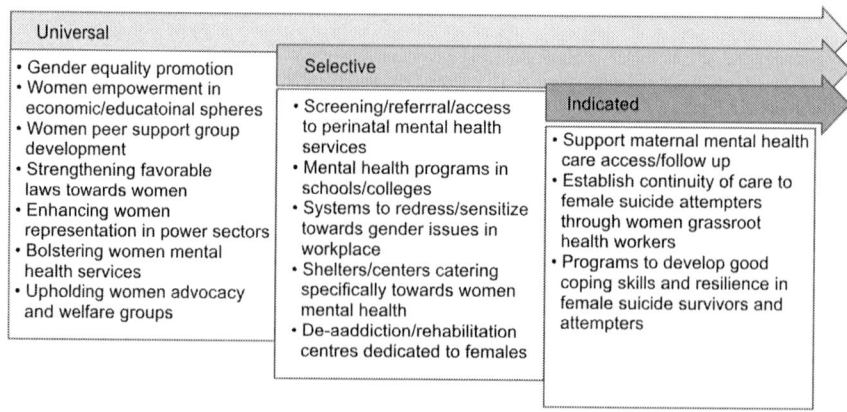

Fig. 2: Interventions for suicidal prevention with a gendered approach.

CONCLUSION

Suicide and self-harm are complex human behaviors which could end fatally if timely preventive interventions are not in place. Women are particularly more at risk, taking into account the variability of gender, age, and cultural contexts across the spectrum of suicidal behavior. Gender-related vulnerability to psychopathology and psychosocial stressors lead to greater vulnerability in women toward suicidal behavior, thus indicating an urgent need for more gendered research on suicidal behavior, especially in developing countries.[44] More sex disaggregated data in trials of suicide prevention that try to provide evidence-based interventions specifically for women are needed. Along with the study of the magnitude of the problem, a deeper understanding of the complex gender and sociocultural underpinnings in the context of suicidal behavior in women, will force us to recognize the need for a more nuanced, gendered approach while trying to implement the recommended preventive strategies along the lines of universal, selective, and indicated interventions.

KEY POINTS

- Suicidal behaviors, which include both self-harm and suicides, are found to be significantly higher in women, more so in the younger age groups and in low- and middle-income countries.
- Gender and sociocultural factors interact with mental health antecedents and consequences among women, hence playing a significant role in the unfolding of the suicidal behaviors in females.
- Suicide prevention strategies to be appropriate, effective, and relevant to women need to consider risk factors and protective factors specific to women and aim to mitigate risk factors and bolster protective factors, which might vary across cultures.
- A culturally-sensitive, regionally-specific, and a more nuanced and gendered approach while trying to implement the recommended preventive strategies along the lines of universal, selective, and indicated interventions would go a long way in effective prevention of suicidal behaviors in women globally.

Acknowledgment: Much of the content of the prevention strategies has been borrowed from an earlier chapter authored by the same authors as of this chapter and permission for same has been obtained from the authors and editors of the book where the said chapter was published (see Reference no. 6).

Conflict of interest: Nil.

REFERENCES

1. Global Burden of Disease Collaborative Network. Global Burden of Disease study 2019 (GBD 2019) results. Seattle, WA: Institute for Health Metrics and Evaluation; 2020.
2. Knipe D, Padmanathan P, Newton-Howes G, Chan LF, Kapur N. Suicide and self-harm. The Lancet. 2022;399(10338):1903-16.

3. Vijayakumar L, Chandra PS, Kumar MS, Pathare S, Banerjee D, Goswami T, et al. The national suicide prevention strategy in India: context and considerations for urgent action. The Lancet Psychiatry. 2022;9(2):160-8.
4. World Health Organization. (2019). Suicide in the world: Global health estimates. World Health Organization. WHO/MSD/MER/19.3. [online] Available from https://platform.who.int/docs/librariesprovider20/default-document-library/resources/who-msd-mer-19-3-eng.pdf?sfvrsn=1fef22be_2 [Last accessed December, 2023].
5. Bertolote JM, Fleischmann A. A global perspective on the magnitude of suicide mortality. In: Wasserman D, Wasserman C)+(Eds). Oxford textbook of Suicidology and Suicide Prevention. Oxford, UK: Oxford University Press; 2009. pp. 91-8.
6. Yadiyal A, Chandra PS. Suicide prevention strategies to protect young women at risk. In: Alfonso CA, Chandra PS, Schulge TG (Eds). Suicide by Self-Immolation: Biopsychosocial and Transcultural Aspects. Switzerland AG: Springer Nature; 2021.pp. 247-64.
7. Patel V, Ramasundarahettige C, Vijayakumar L, Thakur JS, Gajalakshmi V, Gururaj G, et al. Suicide mortality in India: a nationally representative survey. Lancet. 2012;379:2343-51.
8. India State-Level Disease Burden Initiative Suicide Collaborators: Dandona R, Kumar GA, Dhaliwal RS, Naghavi M, Vos T, Shukla DK, et al. Gender differentials and state variations in suicide deaths in India: the Global Burden of Disease Study 1990–2016. Lancet Public Health. 2018;3:e478-89.
9. GBD 2019 Diseases and Injuries Collaborators, Vos T, Lim SS, Abbafati C, Abbas KM, Abbasi M, Abbasifard M, et al. Global burden of 369 diseases and injuries in 204 countries and territories, 1990–2019: a systematic analysis for the Global Burden of Disease Study 2019. Lancet. 2020;396:1204-22.
10. Mew EJ, Padmanathan P, Konradsen F, Eddleston M, Chang SS, Phillips MR, et al. The global burden of fatal self-poisoning with pesticides 2006-15: systematic review. J Affect Disord. 2017;219:93-104.
11. Ajdacic-Gross V, Weiss MG, Ring M, Hepp U, Bopp M, Gutzwiller F, et al. Methods of suicide: international suicide patterns derived from the WHO mortality database. Bull World Health Organ. 2008;86:726-32.
12. National Crimes Record Bureau. Accidental deaths and suicides in India—2019. New Delhi: Government of India; 2020.
13. Canetto SS, Pouradeli S, Khan MM, Rezaeian M. Suicidal Self-Burning in Women and Men Around the World: A Cultural and Gender Analysis of Patterns and Explanations. In: Pompili M (ed). Suicide Risk Assessment and Prevention. Switzerland: Springer, Cham; 2022.
14. Kumar KK, Sattar FA, Bondade S, Hussain M, Munnawar S, Priyadarshini M. A Gender-Specific Analysis of Suicide Methods in Deliberate Self-Harm. Indian J Social Psychiatry. 2017;33(1):7-21.
15. Garg R, Trivedi JK, Dhyani M. Suicidal behavior in special population: Elderly, women and adolescent in special reference to India. Delhi Psychiatry J. 2007;10(2):106-18.
16. Murphy GE. Why women are less likely than men to commit suicide? Compr Psychiatry. 1998;39(4):165-75.

17. Ping Q, Mortensen PB, Agerbo E. Gender differences in risk factors for suicide in Denmark. Br J Psychiatry. 2000;177:546-50.
18. Värnik A, Kõlves K, Allik J, Arensman E, Aromaa E, van Audenhove C, et al. Gender issues in suicide rates, trends and methods among youth aged 15-24 in 15 European countries. J Affect Disord. 2009;113(3):216-26.
19. Hawton K. Sex and Suicide: Gender differences in suicidal behavior. Br J Psychiatry. 2000;177:484-85.
20. Mayer P, Ziaian T. Suicide, gender and age variations in India. Are women in Indian Society protected from suicide? Crisis. 2002;23:98-103.
21. Abdalla SM, Galea S. Is female genital mutilation/cutting associated with adverse mental health consequences? A systematic review of evidence. BMJ Global Health. 2019;4(4):e001553.
22. Devries K, Watts C, Yoshihama M, Kiss L, Schraiber LB, Deyessa N, et al. Violence against women is strongly associated with suicide attempts: Evidence from the WHO multi-country study on women's health and domestic violence against women. Soc Sci Med. 2011;73:79-86.
23. Esang M, Ahmed S. A closer look at substance use and suicide. Am J Psychiatry Res J. 2018; 13(6):6-8.
24. Khalifeh H, Hunt IM, Appleby L, Howard LM. Suicide in perinatal and non-perinatal women in contact with psychiatric services: 15 year findings from a UK national inquiry. Lancet Psychiatry. 2016;3:233-42.
25. Austin MP, Kildea S, Sullivan E. Maternal mortality and psychiatric morbidity in the perinatal period: Challenges and opportunities for prevention in the Australian setting. MJA. 2007;186:364-7.
26. Seponski DM, Somo CM, Kao S, Lahar CJ, Khann S, Schunert T. Family, Health and Poverty factors impacting suicide attempts in Cambodian Women. Crisis. 2019;40(2):141-5.
27. Cavanaugh CE, Messing JT, Eyzerovich E, Campbell JC. Ethnic differences in correlates of suicidal behaviour among women seeking help for intimate partner violence. Crisis. 2015;36(4):257-66.
28. Parkar SR, Nagarsekar B, Weiss MG. Explaining suicide in an urban slum of Mumbai, India: A sociocultural autopsy. Crisis. 2009;30(4):192-201.
29. Vijayakumar L. Hindu religion and suicide in India: In: Wasserman D, Wasserman C (eds). Oxford Textbook of Suicidology and Suicide Prevention. Oxford, UK: Oxford University Press; 2009. pp. 19-26.
30. Maselko J, Patel V. Why women attempt suicide: The role of mental illness and social disadvantage in a community cohort study in India. J Epidemiol Community Health. 2008;62:817-22.
31. Rezaeian M. Suicide among young Middle Eastern Muslim females. The perspective of an Iranian Epidemiologist. Crisis. 2010;31(1):36-42.
32. Canetto SS, Chen J. Women and suicidal behavior: Paradigm-shift lessons from China. In: Cheung FM, Halpern DF (Eds). Cambridge Handbook of the International Psychology of Women. Cambridge: Cambridge University Press; 2020. pp. 497-513.
33. Oquendo MA, Bongiovi-Garcia ME, Galfalvy H, Goldberg PH, Grunebaum MF, Burke AK, et al. Sex differences in clinical predictors of suicidal acts after major depression: A prospective study. Am J Psychiatry. 2007;164:134-41.

34. Cougle JR, Resnick H, Kilpatrick DG. PTSD, Depression and their comorbidity in relation to suicidality: Cross-sectional and prospective analyses of a national probability of women. Depress Anxiety. 2009;26:1151-7.
35. Hawton K, Taylor T. Treatment of suicide attempters and prevention of suicide and attempted suicide. In: Gelder MG, Nancy AC, Lopez-Ibor Jr JJ, Geddes JR (Eds). New Oxford Textbook of Psychiatry, 2nd edition, Volume 1. Oxford, UK: Oxford University Press; 2009. 969-78.
36. Cai Z, Canetto SS, Chang Q, Yip PS. Women's suicide in low-, middle-, and high-income countries: Do laws discriminating against women matter? Soc Sci Med. 2021;282:114035.
37. Canetto SS. Prevention of suicidal behaviour in females: opportunities and obstacles. In: Wasserman D, Wasserman C (eds). Oxford textbook of suicidology and suicide prevention: a Global Perspective. Oxford: Oxford University Press; 2009. pp. 241-7.
38. Zalsman G, Hawton K, Wasserman D, van Heeringen K, Arensman E, Sarchiapone M, et al. Suicide Prevention strategies revisited: 10 year systematic review. Lancet Psychiatry. 2016;3:646-59.
39. Bhadra S. Women in disasters and conflicts in India: Intervention in view of the Millenium Development Goals. Int J Disaster Risk Sci. 2017;8:196-207.
40. Arya V, Page A, Vijayakumar L, Onie S, Tapp C, John A, et al. Changing profile of suicide methods in India: 2014–2021. J affect disord. 2023;340:420-6.
41. Vijayakumar L, Lamech N. Suicide and suicidal behavior in women. Ment Health Ill Women. 2020:35-56.
42. Healey C, Morriss R, Henshaw C, Kinderman P. Self-harm in postpartum depression and referrals to a perinatal mental health team: an audit study. Arch Womens Ment Health. 2013;16(3):237-45.
43. Lega I, Maraschini A, D'Aloja P, Andreozzi S, Spettoli D, Giangreco M, et al. Maternal suicide in Italy. Arch Womens Ment Health. 2020;23:199-206.
44. Vijayakumar L. Suicide in women. Indian J Psychiatry. 2015;57:233-8.

CHAPTER 7

Substance Use and Externalizing Disorders in Women: The Indian Context

Venkata Lakshmi Narasimha, Shalini Kumari

ABSTRACT

The prevalence of substance use among women in India is less than among men. While the prevalence of tobacco use among women has reduced in the last decade, the change in patterns of other substances is unknown. Differences in biological, genetic, environmental, and psychosocial factors determine the vulnerability to substance use disorders (SUDs). Women suffer greater medical and psychiatric comorbidities compared to men. Externalizing disorders, particularly attention deficit hyperactivity disorder (ADHD) increase the vulnerability to SUDs and are often undetected in women due to differences in presentation. Substance use patterns among women differ from men in terms of delayed age of onset, negative affective state as a common reason for initiation, telescoping effect, and poor treatment seeking. Many screening tools have been validated for women using substances, including during pregnancy. Women suffer barriers at an individual, societal, and systemic level in their pathways to care. While regular psychosocial interventions are effective, gender-specific, and sensitive interventions are useful compared to traditional treatment. Management of SUDs and ADHD during pregnancy requires special considerations. Treatment outcomes in the Indian context were poor, and more research needs to be done to understand various dimensions of substance use among women.

Keywords: Substance use disorders, attention deficit hyperactivity disorder (ADHD)

INTRODUCTION

Substance use disorders (SUDs) are chronic, relapsing medical conditions that affect both men and women. Substance use is linked to harm to oneself and others, resulting in significant morbidity and mortality. Earlier epidemiological surveys indicated higher rates of substance use and dependence in men compared to women. However, recent observation suggests that the narrowing of this gap reflects changing trends in substance use patterns among genders.[1] Although women have a lower prevalence of SUDs than men, they experience significantly higher morbidity.[2] Women and men differ in substance use epidemiology, vulnerability, patterns, course, and treatment outcomes.[3] In this chapter, the focus is on SUDs among women in India, understanding gender differences in substance use, and emphasis on externalizing disorders, particularly attention deficit hyperactivity disorder (ADHD). Additionally, the management of SUDs and ADHD during the perinatal period has been discussed.

EPIDEMIOLOGY OF SUBSTANCE USE DISORDERS IN INDIA

Substance use is a significant concern in India, especially among women. Tobacco is the most used substance among women, followed by alcohol and other drugs **(Table 1)**. According to the Magnitude of Substance Use in India Report 2019, for every woman who drinks alcohol, 17 men consume alcohol. Additionally, one in 16 women who use alcohol are dependent on it, while the figure is one in five for men.[4] Alcohol use among women exists in all states of the country. Among them, Arunachal Pradesh, and Chhattisgarh have the largest population of women using alcohol. Longitudinal data is lacking in India regarding the reduction in the prevalence gap between substance use among men and women, despite global studies suggesting such a reduction. Read Lal et al. for previous epidemiological studies and their findings.[5] In Global Adult Tobacco Survey-2 (GATS-2), smoking and smokeless tobacco use among women reduced significantly compared to GATS-1.[6] Similar observations could not be made for alcohol and other drugs due to the unavailability of methodologically similar previous studies. Among treatment-seeking populations, alcohol, and opioids are commonly reported drugs.[7-10]

VULNERABILITY

While environmental factors increase the likelihood of drug initiation, genetic factors increase the likelihood of addiction. Various factors contribute to the vulnerability of SUDs among women.

TABLE 1: Prevalence of substance use among women in India [Global Adult Tobacco Survey (GATS-2) for tobacco and magnitude of substance use in India 2019 for other substances].

Substance	Prevalence
Tobacco	14.2%
Alcohol	1.6%
Cannabis	0.6%
Opioids	0.2%
Inhalants	0.07%
Cocaine	0.01%

Biological (Pharmacokinetic) Differences

Inherent pharmacokinetic differences in how drugs are metabolized result in differential effects of substances in men and women **(Table 2)**.[2,3] Physiological differences in alcohol metabolism are described separately. Further, the neural response to drugs differs between men and women. For example, among cocaine users, women are more susceptible to neural dysregulation compared to men. In contrast, men respond with a greater brain reward system activation than women.[11]

Genetic

While genetics contribute to 50% of vulnerability to SUDS, the genetic vulnerability of substance use among women is different from that of men. While men have a greater genetic vulnerability, environmental factors contribute to SUDs in women.[12,13] Some studies on alcohol dependence did not observe differences in genetic vulnerability between genders.[14]

Environmental

Location of residence, availability of drugs, peer group, economic situation, and family environment are the shared environmental vulnerability for SUDs.[12] Unemployment, lack of formal education, and women belonging to lower socioeconomic populations are the risk factors for tobacco use.[15]

Psychosocial

Women using alcohol or drugs attributed to stress, trauma, physical, or sexual abuse for their substance use.[16] Among the elderly, widowhood has been associated with an increased risk of alcohol and tobacco use.[17]

Comorbidity

Childhood trauma, depression, anxiety, post-traumatic stress disorders (PTSDs), and eating disorders are commonly reported comorbidities among women using substances.[5] A bidirectional relationship has been observed between both disorders.

TABLE 2: Differences in pharmacokinetics of substances between women and men.

Drug	Differences
Tobacco	Due to the effect of estrogen on CYP2A6 nicotine is metabolized quickly in women compared to men, greater risk of addiction
Cocaine and methamphetamine (stimulants)	During the follicular phase (estrogen levels are relatively higher), greater plasma concentrations, along with increased subjective reinforcement, were observed

PHYSIOLOGICAL DIFFERENCES IN THE METABOLISM AND EFFECTS OF ALCOHOL

There are several physiological differences between men and women, and these differences can influence factors, such as body composition **(Table 3)**.

TABLE 3: Physiological differences in alcohol metabolism in women compared to men.

Factors	Men	Women
Gastric emptying	Quick	Delayed compared to men and is 42% lower in women
First pass metabolism	Higher than women	Lower
Volume of distribution	Males have lower body fat and higher body water resulting in a high volume of distribution of alcohol	Females have more body fat and lower body water resulting in a low volume of distribution of alcohol
ADH activity	Higher level of alcohol dehydrogenase (ADH) activity	Lower level of ADH activity
Blood alcohol concentration	Lower than women	Higher blood alcohol concentration
Blood alcohol level	150 lbs is expected to reach a blood alcohol level of around 0.10 g% after consuming 4 ounces of 100-proof spirits (50% alcohol)	150 lbs is expected to reach a blood alcohol level of around 0.12 g% after consuming 4 ounces of 100-proof spirits (50% alcohol)
Time to develop dependence	More compared to female	Less time to develop dependence
Severity and rate of complication	The severity and rate of development of complications less compared to women	More severity and faster rate of complication
Organ damage	Less compared to women	More susceptible for alcohol-related organ damage over a short period of time compared to men
Liver injury	Less compared to women	Alcohol-induced liver disease develops over a shorter period of time and after consuming less alcohol
Neurological effects	Less compared to women	More vulnerable to alcohol-induced brain damage than men
Cognitive impairment	Less compared to women	More cognitive impairment

Women typically have a higher percentage of body fat and lower volume of body water than men of similar weight.[18] This difference in body composition is influenced by hormonal differences, primarily the higher levels of estrogen in women.[19] This results in an increased concentration of alcohol in women's blood and organs when drinking the same amount of alcohol as men.[20] The volume of distribution in women is lower by 7.3% in women compared to men.[21] There are also differences in the metabolism of alcohol between men and women. Women typically have lower concentrations of alcohol dehydrogenase, an enzyme responsible for the initial metabolism of alcohol in the stomach.[22] This leads to a smaller amount of alcohol being broken down in the stomach before it enters the bloodstream. As a result, more alcohol reaches the bloodstream intact, leading to a higher blood alcohol concentration (BAC) in women compared to men. Additionally, gastric emptying is 42% lower in women with a 10% higher rate of oxidation and elimination occurring in the liver.[21] Typically, a male weighing 150 lbs is expected to reach a blood alcohol level of around 0.10 g% after consuming 4 ounces of 100-proof spirits (50% alcohol), four glasses of wine, or four beers. In contrast, a female of the same weight is projected to have a blood alcohol level of 0.12 g% when consuming equivalent amounts of alcohol.[23] The combination of a slower metabolism, and higher BAC makes women more vulnerable to the long-term effects of alcohol on major organs, such as the liver, heart, and brain.

■ COMORBIDITY AND EXTERNALIZING DISORDERS

Psychiatric illnesses that occur alongside SUDs often remain undetected, and the same is valid for SUDs in patients with psychiatric illnesses. Women with SUDs have a two to three times greater risk of psychiatry comorbidity compared to men.[2] About one in four women who have SUDs suffer from comorbid depression or anxiety.[24] About 40–70% of women using alcohol experience intimate partner violence, which increases the risk of PTSD. Women who use substances have a higher risk of medical comorbidity than men who use the same amount **(Table 3)**.

Externalizing problems during childhood have been associated with substance use during adolescence.[25] Externalizing disorders encompass a range of behaviors associated with self-regulation, such as aggression, hostility, violence, addictive tendencies, and disruptive or risk-taking behaviors.[26] The symptoms typically emerge in childhood or early adolescence. Common externalizing disorders include ADHD, oppositional defiant disorder, conduct disorder in childhood; SUDs, and antisocial personality disorder (ASPD) in adults.[27] Maternal and paternal substance use increases the risk of substance use in children along with an increase in externalizing and internalizing problems.[28]

In females, the clinical presentation of externalizing disorders differs from that observed in males. Females with ADHD exhibit a distinct set of behaviors and symptoms in comparison to males. In community samples, there is an indication of a higher prevalence of the inattentive type of ADHD in girls compared to boys.[22] It is important to consider gender differences in ADHD presentation as the symptom severity for hyperactive-impulse symptoms may be lower in females.[29] As hyperactivity and impulsivity are more likely to receive recognition and drive referrals, this contributes to underdiagnosis in females with the inattentive type of ADHD, especially when symptoms are less severe. Additionally, girls with ADHD are less prone than boys with ADHD to display conduct disorder, aggression, or delinquency, making them less likely to be referred for disruptive behavior assessments.[30] The less overt presentation in females compared to males often results in misdiagnosis as internalizing or personality disorders. Attention deficit hyperactivity disorder symptoms in females frequently become more noticeable at later ages, prompting them to engage in self-presentation. These symptoms are also exacerbated by hormonal changes during the menstrual cycle, pregnancy, and menopause.[31] When compared to males, females have more comorbidities and these appear to be more internalized disorders, such as anxiety and depression.[29] These internalizing symptoms are often misinterpreted as primary diagnosis leading to delays in diagnosis and management. Challenges related to emotional lability and emotional dysregulation are more prevalent and severe in girls and women with ADHD. Borderline personality traits become associated in women with hyperactivity or impulsivity.[32] Females with ADHD experience greater impairments in overall intellectual functioning compared to males.[33] They tend to engage in sexual activity at an earlier age compared to their peers, and they may also have a higher number of sexual partners. Additionally, there is an elevated risk of contracting sexually transmitted infections as well as increased rates of teenage, early, and unplanned pregnancies.[34] These females encounter bullying, heightened rates of school dropout, and poor self-esteem. They often resort to dysfunctional coping strategies, such as alcohol consumption or cannabis use, as a means of dealing with emotional distress, social isolation, and feelings of rejection.[29] Attention deficit hyperactivity disorder increases the risk of substance use (2–4x), delays treatment seeking, and prolongs the duration of SUD in adulthood.[35] Women are at a higher risk of developing SUDs compared to men with ADHD.[36] Females with ADHD, without any comorbidities, are at a higher risk of alcohol and cannabis abuse compared to males.[37] Teenage girls with ADHD who exhibit exclusion, truancy, and school phobia are at an increased risk for substance abuse, criminal activity, and early pregnancy.[29] Women with ADHD may experience anxiety and low mood due to failure to plan and achieve meaningful accomplishments, which can lead to harmful coping mechanisms such as self-harm and substance use.[38]

The assessment process for ADHD typically involves the use of rating scales, a clinical interview, and gathering objective information from family or organization. The drawback of many rating scales is that they often come with norms derived from male populations, posing a limitation when assessing females. In situations where specific norms for females are not available, relying on parental and school reports proves essential to ensure a more comprehensive assessment. One valuable assessment tool in this context is the Women's ADHD Self-Assessment Symptom Inventory (SASI).[39] It investigates childhood patterns and issues, as well as commonly observed adult symptoms associated with ADHD. The scale specifically explores childhood patterns of inattention, hyperactivity, learning, social and interpersonal issues, psychological aspects, and problematic behaviors, such as low frustration tolerance, oppositional defiant disorder (ODD), and disordered eating. It also encompasses challenges related to adult life, including aspects; such as parenting, workplace dynamics, and daily life maintenance tasks, such as housework, difficulties related to learning disabilities, hormonal issues, and experiences of abuse and trauma. As timely intervention results in long-term functional benefits, prompt identification is crucial. Specific barriers, including differences in symptom presentation, gender biases, comorbidities, and compensatory functions, impede the recognition of ADHD in girls and women. Recognizing how ADHD manifests in females is crucial for improving identification, assessment, and treatment processes and ultimately enhancing long-term outcomes for this population. It is important to consider how substance use can interact with medication used for ADHD treatment. Treatment of ADHD resulted in a reduction in criminality by 41%, which included substance-related crimes.[40]

Females with ASPD exhibit a higher tendency to engage in runaway behavior, and impulsivity, and display a lack of remorse in contrast with males who report more aggressive behaviors, including initiating fights, using weapons, cruelty to animals, setting fires, and reckless disregard for the safety of others.[41] Furthermore, females are more likely to have multiple sexual partners and experience higher rates of victimization and impairment whereas males are more prone to engaging in traffic offenses and arrests.[42] In conduct disorder, the age of onset is later in females with less aggressive behavior compared to males.[43] They exhibit relational aggression, which is defined as causing harm to others through purposeful manipulation.[44]

SUBSTANCE USE PATTERNS

The natural history, course, and response to treatment are distinct in women with SUD. When it comes to the initiation of substance use, women typically start at a later age compared to men. The reason for initiation in men is to enhance positive emotions or for recreation, while for women, it is to cope with negative emotions and stress.[45] Indian research suggests that the need to alleviate stress or frustration and curiosity are the common reasons for the initiation of substance use among women.[8] Further, older males serve as initiators of alcohol use in women.[8] The initiation of tobacco use in women is attributed to advertisements by the tobacco industry that promote weight loss as a perceived benefit.[46]

However, once initiated, there is a distinctive pattern seen in women as they display an accelerated progression in the rate of substance consumption. This phenomenon is known as "telescoping," signifying a rapid advancement from the initiation of substance use to the development of SUD.[47,48]

Women get intoxicated with smaller amounts of alcohol and have a higher risk of experiencing blackouts compared to men.[49] Moreover, there is an observation that women from higher socioeconomic backgrounds and with greater educational attainment are more prone to engaging in high-risk drinking, which includes heavy drinking.[50]

In India, tobacco use among women predominantly takes the form of smokeless tobacco, often in the application form and used to improve oral health and as a remedy for gastric problems. The form of tobacco used varies on the socioeconomic status of women, where smoked form is prevalent among women belonging to affluent status while smokeless in lower socioeconomic strata.[51]

In the case of opioid use, it has been observed that women typically initiate opioid usage following prescriptions from medical practitioners, as well as being influenced by husbands who use opioids for pain management.[52] Studies indicate that in comparison to men, women typically use smaller amounts of heroin, predominantly in inhalational form rather than injectable, and for shorter durations.[53] In India, among injectable drug users, the pattern of use among women is different compared to men.[54] A more significant proportion of women switched to injection drug use (IDU) faster compared to men. A higher proportion were sex workers, uneducated and unemployed. The choice of opioid and concomitant nonopioid is different compared to men. The needle sharing has been observed in more than half of the women.

Similar to International data, Indian women experience complications in multiple domains—physical, family, and social domains.[8] Some research suggests women experience more physical and psychiatric complications than social consequences.[48] Women using drugs, both injectable and noninjecting, were exposed to multiple sexual partners and unsafe sexual practices like less usage of contraceptive methods. This harms the sexual and reproductive health of women.[55] Alcohol and drug use among women is associated with an increased risk of transmission of human immunodeficiency virus (HIV).[56]

Compared to men, gender-based violence (GBV) is significantly higher in frequency and intensity among women using substances, which include sexual violence, internal personal violence, and trauma. This problem is often hidden in the substance-using population.[57] The prevalence rates of lifetime IPV in women with SUDs range between 40 and 70% compared to 17–35% in the general population.[58] Drug use results in loss of consciousness and inability to defend making them vulnerable to physical and sexual violence.[59] This violence increases the risk of incidence of physical (sexually transmitted infections) and mental illness (depression and anxiety). Women using substances usually are engaged in relationships with substance-using partners. They initiate women into drug use and sometimes are forced to use drugs with their partners. Addicted partners also support their drug use through their indulgence in prostitution. Hence, they suffer a higher prevalence of intimate partner violence.

Alcohol plays an important role in the perpetuation of GBV and in coping with victimization among women.[60] Alcohol acts as a proximal factor along with distal factors like relationship problems in the perpetuation of GBV. Additive use of drugs further increases the risk of violence. A recent meta-analysis suggests that drug use has a significantly stronger association with victimization, compared with alcohol use.[61] Although minimal research is available, integrated gender-sensitive interventions are required for the management of gender-based violence among women using substances.[62]

SCREENING AND DIAGNOSIS OF SUBSTANCE USE DISORDERS IN WOMEN

Screening is an essential process that helps identify potential risks associated with harmful or hazardous substance use. It also educates patients to prevent the progression of SUD. Primary healthcare providers play a vital role in screening and referring women for substance use.[19] Several screening instruments have been created, each varying in the substance they assess, the method of administration, and the specific population they target **(Table 4)**. Screening tools such as Alcohol Use Disorders Identification (AUDIT), AUDIT-C, and cut, annoyed, guilty, and eye (CAGE) are used for alcohol use. AUDIT-C is a three-question screening tool used to screen for alcohol use. It has a cutoff of 0 for pregnant women and ≥3 for nonpregnant women. Screening for tobacco use can be done through the Fagerstrom Test for Nicotine Dependence (FTND) and the Fagerstrom Test for Nicotine Dependence-Smokeless tobacco (FTND-ST) for smokeless tobacco.[63] Alcohol, Smoking, and Substance Involvement Screening Test (ASSIST) and the National Institute on Drug Abuse (NIDA) Quick Screen have been used to screen for overall drug use.[64] Apart from this, screening should include other comorbidities like depression, PTSD, violence, and other medical issues. For screening for violence, tools such as the Intimate Partner Violence Screening Tool (STaT) and the Indian Family Violence and Control Scale (IFVCS) are

TABLE 4: Medical and psychiatric comorbidities among women with SUDs.

Medical comorbidities	Psychiatric comorbidities
• Liver disease (cirrhosis) • Cardiovascular diseases • Diabetes Mellitus • Gastrointestinal diseases • Breast and cervical cancer • Vaginal infection • HIV and HCV	• Depression • Anxiety • Eating disorders • PTSD • ADHD

(ADHD: attention deficit hyperactivity disorder; HCV: hepatitis C virus; HIV: human immunodeficiency virus; PTSD: post-traumatic stress disorder)

TABLE 5: Screening tools for substance use among women.

Alcohol	• (Alcohol Use Disorder Identification Test (AUDIT) • Cut-down, Annoyed, Guilty, and Eye-opener (CAGE) • Michigan Alcoholism Screening Test (MAST)
Cannabis	• Cannabis Use Disorder Identification Test (CUDIT) • Cannabis Use Disorder Identification Test-Revised (CUDIT-R) • Cannabis-Abuse Screening Test (CAST) • Marijuana Screening Inventory
Tobacco	• Fagerstrom Test for Nicotine Dependence (FTND) • Fagerstrom Test for Nicotine Dependence-Smokeless Tobacco (FTND-ST)
Prenatal women	• Substance Use Risk Profile- Pregnancy Scale (SURPPS) • Tolerance, Worried, Eye-openers, Amnesia, (K) Cut down (TWEAK) • T-ACE screening tool • Prenatal Substance Abuse Screen (5Ps) • Wayne Indirect Drug Use Screener (WIDUS) • Substance Use Risk Profile-Pregnancy (SURP-P)

available.[65,66] Specifically in pregnancy, Take (Number of Drinks), Annoyed, Cut Down, Eye-Opener (T-ACE), Tolerance, Worried, Eye-opener, Amnesia, Kut down (TWEAK), and Wayne Indirect Drug Use Screener (WIDUS) have been validated. Substance Use Risk Profile-Pregnancy Scale (SURP-P) and WIDUS are screening tools **(Table 5)** that can be utilized to assess substance use, encompassing a broader spectrum beyond alcohol alone.[67] While screening is used to evaluate the presence of substance use, diagnosis is essential as it defines the severity of the problem and has a role in formulating treatment. Diagnostic and Statistical Manual of Mental Disorders, Fifth Edition (DSM-5) and International Classification of Diseases-10/11th edition (ICD-10/11) are commonly used tools for diagnostic purposes.

PATHWAYS TO CARE, ACCESSIBILITY, AND TREATMENT SEEKING

Accessing treatment becomes more challenging for women with SUD, as they encounter multiple barriers resulting in reduced rates of treatment seeking. In a study conducted by Basu et al., it was reported that <1% of women in India sought treatment for substance use.[68] The reasons for low treatment seeking are systemic barriers; such as lack of gender-specific services for women, limited decision-making authority, and restricted knowledge of professionals due to inadequate research; structural barriers such as poor knowledge about treatment location and concerns related to costs, inadequate awareness about the availability of treatment facilities, limited knowledge about the necessity for treatment, and fear of losing child custody **(Fig. 1)**. Moreover, social factors like insufficient support from family, stigma, and lower education levels further contribute to the challenges. Among all these factors, stigma is the most important barrier.

Additionally, vulnerable populations such as commercial sex workers, immigrant women, and HIV-positive women are the most disadvantaged among all. Targeted interventions focused on the hidden population are essential.[56] Upon entering treatment, women frequently exhibit a more severe clinical profile characterized by a heightened prevalence of comorbidities spanning both physical and psychiatric disorders. Furthermore, beyond these comorbidities, the additional impact of the partner's substance use and violence accentuates the complexity. Thus, the treatment needs of women should be tailored according to sociocultural, parenting status, and presence of comorbidities **(Table 6)**.

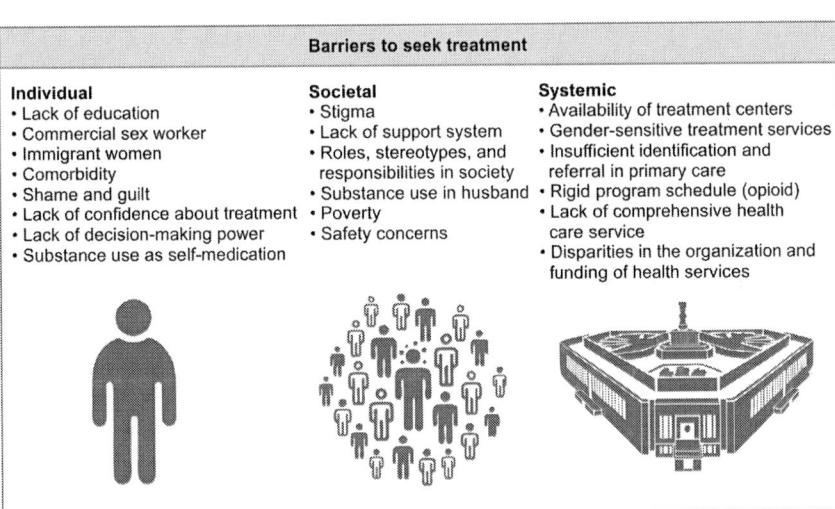

Barriers to seek treatment		
Individual	**Societal**	**Systemic**
• Lack of education	• Stigma	• Availability of treatment centers
• Commercial sex worker	• Lack of support system	• Gender-sensitive treatment services
• Immigrant women	• Roles, stereotypes, and responsibilities in society	• Insufficient identification and referral in primary care
• Comorbidity	• Substance use in husband	• Rigid program schedule (opioid)
• Shame and guilt	• Poverty	• Lack of comprehensive health care service
• Lack of confidence about treatment	• Safety concerns	
• Lack of decision-making power		• Disparities in the organization and funding of health services
• Substance use as self-medication		

Fig. 1: Barriers to seeking treatment among women with substance use disorders.

TABLE 6: Summary of differences between substance use patterns among men and women.

Category	Men	Women
Onset	The peak risk period is late adolescence	Later age compared to men
Reason for initiation	To enhance positive emotion or for recreation	To cope with negative emotions or stress
Binge drinking	Higher rate	A lower rate than men
Tobacco	Smoked form is more common	The smokeless form is more common
Opioid	Injection drug use is more common	More prescription drug use and inhalational form
Illicit drug	More prevalent in men	Less prevalent compared to men
Telescoping	Not common	Common
Consequences	Less compared to women with the same duration of use	More physical and psychiatric complications
Psychiatric comorbidities	Higher rates of externalizing disorders such as conduct disorder and antisocial personality	Higher rate of anxiety and depressive disorders
Social impairment	Less common compared to women	More social impairment
Legal problem	More common	Less common compared to men
Quality of life	Better compared to women	Poorer compared to men
Mortality	3-fold greater mortality rate relative to the general population	5-fold greater mortality rate relative to the general population
Treatment entry	More likely to seek treatment than women	Less likely to seek treatment
The time duration between initiation and disorder onset for seeking treatment	Seek treatment less quickly after substance use initiation and disorder onset	Seek treatment more quickly after substance use initiation and disorder onset
Access to treatment	Better	Poorer
Treatment setting	More likely to receive specialized SUD treatment	More likely to seek treatment in mental health treatment settings
Barrier to treatment	Less	Greater perceived stigma, childcare responsibilities, and lack of family support
Outcome of treatment	Better relative to women	Worse relative to men

MANAGEMENT OF SUBSTANCE USE DISORDERS IN WOMEN AND TREATMENT OUTCOMES

Compared to men, women are less likely to enter treatment.[69] It has been observed at the time of entry into treatment, women have greater severity of problems. Women's engagement and retention to treatment is low compared to men.[2] A single-center study found that women seeking substance use treatment generally have poor follow-up and treatment outcomes.[8] Some studies reported women who completed treatment had better outcomes, and addressing the unique needs of women is important. Women with comorbidities were found to have poor treatment outcomes.

Cognitive behavioral therapy, motivational interviewing, contingency management, couples therapy, and alcohol anonymity were found to be effective.[2,70,71] According to earlier research, the gender of a patient has no impact on treatment outcomes.[69] Gender-specific and sensitive treatment programs are effective compared to traditional treatment programs initially developed for men.[72,73] In patients with cooccurring mental concerns, a recent review suggests the usefulness of integrated gender-responsive treatments.[74] The treatment needs of women with SUDs are different from those of men. The quality of therapeutic relationships, addressing stigma and discrimination from the health care system, and support and informational needs were identified in the Indian context.[75] Women empowerment has been associated with a reduction in intimate partner violence.[76] Furthermore, sociocultural factors should be integrated as a part of management to improve treatment outcomes.[2]

In comparison to men, women face more challenges in quitting smoking, and the relapse rate is also higher, often attributed to concerns related to weight gain. The role of gonadal steroid hormones has also been suggested, and it has been found that women who attempt to quit during the follicular phase have a higher success rate than those attempting in the luteal phase of the menstrual cycle.[77] Among inpatient females with opioid use disorder, opioid use onset > 25 years, use of opioids for pain relief, and having a medical comorbidity are associated with a higher likelihood of treatment completion.[78]

SUBSTANCE USE DISORDERS AND PREGNANCY

Substance use during pregnancy is a significant health concern, resulting in various deleterious outcomes for both the mother and the fetus.[79] In vulnerable populations and indigenous tribals, substance use is woven into the cultural fabric.[80] Tobacco is the most commonly used substance in the perinatal period, followed by alcohol, cannabis, and other illicit substances.[81] According to a study conducted in India, 4.3% of preconception women used alcohol and tobacco.[82] Risk factors associated with substance use during pregnancy include a history of trauma or sexual abuse, domestic violence, familial substance use, low education levels, and comorbidities, such as depressive and anxiety disorders. Perinatal substance use is linked to a spectrum of effects on fetal development, including miscarriage, stillbirth, preterm birth, intrauterine growth restriction (IUGR), teratogenicity, and fetal alcohol syndrome due to alcohol exposure.

Given the complexity of perinatal substance use and its associated complications, screening of pregnant women is essential. Screening for substance use should be a part of comprehensive obstetric care starting from the first prenatal visit. A nonjudgmental approach should be practiced by healthcare professionals during the screening. Screening should also evaluate for conditions such as endocarditis, HIV, hepatitis C, history of sexual and/or physical abuse, and psychiatric disorders. Some commonly used screening instruments are NIDA Quick Screen, Prenatal Substance Abuse Screen (5Ps), T-ACE, TWEAK, and SURPPS.[83] Early identification and intervention are crucial for the well-being of both the mother and the fetus. If the evaluation indicates substance use, the next crucial step is to assess whether the patient engages in single or polysubstance use. This differentiation is vital as the consequences and the approach to treatment vary based on the specific substances involved. Abstinence and treatment lead to improved outcomes both for the mother and fetus. Patient education concerning the maternal and neonatal complications associated with substance use during pregnancy is crucial. In resource-limited settings, the use of technology can reduce the treatment gap. E-health interventions for SUDs during pregnancy are effective.[84] While psychosocial interventions remain the first line of management, pharmacotherapy is recommended for the management of conditions, such as opioid withdrawal, opioid agonist maintenance, and alcohol withdrawal **(Table 7)**. Clinicians should carefully consider the risks and benefits of prescribing pharmacological interventions, as there is insufficient evidence on the safety of agents found effective in nonpregnant women.

Alcohol Dependence

Alcohol consumption while breastfeeding can lead to the presence of alcohol in breast milk equivalent to the amount of alcohol in the bloodstream.[85] It also affects the production of breast milk through its impact on oxytocin and prolactin. Alcohol use during breastfeeding increases the risk of neurodevelopmental disorders like ADHD.

Alcohol withdrawal is a clinical emergency and untreated withdrawal can lead to placental abruption, preterm delivery, fetal distress, or death.[86] It is recommended to manage withdrawals in an inpatient setting.

TABLE 7: Different types of needs/services among women seeking treatment for substance use disorders.

Needs/services	Types of services
Gender-specific needs	• Gynecological care • Prenatal-care
Medical services	• Treatment of infectious diseases • HIV/AIDS services
Psychoeducation	• Education on the effects of alcohol and other substances on prenatal and child development • Education about STDs and other infectious diseases
Cultural and language needs	• Availability of treatment services in the native language • Addressing the cultural factors influencing substance intake
Mental health services	• Trauma-informed and trauma-specific services • Services for comorbid disorders, such as mood, anxiety, and PTSD
Family and child-related services	• Treatment focused on child-rearing • Stress reduction and coping skills

(AIDS: acquired immunodeficiency syndrome; HIV: human immunodeficiency virus; PTSD: post-traumatic stress disorder; STDs: sexually transmitted diseases)

Population-based cohort studies do not suggest a causal relationship between gestational benzodiazepines and z-drugs exposure with preterm birth, small for gestational age, autism spectrum disorder, and ADHD.[87,88] Evidence indicates toward the use of diazepam and chlordiazepoxide compared to the other agents.[89] Though controversial, benzodiazepine use during the first trimester is associated with an elevated risk of cleft palate, and use during the last trimester is associated with floppy infant syndrome.[89,90] Some clinicians recommend the use of lorazepam in the third trimester due to its shorter action and reduced neonatal benzodiazepine withdrawal.[91] Although the British Association of Pharmacology (BAP) does not recommend the use of any relapse prevention medication, acamprosate or naltrexone can be considered in women with a high risk of relapse **(Table 7)**.[92]

Tobacco Dependence

Tobacco use is associated with low birth weight, stillbirth, IUGR, sudden unexplained infant death, and prematurity. Nicotine replacement therapy (NRT) (gums, lozenges, and patches) is effective in pregnant women. Though NRT poses a risk to the fetus, it is less harmful compared to smoking. Varenicline, bupropion, and e-cigarettes do not have sufficient evidence for use during pregnancy. Population-based cohort studies found that smoking cessation pharmacotherapies (NRT, varenicline, and bupropion) are not associated with adverse perinatal events or major congenital malformations.[93]

Opioid Dependence

Women dependent on opioids (heroin crosses the placenta) experience a six-fold increase in maternal obstetric complications, such as low birth weight, toxemia, third-trimester bleeding, malpresentation, puerperal morbidity, fetal distress, and meconium aspiration.[94] Neonatal complications include withdrawal, postnatal growth deficiency, microcephaly, neurobehavioral problems, increased neonatal mortality, and a 74-fold increase in sudden infant death syndrome.

Women dependent on opioids should be started on opioid agonist maintenance treatment with buprenorphine or methadone to reduce harm and prevent relapses.[95] Methadone and buprenorphine have similar efficacy and safety for mother and baby. Though there are no teratogenic effects, there is a risk of neonatal abstinence syndrome (NAS) in >70% of neonates.[96] Therefore, neonates need to be managed in a neonatal intensive care unit with morphine or methadone along with non-pharmacological management. Buprenorphine may be associated with less NAS.[92] Women on either buprenorphine or methadone are encouraged to breastfeed and it is safe.[96]

Cannabis Dependence

Cannabis use in pregnancy is associated with a wide range of adverse outcomes in pregnancy and offspring.[97,98] Tetrahydrocannabinol (THC), the primary psychoactive component of cannabis readily crosses the placental barrier. No pharmacological agents are approved for the management of cannabis use, predominant approach is through psychosocial interventions to promote abstinence.[99] While a randomized controlled trial suggests cannabidiol to be safe and efficacious in the management of cannabis dependence, its utility, and adversity in pregnancy and breastfeeding is unknown.[100]

Benzodiazepine Dependence

During pregnancy, benzodiazepine dependence leads to NAS and floppy infant syndrome.[99] It is unclear about the duration of exposure and development of this syndrome. Benzodiazepine withdrawal can result in seizures and delirium. Therefore, it is important to manage with long-acting drugs like diazepam with a minimum effective dose and gradual tapering. It is preferable to manage in an inpatient setting. Though benzodiazepines are transferred through breast milk, it is less concerning at therapeutic doses; however, at higher doses, it can result in sedation in infants.

Stimulant Dependence and Others

The use of stimulants during pregnancy, such as cocaine, methamphetamines, ecstasy, and prescription stimulants is increasing. Stimulants are also used for the treatment of various conditions, such as ADHD and sleep disorders. Prenatal exposure to methamphetamine leads to withdrawal symptoms such as drowsiness, respiratory distress, and jitteriness and it also affects the serotonergic development of the brain.[101,102] There are reports of congenital anomalies such as limb reduction, cardiac defects, and neural tube defects[103,104] with methamphetamine. In a meta-analysis, there was a correlation between the use of methamphetamine during pregnancy and preterm delivery, low birth weight, and smaller head circumference.[101] The effect of cocaine on pregnant mothers is mostly cardiovascular, such as hypertension, myocardial infarction, and ischemia.[105] The cardiovascular complication is linked to increased susceptibility of the myocardium to elevated progesterone levels.[106] Perinatal effects are preterm birth, low birth weight, small for gestational age, and perinatal infection (HIV, hepatitis, and syphilis).[107,108] Cocaine also leads to structural anomalies, such as limb reduction and genitourinary defects.[109] Prenatal exposure to 3,4-methylenedioxymethamphetamine (MDMA), commonly known as ecstasy, leads to delayed gross and fine motor milestone attainment and impairment in long-term memory and learning.[110,111]

A comprehensive, multidisciplinary approach to clinical care, coupled with access to psychosocial support services, can significantly enhance the likelihood of treatment success for women dealing with SUDs[112] **(Table 8)**.

TREATMENT OF ATTENTION DEFICIT HYPERACTIVITY DISORDER IN PREGNANCY

Treatment of ADHD in nonpregnant women include stimulants such as methylphenidate, dexmethylphenidate, amphetamine, and dextroamphetamine; and nonstimulant drugs atomoxetine (norepinephrine reuptake inhibitor), clonidine (alpha-2 norepinephrine agonist), and guanfacine (alpha-2 norepinephrine agonist). Discontinuation of medication in women with ADHD can result in significant functional impairment. Due to the unavailability of systematic data, there is a lack of guidelines to recommend the use of ADHD medication during pregnancy and postpartum.[120] In general, all drugs used for the treatment of ADHD can cross the placenta, thereby exposing the developing embryo and fetus to these drugs when taken by the mother during pregnancy. While the available evidence does not confirm the major congenital malformations with stimulant medications, the long-term effects on neurocognitive development if unknown. A small increased risk of cardiovascular malformations is reported with methylphenidate, not with amphetamine. Modafinil may be associated with an increased risk of

TABLE 8: Management of substance use disorders among pregnant women.

Substance	Psychological intervention	Pharmacological intervention
Tobacco	• Screening, brief intervention, and referral to treatment (SBIRT) should be part of the protocol for all substance-using pregnant women • Smoking cessation counseling and other psychosocial interventions are recommended as first-line treatment and are found to be effective[113]	• Nicotine replacement therapy with behavioral support was effective[114] • No positive or negative impacts on birth outcomes • Varenicline did not establish safety during pregnancy or breastfeeding • Insufficient evidence for the use of Bupropion or e-cigarettes
Cannabis	Cognitive behavioral therapy (CBT), motivational enhancement therapy (MET), and combination were found to be effective[115]	None
Alcohol	Brief interventions and motivational interviewing are effective[116]	• Clinical significant withdrawal symptoms can be managed with benzodiazepines estimating the risk-benefits[90] • Acamprosate or Naltrexone can be considered.[117,118] Disulfiram is to be avoided
Opioid	• Screening, brief intervention, and referral to treatment have been found to be effective • Contingency management has been studied with mixed results[119]	• Methadone and Buprenorphine have similar efficacy and safety as opioid agonist maintenance treatment for pregnant women and babies[95] • A buprenorphine monoproduct is advisable compared to buprenorphine–naloxone combination[94] • Neonatal abstinence syndrome (NAS) requires a neonatal intensive care unit management with morphine or methadone, along with nonpharmacological management[119]

congenital malformations (including congenital heart defects, hypospadias, and orofacial clefts). Therefore, modafinil should not be initiated in pregnancy. Women of childbearing age should be advised to use effective contraception during treatment with modafinil and for 2 months after discontinuing treatment. Therefore, the use of these medications may be a consideration, and careful discussions with healthcare professionals are essential to assess potential risks and benefits during pregnancy. In addition to having a grasp of the overall risks and benefits associated with ADHD medications during pregnancy, it is crucial to pay specific attention to the link between untreated ADHD and substance use. The information on the use of atomoxetine, guanfacine, and clonidine during pregnancy is limited. Limited data is available to guide regarding the use of stimulants during breastfeeding. Transmission through breast milk can negatively affect fetal growth, sleep, and appetite.[121] Nonpharmacological strategies like cognitive behavior therapy should be encouraged for the management of ADHD during pregnancy.

In summary, if functional impairment is severe, the benefit of stimulant medication use can outweigh the risks of medication exposure (both known and unknown).[121] If a decision is made to take ADHD medication, women should be informed of the known risks and benefits of the medication use in pregnancy and take the lowest therapeutic dose possible; nonpharmacologic approaches should be maximized.

CONCLUSION

Substance use is a significant concern in India, especially among women. Tobacco is the most used substance among women, followed by alcohol and other drugs. While the prevalence of tobacco use among women has reduced in the last decade, the change in patterns of other substances is unknown. Differences in biological, genetic, environmental, and psychosocial factors determine the vulnerability to SUDs. Physiologically women develop higher intoxicating effects, faster dependence, and greater complications with similar doses of alcohol. Women suffer greater medical and psychiatric comorbidities compared to men. Externalizing disorders particularly ADHD increase the vulnerability to SUDs and have an important role in their management. Substance use patterns among women differ from men in terms of delayed age of onset, negative affective state as a common reason for initiation, telescoping effect, and poor treatment seeking. Many screening tools have been validated for women using substances, including during pregnancy. Management of SUDs during pregnancy and lactation poses unique challenges and requires an individualized multi-disciplinary approach. Women suffer barriers at an individual, societal, and systemic level in their pathways to care. While regular psychosocial interventions are effective, gender-specific and sensitive interventions are useful compared to traditional treatment. Treatment outcomes in the Indian context were poor, and more research needs to be done to understand various dimensions of substance use among women.

> **KEY POINTS**
> - In India, women have a lower prevalence of substance use than men.
> - Externalizing disorders, particularly ADHD increase the vulnerability to SUDs.
> - Individual, societal, and systemic barriers exist in the pathways to care.
> - The outcomes of treatment in India are not satisfactory and require further research.

REFERENCES

1. Seedat S, Scott KM, Angermeyer MC, Berglund P, Bromet EJ, Brugha TS, et al. Cross-National Associations Between Gender and Mental Disorders in the World Health Organization World Mental Health Surveys. Arch Gen Psychiatry. 2009;66(7):785-95.
2. Polak K, Haug NA, Dillon P, Svikis DS. Substance Use Disorders in Women. Psychiatr Clin North Am. 2023;46(3):487-503.
3. Polak K, Haug NA, Drachenberg HE, Svikis DS. Gender Considerations in Addiction: Implications for Treatment. Curr Treat Options Psychiatry. 2015;2(3):326-38.
4. Ambekar A, Agrawal A, Rao R, Mishra AK, Khandelwal SK, Chadda R. Magnitude of substance use in India. New Delhi: Minist Soc Justice Empower Gov India; 2019.
5. Lal R, Deb KS, Kedia S. Substance use in women: Current status and future directions. Indian J Psychiatry. 2015;57(Suppl 2):S275-85.
6. Ghosal S, Sinha A, Kanungo S, Pati S. Declining trends in smokeless tobacco use among Indian women: findings from global adult tobacco survey I and II. BMC Public Health. 2021;21(1):2047.
7. Khanra S, Singh U, Munda SK, Das B. Demographic and clinical profile of women receiving inpatient treatment at a deaddiction unit of a psychiatric hospital in India: Five years' observation. Ind Psychiatry J. 2022;31(1):177-80.
8. Nebhinani N, Sarkar S, Gupta S, Mattoo SK, Basu D. Demographic and clinical profile of substance abusing women seeking treatment at a de-addiction center in north India. Ind Psychiatry J. 2013;22(1):12-6.
9. Ambekar A, Parmar A, Therthani S, Mandal P. Profile of women substance users seeking treatment at a tertiary care treatment center in India: A retrospective chart review study. J Subst Use. 2017;22(5):507-10.
10. Supriya S, Shanmugam SB, Ezhumalai S. Profile of Women Seeking Treatment for Substance Use Disorder. J Psychos Wellbeing. 2(1):68-75.
11. Andersen ML, Sawyer EK, Howell LL. Contributions of neuroimaging to understanding sex differences in cocaine abuse. Exp Clin Psychopharmacol. 2012;20(1):2-15.
12. van den Bree MBM, Johnson EO, Neale MC, Pickens RW. Genetic and environmental influences on drug use and abuse/dependence in male and female twins. Drug Alcohol Depend. 1998;52(3):231-41.
13. Maes HH, Neale MC, Ohlsson H, Sundquist J, Sundquist K, Kendler KS. Genetic and Cultural Transmission of Alcohol Use Disorder in Swedish Twin Pedigrees. J Stud Alcohol Drugs. 2023;84(3):368-77.
14. Heath AC, Bucholz KK, Madden PA, Dinwiddie SH, Slutske WS, Bierut LJ, et al. Genetic and environmental contributions to alcohol dependence risk in a

national twin sample: consistency of findings in women and men. Psychol Med. 1997;27(6):1381-96.
15. Kathirvel S, Thakur J, Sharma S. Women and tobacco: A cross sectional study from North India. Indian J Cancer. 2014;51(Suppl 1):S78-82.
16. Malhotra S, Shah R. Women and mental health in India: An overview. Indian J Psychiatry. 2015;57(Suppl 2):S205.
17. Perkins JM, Lee HY, Lee JK, Heo J, Krishna A, Choi S, et al. Widowhood and Alcohol, Tobacco, and Other Drug Use Among Older Adults in India. J Gerontol B Psychol Sci Soc Sci. 2018;73(4):666-74.
18. Bredella MA. Sex Differences in Body Composition. Adv Exp Med Biol. 2017;1043:9-27.
19. Substance Abuse Treatment: Addressing the Specific Needs of Women. Rockville (MD): Substance Abuse and Mental Health Services Administration (US); 2009.
20. Mumenthaler MS, Taylor JL, O'Hara R, Yesavage JA. Gender Differences in Moderate Drinking Effects. Alcohol Res Health. 1999;23(1):55-64.
21. Baraona E, Abittan CS, Dohmen K, Moretti M, Pozzato G, Chayes ZW, et al. Gender Differences in Pharmacokinetics of Alcohol. Alcohol Clin Exp Res. 25(4):502-7.
22. Mowlem FD, Rosenqvist MA, Martin J, Lichtenstein P, Asherson P, Larsson H. Sex differences in predicting ADHD clinical diagnosis and pharmacological treatment. Eur Child Adolesc Psychiatry. 2019;28(4):481-9.
23. Koob GF, Arends MA, Le Moal M. Alcohol. In: Koob GF, Arends MA, Le Moal M, (Eds). Drugs, Addiction, and the Brain, 1st edition. San Diego: Academic Press; 2014.
24. Goldstein R. In: Brady KT, Back SE, Greenfield SF (Eds). Women and Addiction: A Comprehensive Handbook; 2009.
25. Miettunen J, Murray GK, Jones PB, Mäki P, Ebeling H, Taanila A, et al. Longitudinal associations between childhood and adulthood externalizing and internalizing psychopathology and adolescent substance use. Psychol Med. 2014;44(8):1727-38.
26. Samek DR, Hicks BM. Externalizing Disorders and Environmental Risk: Mechanisms of Gene-Environment Interplay and Strategies for Intervention. Clin Pract (Lond). 2014;11(5):537-47.
27. Huberty TJ. Emotional and Behavioral Problems, Students with. In: Spielberger CD (Ed). Encyclopedia of Applied Psychology. New York: Elsevier; 2004. pp. 723-30.
28. McGovern R, Bogowicz P, Meader N, Kaner E, Alderson H, Craig D, et al. The association between maternal and paternal substance use and child substance use, internalizing and externalizing problems: a systematic review and meta-analysis. Addiction. 2023;118(5):804-18.
29. Young S, Adamo N, Ásgeirsdóttir BB, Branney P, Beckett M, Colley W, et al. Females with ADHD: An expert consensus statement taking a lifespan approach providing guidance for the identification and treatment of attention-deficit/hyperactivity disorder in girls and women. BMC Psychiatry. 2020;20(1):404.
30. Biederman J, Mick E, Faraone SV, Braaten E, Doyle A, Spencer T, et al. Influence of Gender on Attention Deficit Hyperactivity Disorder in Children Referred to a Psychiatric Clinic. Am J Psychiatry. 2002;159(1):36-42.

31. Antoniou E, Rigas N, Orovou E, Papatrechas A, Sarella A. ADHD Symptoms in Females of Childhood, Adolescent, Reproductive and Menopause Period. Mater Sociomed. 2021;33(2):114-8.
32. Ende G, Cackowski S, Van Eijk J, Sack M, Demirakca T, Kleindienst N, et al. Impulsivity and Aggression in Female BPD and ADHD Patients: Association with ACC Glutamate and GABA Concentrations. Neuropsychopharmacology. 2016;41(2):410-8.
33. Attoe DE, Climie E. Miss. Diagnosis: A Systematic Review of ADHD in Adult Women. J Atten Disord. 2023;27(7):645-57.
34. Barkley RA, Fischer M, Smallish L, Fletcher K. Young adult outcome of hyperactive children: adaptive functioning in major life activities. J Am Acad Child Adolesc Psychiatry. 2006;45(2):192-202.
35. Zulauf CA, Sprich SE, Safren SA, Wilens TE. The Complicated Relationship Between Attention Deficit/Hyperactivity Disorder and Substance Use Disorders. Curr Psychiatry Rep. 2014;16(3):436.
36. Dalsgaard S, Mortensen PB, Frydenberg M, Thomsen PH. ADHD, stimulant treatment in childhood and subsequent substance abuse in adulthood - a naturalistic long-term follow-up study. Addict Behav. 2014;39(1):325-8.
37. Ottosen C, Petersen L, Larsen JT, Dalsgaard S. Gender Differences in Associations Between Attention-Deficit/Hyperactivity Disorder and Substance Use Disorder. J Am Acad Child Adolesc Psychiatry. 2016;55(3):227-34.e4.
38. Young S, Heptinstall E, Sonuga-Barke EJS, Chadwick O, Taylor E. The adolescent outcome of hyperactive girls: self-report of psychosocial status. J Child Psychol Psychiatry. 2005;46(3):255-62.
39. Nadeau K, Quinn P. Self-Assessment Symptom Inventory (SASI). [online] http://www.merkercounseling.com/ADHDSelfAssessmentWomen.pdf [Last accessed December, 2023].
40. Lichtenstein P, Halldner L, Zetterqvist J, Sjölander A, Serlachius E, Fazel S, et al. Medication for Attention Deficit-Hyperactivity Disorder and Criminality. N Engl J Med. 2012;367(21):2006-14.
41. Goldstein RisëB, Powers SI, McCusker J, Mundt KA, Lewis BF, Bigelow C. Gender differences in manifestations of antisocial personality disorder among residential drug abuse treatment clients. Drug Alcohol Depend. 1996;41(1):35-45.
42. Mikulich-Gilbertson SK, Salomonsen-Sautel S, Sakai JT, Booth RE. Gender similarities and differences in antisocial behavioral syndromes among injection drug users. Am J Addict. 2007;16(5):372-82.
43. Lindner P, Savic I, Sitnikov R, Budhiraja M, Liu Y, Jokinen J, et al. Conduct disorder in females is associated with reduced corpus callosum structural integrity independent of comorbid disorders and exposure to maltreatment. Transl Psychiatry. 2016;6(1):e714.
44. Gelhorn H, Hartman C, Sakai J, Mikulich-Gilbertson S, Stallings M, Young S, et al. An Item Response Theory Analysis of DSM-IV Conduct Disorder. J Am Acad Child Adolesc Psychiatry. 2009;48(1):42-50.
45. Annis HM, Graham JM. Profile types on the Inventory of Drinking Situations: Implications for relapse prevention counseling. Psychol Addict Behav. 1995;9(3):176-82.

46. Saladin ME, Gray KM, Carpenter MJ, LaRowe SD, DeSantis SM, Upadhyaya HP. Gender Differences in Craving and Cue Reactivity to Smoking and Negative Affect/Stress Cues. Am J Addict. 2012;21(3):210-20.
47. Randall CL, Roberts JS, Del Boca FK, Carroll KM, Connors GJ, Mattson ME. Telescoping of landmark events associated with drinking: a gender comparison. J Stud Alcohol. 1999;60(2):252-60.
48. Selvaraj V, Suveera P, Ashok MV, Appaya MP. Women alcoholics : are they different from men alcoholics ? Indian J Psychiatry. 1997;39(4):288-93.
49. Brienza RS, Stein MD. Alcohol Use Disorders in Primary Care: do gender-specific differences exist? J Gen Intern Med. 2002;17(5):387-97.
50. Shiri SS, Shanmugam B, Ezhumalai S. Profile of Women Seeking Treatment for Substance Use Disorder in Tertiary Care Government De-Addiction Centre. J Psychosoc Well Being. 2021;2(1):68-75.
51. Goyal LD, Verma M, Garg P, Bhatt G. Variations in the patterns of tobacco usage among indian females - findings from the global adult tobacco survey India. BMC Womens Health. 2022;22(1):442.
52. Cicero TJ, Lynskey M, Todorov A, Inciardi JA, Surratt HL. Co-morbid pain and psychopathology in males and females admitted to treatment for opioid analgesic abuse☆. PAIN. 2008;139(1):127-35.
53. Greenfield SF, Back SE, Lawson K, Brady KT. Substance Abuse in Women. Psychiatr Clin North Am. 2010;33(2):339-55.
54. Ambekar A, Rao R, Agrawal A, Goyal S, Mishra A, Kishore K, et al. Pattern of Drug Use and Associated Behaviors Among Female Injecting Drug Users From Northeast India: A Multi-Centric, Cross-Sectional, Comparative Study. Subst Use Misuse. 2015;50(10):1332-40.
55. Sharma V, Sarna A, Tun W, Saraswati LR, Thior I, Madan I, et al. Women and substance use: a qualitative study on sexual and reproductive health of women who use drugs in Delhi, India. BMJ Open. 2017;7(11):e018530.
56. Kumar MS, Sharma M. Women and Substance Use in India and Bangladesh. Subst Use Misuse. 2008;43(8-9):1062-77.
57. Moir E, Gwyther S, Wilkins H, Boland G. Hidden GBV: Women and substance use. Front Psychiatry. 2022;13:939105.
58. Fonseca F, Robles-Martínez M, Tirado-Muñoz J, Alías-Ferri M, Mestre-Pintó JI, Coratu AM, et al. A Gender Perspective of Addictive Disorders. Curr Addict Rep. 2021;8(1):89-99.
59. Costa YRS, Lavorato SN, Baldin JJCMC. Violence against women and drug-facilitated sexual assault (DFSA): A review of the main drugs. J Forensic Leg Med. 2020;74:102020.
60. Shiva L, Shukla L, Chandra PS. Alcohol Use and Gender-Based Violence. Curr Addict Rep. 2021;8(1):71-80.
61. Cafferky BM, Mendez M, Anderson JR, Stith SM. Substance use and intimate partner violence: A meta-analytic review. Psychol Violence. 2018;8(1):110-31.
62. Romo-Avilés N, Tarriño-Concejero L, Pavón-Benítez L, Marín-Torres J. Addressing Gender-Based Violence in Drug Addiction Treatment: a Systematic Mapping Review. Int J Ment Health Addict. https://link.springer.com/article/10.1007/s11469-023-01072-4 [Last accessed December, 2023].

63. Wright TE. Screening, brief intervention, and referral to treatment for opioid and other substance use during infertility treatment. Fertil Steril. 2017;108(2):214-21.
64. Polak K, Kelpin S, Terplan M. Screening for substance use in pregnancy and the newborn. Semin Fetal Neonatal Med. 2019;24(2):90-4.
65. Kalokhe AS, Stephenson R, Kelley ME, Dunkle KL, Paranjape A, Solas V, et al. The Development and Validation of the Indian Family Violence and Control Scale. Plos One. 2016;11(1):e0148120.
66. Paranjape A, Liebschutz J. STaT: a three-question screen for intimate partner violence. J Womens Health (Larchmt). 2003;12(3):233-9.
67. Chang G, Ondersma SJ, Blake-Lamb T, Gilstad-Hayden K, Orav EJ, Yonkers KA. Identification of substance use disorders among pregnant women: A comparison of screeners. Drug Alcohol Depend. 2019;205:107651.
68. Basu D, Aggarwal M, Das PP, Mattoo SK, Kulhara P, Varma VK. Changing pattern of substance abuse in patients attending a de-addiction centre in north India (1978-2008). Indian J Med Res. 2012;135(6):830-6.
69. Greenfield SF, Brooks AJ, Gordon SM, Green CA, Kropp F, McHugh RK, et al. Substance abuse treatment entry, retention, and outcome in women: A review of the literature. Drug Alcohol Depend. 2007;86(1):1-21.
70. McCrady BS, Epstein EE, Hallgren KA, Cook S, Jensen NK. Women with alcohol dependence: A randomized trial of couple versus individual plus couple therapy. Psychol Addict Behav. 2016;30(3):287-99.
71. Kelly JF, Hoeppner BB. Does Alcoholics Anonymous work differently for men and women? A moderated multiple-mediation analysis in a large clinical sample. Drug Alcohol Depend. 2013;130(1-3):186-93.
72. Schamp J, Simonis S, Roets G, Van Havere T, Gremeaux L, Vanderplasschen W. Women's views on barriers and facilitators for seeking alcohol and drug treatment in Belgium. Nord Stud Alcohol Drugs. 2021;38(2):175-89.
73. Kissin WB, Tang Z, Campbell KM, Claus RE, Orwin RG. Gender-Sensitive Substance Abuse Treatment and Arrest Outcomes for Women. J Subst Abuse Treat. 2014;46(3):332-9.
74. Johnstone S, Dela Cruz GA, Kalb N, Tyagi SV, Potenza MN, George TP, et al. A systematic review of gender-responsive and integrated substance use disorder treatment programs for women with co-occurring disorders. Am J Drug Alcohol Abuse. 2023;49(1):21-42.
75. Thomas R, Pandian RD, Murthy P. Treatment service related needs and concerns of women with substance use disorders: a qualitative study. Int J Cult Ment Health. 2018;11(2):123-33.
76. Parekh A, Tagat A, Kapoor H, Nadkarni A. The Effects of Husbands' Alcohol Consumption and Women's Empowerment on Intimate Partner Violence in India. J Interpers Violence. 2022;37(13-14):NP11066-88.
77. Wetherill RR, Franklin TR, Allen SS. Ovarian Hormones, Menstrual Cycle Phase, and Smoking: a Review with Recommendations for Future Studies. Curr Addict Rep. 20161;3(1):1-8.
78. Dayal P, Sarkar S, Balhara YPS. Predictors of Inpatient Treatment Completion among Females with Opioid Use Disorder: Findings from a Tertiary Care Drug Dependence Treatment Centre of India. Indian J Psychol Med. 2017;39(4): 464-8.

79. Ruisch IH, Dietrich A, Glennon JC, Buitelaar JK, Hoekstra PJ. Maternal substance use during pregnancy and offspring conduct problems: A meta-analysis. Neurosci Biobehav Rev. 2018;84:325-36.
80. Pati S, Chauhan AS, Mahapatra P, Hansdah D, Sahoo KC, Pati S. Weaved into the cultural fabric: a qualitative exploration of alcohol consumption during pregnancy among tribal women in Odisha, India. Subst Abuse Treat Prev Policy. 2018;13(1):9.
81. Prince MK, Daley SF, Ayers D. Substance Use in Pregnancy. In: StatPearls [Internet]. Treasure Island (FL): StatPearls Publishing; 2023.
82. Biradar RA, Halli SS. Alcohol and tobacco use among preconception women in India. J Subst Use. 2023;28(3):320-4.
83. Coleman-Cowger VH, Oga EA, Peters EN, Trocin KE, Koszowski B, Mark K. Accuracy of Three Screening Tools for Prenatal Substance Use. Obstet Gynecol. 2019;133(5):952-61.
84. Silang K, Sanguino H, Sohal PR, Rioux C, Kim HS, Tomfohr-Madsen LM. eHealth Interventions to Treat Substance Use in Pregnancy: A Systematic Review and Meta-Analysis. Int J Environ Res Public Health. 2021;18(19):9952.
85. Dejong K, Olyaei A, Lo Jo. Alcohol Use in Pregnancy. Clin Obstet Gynecol. 2019;62(1):142-55.
86. Manning V, Wanigaratne S, Best D, Hill RG, Reed LJ, Ball D, et al. Changes in neuropsychological functioning during alcohol detoxification. Eur Addict Res. 2008;14(4):226-33.
87. Chan AYL, Gao L, Howard LM, Simonoff E, Coghill D, Ip P, et al. Maternal Benzodiazepines and Z-Drugs Use during Pregnancy and Adverse Birth and Neurodevelopmental Outcomes in Offspring: A Population-Based Cohort Study. Psychother Psychosom. 2023;92(2):113-23.
88. Huitfeldt A, Sundbakk LM, Skurtveit S, Handal M, Nordeng H. Associations of Maternal Use of Benzodiazepines or Benzodiazepine-like Hypnotics During Pregnancy With Immediate Pregnancy Outcomes in Norway. JAMA Netw Open. 2020;3(6):e205860.
89. Bellantuono C, Tofani S, Di Sciascio G, Santone G. Benzodiazepine exposure in pregnancy and risk of major malformations: a critical overview. Gen Hosp Psychiatry. 2013;35(1):3-8.
90. DeVido J, Bogunovic O, Weiss RD. Alcohol Use Disorders in Pregnancy. Harv Rev Psychiatry. 2015;23(2):112-21.
91. Day E, Daly C. Clinical management of the alcohol withdrawal syndrome. Addiction. 2022;117(3):804-14.
92. Lingford-Hughes A, Welch S, Peters L, Nutt D. BAP updated guidelines: evidence-based guidelines for the pharmacological management of substance abuse, harmful use, addiction and comorbidity: recommendations from BAP. J Psychopharmacol (Oxf). 2012;26(7):899-952.
93. Tran DT, Preen DB, Einarsdottir K, Kemp-Casey A, Randall D, Jorm LR, et al. Use of smoking cessation pharmacotherapies during pregnancy is not associated with increased risk of adverse pregnancy outcomes: a population-based cohort study. BMC Med. 2020;18(1):15.
94. Cook JL, Green CR, de la Ronde S, Dell CA, Graves L, Ordean A, et al. Epidemiology and Effects of Substance Use in Pregnancy. J Obstet Gynaecol Can. 2017;39(10):906-15.

95. Minozzi S, Amato L, Jahanfar S, Bellisario C, Ferri M, Davoli M. Maintenance agonist treatments for opiate-dependent pregnant women. Cochrane Database Syst Rev. 2020;(11):CS006318.
96. Reddy UM, Davis JM, Ren Z, Greene MF; Opioid Use in Pregnancy, Neonatal Abstinence Syndrome, et al. Opioid Use in Pregnancy, Neonatal Abstinence Syndrome, and Childhood Outcomes: Executive Summary of a Joint Workshop by the Eunice Kennedy Shriver National Institute of Child Health and Human Development, American College of Obstetricians and Gynecologists, American Academy of Pediatrics, Society for Maternal-Fetal Medicine, Centers for Disease Control and Prevention, and the March of Dimes Foundation. Obstet Gynecol. 2017;130(1):10-28.
97. Grant KS, Petroff R, Isoherranen N, Stella N, Burbacher TM. Cannabis use during pregnancy: Pharmacokinetics and effects on child development. Pharmacol Ther. 2018;182:133-51.
98. Paul SE, Hatoum AS, Fine JD, Johnson EC, Hansen I, Karcher NR, et al. Associations Between Prenatal Cannabis Exposure and Childhood Outcomes: Results From the ABCD Study. JAMA Psychiatry. 2021;78(1):64-76.
99. Wilson CA, Finch E, Kerr C, Shakespeare J. Alcohol, smoking, and other substance use in the perinatal period. BMJ. 2020;369:m1627.
100. Freeman TP, Hindocha C, Baio G, Shaban ND, Thomas E, Astbury D, et al. Cannabidiol for the treatment of cannabis use disorder: a phase 2a, double-blind, placebo-controlled, randomised, adaptive Bayesian trial. Lancet Psychiatry. 2020;7(10):865-74.
101. Kalaitzopoulos DR, Chatzistergiou K, Amylidi AL, Kokkinidis DG, Goulis DG. Effect of Methamphetamine Hydrochloride on Pregnancy Outcome: A Systematic Review and Meta-analysis. J Addict Med. 2018;12(3):220-226.
102. Won L, Bubula N, Heller A. Fetal exposure to methamphetamine in utero stimulates development of serotonergic neurons in three-dimensional reaggregate tissue culture. Synapse. 2002;43(2):139-44.
103. Nora J, Vargo T, Nora A, Love K, Mcnamara D. Dexamphetamine: A possible environmental trigger in cardiovascular malformations. The Lancet. 1970;295(7659):1290-1.
104. Matera RF, Zabala H, Jimenez AP. Bifid exencephalia. Teratogen action of amphetamine. Int Surg. 1968;50(1):79-85.
105. Lange RA, Hillis LD. Cardiovascular complications of cocaine use. 2001;345(5):351-8.
106. Woods JR, Plessinger MA. Pregnancy increases cardiovascular toxicity to cocaine. Am J Obstet Gynecol. 1990;162(2):529-33.
107. Bauer CR, Langer JC, Shankaran S, Bada HS, Lester B, Wright LL, et al. Acute Neonatal Effects of Cocaine Exposure During Pregnancy. Arch Pediatr Adolesc Med. 2005;159(9):824-34.
108. Gouin K, Murphy K, Shah PS; Knowledge Synthesis group on Determinants of Low Birth Weight and Preterm Births. Effects of cocaine use during pregnancy on low birthweight and preterm birth: systematic review and metaanalyses. Am J Obstet Gynecol. 2011;204(4):340.e1-2.
109. Chávez GF, Mulinare J, Cordero JF. Maternal Cocaine Use During Early Pregnancy as a Risk Factor for Congenital Urogenital Anomalies. JAMA. 1989;262(6):795-8.

110. Singer LT, Moore DG, Min MO, Goodwin J, Turner JJD, Fulton S, et al. Developmental outcomes of 3,4-methylenedioxymethamphetamine (ecstasy)-exposed infants in the UK. Hum Psychopharmacol. 2015;30(4):290-4.
111. Skelton MR, Williams MT, Vorhees CV. Developmental effects of 3,4-methylenedioxymethamphetamine: a review. Behav Pharmacol. 2008;19(2):91-111.
112. Forray A. Substance use during pregnancy. F1000Res. 2016;5:F1000 Faculty Rev-887.
113. Chamberlain C, O'Mara-Eves A, Porter J, Coleman T, Perlen SM, Thomas J, et al. Psychosocial interventions for supporting women to stop smoking in pregnancy. Cochrane Database Syst Rev. 2017;2(2):CD001055.
114. Claire R, Chamberlain C, Davey MA, Cooper SE, Berlin I, Leonardi-Bee J, et al. Pharmacological interventions for promoting smoking cessation during pregnancy. Cochrane Database Syst Rev. 2020;3(3):CD010078.
115. Groff D, Bollampally P, Buono F, Knehans A, Spotts H, Bone C. Interventions Addressing Cannabis Use During Pregnancy: A Systematic Review. J Addict Med. 2023;17(1):47-53.
116. Popova S, Dozet D, Pandya E, Sanches M, Brower K, Segura L, et al. Effectiveness of brief alcohol interventions for pregnant women: a systematic literature review and meta-analysis. BMC Pregnancy Childbirth. 2023;23(1):61.
117. Kelty E, Terplan M, Greenland M, Preen D. Pharmacotherapies for the Treatment of Alcohol Use Disorders During Pregnancy: Time to Reconsider? Drugs. 2021;81(7):739-48.
118. Reus VI, Fochtmann LJ, Bukstein O, Eyler AE, Hilty DM, Horvitz-Lennon M, et al. The American Psychiatric Association Practice Guideline for the Pharmacological Treatment of Patients With Alcohol Use Disorder. Am J Psychiatry. 2018;175(1):86-90.
119. Tobon AL, Habecker E, Forray A. Opioid use in pregnancy. Curr Psychiatry Rep. 2019;21(12):118.
120. Freeman MP. ADHD and Pregnancy. Am J Psychiatry. 2014;171(7):723-8.
121. Baker AS, Freeman MP. Management of Attention Deficit Hyperactivity Disorder During Pregnancy. Obstet Gynecol Clin North Am. 2018;45(3):495-509.

CHAPTER 8

Sexual Problems and Management

Adarsh Tripathi, Mohita Joshi

■ ABSTRACT

Female sexual dysfunction is not merely a medical issue; it is a deeply personal and often silent struggle that deserves understanding, empathy, and effective solutions. This chapter provides an in-depth exploration of female sexual problems. It begins by creating a clear framework to classify different types of female sexual dysfunctions and then proceeds to examine each disorder closely. A significant part of the chapter is focused on assessment of female sexual dysfunctions, followed by a holistic approach involving both pharmacological and nonpharmacological interventions to provide comprehensive and personalized care. In summary, this chapter serves as a comprehensive guide to understanding and managing female sexual issues.

Keywords: Women, sexual functioning, psychosocial interventions, female sexual dysfunction

■ INTRODUCTION

Evolution of the Concept of Female Sexual Dysfunction

The conceptualization of female sexual dysfunction (FSD) has undergone a historical evolution that reflects changing attitudes toward female sexuality.

In the late 19th century, a significant shift occurred in medical discourse when FSD was first recognized as a clinical concern. This coincided with the emergence of psychoanalytic theory pioneered by Freud.[1] However, during this period Freud's work on female sexuality mainly faced criticism for perpetuating myths and biases. Prior to this pivotal period, female sexuality remained largely disregarded and considered unimportant. The terms such as frigidity and sexual aversion syndrome were used in this period to describe a range of sexual problems in women, including a lack of sexual desire or interest, difficulty becoming aroused or achieving orgasm, and negative sexual experiences or associations.[2]

Masters and Johnson introduced the concept of "sexual dysfunction," in their book, "Human Sexual Inadequacy," which they defined as any persistent difficulties related to sexual functioning. They delineated a four-phase model known as the human sexual response cycle, which includes excitement, plateau, orgasm, and resolution. Additionally, they identified three distinct sexual disorders in females—dyspareunia, vaginismus, and orgasmic dysfunction, categorized as primary and secondary.[3] In 1979, Kaplan added the concept of desire as the first step in sexual response cycle.[4]

In the 1990s, the development of new diagnostic tools and treatments for sexual dysfunction led to an increased awareness of the importance of addressing women's sexual health concerns.[5]

In the early 1990s, Rosemary Basson challenged the traditional model of spontaneous sexual desire in women, which was based on the assumption that women experience sexual desire in the same way as men and that sexual stimuli are the primary source of desire. Basson gave the "circular model" of female sexual response, which emphasizes the interconnected nature of psychological, emotional, and physical factors in women's sexual functioning. This model emphasizes the importance of sexual context, including relationship dynamics, communication, and emotional intimacy, as well as the physical sensations of arousal.[6]

Overall, the understanding of FSD has evolved from a narrow, pathologizing perspective of women's sexual experiences to a more nuanced, contextualized view that recognizes the significance of individual differences and the multitude of complex factors that can influence a woman's sexual health and well-being.

Development of the Concept in International Classification of Diseases and Diagnostic and Statistical Manual of Mental Disorders

The classificatory system of FSD has undergone significant evolution over the years, with changes reflecting a growing understanding of the complexities of female sexuality and the need for more accurate diagnosis and treatment. The changes in classification systems for FSD have been driven by a deeper understanding of the complex interplay between psychological, physiological, and relational factors that contribute to sexual health mentioned in **Tables 1 and 2**.

It is worth noting that the field of FSD continues to evolve and future revisions of diagnostic classification systems may refine and further tailor the categories to better reflect the diverse experiences of women.

COMMON SEXUAL PROBLEMS IN FEMALES

Female Sexual Interest/Arousal Disorder

Female sexual interest/arousal disorder (FSIAD) emerged from the merger of female hypoactive sexual desire disorder (HSDD) and female arousal disorder (FSAD) in the DSM-5 [American Psychiatric Association (APA), 2013]. A comparison of FSIAD terminology in DSM-5 and International Classification of Diseases (ICD) is mentioned in **Table 3**.

TABLE 1: Evolution of female sexual dysfunction classification in the "Diagnostic and Statistical Manual of Mental Disorders."[7-11]

DSM-III	DSM-III-R (psychosexual dysfunctions)	DSM-IV (sexual dysfunctions)	DSM-5 (sexual dysfunctions)
Released in 1980, first included sexual problems as a separate category	• Sexual desire disorder/HSDD • Sexual aversion • Female sexual arousal disorder • Inhibited female orgasm • Dyspareunia • Vaginismus • Sexual dysfunction not otherwise specified	• Sexual desire disorder/HSDD • Sexual aversion • Female sexual arousal disorder • Orgasmic disorder • Dyspareunia • Vaginismus • Sexual dysfunction not otherwise specified • Sexual dysfunction due to a general medical condition and substance-induced sexual dysfunction	• FSIAD acknowledges that sexual desire and arousal are closely linked and that problems in one domain can impact the other • Genito-pelvic pain/penetration disorder encompassing dyspareunia and vaginismus • Female orgasmic disorder • Sexual dysfunction due to a general medical condition and substance-induced sexual dysfunction
The categories were more compartmentalized and did not account for the interplay of multiple factors in female sexual functioning			DSM-5, released in 2013, adopted a more comprehensive approach to diagnosing female sexual dysfunction

(FSIAD: female sexual interest/arousal disorder; HSDD: hypoactive sexual desire disorder)

Female sexual interest/arousal disorder is characterized by a lack of, or significantly reduced, sexual interest and/or arousal, requiring the presence of at least three of six symptoms. These symptoms include:
- Loss of interest in sexual activities
- Decreased occurrence of erotic thoughts or fantasies
- Hesitation to initiate sexual activities
- Lowered satisfaction from sexual experiences

CHAPTER 8: Sexual Problems and Management

TABLE 2: Evolution of female sexual dysfunction classification in the International Classification of Diseases (ICD).[7-11]

ICD-6	ICD-9	ICD-10	ICD-11
• First recognized in ICD-6, which was published in 1948, a classification for "frigidity" was introduced • The term "frigidity" was used to describe a lack of sexual desire in women, which was believed to be a psychological issue	• Introduced a classification for "sexual dysfunction, not caused by organic disorder or disease" • This classification included subcategories for male and female sexual dysfunction	• Category F52, which followed Cartesian dualism, dichotomizes disorders into "organic" and "nonorganic" categories • Organic sexual dysfunctions are included under diseases of the genitourinary system • "Nonorganic" sexual dysfunctions are categorized under the chapter on mental and behavioral disorders within the ICD-10	• Female sexual dysfunction is categorized under the section titled "Conditions related to sexual health" • ICD-11 also uses specifiers for life-long and acquired, situational, and generalized sexual dysfunctions • Includes information about co-occurring disorders, such as depression and anxiety, that could be contributing to sexual health problems

TABLE 3: A comparison of FSIAD terminology.[7-9]

DSM-5	ICD-10	ICD-11
FSIAD	F52.0—lack or loss of sexual desire F52.2—failure of genital response	HA00 hypoactive sexual desire dysfunction HA01 sexual arousal dysfunctions • HA01.0 female sexual arousal dysfunction • HA01.Y other sexual arousal dysfunctions

(DSM: Diagnostic and Statistical Manual of Mental Disorders; FSIAD: female sexual interest/arousal disorder; ICD: International Classification of Diseases)

- Weakened arousal in response to stimuli
- Lessened sensations, both genital and nongenital.

For a diagnosis, these symptoms must persist for approximately 6 months, cause significant distress, not be better explained by nonsexual mental disorders or relationship issues, and not exclusively result from medical conditions or substance use.

It is noteworthy that the DSM acknowledges age-related declines in sexual thoughts and response. The DSM-5 explicitly states that a mere desire discrepancy between partners is not sufficient to diagnose FSIAD and diagnosis relies heavily on subjective clinical judgment, considering factors such as gender and age.[7]

Prevalence

As FSIAD is new to the DSM, prevalence studies have not yet been published. However, previous work has examined the prevalence of low sexual interest (HSDD) and low sexual arousal (FSAD) in women. In a global survey involving women from 29 countries, reported instances of low sexual interest varied between 26% and 43%. Clinical diagnoses of HSDD, which consider distress levels, show prevalence rates ranging from 7.3% to 23%. These rates depend on factors such as a woman's age, cultural background, and reproductive status.[10]

Etiology

Sexual interest and arousal are influenced by a multitude of factors **(Fig. 1)**. Understanding these complexities is crucial for effective treatment and intervention.

Treatment

In addressing FSIAD, various therapeutic options are available to tackle low sexual desire in women. These approaches encompass hormonal therapies, including off-label use of testosterone through patches or pills, as well as estrogen treatment for conditions such as vulvovaginal atrophy and tibolone therapy.[11]

Medications such as flibanserin (Addyi) have gained Food and Drug Administration (FDA) approval due to their efficacy in increasing subjective reports of satisfying sexual events.[12] Additionally, the FDA-approved Eros clitoral therapy device increases blood flow to clitoris by gentle suction and offers a nonpharmaceutical option for women's sexual arousal concerns, which is an FDA-approved device for FSAD.[13]

It is noteworthy that vasodilator drugs, while under investigation, have shown a substantial placebo effect on women's sexual arousal. Bupropion, employed to counteract sexual dysfunction resulting from selective serotonin reuptake inhibitor (SSRI) treatment, has modestly improved sexual interest and arousal in nondepressed premenopausal women and those experiencing low sexual desire.[14]

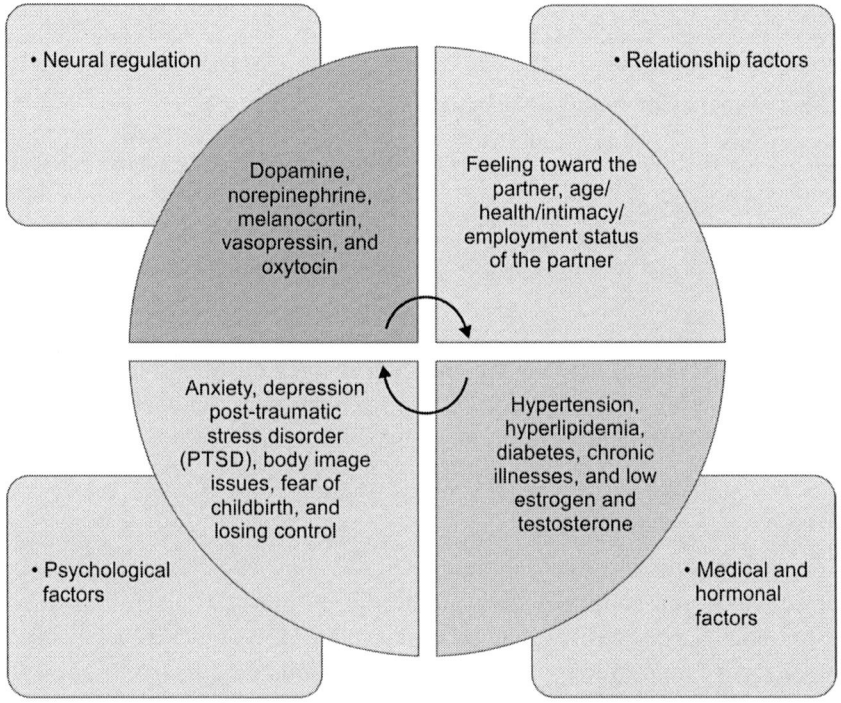

Fig. 1: Etiology of female sexual interest/arousal disorder (FSIAD).[11-13]

Orgasmic Disorder

Orgasm is characterized by intense pleasure creating an altered consciousness state, including pelvic muscle contractions and uterine contractions, leading to a sense of well-being. It can be induced by various forms of stimulation, including genital and nongenital sites, such as the clitoris, vagina, G-spot, breasts, mental imagery, or fantasy. Mechanical stimulation of the vagina, direct clitoral stimulation, or a combination of both can trigger female orgasms.[15]

Female orgasmic disorder (FOD) is defined as a persistent or recurrent delay in or absence of orgasm following normal sexual excitement, causing significant distress. This definition is consistent with the DSM-5 criteria, where the core issue is difficulty achieving orgasm, reduced intensity, or both. Diagnosis requires the presence of these symptoms in 75–100% of sexual encounters.[7] A comparison of orgasmic disorders in DSM-5 and ICD is mentioned in **Table 4**.

Prevalence

Limited prevalence studies on FSD exist due to sociocultural factors. In the United States (US), the PRESIDE (Female Sexual Problems Associated with

TABLE 4: A comparison of orgasmic disorders in DSM-5 and ICD.[7-9]

DSM-5	ICD-10	ICD-11
Female orgasmic disorder	F52.3 orgasmic dysfunction	• HA02 orgasmic dysfunctions • HA02.0 anorgasmia • HA02.Y other specified orgasmic dysfunctions

(DSM: Diagnostic and Statistical Manual of Mental Disorders; ICD: International Classification of Diseases)

Distress and Determinants of Treatment Seeking) study reported 20.5% with low orgasm and 4.7% distressed.[16] In India, a cross-sectional study found a 55.55% prevalence among reproductive-age women.[17]

Types

Female orgasmic disorder can manifest in various ways, including lifelong or acquired and generalized or situational. Primary FOD signifies never experiencing an orgasm, while secondary FOD develops after a period of normal orgasmic functioning. These distinctions emphasize the diverse presentations and the need for tailored interventions.[18]

Etiology

Sexual dysfunction arises from a multitude of factors, explained in **Figure 2**.

Treatment

Psychoeducation and behavioral interventions such as directed masturbation, sensate focus, along with cognitive behavioral therapy (CBT), have demonstrated efficacy in treating FOD, with higher success rates for lifelong or generalized cases.[20]

Other approaches such as systematic desensitization have limited evidence. Successful treatment often requires addressing both psychological and relational factors, acknowledging the intricate connection between mind and body in female orgasmic response.[21]

Genito-pelvic Pain/Penetration Disorder

Genito-pelvic pain penetration disorder (GPPPD) is a complex condition that encompasses various difficulties related to vaginal penetration during sexual activity. A comparison of genito-pelvic pain/penetration disorders in DSM-5 and ICD is mentioned in **Table 5**.

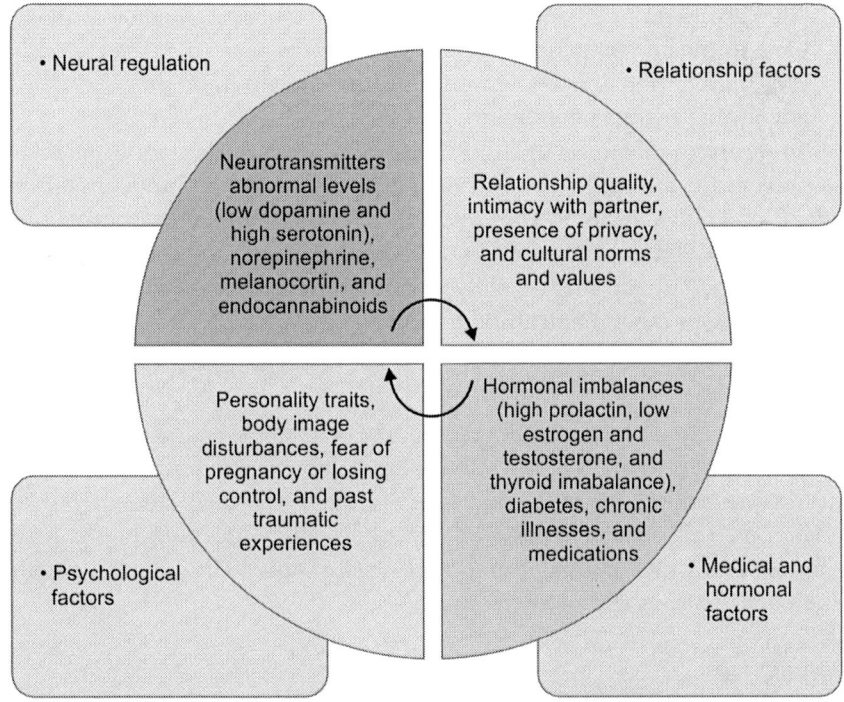

Fig. 2: Etiology of female orgasmic disorders.[19]

TABLE 5: A comparison of genito-pelvic pain/penetration disorders in DSM-5 and ICD.[7-9]		
DSM-5	**ICD-10**	**ICD-11**
• Consolidated dyspareunia or vaginismus, mentioned in prior DSM editions into a single disorder known as genito-pelvic pain penetration disorder • Should be for "at least 6 months"	Classifies female sexual penetration disorders into two broad categories: • F52.5 nonorganic vaginismus • F52.6 nonorganic dyspareunia	• Under "conditions related to sexual health" • HA20 sexual pain-penetration disorder • Should be for "at least several months"

(DSM: Diagnostic and Statistical Manual of Mental Disorders; ICD: International Classification of Diseases)

The diagnostic criteria for GPPPD, as outlined in DSM-5, include the presence of persistent or recurrent difficulties in one or more of the following areas:
- Penetration of the vagina during intercourse
- Noticeable pain in the vulvovaginal or pelvic region during attempts at vaginal intercourse or penetration

- Significant fear or anxiety related to the anticipation of vaginal or pelvic pain during or after penetration
- Pronounced tension or tightening of the pelvic floor muscles when attempting vaginal penetration.

To receive a diagnosis of GPPPD, at least one of these symptoms must be present for a duration of approximately 6 months and must result in significant clinical distress. These symptoms should not be better explained by a nonsexual mental disorder, relationship distress, or other significant stressors and should not be solely attributed to the effects of substances, medications, or other medical conditions.[7]

Types

Genito-pelvic pain penetration disorder is classified based on whether it is lifelong (present since the individual's sexual debut) or acquired (developed after a period of normal sexual functioning). It is also categorized as generalized (affecting all types of vaginal penetration, including intercourse, tampons, and medical examinations) or situational (limited to specific situations, typically sexual intercourse).[22]

Prevalence

Studies conducted prior to the implementation of DSM-5 typically assessed the occurrence of dyspareunia and vaginismus as separate entities. In a recent cross-sectional study by Alizadeh et al., 2019, involving 590 healthy married women aged 18–70 years, the reported prevalence of GPPPD was 10.5% when employing stricter criteria and 25.8% when using more relaxed criteria.[23]

However, there is limited available data regarding the prevalence of female sexual pain disorders (FSPD) in India and other developing Southeast Asian countries.

Etiology

Various factors can contribute to GPPPD **(Table 6)**, including heightened resting muscle tone in the pelvic floor muscles, which may exacerbate pain and discomfort.

Before diagnosing GPPPD, it is crucial to rule out organic factors that could cause genital pain, such as infections (e.g., genital herpes and candidiasis), dermatological conditions (e.g., lichen planus and lichen sclerosus), hormonal changes (e.g., menopause), tissue lesions, or anatomical anomalies (e.g., imperforate hymen and vaginal agenesis).[27]

A genito-pelvic examination is crucial, including pain mapping, vaginal pH measurement, and pelvic floor tonus evaluation. Additional exams such as biopsies or ultrasounds may be required based on history and physical examination findings.[28]

TABLE 6: Factors responsible for genito-pelvic pain/penetration disorders.[24-26]

Increased pelvic floor tone	Decreased vaginal blood flow, causing decreased lubrication, inadequate genital arousal, and increased penetration pain
Stress-induced central nervous system dysregulation	Amplify pain perception
Emotional factors such as anxiety	Trigger reflex contractions of the pelvic muscles
Hypervigilance and catastrophization	Individuals constantly monitor genital sensations and anticipate the worst possible outcome—play an important role in the fear-avoidance model
Psychological, relationship, and cultural factors: • Conservative religious upbringing • Abstinence until marriage • Negative sexual attitudes • Ignorance • Dysfunctional relationships or past abuse • Lack of sexual education	Might contribute, evidence supporting these associations is limited

Treatment

Addressing both physical and psychological aspects is often necessary for effective management and improved quality of life for those with GPPPD.

Throughout the 20th century and beyond, various treatment modalities have been employed for GPPPD. These include psychotherapy (e.g., psychoanalysis and couple therapy) and pharmacotherapy (e.g., local anesthetics, anxiolytic medications, and botulinum toxin).[29]

Recent studies indicate the efficacy of therapist-aided exposure for women with lifelong vaginismus, helping to reduce penetration fears, and avoidance behaviors. CBT aims to challenge common cognitive distortions such as hypervigilance and catastrophic pain. Encouraging the use of sexual fantasies, expressing emotions, and displaying physical affection help reduce anticipatory anxiety.[30]

Electromyographic biofeedback, pelvic floor physiotherapy, and electrostimulation are popular interventions. The combination of these modalities, including graded dilation and biofeedback, have shown some promise.[31]

SEXUAL PROBLEMS AND PSYCHIATRIC ILLNESS

Sexual problems among women with psychiatric illnesses remain a relatively under-recognized area of concern, particularly within the context of India.

These sexual dysfunctions can significantly impact an individual's recovery and overall quality of life, primarily because of unmet needs regarding sexuality and intimacy in those dealing with psychiatric conditions such as psychosis. Depression, a common psychiatric disorder, elevates the risk of developing sexual dysfunction by 50-70%, while in turn, sexual dysfunction increases the likelihood of depression by 130-210%.[32] Additionally, the disruptions in the hypothalamic–pituitary–adrenal axis, sympathetic nervous system, and inflammatory response systems triggered by depression can lead to conditions such as type 2 diabetes, further adversely affecting sexual function.[33] Patients with bipolar disorder often report a decrease in desire, arousal, and orgasm, with sexual dysfunction persisting as a residual symptom even when they achieve euthymic states. Furthermore, it can lead to poor adherence to prescribed medications, thereby complicating treatment outcomes.[32]

Anxiety and other prevalent psychiatric conditions can affect all phases of the sexual response cycle. It impedes arousal by increasing sympathetic tone, leading to issues such as erectile dysfunction in men and reduced lubrication and clitoral tumescence in women. Premature ejaculation is strongly linked to anxiety and is mediated by heightened sympathetic system activity. In women, excessive sympathetic activity during sexual arousal can create both genital congestion and nongenital sensations, which may be erroneously perceived as threatening by anxious individuals, ultimately diminishing sexual pleasure.[34]

In summary, sexual dysfunction and psychiatric illnesses often exist in a complex interplay, with each potentially exacerbating the other, ultimately leading to the perpetuation of illness and a decrease in overall quality of life.

SEXUAL PROBLEMS AND SUBSTANCE ABUSE

Substance use disorders play a pivotal role in impacting female sexual functioning, contributing to sexual dysfunctions through a complex biopsychosocial relationship. Psychoactive substances are frequently employed to initiate or enhance sexual encounters, but their effects vary. Alcohol use has a dose-dependent impact on sexual functioning, often manifesting as arousal problems, while opioids are linked to anorgasmia in females.

They themselves can precipitate or perpetuate sexual dysfunction. Patients with substance use disorders frequently experience co-occurring conditions such as depression and anxiety, which can significantly impact sexual functioning. Additionally, factors such as high levels of marital discord, delusional jealousy, and poor mutual understanding between partners are often prevalent and can either trigger or perpetuate sexual problems in this population.

Understanding the genesis of sexual dysfunction in individuals with substance use disorders necessitates careful examination of biological, psychological, and social factors. The causality between substance use disorder and sexual dysfunction calls for closer scrutiny, prompting questions about whether substance use leads to dysfunction or if preexisting dysfunction triggers substance use—a nuanced consideration in crafting effective interventions.[35,36]

It is crucial to address both substance-related issues and sexual dysfunction simultaneously in treatment. Additionally, healthcare providers should proactively look upon the potential sexual adverse effects of medications used for relapse prevention in these individuals to provide comprehensive care.

ASSESSMENT

Most women present with a complex combination of the aforementioned etiological factors, necessitating a comprehensive assessment that incorporates relevant biopsychosocial elements. Comprehensive management of FSD involves evaluating the points mentioned in **Table 7**.

TABLE 7: Factors to be evaluated while assessing female sexual dysfunctions.[37,38]

Organic factors	A complete medical history along with physical examination and relevant diagnostic tests can uncover underlying organic causes of sexual dysfunction due to conditions such as diabetes, cardiovascular problems, hormonal imbalances, and medication side effects
Presence of comorbid psychiatric conditions	• Psychiatric symptoms, both current and past, should be evaluated as they may be connected to sexual disorders • Comorbid psychiatric conditions, such as depression, anxiety, or post-traumatic stress disorder (PTSD), can also have a significant impact on sexual desire and satisfaction
Comorbid sexual dysfunction	Female sexual dysfunctions are related and identifying and treating comorbid sexual dysfunctions are critical for effective management
Marital disharmony	Recognizing the impact of relationship dynamics and marital disharmony on sexual satisfaction is crucial for resolving concerns and enhancing overall sexual well-being and intimate connection
Psychosocial history	• Understand the woman's age, culture, and religious beliefs as they can impact her sexual experiences and expectations • Discuss her sexual history, education, self-esteem, orientation, and awareness of her anatomy. Investigate her thoughts and emotions during sexual activity, identifying any misconceptions and anxiety triggers
Contextual factors	Also look for lack of privacy or lack of time during foreplay, stress, fatigue, unemployment, infertility, childbirth, or partner infidelity as important concerns, which may affect desire and arousal

Rating Scales

A few of the commonly applied rating scales are mentioned in **Table 8**.

Examination

A thorough general physical examination should be performed along with the local examination to assess signs for:
- Vaginal atrophy, such as dryness, loss of rugae, mucosal thinning, pale hue, and lack of shiny vaginal secretions which can indicate hormonal changes related to menopause
- To identify signs of local infection
- Assess the tension in the genital muscles, including involuntary contractions, either by palpation.[37]

Laboratory Investigations

- Vaginal secretions—pH, potassium hydroxide (KOH) mount, bacterial culture, sensitivity, etc.
- Diabetes screening, lipid levels, thyroid hormone, and prolactin levels should be done if there is history of an endocrine illness.
- Hormonal levels—testosterone, estrogen, and progesterone levels, when indicated
- Genital blood flow can be measured with vaginal photoplethysmography.[42]

■ MANAGEMENT—NONPHARMACOLOGICAL

The effective management of FSD requires a holistic, multidisciplinary approach that incorporates psychological and relational interventions alongside medical interventions.

There are some general strategies that have to be done with all the females presenting with sexual dysfunctions, as they improve overall well-being of the sexual life and some are specific strategies which are discussed later.

TABLE 8: Commonly used rating scales in the evaluation of female sexual dysfunction.[39-41]

Sexual problems	Rating scales
Female interest/arousal disorder	Female sexual function index (FSFI) (desire, arousal, orgasm, satisfaction, the relational aspect with a partner)
Orgasmic disorder	• FSFI • Arizona sexual experience scale-18 (ASEX)—assess multiple domains • Change in Sexual Functioning Questionnaire-20 (CSFQ)—assess multiple domains
Genito-pelvic/penetration disorder	McGill pain questionnaire, subjective rating of pain severity (numerical grading from 1 to 10) scales

General Strategies

Psychoeducation

- Exercises such as scheduling physical and emotional intimacy times
- Communication training to discuss sexual needs and concerns openly
- Balanced lifestyle and exercises
- Behavioral techniques to establish positive associations with sexual experiences
- Identifying and addressing distracting/negative thoughts during sexual activity
- Education about factors affecting sexual desire and relationship-building
- Addressing negative emotions, body image concerns, and performance anxiety
- Addressing prevailing myths is crucial for a healthier sexual mindset.

Kegel Exercises

Kegel exercises improve muscle tone and blood flow to the genital area, enhancing sexual pleasure, lubrication, and control during sex. Identify the right muscles (such as stopping urination midstream), contract for 5 seconds, relax for 5 seconds, repeat for sets of 10, and do it three times a day for better results. Consistency can lead to improved pelvic floor strength, bladder control, and reproductive health benefits.[39]

Sensate Focus

Sensate focus, introduced by Masters and Johnson, focuses on pleasurable touch rather than achieving orgasm. It involves gradual progression from nonsexual to sexual touch, creating a comfortable environment for couples to explore sensuality. Communication and gentle exploration of erogenous zones are key. This exercise strengthens emotional and physical bonds, reinvigorating relationships.[43]

Dual Sex Therapy

Dual sex therapy involves both partners collaborating to improve sexual communication and experiences. It helps with issues such as low desire, arousal problems, or pain during sex. The goal is open dialogue to identify and overcome barriers. Therapy includes tailored strategies, intimacy-building exercises, and education. It strengthens relationships and intimacy. Sessions are short-term and should be guided by a qualified therapist specializing in sexual therapy. It can effectively enhance sexual function and satisfaction for both partners.[44]

Specific Strategies

Directed Masturbation

Directed masturbation is a sex-positive education and self-awareness program, aiming to teach individuals self-stimulation and orgasm, even through partnered sex. It starts with self-exploration, identifying pleasure zones, and direct stimulation. It can include aids such as erotic material or vibrators. It is effective, particularly for women with orgasmic disorders. The program typically spans 4–6 weekly sessions, but it is crucial for individuals to engage voluntarily, with communication, consent, and boundaries respected in solo or partnered activities.

It is highly effective based on findings in the literature. Numerous small-scale randomized trials have highlighted the effectiveness of directed masturbation, particularly for women with primary female orgasmic disorder. These trials consistently demonstrate superior outcomes when compared to other psychosocial interventions or control conditions.[42]

Good Enough Sex

Embracing "good enough sex" emphasizes realistic age-appropriate expectations, relaxation, diverse sources of pleasure, variability, and playfulness. It promotes understanding changing desires with age, prioritizing relaxation, expanding pleasure beyond intercourse, embracing variability, and maintaining playfulness for intimacy and communication.[45]

Coital Alignment Techniques

The coital alignment technique (CAT) enhances pleasure and connection by synchronizing movements during sex. It intensifies clitoral stimulation, nurtures emotional intimacy, and encourages exploration and communication between partners. CAT can be applied to different positions such as spooning CAT, modified cowgirl CAT, and reverse CAT for variety and pleasure.[46]

Physical Therapy

Physical therapy, including pelvic muscle physiotherapy, vaginal dilators, and mindfulness techniques, helps address FSD by promoting pelvic muscle health and overall well-being. Pelvic muscle physiotherapy targets muscle tension to alleviate sexual pain. Vaginal dilators aid in gradual progression to improve comfort during penetration. Mindfulness techniques complement physical therapy by addressing emotional aspects. This integrated approach enhances both physical and emotional well-being, contributing to improved sexual health and satisfaction.[45-48]

Other Techniques

Mindfulness

Mindfulness enhances sexual desire and responsiveness, especially in group settings, with a recommended daily practice of 45 minutes, 6 days a week. Benefits include stress and pain reduction and improvements in desire, arousal, lubrication, orgasm, and satisfaction. Mindfulness heightens self-body awareness and pleasurable sexual experiences.

Two types of mindfulness interventions exist: First-generation, [first-generation, mindfulness-based interventions (FG-MBIs)] such as mindfulness-based stress reduction and mindfulness-based cognitive therapy, and second-generation, [second-generation, mindfulness-based interventions (SG-MBIs)] such as mindfulness awareness training, which integrate more meditation techniques and a spiritual aspect.

Mindfulness improves sexual function by increasing awareness of physical sensations, redirecting focus from performance to partner connection, fostering healthier and more satisfying sexual encounters.[47]

Cognitive Behavior Therapy

Cognitive behavioral therapy can be a valuable option when traditional sex therapy and education alone prove ineffective or inappropriate for addressing FSD. In the context of FSD, CBT embodies a collaborative, short-term, and goal-focused approach.

Cognitive behavioral therapy sessions are designed to be a partnership between the therapist and the individual seeking help. Goals are established following the SMART (Specific, Measurable, Achievable, Relevant, Time-bound) framework, ensuring precise and clear objectives for addressing the issues at hand.

A key characteristic of CBT is the utilization of Socratic dialogue and guided discovery. In this approach, the therapist's role is not to impart knowledge but rather to facilitate a collaborative journey of self-exploration and understanding, empowering individuals to make positive changes in their sexual functioning and overall well-being.[48]

■ MANAGEMENT—PHARMACOLOGICAL

The pharmacological management of FSD encompasses a range of options, including hormonal and nonhormonal medications, as well as the use of lubricants and vaginal moisturizers. Estrogen has been shown to improve vaginal dryness and irritation in postmenopausal women. Currently, there are no FDA-approved nonhormonal medications for treatment of FOD. Numerous nonhormonal treatment alternatives are accessible for addressing FSD such as vasorelaxants. Among the recent pharmaceutical options, flibanserin gained FDA approval in 2015 for its effectiveness in HSDD in women. Also, bremelanotide was approved by FDA in 2019 as a groundbreaking medication in premenopausal women Additionally, for concerns related to vaginal dryness and vulvovaginal pain syndrome, treatments such as vaginal lubricants and moisturizers have been employed with favorable outcomes.[49]

Vasorelaxants—Increasing Genital Blood Flow

Vasorelaxant effects increase vaginal blood flow. Vasorelaxants hold promise as one of the potential treatments for various forms of FSD. While some have shown positive effects in improving sexual function, more research and clinical evidence are needed to fully understand their mechanisms of action and determine their efficacy in addressing the complex issues surrounding female sexual health. Details of various vasorelaxants are mentioned in **Table 9**.

Hormones

During menopause, a decline in estrogen levels may result in various challenges, such as vaginal dryness, thinning and atrophy of the vaginal walls, increased vulnerability to vaginal infections, and a decrease in libido. For patients experiencing these symptoms, hormonal therapy is often recommended as a suitable intervention **(Table 10)**.[54]

Topical Applicants

Various topical applicants which are used to improve vaginal dryness and pain are mentioned in **Table 11**.

Flibanserin

Flibanserin, marketed as Addyi, was originally developed as an antidepressant. It was later repurposed due to its effects on sexual desire. It gained FDA approval in 2015 as the first medication aimed at treating HSDD in premenopausal women. Its various details are mentioned in **Table 12**.

Dopaminergic Agonists

These medications work by stimulating dopamine receptors in the brain, which can increase sexual response and desire. They have also shown promise in improving sexual function in women with HSDD. More research is needed in this area to fully understand the potential benefits and risks of using dopamine agonists for FSD. Commonly used dopaminergic agents are mentioned in **Table 13**.

TABLE 9: Different types of vasorelaxants.[50-53]

PDE5i	Prostaglandins inhibitors	NO donor and combination therapy	VIP
These medications increase pelvic blood flow to the clitoris and vagina through smooth muscle relaxation and the subsequent increase in intracellular cGMP levels	PGE1 initiates adenylate cyclase activity to convert ATP to cAMP, decreasing intracellular calcium ions in the cavernosal smooth muscle cells	L-arginine is converted to NO via NOS, causing an increase in NO and cGMP, which ultimately affects circulation and sexual function	VIP is a polypeptide hormone, containing 28 amino acid residues and is produced in many areas of the human body. VIP has potent vasorelaxant effects and has been suggested to contribute to vaginal blood flow control
Effective in increasing sexual arousal, satisfaction, and orgasm (Khashaba et al., 2023). Beneficial effects of PDE5i are seen in the setting of adverse side effects of SSRI use on orgasm	Although topical alprostadil is a potential new therapy for the treatment of FSAD. *More conclusive results from ongoing clinical studies are needed to further validate the use of topical alprostadil in the treatment of FSAD*	L-arginine, as part of a combination product, may be considered for the treatment of HSDD in women, regardless of age. *Additional research is warranted to determine the efficacy of L-arginine monotherapy in women with HSDD*	There is currently no conclusive data demonstrating its effectiveness in improving clitoral or vaginal blood circulation. Further research is required
Dosage: Sildenafil—25–100 mg daily over 4–12 weeks. Tadalafil—10/20 mg on demand or 5 mg once daily for 12 weeks	Topical alprostadil can have a vasodilating effect within 20 minutes of application that leads to enhancement of sexual functions		

(ATP: adenosine triphosphate; cAMP: cyclic adenosine monophosphate; cGMP: cyclic guanosine monophosphate; FSAD: female sexual arousal disorder; HSDD: hypoactive sexual desire disorder; NO: nitric oxide; NOS: nitric oxide synthase; PDE5i: phosphodiesterase 5 inhibitors; PGE1: prostaglandin E1; SSRI: selective serotonin reuptake inhibitors; VIP: vasoactive intestinal peptide)

TABLE 10: Hormonal treatment in treatment of female sexual dysfunction.[54,55]

Hormonal treatment	Mechanism of action	Indications	Dosage and administration	Potential side effects
Testosterone (oral, transdermal)	Increases testosterone levels in women, which can enhance sexual desire and arousal	• Hypoactive sexual desire disorder (HSDD) in premenopausal and postmenopausal women • Before starting oral testosterone therapy, testosterone levels should be measured at baseline and after 3–6 weeks to avoid supraphysiologic concentrations	• 300 mg/day patch has been reported effective in improving the desire women • Testosterone patches—applied to the skin once daily, typically on the lower abdomen or buttocks	• Alterations in mood or behavior • Potential cardiovascular risks (monitoring may be required) • Skin irritation or allergic reactions at the application site (more common with patches) • Changes in menstrual patterns (e.g., irregular periods) • Virilization in cases of excessive dosing (e.g., voice deepening, clitoral enlargement)
Estrogen (oral, intramuscular, transdermal, and intravaginal creams)	Increases estrogen levels in women, which can enhance sexual desire and arousal	Improve vaginal dryness and irritation in postmenopausal women, improves lubrication and desire, and decreases pain	Those with estrogen deficiency during menopause, 0.625 mg of estrogen or equivalent	• Dose-dependent increased risk of endometrial cancer with estrogen use (can lower with use of progesterone) • Lowered free testosterone

TABLE 11: Different topical applicants to treat female sexual dysfunction.[56-59]

Local anesthetics	• Decreases sensitization of the vulvovestibular nociceptive receptors, may help in GPPPD • Considered to be effective, placebo-controlled RCT has shown negative results
Capsaicin	• Acts on the vanilloid receptor and causes long-term desensitization of the nociceptor, may help in GPPPD • Efficacy data is limited
Estradiol (0.01%), testosterone (0.1%)	Improve the subjective-pain rating in women with GPPPD
Vaginal DHEA	Improves vaginal dryness and irritation and helps in increasing sexual desire
Vaginal lubricants and moisturizer	• For complaints of vaginal dryness, various vaginal moisturizers and lubricants can be used • They can provide short-term relief from vaginal dryness by reducing friction, thus relieving pain during sex

(DHEA: dehydroepiandrosterone; GPPPD: genito-pelvic pain/penetration disorder; RCT: randomized controlled trial)

TABLE 12: Flibanserin for hypoactive sexual desire disorder.[12,60]

Mechanism	Pharmacokinetics	Interactions	Indications	Dosage	Side effects
It is non-hormonal; it is 5-HT$_{1A}$ agonist and 5-HT$_{2A}$ antagonist, and moderate agonistic activity in 5-HT$_{2B}$, 5-HT$_{2C}$ and dopamine D$_4$ receptors Flibanserin functions by decreasing serotonin levels and increasing both dopamine and norepinephrine levels	Peak plasma concentration—1–4 hours Its oral bioavailability is 33% It has a half-life of around 11 hours, necessitating daily dosing With mild hepatic impairment, half-life increases to 26 hours	Interaction with strong CYP3A4 inhibitors can increase flibanserin concentrations, influencing its efficacy and potential side effects Notably, it interacts with alcohol, causing a heightened risk of hypotension and fainting	Indicated for premenopausal women diagnosed with hypoactive sexual desire disorder (HSDD), characterized by persistently low sexual desire, causing distress	Dose—100 mg once daily at bedtime It is discontinued after 8 weeks if no improvement occurs It is crucial to acknowledge that the benefits may take several weeks to manifest, necessitating patient commitment	Somnolence, sedation, fatigue, and dry mouth are the most common side effects

TABLE 13: Commonly used dopaminergic agents.[11,61]

Bupropion	Apomorphine
Bupropion is a dopamine and serotonin reuptake inhibitor	Dopamine agonist
In the context of FSD, it is considered an off-label treatment and may have a beneficial effect on women with FOD and HSDD	Apomorphine is not commonly used in the treatment of female sexual dysfunction and is more often associated with male sexual dysfunction (specifically, erectile dysfunction)
Bupropion has been found to have a lower incidence of sexual dysfunction in patients with major depressive disorder	Its use in female sexual dysfunction is less established and more research is needed to determine its effectiveness and indications in this context
Dosage: 150 mg twice a day, although lower doses, such as 75 mg twice a day, can also achieve optimal improvement in sexual arousal potential in some cases	*Dosage:* Sublingual apomorphine (2 and 3 mg) was found to be useful in some women with HSDD and FSAD

(FOD: female orgasmic disorder; FSAD: female sexual arousal disorder; FSD: female sexual dysfunction; HSDD: hypoactive sexual desire disorder)

TABLE 14: Bremelanotide in hypoactive sexual desire disorder.[62]

Mechanism	Pharmacokinetics	Interactions	Indications	Dosage	Side-effects
Agonists at melanocortin receptors, particularly MC4R and MC3R, stimulate dopamine in the medial preoptic area	• Peak plasma concentration—1 hour • Subcutaneous injection—100% bioavailability • Its half-life is 2.5 hours • The fast onset of action and relatively short half-life make bremelanotide suitable for on-demand use	Caution should be exercised when coadministering with potent CYP3A4 inhibitors due to potential effects on metabolism	It is indicated for premenopausal women diagnosed with HSDD, characterized by persistently low sexual desire causing distress The effect is even smaller than the reported effect of flibanserin	Administered intranasally or as a subcutaneous injection *Dosage:* 1.75 mg injected subcutaneously in the abdomen or thigh at least 45 minutes before sexual activity	• Nausea, vomiting, and flushing • Activation of MC1R receptors may contribute to the adverse effect of hyperpigmentation in 1%, limiting its use to eight doses per month • Contraindicated in individuals with uncontrolled hypertension or cardiovascular disease

(HSDD: hypoactive sexual desire disorder; MC4R: melanocortin 4 receptor)

TABLE 15: Other novel treatments in the treatment of female sexual dysfunctions.[61,63-66]

Other novel treatment	Mechanism of action	Administration	Side effects
BP101	Synthetic peptide molecule under investigation	Nasal spray in clinical trials	Promising results in female rats, significant impact on solicitation behavior when administered in the medial preoptic area (MPOA) of the brain. In phase II study level for hypoactive sexual desire disorder (HSDD)
Testosterone intranasal gel	Testosterone-based intranasal gel	Intranasal application	Improved genital and subjective sexual arousal in women with HSDD or anorgasmia. Safety and testosterone levels within normal limits
Oxytocin	Hormone released through posterior pituitary	Sublingual lozenges, with a dosage of 250 IU, typically taken 30 minutes to an hour before engaging in sexual activity	Emerging research suggests potential for enhancing libido, improving orgasms, and overall sexual satisfaction
Zestra	Blend of natural ingredients, including borage seed oil, angelica extract, evening primrose oil, coleus extract, and vitamins C and E	Topical application	Aims to enhance sexual arousal and pleasure in women by increasing sensitivity and improving overall sexual satisfaction

Bremelanotide

Bremelanotide, a synthetic peptide analog of the melanocortin alpha-melanocyte-stimulating hormone (α-MSH), has made significant strides in the realm of female sexual health. It gained FDA approval in 2019 as a groundbreaking medication for HSDD in premenopausal women.[62] Details of bremelanotide are mentioned in **Table 14**.

The journey through this chapter has illuminated the diverse spectrum of these issues, offering a clear framework for classification and a close examination of each disorder **Table 15**. The emphasis on assessment underscores the importance of tailored approaches.

> **KEY POINTS**
> - Recent classification emphasizes a biopsychosocial approach to female sexual health and recognizes the multifaceted nature of sexual disorders.
> - Understanding the interaction between psychological causes and organic factors is the key. Even when an organic cause is present, psychological factors can influence sexual interest. Acknowledging this interplay guides tailored treatment plans.
> - Nonpharmacological approaches such as psychotherapy, counseling, lifestyle changes, sexual education and enhanced sexual well-being. Open communication, a supportive environment, and tailored interventions addressing both physical and emotional factors are crucial for the successful management of FSD.
> - Effective pharmacological treatment for FSD, including vasorelaxants, FDA-approved options such as flibanserin and melanocortin, requires a thorough assessment, considering individual needs and potential side effects.

REFERENCES

1. Freud S, Freud A, Strachey A, Strachey J, Tyson AW (Eds).The Ego and the Id, and Other Works. London: Hogarth Press; 1961.
2. Freud S, Strachey J, Freud A. The Standard Edition of the Complete Psychological Works. London: Hogarth Press; 1955.
3. Masters WH, Johnson VE (Eds). Human Sexual Inadequacy. University of Michigan: Little, Brown; 1970.
4. Rosen RC, Barsky JL. Normal sexual response in women. Obstet Gynecol Clin. 2006;33(4):515-26.
5. Rosen RC, Leiblum SR. Treatment of sexual disorders in the 1990s: an integrated approach. J Consult Clin Psychol. 1995;63(6):877.
6. Basson R. Women's sexual dysfunction: revised and expanded definitions. CMAJ. 2005;172(10):1327-33.
7. DSM Library. (2022). Diagnostic and Statistical Manual of Mental Disorders, 5th edition. [online] Available from https://dsm.psychiatryonline.org/doi/book/10.1176/appi.books.9780890425596 [Last accessed December, 2023].
8. First MB. Harmonisation of ICD-11 and DSM-V: opportunities and challenges. Brit J Psychiatry. 2009;195(5):382-90.
9. World Health Organization (WHO). The ICD-10 Classification of Mental and Behavioural Disorders: Diagnostic Criteria for Research. Geneva: World Health Organization; 1993.
10. Bancroft J, Loftus J, Long JS. Distress About Sex: A National Survey of Women in Heterosexual Relationships. Arch Sex Behav. 2003;32(3):193-208.
11. Fooladi E, Davis SR. An update on the pharmacological management of female sexual dysfunction. Expert Opin Pharmacother. 2012;13(15):2131-42.
12. Stahl SM, Sommer B, Allers KA. Multifunctional pharmacology of flibanserin: possible mechanism of therapeutic action in hypoactive sexual desire disorder. J Sex Med. 2011;8(1):15-27.
13. Josefson D. FDA approves device for female sexual dysfunction. BMJ. 2000;320(7247):1427.

14. Stahl SM, Pradko JF, Haight BR, Modell JG, Rockett CB, Learned-Coughlin S. A review of the neuropharmacology of bupropion, a dual norepinephrine and dopamine reuptake inhibitor. Prim Care Companion J Clin Psychiatry. 2004;6(4):159.
15. Meston CM, Levin RJ, Sipski ML, Hull EM, Heiman JR. Women's orgasm. Ann Rev Sex Res. 2004;15(1):173-257.
16. Shifren JL, Monz BU, Russo PA, Segreti A, Johannes CB. Sexual problems and distress in United States women: prevalence and correlates. Obstet Gynecol. 2008;112(5):970-8.
17. Mishra VV, Nanda S, Vyas B, Aggarwal R, Choudhary S, Saini SR. Prevalence of female sexual dysfunction among Indian fertile females. J Midlife Health. 2016;7(4):154-8.
18. Parish SJ, Cottler-Casanova S, Clayton AH, McCabe MP, Coleman E, Reed GM. The evolution of the female sexual disorder/dysfunction definitions, nomenclature, and classifications: a review of DSM, ICSM, ISSWSH, and ICD. Sex Med Rev. 2021;9(1):36-56.
19. Pfaus JG. Pathways of sexual desire. J Sex Med. 2009;6(6):1506-33.
20. Heiman JR. Psychologic treatments for female sexual dysfunction: Are they effective and do we need them? Arch Sex Behav. 2002;31:445-50.
21. Brotto LA, Erskine Y, Carey M, Ehlen T, Finlayson S, Heywood M, et al. A brief mindfulness-based cognitive behavioral intervention improves sexual functioning versus wait-list control in women treated for gynecologic cancer. Gynecol Oncol. 2012;125(2):320-5.
22. Faubion SS, Rullo JE. Sexual dysfunction in women: a practical approach. Am Fam Physician. 2015;92(4):281-8.
23. Alizadeh A, Farnam F, Raisi F, Parsaeian M. Prevalence of and risk factors for genito-pelvic pain/penetration disorder: a population-based study of Iranian women. J Sex Med. 2019;16(7):1068-77.
24. Dias-Amaral A, Marques-Pinto A. Female Genito-Pelvic Pain/Penetration Disorder: Review of the Related Factors and Overall Approach. Rev Bras Ginecol Obstet. 2018;40(12):787-93.
25. Azim KA, Happel-Parkins A, Moses A, Haardoerfer R. Exploring Relationships Between Genito-Pelvic Pain/Penetration Disorder, Sex Guilt, and Religiosity Among College Women in the U.S. J Sex Med. 2021;18(4):770-82.
26. Berenguer-Soler M, Navarro-Sánchez A, Compañ-Rosique A, Luri-Prieto P, Navarro-Ortiz R, Gómez-Pérez L, et al. Genito Pelvic Pain/Penetration Disorder (GPPPD) in Spanish Women—Clinical Approach in Primary Health Care: Review and Meta-Analysis. J Clin Med. 2022;11(9):2340.
27. Revicky V, Mukhopadhyay S, Morris E. Dyspareunia in gynaecological practice. Obstet, Gynaecol Reprod Med. 2012;22(6):148-54.
28. Phillips NA. The clinical evaluation of dyspareunia. Int J Impot Res. 1998;10:S117-20.
29. Padoa A, McLean L, Morin M, Vandyken C. The overactive pelvic floor (OPF) and sexual dysfunction. Part 2: evaluation and treatment of sexual dysfunction in OPF patients. Sex Med Rev. 2021;9(1):76-92.
30. Conforti C. Genito-Pelvic Pain/Penetration Disorder (GPPPD): An overview of current terminology, etiology, and treatment. Womens Health. 2017;7(2):48.

31. da Silva Nunes AC, Lemos CIL, dos Santos Araújo N, Nunes EFC, Rodrigues CNC. Physiotherapeutic approach in genito-pelvic pain/penetration disorder. Man Ther Posturology Rehabil J. 2019;1-5.
32. Waldinger MD. Psychiatric disorders and sexual dysfunction. Handb Clin Neurol. 2015;130:469-89.
33. Hartmann U. Depression and sexual dysfunction: aspects of a multi-faceted relationship. Psychiatr Prax. 2007;34 Suppl 3:S314-7. [German].
34. Halvorsen JG, Metz ME. Sexual dysfunction, Part I: Classification, etiology, and pathogenesis. J Am Board Fam Pract. 1992;5(1):51-61.
35. Sarkar S, Chawla N, Tom A, Pandit PM, Sen MS. A systematic review of Indian studies on sexual dysfunction in patients with substance use disorders. Indian J Psychiatry. 2021;63(4):326-34.
36. Sakaluk JK, Kim J, Campbell E, Baxter A, Impett EA. Self-esteem and sexual health: a multilevel meta-analytic review. Health Psychol Rev. 2020;14(2):269-93.
37. Rosen RC. Assessment of female sexual dysfunction: review of validated methods. Fertil Steril. 2002;77:89-93.
38. Latif EZ, Diamond MP. Arriving at the diagnosis of female sexual dysfunction. Fertil Steril. 2013;100(4):898-904.
39. Rosen R. The Female Sexual Function Index (FSFI): a multidimensional self-report instrument for the assessment of female sexual function. J Sex Marital Ther. 2000;26(2):191-208.
40. Weinfurt KP, Lin L, Bruner DW, Cyranowski JM, Dombeck CB, Hahn EA, et al. Development and initial validation of the PROMIS˚ sexual function and satisfaction measures version 2.0. J Sex Med. 2015;12(9):1961-74.
41. Melzack R, Raja SN. The McGill pain questionnaire: from description to measurement. J Am Soc Anesthesiol. 2005;103(1):199-202.
42. Basson R, Althof S, Davis S, Fugl-Meyer K, Goldstein I, Leiblum S, et al. Summary of the recommendations on sexual dysfunctions in women. J Sex Med. 2004;1(1):24-34.
43. Regev L, Schmidt J. Sensate focus. In: O'Donohue WT, Fisher JE (Eds.). Cognitive Behavior Therapy: Applying Empirically Supported Techniques in your Practice. Washington, DC: John Wiley & Sons, Inc.; 2008. pp. 486-92.
44. Master WH, Johnson VE. Principles of the new sex therapy. Am J Psychiatry. 1976;133(5):548-54.
45. Metz ME, McCarthy BW. The "Good-Enough Sex" model for couple sexual satisfaction. Sex Relation Ther. 2007;22(3):351-62.
46. Pierce AP. The coital alignment technique (CAT): An overview of studies. J Sex Marital Ther. 2000;26(3):257-68.
47. Stephenson KR, Kerth J. Effects of mindfulness-based therapies for female sexual dysfunction: A meta-analytic review. J Sex Res. 2017;54(7):832-49.
48. Metz M, Epstein N, McCarthy B. Cognitive-behavioral therapy for sexual dysfunction. New York: Routledge; 2017.
49. Burton CS, Mishra K. Pharmacologic therapeutic options for sexual dysfunction. Curr Opin Obstet Gynecol. 2022;34(6):402-8.
50. Chen L, Staubli SE, Schneider MP, Kessels AG, Ivic S, Bachmann LM, et al. Phosphodiesterase 5 inhibitors for the treatment of erectile dysfunction: a trade-off network meta-analysis. Eur Urol. 2015;68(4):674-80.

51. Kielbasa LA, Daniel KL. Topical alprostadil treatment of female sexual arousal disorder. Ann Pharmacother. 2006;40(7-8):1369-76.
52. Wimalawansa SJ. Nitric oxide: new evidence for novel therapeutic indications. Expert Opin Pharmacother. 2008;9(11):1935-54.
53. Segraves RT. Emerging therapies for female sexual dysfunction. Expert Opin Emerg Drugs. 2003;8(2):515-22.
54. Kronawitter D, Gooren LJ, Zollver H, Oppelt PG, Beckmann MW, Dittrich R, et al. Effects of transdermal testosterone or oral dydrogesterone on hypoactive sexual desire disorder in transsexual women: results of a pilot study. Eur J Endocrinol. 2009;161(2):363-8.
55. Santoro N, Worsley R, Miller KK, Parish SJ, Davis SR. Role of estrogens and estrogen-like compounds in female sexual function and dysfunction. J Sex Med. 2016;13(3):305-16.
56. Burrows LJ, Goldstein AT. The treatment of vestibulodynia with topical estradiol and testosterone. Sex Med. 2013;1(1):30-3.
57. Edwards D, Panay N. Treating vulvovaginal atrophy/genitourinary syndrome of menopause: how important is vaginal lubricant and moisturizer composition? Climacteric. 2016;19(2):151-61.
58. Andelloux M. Products for sexual lubrication: understanding and addressing options with your patients. Nursing for Women's Health. 2011;15(3):253-7.
59. Sinha A, Ewies AAA. Non-hormonal topical treatment of vulvovaginal atrophy: an up-to-date overview. Climacteric. 2013;16(3):305-12.
60. Dooley EM, Miller MK, Clayton AH. Flibanserin: from bench to bedside. Sex Med Rev. 2017;5(4):461-9.
61. Fourcroy JL. Female sexual dysfunction: potential for pharmacotherapy. Drugs. 2003;63:1445-57.
62. Dhillon S, Keam SJ. Bremelanotide: first approval. Drugs. 2019;79(14):1599-606.
63. Nemenov D, Lomonosov M, Golikov D. 150 BP101 new molecule for HSDD treatment-results of proof-of-concept phase 2a study. J Sex Med. 2018;15(2):S41-2.
64. Krychman ML. Female sexual disorders: Treatment options in the pipeline. Formulary. 2013;48(3):113.
65. Muin DA, Wolzt M, Marculescu R, Rezaei SS, Salama M, Fuchs C, et al. Effect of long-term intranasal oxytocin on sexual dysfunction in premenopausal and postmenopausal women: a randomized trial. Fertil Steril. 2015;104(3):715-23.
66. Ferguson DM, Singh GS, Steidle CP, Alexander JS, Weihmiller MK, Crosby MG. Randomized, placebo-controlled, double-blind, crossover design trial of the efficacy and safety of Zestra for Women in women with and without female sexual arousal disorder. J Sex Marital Ther. 2003;29(Suppl 1):33-44.

Psychiatric Disorders in Older Women

CHAPTER 9

Debadatta Mohapatra, Tathagata Biswas, Shree Mishra

ABSTRACT

In older women, aging can pose new psychological challenges including role reversal, general discontentment about life, menopause, bereavement, social isolation, and a plethora of medical illnesses. Understandably, globally as well as in India, psychiatric morbidity among older women is common, notably mood disorders. This chapter primarily focuses on the impact of psychiatric disorders in older women and the pertinent risk and protective factors. Specific psychiatric disorders such as dementia, psychotic disorders, mood disorders, sleep and sexual disorders, and suicide, in the context of elderly women, are highlighted. Lastly, assessment and treatment considerations are discussed.

Keywords: Geriatric psychiatry, late life

INTRODUCTION

The Normal Aging Process in Women

Aging is a complex multifactorial process, largely influenced by one's genetics, lifestyle, and environment, involving physical, physiological, and psychological changes. Aging can affect all organ systems with a declining efficacy of the heart, lungs, muscles, and bones. The digestive and absorptive functions of the gut decrease causing low appetite and altered bowel habits. Hormonal fluctuations can result in a disrupted sexual life. Age-related changes in hormonal milieu, sleep, and sexual cycle have been described in the specific sections below, with a special focus on elderly women. Neuroimaging studies have shown global atrophic changes and volume loss in basal ganglia, thalamus, and limbic system. These changes are however slower in aging females, compared to males.[1]

The growing physical weakness and diminishing functionality with aging directly affect one's confidence and self-esteem. Older adults are haunted by fears of loss of control, perceived burdensomeness, and health-related worries. For traditional women, who had been catering to the needs of the family members for most part of her life, there occurs a gradual role reversal where she is in need of most care. This along with other psychosocial factors described below has immense psychological impact often leading to psychiatric disorders.[2]

Psychological Changes Associated with Aging

The psychological demands and sources of stress among women have been found to differ across their lifetimes. Although some studies found that middle-aged females at greater risk of stress due to "general life dissatisfaction", others reported favorable psychological health in them, especially in traditional women. Nevertheless, Schlossberg and Waters found women in their mid-life distressed over factors such as separation or divorce, loneliness, "empty nest," having dependent parents, role reversal with aging, and menopause. In contrast, a woman in late life is faced with higher risks of poverty, isolation, widowhood, and retirement. However, they also showed a greater psychological strength to survive.[3] Thus, the associations are not direct and it is a complex interplay among various psychosocial factors that dictates the final mental health outcome in elderly women.

■ IMPACT OF PSYCHIATRIC DISORDERS IN OLDER WOMEN

The global population of persons above the age of 60 years was 900 million in 2015, and is estimated to cross 2 billion in 2050.[4] Similar trend is also reflected in India, where the elderly population, which was about 140 million in 2021 is expected to cross 300 million (i.e., 20% of the total population) by 2050.[5] Such a demographic transition is a result of declining birth rate, increasing life expectancy, and decreasing mortality rate. Currently, most aging Indian citizens (80%) are residing in rural areas with poor accessibility to healthcare services. Moreover, almost a third of the elderly population in India are below the poverty line. Additionally, in both Western and Indian population, the ratio of women to men increases with aging.[5,6]

Globally, an estimated 6.6% of the total disability-adjusted life years (DALYs) and 17.4% of years lived with disability (YLD) for older persons are caused by mental and neurological disorders. The common mental illnesses among the elderly include depression, dementia, anxiety, and substance use (affecting 7%, 5%, 3.8%, and 1% of the world's older population, respectively).[7] Notably, elderly women are more affected by mental health problems than elderly men.[6] A study in a rural community in West Bengal, India, estimated 60% of the elderly population with mental illness, with higher morbidity among women (77.6%) versus men (42.4%). Morbidity was significantly higher above the age of 70 years.[8] Another study in Uttar Pradesh, India, estimated higher psychiatric morbidity in the geriatric group (43.32%) compared to the nongeriatric group (4.66%). The most common psychiatric disorder in the geriatric group was neurotic depression, followed by manic-depressive psychosis and anxiety states.[9] Mood disorders were also found as the most common psychiatric morbidity among the elderly in several other Indian studies.[10]

The functioning of elderly people is usually compromised due to the presence of chronic medical disorders. The presence of psychiatric disorders not only adds to the burden but also reduces their quality of life, further compromising their functioning, which in turn increases their dependence on a caregiver, leading to more caregiver burden.

Risk Factors for Psychiatric Disorders Specific to Older Women

In most societies today, women live significantly longer than men. Life expectancy at birth in India is 66.9 years among males and 70.0 years among females.[11] A longer lifespan inadvertently means a higher chance of developing and suffering from chronic illnesses. The complications of prolonged hypertension, diabetes, dyslipidemia, chronic heart-lung-kidney- and-liver diseases, and dementia increases with age. Also, greater longevity increases the chances of experiencing loss and loneliness. Unemployment, financial constraints, and inadequate access to services are common problems. Being a vulnerable group, elderly women are easy victims of abuse and neglect. Moreover, some mental illnesses such as depression, anxiety, and psychosis are more common in older women than male counterparts. Also, some conditions such as substance abuse and prescription medication abuse are understudied in elderly women.[12]

Menopause

The "climacteric" period in women coincides with the so-called "middle age", corresponds with progressive ovarian failure, is characterized by menstrual irregularities, and concludes with cessation of menses.[13] On average, women from Western countries attain menopause at the age of 51, much later than Indian women (average 46.2 years).[14] To an aging woman, menopause may symbolize loss of fertility and womanhood. The psychological impact may vary from reduced self-esteem to severe body image issues.[15] Additionally, the changing hormonal milieu may cause irritability, mood fluctuations, hot flashes, headache, and loss of libido.[13,15] Several studies have concluded menopausal women report higher rates of distress, anxiety, and depression.[16] This has traditionally been attributed to an imbalance in the hypothalamic-pituitary-gonadal axis and a fall in estrogen levels. Furthermore, hormonal replacement therapy (HRT) has shown beneficial effects in alleviating their depressive and anxiety symptoms. However, recent studies have demonstrated prior depressive episodes, increased stress, interpersonal issues, and other socioeconomic factors as more predictive of mood dysfunction in perimenopausal women.[15]

Bereavement and Loneliness

The loss of a spouse is a "major disruptive crisis" with a heavy toll on the mental health of the survivor. While grief is a normal process, it may often get complicated with intense, debilitating, and persistent (beyond 12 months) symptoms, inadequate integration, psychosis, and suicidality. Studies have reported that widowed females experience greater distress than their married counterparts,[3] attributable to the loss of financial and family support.[3] The stressful changes of widowhood were associated with a higher risk of death.[17] Literature suggests that widows missed various aspects of their previous relationship, such as having a companion, a love object, a person to share their time, and a state of being loved.[18]

The likelihood of becoming a widow is increased by the higher longevity in women and their tendency to marry older men. In one study, almost 20% of elderly women over 75 years reported widowhood.[19] Additionally, various situations may contribute to loneliness or isolation of elderly women such as neglect from children, severe dementia in spouse, and living in a nursing home with inadequate care. Also, social situations such as restrictions imposed during the coronavirus pandemic may increase isolation of the elderly persons. It has been found that 10% of people aged 65 years, mostly women, reported loneliness as a significant problem affecting their lives.[18]

Elder Abuse

It involves single or repetitive acts of commission or omission by persons within relationships built on trust resulting in harm or distress of an older individual. Elder abuse is a violation of human rights and may take many forms (physical, sexual, psychological, and emotional abuse, abandonment, neglect, disrespect, etc.).[7] A recent systemic review including 52 studies across 28 countries estimated that >15% of people above 60 years were subjected to abuse.[20] In institutional settings such as hospitals, nursing homes, and other facilities, about 64% of staff admitted to some form of elder abuse, the most prevalent being psychological abuse (33.4%).[21] Earlier studies have reported higher cases of elder abuse among older women (75%). Interestingly, the abuser is most likely a person close to the victim, her daughter, caretaker, or a female relative burnt out by the victim's long-term medical or financial issues.[2]

Comorbid Physical Illness

Aging increases the risk of developing various medical illnesses. It is estimated about 80% of people over 65 years of age suffer from at least one chronic medical condition, with women more commonly affected than men.[19] Common medical comorbidities include diabetes mellitus (DM), hypertension, dyslipidemia, hypothyroidism, and nutritional deficiencies. The leading cause of mortality in elderly women is cardiovascular disorders, with death occurring twice as often as men following their first myocardial infarction.[22] Similarly elderly women with orthostatic hypotension are at higher risks of falling and hip fractures than elderly men.[23] Additionally, osteoporosis is a common problem in elderly women partly due to decreased estrogen levels, deficiency in dietary calcium and vitamin D, and reduced physical activities with aging. The reduction in bone density often presents with chronic pain, debility, and frequent fractures of the spine, hip, and wrist.[24] Another important problem in this age group is progressive impairments in vision and hearing. Above one-third of the older US population aged ≥70 years report hearing loss, and about one-fifth report blindness in one or both eyes.[25] Furthermore, several underlying conditions affecting multiple systems may lead to a complex health state, called geriatric syndrome with a poorer prognosis. It is most commonly characterized by frailty, falls, pressure ulcers, incontinence, and delirium.[26]

Also, end-stage illnesses such as organ failures and cancers are common in older age. Malignancies are fourfold more frequent in women above 65 years of age, the most common being breast, colon, and lung cancers. Apart from the primary effects of the illness, surgery, chemotherapy, and radiation add to the patient's physical, mental, and financial burden.[27]

The chronic physical illnesses affect the daily functioning and quality of life, causing mental health problems. Long-term suffering and need for frequent investigations and hospitalizations may result in feelings of helplessness, loss of control, anxiety, depression, and various psychological issues.[27] Sensory deprivation, dyselectrolytemia, infection, and treatment adverse effects may precipitate psychotic symptoms.

■ SPECIFIC PSYCHIATRIC DISORDERS IN OLDER WOMEN

Dementia

Dementia is a major cause of morbidity and mortality among the elderly population. At least 4% of women above the age of 65 years and 20% of those above the age of 85 years are affected by dementia[6,28] with a median survival from onset estimated around 4.6 years.[29] The most common is Alzheimer dementia (AD) (50%) followed by multiinfarct dementia (13–50%).[30] Also, most studies showed women are more likely than men to develop AD.[6] However, older women with dementia are more likely to live within the community under good support care.[18]

The proven risk factors for dementia are old age, apolipoprotein E4, hyperchromocysteinemia, atherosclerotic disease, and trisomy-21. Smoking, depression, posttraumatic stress disorder (PTSD), and antidepressant use has also been associated with increased risks. However, education, physical activity, cognitive stimulating activity, social engagement, and HRT have shown some protective role; although the findings are inconsistent. Early-onset (before the age of 65 years) dementia accounts for <1% of cases, and is usually related to genetic mutations.[6,29] Reversible causes of particular importance at older age are vitamin B_{12} deficiency, depression, hypothyroidism, head injury, normal pressure hydrocephalus, meningoencephalitis, alcohol, chronic organ failure, and medication side effects.[31]

Dementia is a progressive disorder characterized by a global deterioration of intellectual function and increasing difficulties in daily activities of life.[18] It results in severe disability during late life, often necessitating palliative care and hospitalization.[29] Almost 97% of dementia present with heterogeneous noncognitive symptoms and behavioral problems over the course of illness (called behavioral and psychological symptoms of dementia, BPSD). Overall, depression or apathy is the most commonly reported BPSD, while one-third of patients also present with delusions, agitation, or motor abnormalities. Depending on the type of dementia, delusions are common in AD, depression, or apathy in vascular dementia and disinhibition and eating disturbances in frontotemporal dementia.[32] A study found that most elderly bipolar patients had AD, followed by vascular dementia.[33] Among patients with dementia, BPSD is an independent cause of poor outcomes, caregiver discomfort, prolonged hospitalization, caregiver burden, and higher medical costs.[32]

Schizophrenia and Related Psychotic Disorders

The population of elderly women having schizophrenia consists of two distinct cohorts: (1) earlier onset chronic illness and (2) late-onset (after the age of 40 years) or very late-onset (after the age of 60 years) illness. It is shown that the "older chronic group" have poorer self-care and community skills and higher self-care needs. Chronic elderly schizophrenia was also found to have more negative symptoms than younger patients. However, the course of chronic schizophrenia was similar in men and women. The prevalence rates of schizophrenia was estimated to be 0.6% between ages 45–64, and 0.1–0.5% after the age of 65 years. Women, compared to men, are more likely to develop late-onset schizophrenia (LOS) showing a male:female ratio of 1:2-1:4.[6,34] A retrospective chart review study on nonaffective, nonorganic, late-onset psychosis (LOP) at the National Institute of Mental Health and Neurosciences (NIMHANS), India between years 2006–2011 found 67.5% of the sample constituted by elderly females.[35] The higher risks in elderly women have been attributed to the loss of the protective role of estrogen with advancing age. However, the course is similar in both genders with the positive symptoms usually diminishing with age.[6,34]

Late-onset schizophrenia, compared to early-onset schizophrenia, presents with more visual hallucinations, affective blunting, and neuroleptic sensitivity but less formal thought disorders and better neuropsychological performance. In the NIMHANS study, it was observed that the most common psychopathology among the patients with LOP were delusions (88%) followed by hallucinations (63.9%). Among delusions, persecution (80.7%) and reference (38.5%) were most common. Second person accusative/derogatory auditory hallucinations were most common (51.8%).[35] Contrast to the Indian sample, western studies have also reported partition delusions as common in LOP/LOS.[35] Additionally, patients with LOS usually report a better premorbid educational, occupational, and psychosocial functioning. Moreover, the brain changes in LOS as observed in neuroimaging studies are similar to age-related changes in older adults without schizophrenia.[35]

Various medical conditions prevalent in old age such as cerebrovascular accidents, malignancy, and neurodegenerative disorders are associated with secondary psychosis.[36] Certain medications such as steroids, anticholinergics, anti-parkinsonian drugs, beta-blockers, digoxin, quinolones, and chemotherapeutic agents may precipitate or aggravate psychotic symptoms.[37] Therefore, clinicians while approaching patients with LOP must carefully rule out the possibilities of secondary psychosis.

Depression

About 50% of depression among elderly people are late onset (after the age of 65 years). Although epidemiological studies have found lower rates of major depressive disorder in elderly women than in younger women, the depressive symptoms become more prevalent with further aging. Also, the gender differences in the rates, as observed in younger population, tends to diminish among older age groups.[38] According to the estimates of the large-scale Epidemiologic Catchment Area (ECA) study, in women of age ≥65 years, the prevalence of major depressive disorder and dysthymia was 1.5% and 2.3%, respectively.[38,39] Several Indian studies have reported depression as the most common psychiatric morbidity among elderly population.[10] Also, elderly women were found to have higher rates of depression (704/1,000) than elderly men in a rural community study in India.[10]

The development of depressive symptoms in elderly women follows a biopsychosocial model. It is hypothesized that aging causes neurobiological changes, especially reduction in the brain monoamines, increasing the susceptibility to depression. The risks may be further increased by a myriad of comorbid physical illnesses such as diabetes, hypothyroidism, sensory deprivation, etc. A subset of late-onset depression is associated with vascular insults to the brain (vascular depression). Also, about 20% of elderly depression with onset after the age of 70 years was found to be the early manifestation of an underlying progressive dementia. One important psychological factor is depletion of one's coping abilities while grieving the frequent losses occurring during the life span. In this context, Seligman (1975) described a reduction in the active efforts made by an individual to overcome the constant challenges posed by life (learned helplessness). Loneliness, isolation, role transition, lack of social stimulation, and financial problems are other major causes behind elderly depression.[40]

Characteristically, depression in elderly women may present with the Beck's "cognitive triad". However, contrast to depression at younger ages, elderly depression is marked by symptoms cluster, called "depletion syndrome": (1) lack of interest, (2) anergia, (3) hopelessness, (4) helplessness, and (5) psychomotor retardation.[38] Additionally, elderly women commonly present with "masked depression", wherein the usual mood symptoms are either hidden or denied. The emotional distress is expressed indirectly as vague dissatisfaction or somatic complaints.[40] Vascular depression, involving structural brain changes, presents with psychomotor retardation, apathy, neurocognitive deficits, movement disorders, and relative absence of dysphoria with longer course, antidepressant resistance, and poorer outcomes.[38] Interestingly, 80% elderly women with depression show indirect suicidal behaviors (conscious refusal of food, water, or medications).[38,41] A study on prognosis of late-onset depression among Indian samples reported 28% complete recovery, 30% partial recovery, 23% relapse, 6% continuous illness, and 11% death. Another 6% was found to have comorbid dementia. Full recovery and wellness for 1 year, shorter episode duration, and living with joint family were reported as good prognostic factors.[42]

Elderly depression needs careful differentiation from grief and dementia. In normal grief reaction, the depressive symptoms subside as grief resolves. The symptoms fluctuate over time, emotional reactivity and self-esteem are usually preserved, and dysfunctions are less pronounced. Survival guilt and death wishes to reunite with the deceased loved one may be present.[43] However, successive losses causing persistence of symptoms should not be confused with chronicity. Dementia, in contrast to depression, has a vague onset, long progressive course, fluctuating mood symptoms, memory deficits, and prominent cognitive impairments and disorientation.[40] Also, the presence of comorbid medical illnesses in old age may confound the depressive symptoms, wherein the Endicott's approach of substituting the somatic symptoms of depression with useful alternatives can help the diagnosis.[44]

Bipolar Disorder in Late Life

Most bipolar disorders has an onset during early adult life with only 10% of cases accounting for late-onset disease.[6] Distinct phenotypes of bipolar disorder according to the age of onset have been observed.[45,46] Accordingly, three subgroups have been described: early, middle, and late, with mean onset at 17, 27, and 46 years, respectively. Together, older age bipolar disorder (OABD) showed a point prevalence of 1% in the general population. The rates were observed to be higher (3-10%) in hospital settings.[47,48] About a quarter of the bipolar patients were elderly (≥60 years), and among them 70% were females.[48,49] Bipolar disorder is more common in women (male: female ratio of 1:2) with no significant gender differences in presentations.[33]

Traditional views considered that the occurrence of manic episodes diminishes with advancing age. However, a long-term prospective study in 2005 found that about 0.5-1% of cases of unipolar depression progressed to bipolar I every year. Furthermore, the prevalence of "late life mania" was estimated as 44% among elderly inpatients with manic episodes.[50] About 5-10% patients of age ≥50 had first episode mania.[33]

Early-onset bipolar disorder (EOBD) and late-onset bipolar disease (LOBD) have different presentations, attributable to the different duration of illness, progression, and an increased risk for an organic etiology among older patients. A positive family history, higher rates of psychotic symptoms, rapid cycling, and a severe course are usually associated with EOBD, while neurological comorbidities, cognitive deficits, somatic conditions, and treatment resistance are more common in LOBD.[33] Summarizing several studies, about 3% of LOBD patients had reportedly an underlying organic etiology, 17-43% elderly mania had cerebral disorders and 3-32% of OABD patients had developed dementia.[6,33] Also, LOBD is more likely to present as bipolar II with milder manic and more depressive symptoms.[33]

Sleep Disorders

Aging leads to physiological changes in the sleep patterns affecting both sleep structure and circadian rhythm. Polysomnographic studies in elderly have found (1) reduced slow wave (stage 3 and 4) sleep, corresponding to a decline in growth hormone, (2) reduced sleep efficiency, and (3) shorter rapid eye movement (REM) latency. Consequently, the sleep is characterized by nocturnal awakenings, difficulty in falling asleep again, and early morning awakenings. The changes in the sleep structure are less prominent in elderly women than male counterparts. The circadian rhythm in the elderly is marked by reduced amplitude (amount) and phase (timing) advancement. These are caused by factors both endogenous (aging retina causing reduced stimulation of the suprachiasmatic nucleus and global neurodegeneration) and exogenous (reduced exposure to sunlight and daytime napping). Changes in estrogen have also been implicated for altered sleep patterns in elderly women.[51] Overall, sleep problems are more common in elderly women than elderly men.[51]

Women's sleep is further influenced by her household responsibilities and gender roles. Sleep takes a priority second to her duties to ensure the well-being of the others in her family. Subsequently, "poor sleep" often gets neglected as a "normal" feature of her daily life. Women's sleep may get further affected by the problems of her aging spouse (poor health, snoring, and enlarged prostate). Even in widowhood, the lonely nights may prevent her from having a good sleep like before.[51]

About 70% of older people report sleep problem, and 20% report coexisting mental health problem.[52] In elderly, sleep problems can occur independently or secondary to another physical or mental illness. Physical health issues such as chronic disorders, obesity, pain conditions, and delirium can disrupt one's sleep. Medications such as antihypertensives (beta blockers), antiparkinsonian drugs (levodopa), steroids, antihistaminics, antidepressants, and psychostimulants can decrease sleep. Poor sleep can also be a feature of depression, anxiety, psychosis, and substance use disorders.[53] Additionally, poor sleep may have a negative impact on health (physical and mental). For example, fragmented sleep and shorter sleep duration were found to be independent risk factors for falls in women aged ≥70 years.[54]

Insomnia (subjective nonspecific reduction in quality or quantity of sleep) is common in menopausal women (51–77%). Moreover, women aged above 45 years are 1.7 times more likely to have insomnia, with increased risks among those who are separated, divorced, or widowed.[55]

Restless leg syndrome (RLS), characterized by a strong urge to move due to unpleasant sensations in legs, is a major cause of sleep disturbance with a peak prevalence between the age of 50 and 65 years (15.3%).[56] The cause may be idiopathic or secondary to pregnancy, anemia (iron and folate deficiency), and antipsychotic use.[51]

Older people ≥65 years are also more likely than younger individuals to have *obstructive sleep apnea syndrome* (OSAS) (prevalence rate 13–32%). Females are less commonly affected than males (male:female ratio ranging from 10:1 to 2:1 across studies) with the female sex hormones exhibiting some protection against its development. Therefore, postmenopausal women without HRT have higher prevalence rates (2.7%) than those on HRT (<1%).[51] Also, women with OSAS are at higher risks of developing depression and obstructive lung disease than men.

Hypersomnia disorders including *narcolepsy* are typically rare in older age.[53]

In contrast, *REM sleep behavioral disorders* (RSBD) involving enactment of dreams during sleep peaks in 50s and 60s; and may represent early manifestations of neurodegenerative disorders (parkinsonism and Lewy body dementia). However, women are less affected than men (male:female ratio 9:1).[51]

Sexual Problems

Aging results in several anatomic and physiological changes in the women genitourinary system: atrophy of vaginal epithelium and labia majora, loss of fat from mons pubis, reduction of pubic hair, and reduction of elasticity of vaginal wall. A decline in vaginal secretions, epithelial glycogen, and estrogen levels post menopause affect the vaginal microbial environment, making it prone to infections. Also, reduced vaginal blood flow, lubrication, and nerve sensitivity cause changes in women's sexual response cycle affecting sexual performance and pleasure. Most notable changes are delay in reaching excitement and prolongation of plateau phase. However, orgasmic capacity may remain preserved. Hypertonicity of levator ani and perineal membrane secondary to childbirth, uterine prolapse, surgery or aging can cause sexual dysfunction.[57] Also, menopausal women report diminished sexual behaviors such as reduced frequencies of sexual fantasy, foreplay, and intercourse.[58] Sexual dysfunction negatively affects the women's self-esteem, sexual relationships, and quality of life.[59]

Additionally, 60% of cases of sexual dysfunction have some underlying medical risk factors. These include chronic illnesses (liver or kidney disease, tuberculosis, and osteoarthritis), vascular conditions (hypertension, cardiovascular disorders, peripheral vascular disease, etc.), neurogenic problems (multiple sclerosis and spinal injuries), hormonal disorders (DM, metabolic syndrome, hypothyroidism, ovarian failure etc.), and autoimmune disorders (psoriasis and systemic lupus). Also, certain medications (benzodiazepines, antihypertensives, antiepileptics, chemotherapies, opiates, and antidepressants) are associated with sexual side effects.[52,60] Further, Walsh et al. (2004), in the context of sexual problems in older women, described certain "psychosexual red flags" which warrants referral to trained sex therapist. These include sexual issues which are lifelong or situational, any history of abuse or trauma, positive psychiatric history, present mood symptoms, stress, or relationship conflicts.[57] Substance use like alcohol and tobacco are also associated with sexual dysfunction.[52]

The prevalence rates of sexual dysfunctions in women post menopause ranged from 68 to 86.5% across studies.[59] The large National Health and Social Life Survey data estimated 67% of elderly women of 40–59 years with decreased interest in sex, 45% with difficulty achieving orgasm (*anorgasmia*), and 21% with pain during sex (*dyspareunia*). Older women also had more frequent complaints of trouble lubricating.[58,61] A community-based study reported 68% menopausal women with sexual problems, especially pertaining to their sexual desire, response, and behavior.[62] Another 68% of postmenopausal women participating in the Yale midlife study reported sexual problems concerning vaginal dryness, dyspareunia, decreased clitoral sensitivity, and difficulty with orgasm.[63] Also, elderly women with higher premenopausal sexual interest reported greater distress due to the age-related changes in sexual health.[58]

Suicide

Every year, suicides claim the life of over 7 lakh people worldwide. And more than three-fourths of global suicides occur in low- and middle-income countries [World Health Organization (WHO)]. Epidemiological studies have consistently found that women make more suicide attempts than men. However, men have 2-4 times higher suicide related mortality rates than women.[64] Also, Asian women have higher suicide rates than women of other regions.[65] The suicide rates in elderly women were observed to increase with age: 9.7 (45-54 years), 10.6 (55-64 years), 12.3 (65-74 years), and 15.9 (>75 years).[66]

About methods, men are more likely to use a more lethal way to die than women. Drug overdose and pesticide ingestion are the most preferred ways among women of developed and developing countries, respectively. Also, among western elderly women, the most common method was found to be drug overdose for age 50-64 years and firearm use for age ≥65 years.[67] In a study in rural India, 67% of females were found with self-harm by pesticide poisoning. Another preferred method among Indian women was found to be self-immolation (63% of all self-immolation cases). This may be because of the cultural values considering fire as a "purifier", past practices of Sati/Jauhar and easy accessibility to home kerosene.[68]

Depression is the most common mental health risk for suicides in both genders. Moreover, depression is twice more prevalent in women than in men with suicidal behaviors. A prospective study on patients of major depressive disorder (MDD) found that women with "past suicide attempt, higher lethality of the attempt and lower number of reasons for living" are at higher risk for suicide.[69] Presence of PTSD over depression further increases the suicide risk, as observed in a national household probability sample of 3085 US women.[70] Other important contributors to late life suicides include intimate partner violence, substance use, and physical health problems.[67]

ASSESSMENT OF PSYCHIATRIC DISORDERS IN ELDERLY WOMEN

Assessment for psychiatric disorders in elderly women needs a comprehensive approach to identify the underlying risk factors, comorbidities, ongoing medications and possible side effects, severity of the symptoms, level of dysfunction, suicide risk, and family support and other sociocultural factors influencing the illness outcomes. Often opinions and consultation-liaison with other specialties are required for a complete understanding of the presentations and a holistic management. Also, assessment is not a cross-sectional procedure but must be carried at regular intervals as per the clinical and psychological needs of the patient.

The very first step is obtaining an adequate history from reliable sources. In case of an elderly woman, the spouse with whom she had sharing her every day for the last several years is best person to ask a detailed history. In widowed patients' history taking may become a challenge, especially if she is staying alone or has no fixed residence. In such a scenario, bits-and-pieces of the history obtained from several sources or acquaintances and previous prescriptions can help. **Box 1** summarizes the important components of psychiatric assessment and evaluation in elderly women.

As previously stated, differentiating between the psychiatric symptoms in geriatric patients as primary or secondary to a medical condition is a clinical challenge. A premorbid absence of psychiatric illness, acute onset of symptoms, rapid worsening, abnormal vitals, emotional lability, impaired cognition, altered sensorium, and prominent visual hallucinations usually hint toward an underlying medical cause.

■ TREATMENT CONSIDERATIONS

The physiological changes with aging alter the pharmacokinetic and pharmacodynamic properties of most drugs. For instance, the gut motility and gastric secretions decrease with age causing a reduction in the rate of absorption of the drugs. Older adults have more body fat and less body water and plasma albumin. As a result, the volume of distribution of fat-soluble drugs increases and that of albumin-bound drugs decreases. Both metabolism by the liver and excretion by the kidney declines with age, requiring dose reduction of most drugs, particularly in patients with comorbid hepatic or renal diseases. The risk of drug toxicity is also high among older adults. There is also increased chances of drug interactions in older patients, as they are often on multiple medications for the concurrent physical illnesses. Pharmacodynamic studies have shown that receptor sensitivity increases with age. Consequently, older people are at higher risk to develop the common adverse effects of the drugs. For example, antipsychotics are prone to cause extrapyramidal symptoms (EPS), constipation, and sedation. Even serious side effects such as agranulocytosis with clozapine, bleeding, or hyponatremia with antidepressants are higher in older age group. Furthermore, some drugs such as antidepressants may show delay in their therapeutic response.

Thus, the thumb rule of prescription for elderly people is "start low and go slow". Only the required minimum number of drugs should be prescribed, while meticulously avoiding any major drug–drug interaction. Once a daily dose may be preferred for the ease in administration and improved compliance. It is wiser to keep the anticholinergic load low in elderly patients.

CHAPTER 9: Psychiatric Disorders in Older Women

> **BOX 1:** Components of psychiatric assessment and evaluation in an elderly.
>
> - *Sociodemographics:* Education, career (year of retirement/leaving job), marital status (married/separated/widow), religion, cultural milieu, living conditions, financial condition, residence (rural/urban)
> - *History of present illness:* Precipitating event(s), age at onset, duration of illness, course, symptom severity, symptom dimensions, catatonia, suicidal behaviors, altered sensorium, mobility and falls, bladder incontinence, sleep and appetite, self-care, dysfunction in personal, familial and social domains
> - *Past psychiatric history:* Onset, duration and symptom severity, comparison with current presentation, diagnosis, and management
> - *Medical history:* Comorbid conditions (hypertension, hypothyroidism, diabetes mellitus, osteoporosis, arthritis, cardiovascular diseases, liver/kidney diseases, etc.), their course and current severity, association/relationship with the psychiatric symptoms, ongoing treatments, possible side effects (including secondary psychiatric problems), drug interactions
> - *Treatment review:* Past trials and ongoing psychotropics, adherence, response, side-effects, possible drug interactions, electroconvulsive therapy (ECT) in the past (indication, sessions, and response)
> - *Childhood and adulthood history* (the information sources in elderly patients may be limited): Childhood trauma, and sexual abuse
> - *Education and career:* Performance, achievements, and difficulties
> - *Menstrual history:* Age at menopause, postmenopausal symptoms (hot flush, mood swings, headache, and irritability), and bleed per vagina
> - *Marital and sexual history*
> - *Family history:* Medical and psychiatric problems in close relatives, suicides in the family, family knowledge-attitude-and-practice related to patient's illness, resources, caregivers, burnt out and expressed emotions, empty-nest
> - *Substance history:* Substance type, pattern, last intake, withdrawal symptoms, and intoxication
> - *Premorbid personality:* Premorbid functionality, adjustment, and religious/spiritual-based coping
> - Social support system
> - *General physical assessment:* Assessment of vitals, body mass index (BMI), pallor, thyroid-swelling, nutritional deficiency, signs of physical illnesses, sensory deprivation
> - *Mental status assessment:* Special attention to psychopathology, suicidal intentions, cognitive deficits, judgment, and insight
> - *Need for in-patient care:* Self-harm behavior/suicidality, catatonia, severe psychopathology, malnutrition, poor general condition, and difficult to manage at home
> - *Investigations:* Complete hemogram, blood sugar, thyroid profile, lipid profile, liver and renal function test, electrocardiogram, serum B12 (if indicated), neuroimaging (especially in late-onset psychiatric illness, prominent cognitive deficits, abnormal movements, high neuroleptic sensitivity, history of unconsciousness, and scatatonia)
> - *Psychiatric rating scales:* To assess the severity of the symptoms and monitor response **(Table 1)**
> - *Consultations from other specialties:* As relevant for the case

Regular assessments for adverse effects and toxicity must be done. The American Geriatric Society Beers Criteria list the medication guidelines that health professionals can refer for safer treatment decisions in elderly patients.

TABLE 1: Validated tools for assessment of various mental health conditions in elderly.

Consciousness	*Glasgow Coma Scale*
Delirium	• Delirium Rating Scale – Revised-98 • Confusion Assessment Scale
Cognition	• Mini-Cog Instrument • Folstein Mini-mental Status Examination • Montreal Cognitive Assessment • Informant Questionnaire on Cognitive Decline in Elderly
Dementia	Dementia Rating Scale
Neuropsychiatric assessment	Neuropsychiatric Inventory
Psychiatric problems	Brief Psychiatric Rating Scale
Depression	• Geriatric Depression Scale • Patient Health Questionnaire-9 • Beck Depression Inventory • Montgomery–Åsberg Depression Rating Scale • Hamilton Depression Rating Scale
Anxiety	Generalized Anxiety Scale-7
Schizophrenia	• Positive and Negative Syndrome Scale • The Manchester Scale
Sleep problems	
Sexual problems	
Substance abuse	• Clinical Institute Withdrawal Assessment for Alcohol Scale • Clinical Institute Withdrawal Assessment for Benzodiazepine • Clinical Opioid Withdrawal Scale
Suicide	• Sad Person Scale • Beck's Suicidal Inventory • Beck Suicidal Intent Scale • Columbia-Suicide Severity Rating Scale
Elderly abuse	Caregiver Abuse Screen Evaluation
Frailty	Frailty Index
Dysfunction	• Global Assessment of Functioning • Katz Index of Independence in Activities of Daily Living • Lawton Instrumental Activities of Daily Living Scale
Disability	Indian Disability Evaluation and Assessment Scale

In geriatric depression, all antidepressants are effective with no significant gender difference in response. However, selective serotonin reuptake inhibitors (SSRIs) are preferred as tricyclic antidepressants (TCAs) cause intolerable anticholinergic and cardiac side effects. Among SSRIs, escitalopram and sertraline are preferred for fewer drug-drug interactions and better side effect profile. Venlafaxine, bupropion, and mirtazapine are the preferred second-line options.[71] In psychotic disorders, the second-generation antipsychotics such as risperidone and olanzapine are the first choice due to lower risk of EPS. However, olanzapine has higher risk of weight gain, metabolic side effects, hyperglycemia, and dyslipidemia. Depot injections in elderly patients have shown to improve compliance.[72] In elderly patients with treatment-resistant cases, clozapine is still the gold standard. Tardive dyskinesia (TD) is an important treatment challenge especially in older patients on antipsychotics. The incidence rate of TD in older patients on conventional antipsychotics is 20-30% per year, about 4-5 times higher compared to younger patients.[73,74] Among patients of age ≥40 years, the rates were found to be higher among women than men.[75]

A major issue among elderly patients is benzodiazepines overuse. A recent cross-sectional study in US reported the prevalence of home benzodiazepine as 13.5% among older adults at the time of hospital admission. Benzodiazepine use was more prevalent among elderly women with dementia, and the use remained fairly constant with increasing age.[76] A higher prevalence rate (47%) was estimated for benzodiazepine long-term use among elderly population in Europe.[77] In India, benzodiazepines were found to be the most prescribed psychotropic in elderly patients (64% of cases).[78] And, among elderly outpatients, clonazepam was the most commonly prescribed benzodiazepine followed by lorazepam.[79] Chronic benzodiazepine use/overuse can cause lethargy, confusion, cognitive deficits, and increased risks of falls and fractures.[76,80]

Electroconvulsive therapy (ECT) is a safe and viable option in older patients, especially in those with severe symptoms, high suicidality, catatonia, poor nutrition, and drug resistance. However, patients aged above 80 years are at higher risks for delirium and cardiovascular side effects.[6]

KEY POINTS

- Aging is a complex multifactorial process, influenced by one's genetics, lifestyle, and environment with effects on physical and mental health.
- In an elderly woman, aging can pose new psychological challenges including role reversal, general discontentment about life, menopause, bereavement, social isolation, and a plethora of medical illnesses.
- Globally and in India, mood disorders have been reported as the most common psychiatric morbidity among older women.
- The other common psychiatric conditions are dementia, psychosis, sleep disturbances, and sexual problems.
- Suicide is also a major concern among the older population with prevalence increasing with age.
- Diagnosis is often a challenging due to the coexistence of physical conditions and management often requires a holistic multidisciplinary care.

REFERENCES

1. Wang Y, Xu Q, Luo J, Hu M, Zuo C. Effects of age and sex on subcortical volumes. Front Aging Neurosci. 2019;11:259.
2. Beck CM, Pearson BP. Mental health of elderly women. J Women Aging. 1989;1(1-3):175-93.
3. Levy SM. The aging woman: Developmental issues and mental health needs. Prof Psychol. 1981;12(1):92-102.
4. Rangarajan SK, Sivakumar PT, Manjunatha N, Kumar CN, Math SB. Public health perspectives of geriatric mental health care. Indian J Psychol Med. 2021;43(5 Suppl):S1-7.
5. Lodha P, De Sousa A. Geriatric mental health: The challenges for India. J Geriatr Ment Health. 2018;5(1):16.
6. Lehmann SW. Psychiatric disorders in older women. Int Rev Psychiatry. 2003;15(3):269-79.
7. World Health Organization. (2023). Mental health of older adults. [online] Available from https://www.who.int/news-room/fact-sheets/detail/mental-health-of-older-adults [Last accessed December, 2023].
8. Nandi PS, Banerjee G, Mukherjee SP, Nandi S, Nandi DN. A study of psychiatric morbidity of the elderly population of a rural community in West Bengal. Indian J Psychiatry. 1997;39(2):122-9.
9. Tiwari SC. Geriatric psychiatric morbidity in rural northern India: implications for the future. Int Psychogeriatr. 2000;12(1):35-48.
10. Grover S, Dutt A, Avasthi A. An overview of Indian research in depression. Indian J Psychiatry. 2010;52(Suppl1):S178-88.
11. Asaria M, Mazumdar S, Chowdhury S, Mazumdar P, Mukhopadhyay A, Gupta I. Socioeconomic inequality in life expectancy in India. BMJ Global Health. 2019;4(3):e001445.
12. Malatesta VJ (Ed). Mental Health Issues of Older Women: A Comprehensive Review for Health Care, 1st edition. UK: Routledge; 2007.
13. Dennerstein L, Burrows GD. A review of studies of the psychological symptoms found at the menopause. Maturitas. 1978;1(1):55-64.
14. Ahuja M. Age of menopause and determinants of menopause age: A PAN India survey by IMS. J Midlife Health. 2016;7(3):126-31.
15. Deeks AA. Psychological aspects of menopause management. Best Pract Res Clin Endocrinol Metab. 2003;17(1):17-31.
16. Pearlstein T, Rosen K, Stone AB. Mood disorders and menopause. Endocrinol Metab Clin North Am. 1997;26(2):279-94.
17. Rowland KF. Environmental events predicting death for the elderly. Psychol Bull. 1977;84(2):349-72.
18. Roughan PA. Mental health and psychiatric disorders in older women. Clin Geriatr Med. 1993;9(1):173-90.
19. Bogunovic O. Women and aging. Harv Rev Psychiatry. 2011;19(6):321-4.
20. Yon Y, Mikton CR, Gassoumis ZD, Wilber KH. Elder abuse prevalence in community settings: a systematic review and meta-analysis. Lancet Glob Health. 2017;5(2):e147-56.
21. Yon Y, Ramiro-Gonzalez M, Mikton CR, Huber M, Sethi D. The prevalence of elder abuse in institutional settings: a systematic review and meta-analysis. Eur J Public Health. 2019;29(1):58-67.

22. Mosca L, Mochari H, Christian A, Berra K, Taubert K, Mills T, et al. National study of women's awareness, preventive action, and barriers to cardiovascular health. Circulation. 2006;113(4):525-34.
23. Swantek SS, Goldstein MZ. Practical geriatrics: age and gender differences of patients with hip fracture and depression. Psychiatr Serv. 2000;51(12):1501-3.
24. Delmas PD. Treatment of postmenopausal osteoporosis. Lancet. 2002;359(9322):2018-26.
25. Crews JE, Campbell VA. Vision impairment and hearing loss among community-dwelling older Americans: implications for health and functioning. Am J Public Health. 2004;94(5):823-9.
26. Inouye SK, Studenski S, Tinetti ME, Kuchel GA. Geriatric syndromes: clinical, research, and policy implications of a core geriatric concept. J Am Geriatr Soc. 2007;55(5):780-91.
27. Hansen J. Common cancers in the elderly. Drugs Aging. 1998;13(6):467-78.
28. Aloysi A, Van Dyk K, Sano M. Women's cognitive and affective health and neuropsychiatry. Mt Sinai J Med. 2006;73(7):967-75.
29. LoGiudice D, Watson R. Dementia in older people: an update. Intern Med J. 2014;44(11):1066-73.
30. Grau L. Mental health and older women. Women Health. 1989;14(3-4):75-92.
31. Tripathi M, Vibha D. Reversible dementias. Indian J Psychiatry. 2009;51 Suppl 1(Suppl1):S52-55.
32. Cloak N, Al Khalili Y. Behavioral and Psychological Symptoms in Dementia. Treasure Island (FL): StatPearls Publishing; 2023.
33. Arnold I, Dehning J, Grunze A, Hausmann A. Old age bipolar disorder—Epidemiology, aetiology and treatment. Medicina (Kaunas). 2021;57(6):587.
34. Dickerson FB. Women, aging, and schizophrenia. J Women Aging. 2007;19(1-2):49-61.
35. Ramasamy S, Bharath S. Clinical characteristics of patients with non-affective, non-organic, late onset psychosis. Asian J Psychiatr. 2017;25:74-8.
36. Kim K, Jeon HJ, Myung W, Suh SW, Seong SJ, Hwang JY, et al. Clinical approaches to late-onset psychosis. J Pers Med. 2022;12(3):381.
37. Casagrande Tango R. Psychiatric side effects of medications prescribed in internal medicine. Dialogues Clin Neurosci. 2003;5(2):155-65.
38. Gatz M, Fiske A. Aging women and depression. Professional psychology: Research and practice. 2003;34(1):3-9.
39. Jeste DV, Alexopoulos GS, Bartels SJ, Cummings JL, Gallo JJ, Gottlieb GL, et al. Consensus statement on the upcoming crisis in geriatric mental health: research agenda for the next 2 decades. Arch Gen Psychiatry. 1999;56(9):848-53.
40. LaGodna GE. Aging women and depression: Unresolved conceptual, etiologic, and epidemiologic issues. Issues Men Health Nurs. 1988;9(3):285-98.
41. Osgood N, Brant B, Lipman AP. Suicide Among The Elderly In Long-Term Care Facilities. UK: Bloomsbury Academic; 1991.
42. Jhingan HP, Sagar R, Pandey RM. Prognosis of late-onset depression in the elderly: a study from India. Int Psychogeriatr. 2001;13(1):51-61.
43. Widera EW, Block SD. Managing grief and depression at the end of life. Am Fam Physician. 2012;86(3):259-64.
44. Saracino RM, Rosenfeld B, Nelson CJ. Performance of four diagnostic approaches to depression in adults with cancer. Gen Hosp Psychiatry. 2018;51:90-5.

45. Bellivier F, Golmard JL, Rietschel M, Schulze TG, Malafosse A, Preisig M, et al. Age at onset in bipolar I affective disorder: Further evidence for three subgroups. AJP. 2003;160(5):999-1001.
46. Azorin JM, Bellivier F, Kaladjian A, Adida M, Belzeaux R, Fakra E, et al. Characteristics and profiles of bipolar I patients according to age-at-onset: Findings from an admixture analysis. J Affect Disord. 2013;150(3):993-1000.
47. Greenwald BS, Kremen N, Aupperle P. Tailoring adult psychiatric practices to the field of geriatrics. Psych Quart. 1992;63(4):343-66.
48. Depp CA, Jeste DV. Bipolar disorder in older adults: a critical review. Bipolar Disord. 2004;6(5):343-67.
49. Sajatovic M, Gyulai L, Calabrese JR, Thompson TR, Wilson BG, White R, et al. Maintenance Treatment Outcomes in Older Patients with Bipolar I Disorder. Am J Geriatr Psychiatry. 2005;13(4):305-11.
50. Dols A, Kupka RW, van Lammeren A, Beekman AT, Sajatovic M, Stek ML. The prevalence of late-life mania: a review. Bipolar Disord. 2014;16(2):113-8.
51. Dzaja A, Arber S, Hislop J, Kerkhofs M, Kopp C, Pollmächer T, et al. Women's sleep in health and disease. J Psychiatr Res. 2005;39(1):55-76.
52. Thomas KM, Redd LA, Wright JD, Hartos JL. Sleep and mental health in the general population of elderly women. J Prim Prev. 2017;38(5):495-503.
53. Suzuki K, Miyamoto M, Hirata K. Sleep disorders in the elderly: Diagnosis and management. J Gen Fam Med. 2017;18(2):61-71.
54. Stone KL, Ancoli-Israel S, Blackwell T, Ensrud KE, Cauley JA, Redline S, et al. Actigraphy-measured sleep characteristics and risk of falls in older women. Arch Intern Med. 2008;168(16):1768-75.
55. Patel D, Steinberg J, Patel P. Insomnia in the elderly: A review. J Clin Sleep Med. 2018;14(6):1017-24.
56. Aksoy D, Çelik A, Solmaz V, Çevik B, Sümbül O, Kurt S. The prevalence of restless legs syndrome in patients undergoing coronary angiography and its relationship with the severity of coronary artery stenosis. Sleep Breath. 2021;25(1):257-62.
57. Walsh KE, Berman JR. Sexual dysfunction in the older woman: an overview of the current understanding and management. Drugs Aging. 2004;21(10):655-75.
58. Gelfand MM. Sexuality among older women. J Womens Health Gend Based Med. 2000;9 Suppl 1:S15-20.
59. Addis IB, Van Den Eeden SK, Wassel-Fyr CL, Vittinghoff E, Brown JS, Thom DH, et al. Sexual activity and function in middle-aged and older women. Obstet Gynecol. 2006;107(4):755-64.
60. Ambler DR, Bieber EJ, Diamond MP. Sexual function in elderly women: a review of current literature. Rev Obstet Gynecol. 2012;5(1):16-27.
61. Laumann EO, Paik A, Rosen RC. Sexual dysfunction in the United States: prevalence and predictors. JAMA. 1999;281(6):537-44.
62. Sarrel PM, Whitehead MI. Sex and menopause: defining the issues. Maturitas. 1985;7(3):217-24.
63. Sarrel PM. Sexuality and menopause. Obstet Gynecol. 1990;75(4 Suppl):26S-30S.
64. Beautrais AL. Women and suicidal behavior. Crisis. 2006;27(4):153-6.
65. Vijayakumar L, Nagaraj K, Pirkis J, Whiteford H. Suicide in developing countries (1): frequency, distribution, and association with socioeconomic indicators. Crisis. 2005;26(3):104-11.

66. Vijayakumar L. Suicide in women. Indian J Psychiatry. 2015;57(Suppl 2):S233-8.
67. Choi NG, DiNitto DM, Sagna AO, Marti CN. Older women who died by suicide: suicide means, sociodemographic and psychiatric risk factors, and other precipitating circumstances. Int Psychogeriatr. 2018;30(10):1531-40.
68. Vijayakumar L. Hindu religion and suicide in India. In: Wasserman D, Wasserman C (Eds). Oxford Textbook of Suicidology and Suicide Prevention. Oxford: Oxford University Press; 2009.
69. Oquendo MA, Bongiovi-Garcia ME, Galfalvy H, Goldberg PH, Grunebaum MF, Burke AK, et al. Sex differences in clinical predictors of suicidal acts after major depression: a prospective study. Am J Psychiatry. 2007;164(1):134-41.
70. Cougle JR, Resnick H, Kilpatrick DG. PTSD, depression, and their comorbidity in relation to suicidality: cross-sectional and prospective analyses of a national probability sample of women. Depress Anxiety. 2009;26(12):1151-7.
71. Lenze EJ, Ajam Oughli H. Antidepressant treatment for late-life depression: Considering risks and benefits. J Am Geriatr Soc. 2019;67(8):1555-6.
72. Karim S, Byrne EJ. Treatment of psychosis in elderly people. Adv Psychiatr Treat. 2005;11(4):286-96.
73. Jeste DV, Caligiuri MP, Paulsen JS, Heaton RK, Lacro JP, Harris MJ, et al. Risk of tardive dyskinesia in older patients. A prospective longitudinal study of 266 outpatients. Arch Gen Psychiatry. 1995;52(9):756-65.
74. Saltz BL, Woerner MG, Kane JM, Lieberman JA, Alvir JM, Bergmann KJ, et al. Prospective study of tardive dyskinesia incidence in the elderly. JAMA. 1991;266(17):2402-6.
75. Woerner MG, Kane JM, Lieberman JA, Alvir J, Bergmann KJ, Borenstein M, et al. The prevalence of tardive dyskinesia. J Clin Psychopharmacol. 1991;11(1):34-42.
76. Gress T, Miller M, Meadows C, Neitch SM. Benzodiazepine overuse in elders: Defining the problem and potential solutions. Cureus. 2020;12(10):e11042.
77. Kurko TAT, Saastamoinen LK, Tähkäpää S, Tuulio-Henriksson A, Taiminen T, Tiihonen J, et al. Long-term use of benzodiazepines: Definitions, prevalence and usage patterns - a systematic review of register-based studies. Eur Psychiatry. 2015;30(8):1037-47.
78. Sahana DA, Pai K, Rajeshwari S, UllalSheetal D, RathnakarU P, Jaykumar JS. Pattern of psychotropic drug usage in psychiatric illnesses among elderly. 2010.
79. Grover S, Kumar V, Avasthi A, Kulhara P. First prescription of new elderly patients attending the psychiatry outpatient of a tertiary care institute in North India. Geriatr Gerontol Int. 2012;12(2):284-91.
80. Singh S, Sarkar S. Benzodiazepine abuse among the elderly. J Geriatr Mental Health. 2016;3(2):123.

CHAPTER 10

Mood Swings and Mayhem: Personality Disorder in Women

Ashlesha Bagadia, Sowmya Krishna

ABSTRACT

Knowledge on assessment and management of personality disorder in Indian women is still emerging. But enough evidence and guidelines exist to understand the etiological factors, sociodemographic factors and gender related factors that impact on assessment and management. This chapter covers key aspects of assessment and management of one of the most common personality disorder—Borderline Personality Disorder. Consistency of care, structured practice and key therapeutic approaches are highlighted along with the current evidence for various pharmacological approaches.

Keywords: Borderline personality disorder, vulnerable temperament, traumatic childhood, dialectical behavior therapy, mentalization based treatment, schema focused therapy, transference focused therapy, crises management, BPD in adolescents

"*She has mood swings*"—this can be a common presentation of a patient who has reluctantly agreed for a psychiatric assessment after much coaxing by an exhausted and frazzled family member.

"*Mood swings = borderline personality disorder*"—this can be a knee-jerk diagnosis by a psychiatrist in a busy mental health service, ill-equipped to manage an enduring condition like personality disorder.

INTRODUCTION

Despite a large body of emerging research in this area, personality disorder continues to be misunderstood and poorly managed across the globe and especially in low-resource countries, such as India and it is neighboring South Asian regions. We know that there is variability in gender representations of personality disorder. Interestingly, recent studies are now being done on the impact of femininity and masculinity on personality vulnerability rather than preassigned gender roles.[1] Antisocial, narcissistic, paranoid, and schizoid personality disorders are more represented by males, while dependent personality disorder criteria are more represented by females. Prevalence rates for schizotypal, borderline, histrionic, avoidant, and obsessive-compulsive personality disorders are more similar across both genders.[1] Although studies from South Asia are limited, there is an indication this reduced gap between genders for emotionally unstable personality disorder is also being observed in India.[2]

CHAPTER 10: Mood Swings and Mayhem: Personality Disorder in Women

The most common personality disorders in India appear to be "borderline personality disorder and anxious avoidant personality disorder",[3] with more representation of the former in clinical populations and hence the focus of this chapter. We will outline the etiological factors and best practices for assessment, diagnosis, and management. India is also used as a reference country in this chapter but due to cultural similarities, this is also applicable to its neighboring South Asian countries.

■ NORMAL PERSONALITY

Normal personality structure is understood as the integration of three key aspects of life:[4]
1. An integrated sense of self and significant others, which contributes to their core identity and impacts on their personal relationships.
2. A broad spectrum of affective response and regulation that can vary through a complex range of emotions with minimal loss of impulse control.
3. Presence of a well-formed value system that is mature and internalized, not rigidly tied to nor likely to change frequently in response to external relations.

Diagnostic and Statistical Manual of Mental Disorders IV (DSM IV: describes personality disorder as follows "Personality traits are enduring patterns of perceiving, relating to and thinking about the environment and oneself. They are exhibited in various important social and personal contexts. When these traits are significantly maladaptive and cause serious functional impairment or subjective distress, they constitute a personality disorder (PD)".[5] DSM-V has emphasized on presentation of personality disorder on a continuum, ranging from severely debilitated to high functioning. Patients may also shift within their own continuum, functioning at a baseline level through some aspects of their life, presenting as patients when in crisis, and then reverting back to baseline once the crisis is resolved.[6] Personality disorders are classified in various ways, the categorical classification system being the most common and outlined in the DSM-V and International Classification of Diseases (ICD)-10 classification manuals: Cluster A—odd/eccentric—paranoid, schizoid, and schizotypal; cluster B—dramatic—antisocial, borderline, histrionic, and narcissistic; and cluster C—anxious/fearful—avoidant, dependent, and obsessive/compulsive.[6]

Box 1 outlines the diagnostic criteria for borderline personality disorder.[7]

■ DEVELOPMENT PATHWAY OF PERSONALITY DISORDER

Broadly there are three factors that contribute to the development trajectory of personality disorder, they are as follows:[8]
1. Vulnerable temperament
2. Traumatic childhood
3. Triggering event or series of triggering events.

> **BOX 1:** Diagnostic criteria for borderline personality disorder.
>
> A pervasive pattern of instability of interpersonal relationships, self-image and affects, and marked impulsivity beginning by early adulthood and present in a variety of contexts, as indicated by five (or more) of the following:
> 1. Frantic efforts to avoid real or imagined abandonment
>   *Note:* Do not include suicidal or self-mutilating behavior covered in criterion 5.
> 2. A pattern of unstable and intense interpersonal relationships characterized by alternating between extremes of idealization and devaluation
> 3. Identity disturbance: markedly and persistently unstable self-image or sense of self
> 4. Impulsivity in at least two areas that are potentially self-damaging (e.g., spending, sex, substance abuse, reckless driving, and binge eating)
>   *Note:* Do not include suicidal or self-mutilating behavior covered in criterion 5
> 5. Recurrent suicidal behavior, gestures or threats, or self-mutilating behavior
> 6. Affective instability due to a marked reactivity of mood (e.g., intense episodic dysphoria, irritability, or anxiety usually lasting a few hours and only rarely more than a few days)
> 7. Chronic feelings of emptiness
> 8. Inappropriate, intense anger or difficulty controlling anger (e.g., frequent displays of temper, constant anger, and recurrent physical fights)
> 9. Transient, stress-related paranoid ideation or severe dissociative symptoms

When each of these factors is explored further in women, its impact on the development trajectory can become clearer.

Vulnerable Temperament

Although no significant sex difference is found genetically for borderline personality disorder[9] there is sufficient data to suggest that women are more prone to most common mental disorders, which are often comorbid with personality disorder.[10] A more vulnerable temperament puts them at a higher risk of succumbing to adverse environmental factors.

Traumatic Childhood

Identifying the sex of the fetus is still illegal in India because of the ongoing practice of female infanticide. Despite legal barriers, raising girls continues to be perceived as a burden in India.[11] Being unwanted from the time of birth can significantly contribute to the environment girls are raised in. Women are more susceptible to physical, emotional, and sexual abuse,[12] more likely to be invalidated and dismissed as "too sensitive" which are major contributing factors for the development of personality disorder.

Triggering Event or Series of Triggering Events

Women are still the underprivileged gender in India irrespective of their socioeconomic status.[13] Physiologically women navigate many milestones

CHAPTER 10: Mood Swings and Mayhem: Personality Disorder in Women

> **BOX 2:** Personality disorder in adolescent girls.
>
> - Most studies so far have looked at personality disorders in adults in the third to fifth decades of life. Mental health services for adolescents have always been sparse, the girls often falling through the cracks between child-centric and adults only clinics. Pediatricians and gynecologists often being the only health professionals seeing adolescent girls, who may not be well equipped to understand personality disorder. Only girls in the severe end of the spectrum ending up seeing a psychiatrist
> - Even amongst psychiatrists there is varying opinion on when and how a diagnosis should be made. Should it be included under childhood pervasive developmental disorders or should the diagnosis have specific criteria that can be applied irrespective of age? The new ICD 11 and DSM 5 have taken a dimensional approach rather than categorical [American Psychiatric Association (2013) Diagnostic and statistical manual of mental disorders (DSM-5)].[5] They also consider functional impairment, distress associated and symptom profile which helps with planning treatment
> - Gender bias in the prevalence of personality disorder in adolescents is similar to that in older women. However, high prevalence of eating disorders (both typical and atypical) is seen in young girls, especially teenagers. Studies have shown that around 50–60% of people in eating disorder services meet criteria for borderline personality, while males are likely to present more with atypical eating disorders
> - Onset of puberty brings numerous emotional and physical changes which can be confusing without the right kind of support/information. Adolescents are exposed to numerous sources of information—internet, social media, school, peers, and family. Having awareness only reduces the confusion to an extent but adolescents are left feeling unequipped to handle the range of emotions or thoughts
> - Bodily changes can feel both exciting as well as disappointing, depending on how well they fit the social criteria of good appearance. Especially for uncontrollable factors such as acne, weight, development of secondary sexual characters. For adolescents who are unable to fit a certain acceptable profile, this phase can be traumatic being bullied through body shaming or being excluded and can precipitate the onset of personality disorder
> - Menarche in some Indian communities is considered an important milestone. This is celebrated with ceremonies and gifts being showered and prayers being offered for the fertility of the young female. This is often followed by a sense of shame when the regularity of menstrual cycles set in - discussions around menstruation being stigmatized, lack of access to personal hygiene products during menstruation, ridicule directed at females at premenstrual symptoms, being criticized by the society for "using menstrual pain as an excuse" when the adolescent is unable to attend to their usual roles/responsibilities. Some of these may be subtle and some explicit. This is prevalent in both urban and rural India. For the young person, this whole experience can be confusing—from being celebrated to being criticized and made fun of. This can have a significant impact on the young person's mental health

that directly make them more susceptible to mental disorders. Puberty and associated stigma around menstruation, and the development of secondary sexual characteristics are often experienced as traumatic by young women (**Box 2** signifies specific factors to be considered for personality disorder in Adolescence). Lack of autonomy in decision-making about key issues in their life such as education, marriage, career, and conception of children, can be major triggering events. The perinatal period continues to be one of the most vulnerable times in the life cycle of a woman.[14] Inability to conceive is still viewed as primarily a woman's fault leaving her more vulnerable to the range of stressful factors contributed by infertility.[15] Majority of married women in India continue to experience gender-based violence[16] which can precipitate crises events in personality disorder. The presence of a mental disorder further makes them vulnerable to discrimination and stigma perpetuating the environmental stress that contributes to personality disorder.

ASSESSMENT

A thorough and comprehensive assessment is a crucial element of the assessment of personality disorder. A clinical interview, conducted with the woman alone and along with the family and friends can give valuable information that goes beyond diagnosis; it can help understand the barriers to seeking help, rule out comorbidity, and help align the right treatment to the patient.[17]

It gives an opportunity to study the patient's interaction and response to the assessor and any reciprocal emotional response generated by the assessor, all of which can be helpful in understanding the diagnosis, engaging the patient, and setting the foundation for the future therapeutic alliance. Apart from the standard interview schedule some of the key points to remember during the assessment are:

- History should be obtained from the patient preferably in a confidential space, and only one family member's version should not be accepted for diagnosis. Plenty of time should be set aside for the assessment interview. Often a series of interviews may be necessary; it is not recommended to confirm a diagnosis of personality disorder in a cross-sectional interview.
- Collateral from family members, friends, and significant others must be obtained, and attempts must be made to educate and engage them in the treatment plan.
- The interview should include a thorough exploration of the vulnerability factors described above—temperament as a child, environment while growing up, personal experience of the patient of the environment, whether perceived as abusive.
- Gentle exploration of dysfunctional adaptive behaviors, their effect on the individual and others, attitudes and relationships with others, and social functioning in all areas of the person's life over a prolonged period of time.[18]
- Apart from eliciting symptoms, questions should be targeted towards documenting the patient's own understanding of the severity and

what aspect of their life causes them the most distress. This can help in preparing collaborative treatment goals that are realistic and helpful.
- A comprehensive risk assessment should also be completed, that covers the risk of self-harm and harm to others, risks from comorbidities, and potential triggers that could lead to a crisis.
- Involving the patient in understanding their diagnosis and treatment options is proven to be beneficial. Clinicians are often reluctant to directly give patients a diagnosis of personality disorder but evidence suggests that informing them and giving sound psychoeducation can itself help reduce their symptoms and improve long-term engagement.[6]

One of the limitations of a clinical interview is the reliability of the patient's account; some may exaggerate their symptoms while others may minimize them. It is useful to support a clinical interview with an interview tool. There are many interview schedules, structured and semistructured, that have reasonable evidence in the assessment of personality disorders.[6] However, they are time-consuming and are more likely to overdiagnose if used in isolation. Formalized interview schedules can be a barrier to developing a rapport and engaging the patient, so should be used as an adjunct to, and not in place of, the clinical interview. Following are the interview schedules that can be used: International Personality Disorder Examination, Diagnostic Interview for DSM-IV Personality Disorders, Structured Interview for DSM-IV Personality Disorders, Structured Clinical Interview for DSM-IV Axis I Disorders, Personality Disorder Interview-IV, Personality Diagnostic Questionnaire, Standardized Assessment of Personality, Personality Assessment Schedule, Schedule for Normal and Abnormal Personality, Personality Assessment Inventory, Minnesota Multiphasic Personality Inventory-II, Millon Clinical Multiaxial Inventory-III, Eysenck Inventory Questionnaire, NEO Five-Factor Inventory, Rorschach test, and Thematic Apperception Test.

GENERAL PRINCIPLES OF MANAGING PERSONALITY DISORDER

Most of the evidence in managing personality disorders comes from Western studies which may have poor applicability in India. Psychiatrists often work in isolation and can be the sole practitioner looking after the patients and caring for their families. A divided functions approach where psychiatrists work along with psychologists and social workers is possible in an institutional setting or in a group practice.[19] Referral to a specialist team that exclusively works with personality disorders is less commonly available in India.

Whatever the setting is, some basic principles of managing personality disorder should be kept in mind as mentioned underneath.[17]

Treatment Plan

All patients should have a shared treatment plan which includes medication management, a psychotherapy plan, crisis management, and access to acute inpatient care. It is imperative that the care is patient-centered and she is included in the formation of the treatment plan. Clearly outlined steps that will be taken during instances of self-harm or attempted suicide, can reassure the patient and also provide structure to the psychiatrist during a crisis.

Engagement

A considerable part of the initial phase of treatment should be spent on engaging the patient. It may involve helping her to stabilize social aspects of care, such as living arrangements and engaging families. Or addressing comorbid substance abuse or active mental illness. Attempts should be made to ensure that treatment is accessible and appointments are at times acceptable to both the patient and the treatment plan. The roles of each of the clinicians involved should be clearly defined, including what they will not be able to do (e.g., the psychologist will not be involved in medication management, who will be the designated person to contact in crises, etc.). The initial part of the engagement should be spent on formulating her disorder and helping her to recognize and manage her frustration or impulsivity as it arises. A clear pathway to care during a crisis is also crucial to engagement. The crisis plan is enumerated in **Box 3**.

Consistency

Providing consistent care to patients with challenging behaviors can be difficult. Limiting the care of the patient to only those people whose roles

---

BOX 3: Crisis plan name:
- Demographic and contact details: _____
- Contact details of next of kin: _____
- Current self-harming behaviors: _____
- Triggers/stressors: _____
- Examples of crisis situations: _____
- Current coping mechanisms: _____
- Helpful people to contact in crises: _____
- Specified clinician to be contacted in the times of crises: _____
- Plan for support by phone during the crisis: (designated clinician for crisis support, duration of each call, and designated time slots for the call)
- Plan for time-limited hospital admission: (encourage brief hospital stays only in times of extreme crises)

Alternate crisis management plan: (Any other reasonable strategies that have helped the patient in the past)

List of helplines, nearby hospitals, other resources that can be used in times of crises.

and tasks are clear can reduce inconsistency (for example, clearly defining the role of the inpatient psychiatrist from that of the outpatient psychiatrist, designating therapy to a specific clinician, etc.). Steps should be taken to see if there are disagreements in the team that are contributing to the inconsistency. Or whether it is due to the internal pathology of personality disorder which can often result in splitting between the different clinicians.[19] Often these women would have had inconsistent care in their formative years; hence, it becomes even more important to provide consistent care, which can also help in setting boundaries and sustaining engagement.

Constancy

Patients with borderline personality disorder are most sensitive to changes in the professionals. It can reawaken feelings of loss, rejection, and abandonment. As far as possible senior clinicians who are less likely to move between jobs, and have more experience with difficult patients, should take up long-term care of these patients. Even otherwise, clinicians should take extra care in reducing abrupt changes, abrupt termination, or unplanned handover to other clinicians.

Inpatient Care

Despite evidence suggesting that hospital admissions should be avoided at all costs for personality disorders, sometimes they can be the most effective way of managing a crisis. Other indications for hospital admissions are for a comprehensive assessment and diagnosis, managing comorbidity, reducing risk to others, and stabilizing medication. Bateman and Tyrer suggest some guidelines for inpatient care of personality disorders **(Box 4)**.[20]

Medication Management

Although pharmacotherapy is significantly used in personality disorders, indications are mainly for managing crises, behavioral disturbances, and comorbidities. No one medication has any robust evidence for the treatment of specific personality disorders, often the onus is on the psychiatrist to judicially assess and prioritize the reason for prescribing.[20]

> **BOX 4:** Admissions to a general psychiatric ward.
>
> It should be:
> - Informal, with patient-determined admission and discharge
> - Organized around specific goals agreed upon between the patient, psychiatrist, and nursing staff
> - Arranged with the clear agreement of the nursing staff
> - Brief, time-limited and goal-determined—the patient may be discharged if the goals of admission are not met

There is a significant role of pharmacotherapy for the management of personality disorder, but often it is limited to addressing behavioral clusters and comorbidities. There is no robust evidence for any particular medication that is directly indicated for the treatment of a specific personality disorder and psychiatrists must use their clinical judgment to prioritize the problem area that needs to be addressed first. A borderline personality disorder is the most studied for pharmacotherapy as these patients are more likely to seek medications.[21]

One of the major factors to bear in mind is access to medication for those with suicidal ideas. Shorter duration of prescriptions with weekly pickup from their pharmacy, or supervised access with the help of family members, is encouraged. Another important factor is the reproductive stage of the woman, which can be a barrier to compliance if the woman perceives these medications as harmful to her offspring.

ANTIDEPRESSANTS

Selective serotonin reuptake inhibitors (SSRIs) are the most researched and commonly prescribed for borderline personality disorder. Apart from treating comorbid depression or anxiety, there is also evidence to suggest a reduction in aggression, irritability, mood instability, and self-harming behaviors after treatment with SSRIs. However, there are also reports of SSRIs causing an increase in suicidal thoughts, which must be kept in mind while prescribing these drugs.

MOOD STABILISERS

These are also commonly prescribed and help manage emotional dysregulation, irritability, impulsivity, and recurrent depression. Lithium is often used to reduce suicidality and aggressive or combative behavior.[21,22] Small studies show some efficacy with the use of carbamazepine and sodium valproate. But sodium valproate is contraindicated in all women of childbearing age[23] and hence avoided as much as possible in this group.

ANTIPSYCHOTICS

Although the direct evidence of efficacy in personality disorders is very limited, regular use of atypical antipsychotics is also advised in reducing paranoid thoughts, impulsivity, and other psychotic symptoms.[24] Doses of the antipsychotics are usually lower than those used for severe mental disorders, except when indicated by the severity of the psychosis.

SUBSTANCE ABUSE

Appropriate treatment for substance withdrawal, treatment of cravings, and maintaining substitution should be undertaken as indicated.

Benzodiazepines should be prescribed judiciously and only restricted to intermittent use, as there is a high risk of misuse and dependency, and some evidence of increased risk of disinhibition. There is no evidence to prove its efficacy in the management of personality disorders.

PSYCHOTHERAPY

Psychotherapy continues to be the main evidence-based treatment for personality disorder, with the majority of interventions aimed at borderline personality disorder. The longer, traditional therapies that used dynamic principles are now being replaced by shorter, structured, and time-limited therapies that can be more easily adapted to the Indian setting. Evidence from Indian studies on interventions is still very sparse, with most of them describing a dialectical behavior therapy (DBT)-like approach.

DIALECTICAL BEHAVIOR THERAPY

Developed by Marsha Linehan, originally for women who self-harm, DBT evolved into a comprehensive program as a skill-based therapy for borderline personality disorder.[25,26]

Therapy is focused on social skills training that helps to reduce self-harming behaviors, therapy interfering behaviors, and increase behaviors that improve quality of life. Once this is achieved, long-term goals such as reducing post-traumatic stress disorder (PTSD), increasing self-respect, and achieving life goals, are addressed. A comprehensive DBT model includes engagement in individual as well as group therapy for 1–2 years.[27] Group therapy is used to educate the patients in social skills through four modules:
1. Emotional regulation
2. Distress tolerance
3. Interpersonal interaction
4. Mindfulness.

Individual therapy is used to reinforce these skills and reduce self-harming behaviors. Some of the key strategies used in DBT are behavioral chain analysis of self-destructive behavior, looking at alternative more adaptive behaviors; solution analysis, and validation techniques.

MENTALIZATION-BASED THERAPY

Developed by Anthony Bateman a Peter Fonagy, mentalization-based therapy (MBT) is an amalgamation and further development of elements of psychodynamic principles and structured therapy.[28] Children develop internal working models through initial attachment systems. Secure attachment leads to better self-soothing and self-regulation of emotions; a good enough caregiver reflects on the infant's intentions accurately and does not overwhelm the infant. Consistent secure care enables the child to understand others' emotions and learn from them: through contingent marked mirroring (basis for affect regulation). Disorganized/insecure attachment leads to patients vacillating between intimacy and autonomy and a limited ability to understand their own mental states and those of others. Evidence suggests a combination of individual and group therapy along with psychiatric support for at least 12-18 months, has the most favorable outcome for patients.[28]

SCHEMA-FOCUSED THERAPY

Developed by Jeffrey Young combining principles of CBT, Gestalt therapy, and psychoanalytical object relations.[29] Patients with personality disorders develop maladaptive schemas, the identification of which can help change their behavior patterns. If a patient's basic emotional needs (connection, mutuality, reciprocity, flow, and autonomy) are not met in childhood, then schemas, coping styles, and modes (mind states) can develop in a dysfunctional maladaptive manner leading to the personality disorder.[29] Changing cognitive patterns linked to the schema can develop adaptive patterns of behavior. Schema-focused therapy (SFT) uses three basic techniques, that are (1) cognitive, (2) experiential, and (3) behavioral. Experiential techniques expand on Gestalt therapy using empty chair techniques and other forms of psychodrama. The aim is to identify the dysfunctional schema and guide the patient to develop more mature behavioral schemas. Schema-focused therapy is delivered in individual and group therapy format for 1-2 years duration.

TRANSFERENCE-FOCUSED PSYCHOTHERAPY

Conceptualized and developed by Otto Kernberg and his team, this is fundamentally structured around a psychoanalytical and object relations framework.[30] Transference-focused psychotherapy (TFP) is also highly structured and delivered as twice-weekly therapy, where the split sense of self is reintegrated using transference and countertransference to understand the splits and object relations to build a coherent sense of self and others.

GOOD PSYCHIATRIC PRACTICE AND SUPPORTIVE PSYCHOTHERAPY

For the majority of Indian clinical settings, most of the above therapies are yet to become accessible. Considering the huge role played by social determinants on the presentation of personality disorder crises in women, structured psychiatric care and supportive psychotherapy have a strong role to play in management. This is well supported by evidence from senior psychotherapists working in high-resource settings and adapted for various crisis settings.[31,32]

- Robust assessment including confidential enquiry and collateral information.
- Rule out other conditions which can mimic personality disorder when there is a crisis.
- Offer a diagnostic formulation that is personal to the patient rather than a generic diagnosis, avoid using diagnosis as a label to define the patient.
- Apart from eliciting symptoms and risk factors, highlight strengths and factors that can contribute to resilience.
- Good collaboration with all involved clinicians.
- Establishing a structure of regular appointments and adhering to the structure as best as possible.
- Developing the crisis plan early during care and establishing a reliable pathway of contact to only available mental health clinicians during crises.
- Establishing healthy boundaries and encouraging various clinicians to follow the same consistently.
- Noticing and not reinforcing any "splitting" between the various clinicians.
- Attention to transference and countertransference which are most likely to arise in this setting.
- Care during termination of treatment or transfer to other clinicians as they are most likely to trigger feelings of abandonment.
- Psychoeducation of patient and family, engaging them regularly and ensuring any mental disorders in the family members are addressed.
- Empathetic and nonjudgmental stance throughout the assessment and management process, including and especially when patients may slip back during a crisis (for example, when they may self-harm after a long gap or return to an abusive husband).

SELF-CARE FOR PSYCHIATRISTS

Caring for vulnerable women who may be in abusive environments and exhibiting high-risk behaviors can be very challenging even for experienced psychiatrists. This can be even more difficult in the context of unsurmountable larger social issues. Clinicians should also assess their ability and access to resources to manage the same. Clinicians own gender and personal experiences can be both a facilitator and/or a barrier in working with this population. However, working with this population can also be rewarding, and interpersonal factors on both sides can contribute to the same.[33]

Working with good seniors and mentors, frequent reflective discussions, and personal therapy are helpful ways to enable self-care. Marsha M Linehan

> **BOX 5:** Basic assumptions that can help with patient care in personality disorder.
> - Patients want to improve
> - They are doing the best they can
> - They need to do better, try harder, and be more motivated to change
> - Patients may not have caused all their problems but they have to solve them anyway
> - Their lives are unbearable as they are currently being lived
> - They need to learn new behaviors in a relevant context
> - Treatment should be administered as a real relationship between equals
> - Principles of behavior are universal affecting therapists no less than patients
> - Therapists need support
> - Therapists can fail
> - Therapy can fail even when therapists do not

describes basic reminders that can be helpful in continuing to care for women with personality disorders as shown in **Box 5**.[27]

> ### KEY POINTS
> - Understand the nature of personality disorder.
> - Establish diagnosis through a comprehensive assessment.
> - Share and discuss diagnosis and management plan with the patient and key family members.
> - Ensure there is consistency of care with well-structured and well-maintained boundaries.
> - Approach management in adolescents with special care.
> - Apply good practice and evidence-based therapy approaches wherever possible.
> - Ensure team-based approach and self-care to sustain long term care.

■ REFERENCES

1. Klonsky ED, Jane JS, Turkheimer E, Oltmanns TF. Gender role and personality disorders. J Pers Disord. 2002;16(5):464-76.
2. Sharan P. An overview of Indian research in personality disorders. Indian J Psychiatry. 2010;52(Suppl 1):S250-4.
3. Gupta S, Mattoo SK. Personality disorders: prevalence and demography at a psychiatric outpatient in North India. Int J Soc Psychiatry. 2012;58(2):146-52.
4. Yeomans F, Clarkin JF, Kernberg OF. Transference-Focused Psychotherapy for Borderline Personality Disorder: A clinical guide, 1st edition. Washington, DC: American Psychiatric Association Publishing; 2015.
5. American Psychiatric Association. Diagnostic and Statistical Manual of Mental Disorders, 4th edition. Washington, DC: American Psychiatric Association Publishing; 2000.
6. Biskin RS, Paris J. Diagnosing borderline personality disorder. CMAJ. 2012;184(16):1789-94.
7. Tyrer P, Reed GM, Crawford MJ. Classification, assessment, prevalence, and effect of personality disorder. Lancet. 2015;385(9969):717-26.

8. Zanarini MC, Frankenburg FR. Pathways to the Development of Borderline Personality Disorder. J. Pers. Disord. 1997;11(11):39-104.
9. Reichborn-Kjennerud T. The genetic epidemiology of personality disorders. Dialogues Clin Neurosci. 2010;12(1):103-14.
10. Albert PR. Why is depression more prevalent in women? J Psychiatry Neurosci. 2015;40(4):219-21.
11. Office of Registrar General and Census Commissioner of India and UNFPA. (2014). Missing... Mapping the Adverse Child Sex Ratio in India. [online] Available from: https://india.unfpa.org/en/publications/missing-mapping-adverse-child-sex-ratio-india-0 [Last accessed December, 2023].
12. Malhotra S, Shah R. Women and mental health in India: An overview. Indian J Psychiatry. 2015 Jul;57(Suppl 2):S205-11.
13. World Health Organization. Gender disparities and mental health: The Facts. Geneva: World Health Organization; 2001.
14. Fisher J, de Mello MC, Patel V, Rahman A, Tran T, Holton S, et al. Prevalence and determinants of common perinatal mental disorders in women in low- and lower-middle-income countries: a systematic review. Bull World Health Organ. 2012;90(2):139-49.
15. Domar AD, Zuttermeister PC, Friedman R. The psychological impact of infertility: a comparison with patients with other medical conditions. J Psychosom Obstet Gynaecol. 1993;14(Suppl):45-52.
16. Press Trust of India. Two-Third Married Indian Women Victims of Domestic Violence: UN. [online] Available from: https://zeenews.india.com/news/nation/twothird-married-indian-women-victims-of-domestic-violence-un_248394.html [Last accessed December, 2023].
17. Bagadia A. Interventions for Personality Disorders. In: Advancing Frontiers of Psychiatric Therapeutics, 1st edition. New Delhi: Jaypee Brothers Medical Publishers (P) Ltd; 2020. p. 97.
18. Banerjee PJM, Gibbon S, Huband N. Assessment of personality disorder. In: Advances in Psychiatric Treatment. United Kingdom: Cambridge University Press; 2009. Pp. 389-97.
19. Bateman A, Anthony W, Tyrer P. Services for personality disorder: organisation for inclusion. Adv Psychiatr Treat. 2004;10(5):425-33.
20. Tyrer P, Bateman A. Drug treatment for personality disorders. Adv Psychiatr Treat. 2004;10:389-98.
21. Tyrer P. Drug treatment of personality disorder. Psychiatric Bulletin. 1998;22(4):242-4.
22. Davison SE. Principles of managing patients with personality disorder. Adv Psychiatr Treat. 2002;8:1-9.
23. Medicines and Healthcare products Regulatory Authority Valproate use by women and girls: current advice; 2018. [Online] Available from: https://www.gov.uk/guidance/valproate-use-by-women-and-girls. [Last accessed November 2023].
24. Walker C, Thomas J, Allen TS. Treating impulsivity, irritability, and aggression of antisocial personality disorder with quetiapine. Int J Offender Ther Comp Criminol. 2003;47(5):556-67.

25. Linehan MM. Cognitive-behavioral treatment of borderline personality disorder (Diagnosis and Treatment of Mental Disorders), 1st edition. New York: Guilford Press; 1993.
26. Lynch TR, Trost WT, Salsman N, Linehan MM. Dialectical behavioral therapy for borderline personality disorder. Annu Rev Clin Psychol. 2007;3:181-205.
27. Linehan MM. DBT Skills Training Manual, 2nd edition. New York: Guilford Publications; 2014.
28. Bateman A, Fonagy P. Handbook of Mentalizing in Mental Health Practice. Washington, DC: American Psychiatric Publishing; 2012.
29. Jeffrey YE, Janet KS, Marjorie WE. Schema Therapy: a practitioners guide. New York: Guildford Press; 2003.
30. Kernberg OF 1995. [Psychotherapeutic treatment of borderline patients]. Psychother Psychosom Med Psychol 45:73-82.
31. Gunderson J, Masland S, Choi-Kain L. Good psychiatric management: a review. Curr Opin Psychol. 2018;21:127-131.
32. Aviram RB, Hellerstein DJ, Gerson J, Stanley B. Adapting supportive psychotherapy for individuals with Borderline personality disorder who self-injure or attempt suicide. J Psychiatr Pract. 2004;10(3):145-55.
33. Bhola P, Mehrotra K. Associations between countertransference reactions towards patients with borderline personality disorder and therapist experience levels and mentalization ability. Trends Psychiatry Psychother. 2021;43(2):116-25.

SECTION 2

Reproductive Psychiatry

- **Perinatal Psychiatry**
  Prerna Kukreti
- **Gynecological Conditions and Mental Health**
  Sonia Shenoy
- **Menarche, the Menstrual Cycle, and Menopause: Biological Cycles and Women's Mental Health**
  Imon Paul, Anamika Das

CHAPTER 11

Perinatal Psychiatry

Prerna Kukreti

ABSTRACT

Perinatal psychiatry is a branch of psychiatry dealing with diagnosis and management of mental health conditions surrounding pregnancy and postpartum period. Perinatal psychiatrist can assist patients, family members, and reproductive child healthcare providers in planning pregnancy and handle challenges related to management of mental disorders during different phases of pregnancy and lactation, thereby improving maternal and child outcomes. It is essential to be aware about risk mental illness poses for obstetric and neonatal outcome and safety of psychotropic and neuromodulatory treatment modalities. Healthcare providers should conduct regular screening for perinatal mental disorders and evidence-based care should guide the treatment. Shared decision making should involve informing the patient and family about current clinical status, course of illness, effects, and side effects of medication. Alone concerns about teratogenic effect of psychotropic should not lead to denial of due care needed by women with mental disorders. A judicious evidence-based collaborative decision making can help to reduce burden of maternal mental disorders on mother, infant, and family.

Keywords: Perinatal mental illness, postpartum psychosis, suicide in pregnancy, infanticide, substance use disorder management in pregnancy, lactation and psychotropics, Neuromodulation in pregnancy, mother infant attachment disorder, pre conception planning.

LEARNING OBJECTIVES
- Spectrum of perinatal mental health conditions
- Risk benefit assessment for clinical decision making
- Principles of pharmacotherapy prescribing in perinatal period
- Use of neuromodulation in perinatal period
- Managing psychiatry emergencies in perinatal period

INTRODUCTION

"Perinatal psychiatry" is a specialized branch of psychiatry dealing with assessment, diagnosis, and treatment of mental disorders during planning of pregnancy, pregnancy, and postpartum.

Magnitude of perinatal mental disorders is high, pooled prevalence of common mental disorders in this period has been found to be 22% in low- and middle-income countries[1] and it not only increases maternal mental morbidity but also poses risk for obstetric complications, maternal-fetal attachment, and fetal growth and development. Suicide can be a serious consequence, as per report of Global Burden of Diseases, Injuries, and Risk Factors Study (GBD) 2016, suicide remains the leading cause of mortality in women of childbearing age in India from 1990 to 2016.[2] In the United States, suicide is the leading cause of mortality in postpartum period accounting for 20% of maternal deaths.[3]

Scope of perinatal psychiatry expands also beyond maternal psychiatric disorders to other mental health issues related to childbearing like stress, grief related to pregnancy loss and mother-infant attachment disorders.

In this chapter, we have focused on spectrum of perinatal mental health conditions, their impact on obstetric and neonatal outcome, general principles of assessment and management, challenges in usage of psychopharmacological agents/neuromodulation therapies/substance use disorder therapies, managing emergencies such as suicide/infanticide/acute agitation, promoting lactation with ongoing treatment, maternal infant bonding disorder, contraception planning with ongoing treatment, integrating screening in reproductive child healthcare settings and service delivery provisions specific to mother-baby units.

■ PERINATAL MENTAL HEALTH CONDITIONS

Nosological Status of Perinatal Mental Disorders

"Perinatal mental disorder" refers to the psychiatric illnesses occurring during entire period of pregnancy to postpartum period up to 1 year. Description of postpartum time frame is contentious ranging from 4 weeks to 6 weeks to 1 year.[4] Nosological status of perinatal disorders as in standard classificatory systems is mentioned in **Box 1** and clinical features of perinatal mental disorders are similar to nonpregnant state, and details about clinical features and course outcome of various perinatal mental disorders commonly encountered in clinical practice are mentioned in **Table 1**.[5-7]

> **BOX 1:** Nosological status of perinatal mental disorders.
>
> - *International classification of mental and behavioral disorders (ICD-11):* It classifies it under Block L1-6E2 as "mental or behavioral disorders associated with pregnancy, childbirth, and the puerperium" and refers to perinatal mental disorders occurring *during pregnancy or puerperium (commencing within about 6 weeks after delivery)*[5]
> - *Diagnostic and Statistical Manual (DSM5):* No separate category for perinatal disorders rather uses specifiers in different disorders such as brief psychotic disorder, depressive disorder, or bipolar disorder "With postpartum onset", if onset of symptoms is *during pregnancy or within 4 weeks postpartum*"[6]

TABLE 1: Clinical feature, course, and outcome of perinatal mental health conditions.

Mental health condition	Clinical feature, course outcome, and risk factor
Baby blues	• This is a common and temporary experience occurring in up to 80% of new mothers within first week of childbirth characterized by sudden dysphoric mood, irritability, crying spells, lability, and difficulty in focusing • It peaks 3–5 days after delivery and resolves 10–12 days postpartum • It is not a mental illness, just needs assurance and remits spontaneously
Adjustment disorder	• It is a stress-related and shorter-term condition. New mother may have feelings of being overwhelmed and present with an overly intense, irritable, and/or depressed disposition but does not meet clinical criteria for full postpartum depression or anxiety • Identifiable stressful event such as childbirth, sudden demands of parenthood, transition from working professional to stay-at-home mom or going back to work after maternity leave • The disorder is time limited, usually beginning within 3 months of the stressful event, and symptoms lessen within 6 months upon adaptation of the transitional event
Perinatal depressive disorder	• Major depressive disorder can present during pregnancy, just after delivery, or anytime in the first year following childbirth affecting up to 20% of new mothers • Symptoms include excessive worry, difficulty making decisions, feeling overwhelmed, cannot "think straight," sleep disturbance, feelings of sadness, guilt, hopelessness, doom, fear, physical complaints/symptoms with no apparent cause. It may include thoughts of self-harm or harm to others and is longer lasting than a depressed mood during a major life adjustment • Risk factors include past history of psychiatric illness in self or family, childhood abuse, prior traumatic experiences, domestic abuse, substance use, comorbid medical disorder, pressure for birth of a specific gender of child, obstetric violence, or pregnancy losses
Perinatal anxiety disorder	• It includes generalized anxiety disorder (GAD), obsessive-compulsive disorder (OCD), and panic disorder. Sometimes severity of anxiety symptoms (e.g., worry, avoidance, and obsessions) does not rise to the level of diagnosis; nevertheless, it still causes mild-to-moderate levels of distress and impairment • Main focus is on the fear of fetal loss (especially in those with a history of infertility, in vitro fertilization, miscarriage, or stillbirth), of lack of support, of inadequacy as a mother, or of parturition (tocophobia)

Contd...

Contd...

Mental health condition	Clinical feature, course outcome, and risk factor
	• In most cases, past history of anxiety disorder is a known risk factor for perinatal anxiety disorders • 66% of women with postpartum depression also have comorbid anxiety disorder • Any first onset episode panic attack in pregnancy warrants excluding thyroid disorders, anemia, and cardiac arrhythmias • Prevalence of panic disorder ranges from 1.4 to 9.1% in pregnancy to 0.5–2.9% after 6–10 weeks of pregnancy
Postpartum psychosis	• Typical onset for this is 2–3 days after childbirth • It is rare but severe complication, occurs in 1–3 women per 1,000 childbirths • Postpartum psychosis has a 5% suicide rate and 4% infanticide rate • Symptoms include hallucinations, delusional thinking, delirium, and mania • Preexisting bipolar disorder or other psychotic disorder is a risk factor • Delirium, cortical venous thrombosis, and eclampsia need to be ruled out *Note:* "Flag as medical emergency for immediate intervention"
Perinatal obsessive-compulsive disorder (OCD)	• It is associated with unwanted intrusive aggressive obsessive thoughts of "hurting baby" or "extreme concern of psychological well-being of infant" leading to significant distress and is often associated with depressive symptoms. OCD is known to worsen or recur in women with past history of this disorder during perinatal period[8] • Prevalence of obsessive-compulsive disorder (OCD) ranges from 1.2 to 5.2% during pregnancy to 4.0% after 6 months of pregnancy[7] • Past or family history of OCD and other anxiety disorders is a risk factor
Perinatal grief	• Grief following perinatal loss due to miscarriage, intrauterine death, or stillbirth can affect mother as well as partner • It can resolve with emotional support in due course of time or can also be risk factor in some cases for developing PTSD and depressive and anxiety disorders
Perinatal post-traumatic stress disorder (PTSD)	• Symptoms include recurrent nightmares, extreme anxiety, relieving, or having flashbacks of past-traumatic events (i.e., trauma during delivery, miscarriage, loss of child or loved one, past emotional, sexual, or physical trauma) • It affects usually 2–15% of women • Risk factor is difficult labor, child loss, and past traumatic experiences

BIOPSYCHOSOCIAL RISK FACTORS FOR PERINATAL MENTAL DISORDERS

Psychosocial Risk Factors for Perinatal Mental Disorders

Pregnancy and transition to parenthood is often associated with significant biological, psychological, and social changes, which often predisposes the vulnerable women at higher risk of developing mental disorders.

Psychological risk factors include past history of psychiatric disorders, family history of psychiatric disorder, lifetime use of alcohol and tobacco, and poor coping styles.[8]

Obstetric risk factors include primigravida, comorbid medical disorder, unwanted conception, and negative experience during any stage of pregnancy, fear of childbirth, and apprehensions about delivery.[8]

Social risk factors include poor social support, intimate partner violence, past history of childhood abuse, poor socioeconomic status, and significant negative life events.[8,9]

Neurobiological Risk Factors for Perinatal Mental Disorders

Neuroplasticity in Pregnancy

Brain undergoes significant structural and functional neuroplasticity in peripartum phase. Reorganization of brain tissue and functional changes in hippocampus, amygdala, prefrontal cortex, posterior cingulate cortex during pregnancy and reduction in gray matter volume in postpartum brain as compared to prepregnancy stages have been consistently reported in several studies.[10]

These are the areas involved in social cognition and emotional responsiveness, dysfunction in the dynamic changes at this time can predispose to mental illnesses. Cárdenas, Kujawa, and Humphreys hypothesize that hypo- and hyperresponsive brain changes may be associated with decreased and increased risk for psychopathology, respectively. Mothers with PPD have been shown to have aberrant and heightened activity in amygdala, insula, and orbitofrontal cortex leading to dampened reward response and reduced emotional responsiveness to infant.[10]

Neuroendocrine Changes

There occurs a sequential change in hormonal and immunological milieu during pregnancy and postpartum period.

Placenta releases chorionic gonadotropin, which promotes secretion of placental corticotropin-releasing hormone (CRH), progesterone, and estrogen. All three rise during first 3 months of pregnancy, remain elevated during pregnancy, and decrease drastically within 24 hours postpartum, as opposed to prolactin and oxytocin which continue to rise postpartum.

In contrast to negative regulation of hypothalamic–pituitary–adrenal (HPA) axis, glucocorticoids simultaneously upregulate placental CRH production and downregulate stress reactivity at hypothalamic level in peripartum period as adaptive response.[10]

However, in people with altered HPA axis, due to past-traumatic experiences or psychiatric illness or epigenetic modification, this fine balance may be disrupted.

Immunological Changes

There are three discrete immunological phases in peripartum period: (1) Proinflammatory phase during first two trimester of pregnancy, (2) Anti-inflammatory phase conducive for fetal development, and (3) strong immune response in parturition and postpartum phase.

Dysregulated immune activation along with sudden neuroendocrine changes have been linked with postpartum psychosis, blues, and delirium.[10]

IMPACT OF MENTAL ILLNESS ON PREGNANCY AND NEONATAL OUTCOME

Stika and Frederiksen in 2001 stated that pregnant women are the "last true therapeutic orphan"[11] and even after 2 decades it still holds true. On account of reducing fetal exposure and "do no harm" *act of commission* of *withholding drugs for expectant mothers is far more common than act of omission* of *not treating the mothers* on whose well-being depends good health of fetus. Due to such prevalent notions in general masses as well as physicians, psychotropics are discontinued or switched as a knee jerk reaction by mothers as well as practitioners on sudden discovery of pregnancy.

But, it is important to understand that such skewed binary decision is based only on teratogenic risk of psychotropic versus maternal mental morbidity, what is forgotten is the third important fulcrum of pendulum, i.e., the paramount risk untreated mental illness poses on obstetric and neonatal outcome as detailed in **Box 2** in general and **Table 2** for specific mental illnesses.

PSYCHOTROPIC DRUGS USE IN PERINATAL PERIOD

The potential concern for psychotropic peripartum period centers around following domains:
- Teratogenicity or major malformation (first-trimester exposure)
- Neonatal toxicity (third-trimester exposure)
- Longer-term neurobehavioral effects, and
- Increased risk of physical health problems in adult life[18]

BOX 2: Risk untreated mental illness poses on obstetric and neonatal outcome.

- *Risk of relapse:* Pregnancy is not protective against mental illness. Decision to discontinue medications is associated with high risk of relapse. Very high relapse rates are found in depressive disorder up to 70%[12] and bipolar disorder up to 86%.[13] Antenatal mental illnesses are predictor of postpartum onset or continuation of symptoms
- *Impact on antenatal care and family:* Untreated mental disorders may be associated with delayed health seeking for antenatal services, poor follow-ups, poor dietary patterns, self-neglect, smoking, alcohol use, high-risk behaviors like indiscriminate sex, exposure to sexually transmitted infections, and restrained interpersonal relationships with caregivers[14]
- *Impact on pregnancy outcome:* Maternal mental illness during pregnancy has been associated with adverse perinatal outcomes, including placental abnormalities, small-for-gestational-age fetuses, fetal distress, preterm delivery, low birth weight, and neonatal hypoglycemia[15]
- *Effect on infant development:* Untreated mental illnesses have been associated with detrimental effect on infant's neurodevelopmental development. This has been partly attributed to effect of uterine environment and fetal programming during critical period of in-utero development. High-risk behaviors due to untreated mental illness such as smoking, alcohol use, and poor nutrition status may also contribute to it. Poor mother-child bonding and attachment increase rates of emotional and behavioral problems in children born to mothers with mental disorders[16]

TABLE 2: Association of different psychiatric illness with pregnancy and neonatal outcome.[17]

Illness	Teratogenic effect	Association with obstetric outcome	Association with neonatal outcome
Anxiety disorder	N/A	Increased incidence of forceps deliveries, prolonged labor, precipitate labor, fetal distress, preterm delivery, and spontaneous abortion	Decreased developmental scores and inadaptability; slowed mental development at 2 years of age
Depressive disorder	N/A	Increased incidence of low birthweight, decreased fetal growth, and postnatal complications	Increased newborn cortisol and catecholamine levels, increased infant crying and rates of admission to neonatal intensive care units
Schizophrenia	Congenital malformations, especially of cardiovascular system	Increased incidence of preterm delivery, low birthweight, small for gestational age, placental abnormalities, and antenatal hemorrhage	Increased rates of postnatal death

Limitation in interpretation of psychotropic safety data: The safety of psychotropic drugs in pregnancy cannot be clearly established because robust and prospective trials are obviously unethical. Individual decisions on psychotropic use in pregnancy are therefore based on database studies that have many limitations. They are based on isolated case reports or case series with several confounders, e.g., failure to control for the effects of illness, smoking, obesity, other medications, etc.

Table 3 summarizes the psychotropics, different classes they belong to as per old system of Food and Drug Administration (FDA) to classify psychotropics in pregnancy as category A to X and in lactation as Hales category of L1 to L4 and current recommendation based on latest regulation of pregnancy and lactation labeling rule (PLLR).[18-20]

Based on knowledge of psychotropic safety, **Table 4** summarizes different class of psychotropics and management pearls during different stages of pregnancy.[19]

RISK BENEFIT ASSESSMENT: SETTING RIGHT TONE

Clinicians must understand while communicating risk and benefit based on risk posed by mental illness or psychotropics, general tone of the interaction and choice of words used are the key to establish atmosphere of trust and nonjudgmental conversation.

Words like "teratogenic", "psychopathology", "risk" and discussion about "adverse maternal child outcomes" can be extremely anxiety provoking for the mother and family. Instead sensitive terms like "chance" and "likelihood" can be used and also worth emphasizing to client is— these all are relative risks not absolute risks.[16]

Attempt should be made to give a pictorial description of risk percentages against normal pregnancy or untreated cohort with similar illness to give a clear picture. Attempt should be made for shared decision making with patient and family and documenting the choices made.

GENERAL MANAGEMENT GUIDELINES FOR MANAGEMENT OF MENTAL DISORDERS IN DIFFERENT PERINATAL PHASES

A treating psychiatrist may encounter perinatal mental disorders in following situations:
- *Prepregnancy*
  - A patient with mental disorders on medications wanting to conceive
  - A Patient undergoing treatment for infertility referred for evaluation
- *During pregnancy and intrapartum phase*
  - A patient with perinatal mental disorders
  - Acutely symptomatic (first episode or relapse)
  - In remission (with/without medication)

TABLE 3: Psychotropics and safety recommendations for pregnancy and lactation.

Class of drugs and generic name	Old system		New system	Remarks
	FDA category for pregnancy*	Hales category for lactation#	PLLR	
Antidepressants				
Fluoxetine	C	L2 in older infant/L3 if used in neonatal period	• First trimester fluoxetine use is associated with increased risk of cardiovascular malformations; Paroxetine is linked to cardiac malformations (ventricular septal and valve defects) • Consideration should be given to either discontinuing paroxetine use or switching to another antidepressant	• Sertraline is most preferred molecule • Paroxetine is to be avoided
Sertraline	C	L2		
Escitalopram	C	L2		
Venlafaxine	C	L3		
Mirtazapine	C	L3		
Paroxetine	D	L2	—	—
Antiobsessive medication				
Fluvoxamine	C	L2		
Clomipramine	C	L2		

Contd...

Contd...

Class of drugs and generic name	Old system		New system	Remarks
	FDA category for pregnancy*	Hales category for lactation#	PLLR	
Benzodiazepine (BZD)			• Nonteratogenic risks include reports of neonatal flaccidity, respiratory and feeding difficulties, hypothermia, and neonatal withdrawal symptoms during the postnatal period • Use of these drugs in first trimester exposure should almost always be avoided until a matter of urgency	• BZD with short half-life like lorazepam preferred • If using it in last trimester, observe infant for any withdrawal signs
Clonazepam	D	L3		
Alprazolam	D	L3		
Chlordiazepoxide	D	L3		
Lorazepam	D	L3		
Diazepam	D	L3/L4 if used chronically		
Non-BZD sedative				
Zolpidem	B	L3	--	--
Non-BZD Anxiolytic				
Buspirone	B	L3	--	--

Contd...

Contd...

Class of drugs and generic name	Old system		New system	Remarks
	FDA category for pregnancy*	Hales category for lactation#	PLLR	
Antipsychotic			• No teratogenic effects or fetal toxicity have been observed in animal studies involving exposure to clozapine or lurasidone in animals • There are no adequate and well-controlled studies in pregnant women • Third trimester exposure increases risk for neonatal extrapyramidal and/or withdrawal symptoms (EPS)	Women on Olanzapine and clozapine to be worked up for gestational diabetes
Haloperidol	C	L2		
Chlorpromazine	C	L3		
Aripiprazole	C	L3		
Risperidone	C	L3		
Quetiapine	C	L4C		
Olanzapine	C	L2		
Clozapine	B	L3		

Contd...

Contd...

Class of drugs and generic name	Old system		New system	Remarks
	FDA category for pregnancy*	Hales category for lactation#	PLLR	
Mood stabilizer				
Lithium	D	L4	• There are no adequate and well-controlled studies in pregnant women • Lithium may cause Ebstein's anomaly • Carbamazepine is associated with risk to the fetus, including congenital malformations (spinal bifida), and developmental delays • Valproate may produce congenital malformations (e.g., neural tube defects) at a rate higher than other drugs and general population • Valproate should not be used in pregnancy	• Lithium is safest in pregnancy but contraindicated in lactation • Carbamazepine is safe in lactation • Lamotrigine is a good mood stabilizer for maintenance therapy in pregnancy and lactation • Valproate is to be avoided in pregnancy, permissible in lactation
Valproate	D	L2		
Carbamazepine	D	L2		
Lamotrigine	C	L3		

*Food and Drug Administration (FDA) categories: A—controlled study shows no risk; B—No evidence of risk in humans; C—risk cannot be ruled out for humans; D—possible evidence of risk; X—contraindicated
#Hales lactation risk category—L1: safest; L2: safer; L3: moderately safe; L4: possibly hazardous; L5: contraindicated.

CHAPTER 11: Perinatal Psychiatry

TABLE 4: Psychotropics and management issues in different stages of pregnancy.

Medication class	Birth defects	Pregnancy	Delivery	Neonatal	Lactation	Preferred medications
Benzodiazepine	Possible increased incidence of cleft lip or palate	Ultrasonography for facial morphology	Floppy infant syndrome	Withdrawal syndrome	Infant sedation reported	• Lorazepam • Clonazepam • Alprazolam
Antidepressants	None confirmed	Decreased serum concentrations across pregnancy	None	Neonatal, withdrawal syndrome	None	• Sertraline • Fluoxetine
Lithium	Increased incidence of heart defects	Ultrasonography or fetal echocardiography for heart development or both Decreases serum concentrations across pregnancy	Give intravenous fluids to avoid increased risk of lithium toxicity in mother	Be cautious for increased risk of lithium toxicity in premature infant	Monitor infant complete blood count, thyroid-stimulating hormone levels, and lithium levels	Sustained release lithium

Contd...

Contd...

Medication class	Birth defects	Pregnancy	Delivery	Neonatal	Lactation	Preferred medications
Mood stabilizers	Increased incidence of birth defects	• Decreased serum concentrations across pregnancy • Folate supplement • Vitamin K supplement for some antiepileptic drugs	None	Vitamin K for some antiepileptic drugs	Monitor infant complete blood count, thyroid-stimulating hormone levels, and lithium levels	• Lamotrigine • Lithium
Antipsychotics			None	Possible risk for neuroleptic malignant syndrome and intestinal obstruction	Monitor infant complete blood count, liver enzyme levels, antiepileptic drug levels	• Haloperidol • Olanzapine

- *Postdelivery*
  - A patient with perinatal mental disorders
    - Acutely symptomatic (first episode or relapse)
    - In remission (with/without medication)
  - Baby blues
  - Postnatal grief
  - Mother-infant bonding disorders

As a golden dictum, these patients are best managed with a collaborative perinatal mental health team having obstetrician, psychiatrist, and neonatologist who are sensitive to needs of such patients, can collaboratively share documented decisions across departments and convey uniform messages about safety of evidence-based therapeutic options to patient and family.

MANAGEMENT IN PRECONCEPTION PHASE

General Measures

Any person with mental disorder planning to conceive can be offered following management:

- *High-dose of folic acid:* Consider starting such patients on high dose (5 mg) folic acid daily.
- *Healthy lifestyle practices advice:* Work on addressing other modifiable risk factors (if present any) for poor obstetrical outcome, e.g., offering treatment for smoking cessation, alcohol deaddiction, obesity, and diabetes. Referral to social worker for clients reporting history of domestic violence.
- *Avoid unplanned pregnancy:* Practice contraception, preferably barrier methods, and oral contraceptives may have drug interaction with some psychotropics and maintain menstrual calendar.
- *Planning pregnancy* in stable phase of illness preferably.

Specific Issues in Management of Mental Disorders

- *Decision making about treatment:* Any person with any perinatal mental disorder planning to conceive while on medication can be offered following treatment options:
  - Discontinue the treatment prior to conception
  - Continue treatment throughout the pregnancy

  All these decisions would depend on following variables:
  - Frequency and severity of previous episodes
  - Past and current levels of functioning or impairment
  - Past and recent duration of clinical stability, with and without medication

- The nature of prodromal symptoms that indicate an impending relapse, and
- Average time to recovery following reintroduction of treatment
- *Stable patient/mild or infrequent illness:* If there is past history of one or infrequent episodes with long period of remission—pharmacological agents can be tapered off slowly and the women should be closely monitored for conception and relapse of symptoms.
- *Severe illness with frequent episodes or difficult to manage episodes in past with history of self-harm:*
    - Consider continuing medication throughout pregnancy.
    - Prefer to keep patient on monotherapy, if possible.
    - Safer drug to be chosen, but change of medication is usually not advised (except in case of valproate or paroxetine) because it poses patient at increased risk of relapse, exposes infant to two different psychotropic agents.
- *Patient with mental disorder on medications having difficulty in conceiving* should be evaluated for:
    - Ruling out depressive disorder or negative symptoms contributing to it
    - Ruling out sexual dysfunctions primary or secondary to any psychotropic
    - In case of drug-induced amenorrhea/other menstrual abnormality/hyperprolactinemia: For switching on to use of prolactin sparing medications. **Table 5** mentions psychotropics and effect on ability to conceive.[21]

TABLE 5: Psychotropics and effect on ability to conceive.

Medication class	Effect on ability to conceive
Antidepressants	No effect on the ability of women to conceive, although there is some evidence that they may affect male sperm count and morphology.[22]
Anxiolytic and hypnotic	No effect
Antipsychotics	All FGAs and some SGAs (especially risperidone and amisulpride) can cause hyperprolactinemia and impaired fertility[23]
Lithium	Lithium is not known to have significant effects on female fertility but may inhibit sperm motility[24]
Mood stabilizers	Women with epilepsy using valproate have an increased rate of polycystic ovary syndrome/ovaries.[25] Valproate treatment is reported to be associated with adverse spermatogenesis in men[26]

Flowchart 1: Treatment planning for persons with mental disorder on medication planning to conceive.

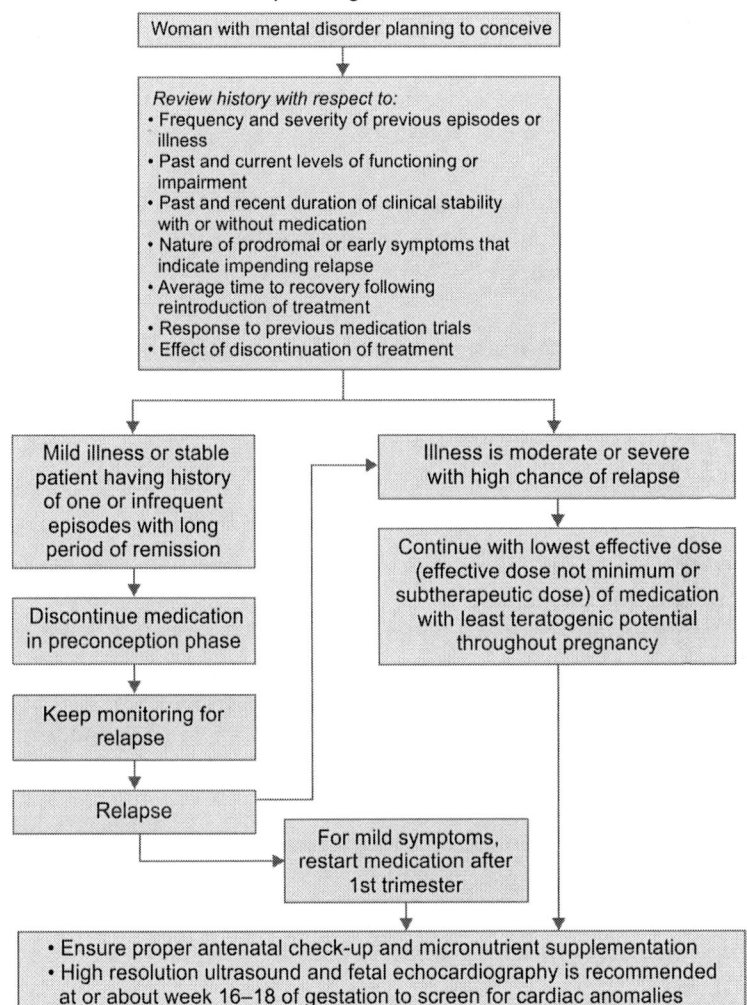

Flowchart 1 details decision making matrix for patients with mental illness planning to conceive.

MANAGEMENT OF PERINATAL MENTAL DISORDERS DURING PREGNANCY[21]

General Measures
- *Flag as high-risk pregnancy:* Manage pregnancy among women with severe mental illness as a high-risk pregnancy requiring more intensive monitoring, with close liaison with obstetrician.

- *High-dose folic acid:* Consider starting such patients on high dose (5 mg) folic acid daily.
- *Healthy lifestyle practices advice:* Work on addressing other modifiable risk factors (if present any) for poor obstetrical outcome, e.g., offering treatment for smoking cessation, alcohol deaddiction, obesity, and diabetes. Referral to social worker for clients reporting history of domestic violence.
- *Excessive weight gain and gestational diabetes:* Monitor for excessive weight gain and gestational diabetes, particularly for women on a second-generation antipsychotic (SGA).

Specific Issues in Management of Mental Disorders

Decision making: For individualized treatment plan to be made weighing risk and benefit based on following clinical situations:

Patient with Mental Disorder in Remission Conceives

- *Single episode of mild illness, currently in remission:* It can be considered for tapering off medicines.
  - *If infrequent episodes/mild illness (pregnancy < 3 months):* It can be considered for tapering off medicines or starting psychotherapeutic options if mild depression or mild anxiety disorders.
  - *If infrequent episodes/mild illness (pregnancy > 3 months):* Do risk assessment for deciding future course of treatment.
  - Continue medications in case of severe illness with frequent episodes or difficult to manage episodes in past with history of self-harm assessing safety of psychotropics.

Symptomatic Patient with Mental Disorder Conceives

- *On treatment:* Consider optimizing preexisting treatment. Avoid switching medications unless risk outweighs benefit, e.g., stopping valproate. In rest all cases, consider continuing patient on monotherapy preferably on agent with the best response in past.
- *First episode/patient off drugs:* Initiate a medicine safe for peripartum period if symptoms are severe, else try to keep patient on nonpharmacological therapies, e.g., psychotherapy for mild depressive disorder or anxiety disorder.
  - *Antipsychotics:* Among first generation antipsychotics (FGAs) haloperidol is preferred among second generation antipsychotics (SGAs) quetiapine or olanzapine is preferred unless risk of metabolic disorders.

- *Antidepressants:* Selective serotonin reuptake inhibitors (SSRIs) are preferred and most data on safety is concerning sertraline followed by on fluoxetine. Paroxetine is to be avoided.
- *Sedatives and hypnotics:* Prefer using non-BZD derivatives like zolpidem as hypnotic. If needed to use BZD, consider using BZD with short half-life like lorazepam. Use before delivery should be cautious and minimal to avoid neonatal withdrawal syndrome.
- *Mood stabilizers:* Lamotrigine and lithium are safer mood stabilizer but still latter carries risk of cardiac anomalies, so fetal echocardiography and second trimester anomaly scans should be planned well. Valproate is contraindicated and should be avoided as much as possible.

Flowchart 2 summarizes the treatment algorithm for management of patients having active symptoms of common mental illnesses (Depression/anxiety/OCD) during pregnancy.

Flowchart 3 summarizes the treatment algorithm for management of patients having active symptoms of severe mental illnesses (psychosis/schizophrenia/mania) during pregnancy.

INTRAPARTUM MANAGEMENT OF PERINATAL MENTAL DISORDERS[21]

- In women with a severe mental illness, it is recommended that delivery should be in tertiary care hospital with round the clock psychiatry services.
- Anticipate potential issues which might arise with perinatal mental health team.
- Clear orders for medication which needs to be reduced or stopped before labor weighing benefit and risk, for example:

Flowchart 2: Management algorithm for persons with symptoms of common mental illnesses (CMI) during pregnancy.

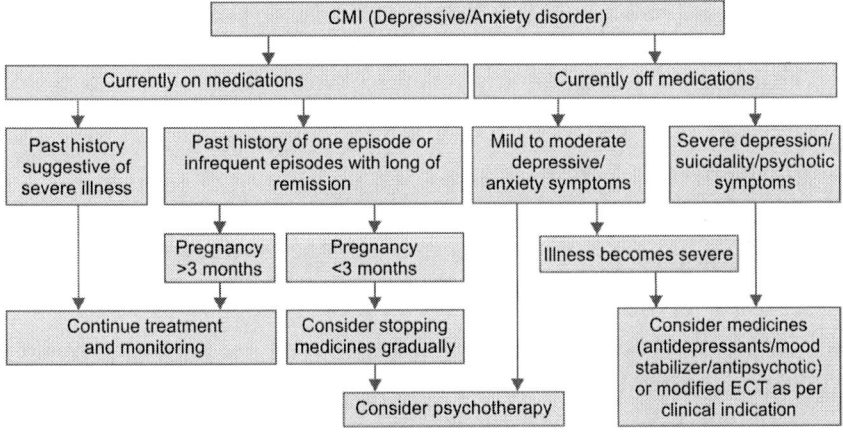

Flowchart 3: Management algorithm for persons with symptoms of severe mental illnesses (SMI) during pregnancy.

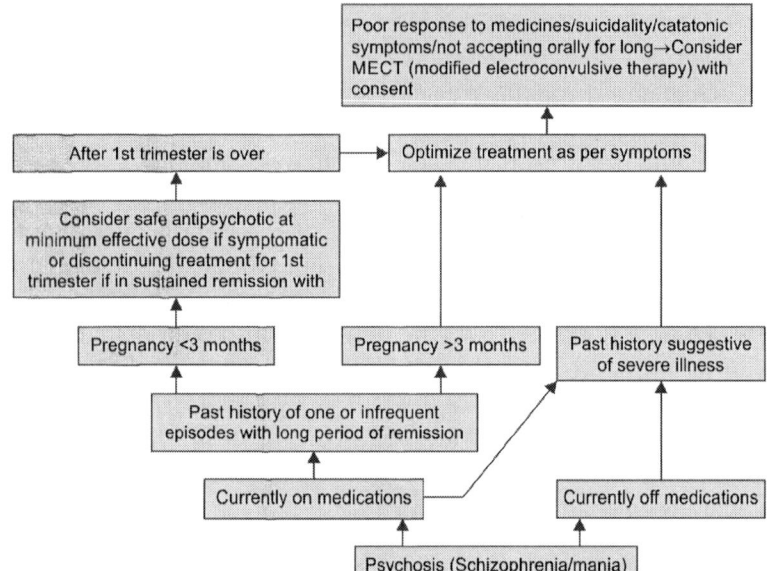

- Considering dose reduction of FGA (like haloperidol), if possible to reduce chance of extrapyramidal symptoms to neonate or if not possible, inform neonatologist to observe for any such signs.[21]
- *Cautious monitoring for lithium:* National Collaborating Center for Mental Health suggests reducing or stopping lithium on day of delivery for reducing neonatal complications.[27] Lithium blood levels should be measured 24 hours before and after delivery in mother and lithium levels and free T4 levels in umbilical cord.[28,29] Hydration should be maintained for preventing lithium toxicity. If cesarean is planned, anesthetist should be informed because lithium potentiates succinylcholine and pancuronium and can be expected to potentiate effect of other depolarizing and nondepolarizing muscle relaxants.[30]
- Ensure good analgesia and sleep to avoid triggers for relapse or exacerbation of mental illnesses.

POSTNATAL MANAGEMENT OF PERINATAL MENTAL DISORDERS[21]

General Measures

Assessment of Mother

- *Baby blues:* Be watchful in stable patients too for postpartum blues, they are transient and can be managed well with assurance, any sustenance of symptoms will warrant close follow-up.

- *Mental disorders new episode or exacerbation:* Postnatal period up to 6 weeks is period for likely exacerbation of mental illnesses. Screen women using standardized rating scale. As in pregnancy, previous treatment response should guide future treatment choices
- *Lactation advice:* Continue breastfeeding on demand as per comfort of mother, there is no need of withholding breastfeeding after each dose of medications, since all the medications achieve steady state after few days of initial treatment. Consider keeping minimum number of medications, prefer monotherapy and less complicated dosing regimen. Medications with low relative infant dose (RID) < 10% (RID is the daily amount of drug ingested by the infant during exclusive breastfeeding per kg bodyweight divided by the maternal daily dose per kg body weight) to be used.[31] If due to poor mental health mother is unable to breastfeed in immediate postpartum period, allow her to express breast milk at regular intervals. Medication safety with respect to lactation is detailed in **Table 6** for use in breastfeeding women.
- *Supportive measures:* Pain and insomnia can be potential triggers for exacerbation, address them well.
- *Adjusting psychotropics:* Take neonatology opinion if it is a premature delivery and mother is breastfeeding. Adjust medicines causing excessive sedation may be needed if hindering baby care and breastfeeding.

Assessment of Neonate

- *Neonate care:* Advise mothers for rooming-in and skin-to-skin contact. If medicines are causing excessive sedation, encourage use of baby crib besides mother's bed. Monitor the infant for adverse effects such as oversedation and poor feeding. Monitor neonate for drug withdrawal syndrome.

TABLE 6: Psychotropic class and safety profile during lactation.[21]

Psychotropic class	Safety profile for lactation
Antidepressants	SSRIs can be used with moderate safety
Antipsychotics	Haloperidol, olanzapine, and quetiapine are preferred. Clozapine is contraindicated owing to risk of infant agranulocytosis and seizure
Mood stabilizers	Valproate and carbamazepine are preferred. Lithium use to be avoided
Sedative and anxiolytic	Benzodiazepines are associated with sedation, lethargy, withdrawal in infant. Consider non-BZD drugs like zolpidem for sleep and buspirone for anxiety

(BZD: benzodiazepine; SSRI: selective serotonin reuptake inhibitors)

- *Maternal-infant attachment disorders:* Presence of psychiatric disorder, specifically severe mental illnesses at times may have bearing on mother-infant relationship. A mother may have difficulty at three levels, inability to perceive infant cues, incorrectly understanding infant cues, or inability to respond consistently and in an appropriate manner. This can lead to mother-infant disorders, which are detailed in **Table 7**.[32]

Psychometric tools specific for perinatal settings like NIMBUS (NIMHANS Maternal Behavioral Scale), maternal fetal attachment scale (MFAS), prenatal fetal attachment scale (PFAS), maternal antenatal attachment scale (MAAS), prenatal attachment inventory (PAI), and postpartum bonding questionnaire (PBQ) can be used to assess mother-infant bonding patterns.

Role of Other Family Members

- *Social support:* Encourage mothers with known past or family history of severe mental illness to have social support for care of neonate and mother and ensure adequate sleep to mother.

TABLE 7: Different manifestations of maternal-infant bonding disorder.

Mild disorders (Delay, ambivalence, or loss in maternal response)	When the mother experiences delay or loss of maternal emotional response, she may express disappointment about her feelings toward her infant (e.g., that she has no feelings, or she feels estranged or distant from him, or she feels that he is not her baby, or that she is baby-sitting for someone else)
Rejection (threatened or established)	It may present with rejection of the infant (when the mother expresses strong negative feelings about the child: dislike, hatred, and regret about his birth). There is absence of affectionate behavior such as kissing, cuddling, cooing, singing, and playing. She feels better when away from the infant; she expresses the feeling of being trapped by motherhood. She may express the wish that the infant care is transferred to someone else. She may have the wish that the infant is stolen or dies and she may have run away to escape the care of the infant
Pathological anger (mild, moderate, or severe)	When a mother experiences pathological anger toward the infant, she may have a milder form (an experience of anger which is controlled with difficulty) or she may have an impulse to harm or kill the child, or she may lose control at a verbal level and shout and scream at the baby. When the presentation of anger is more pronounced, this may result in handling the baby roughly (e.g., throwing it into the cot or jerking his limbs, shaking him, occluding his breathing), or she may strike, beat, bite, burn or throw him or make a deliberate attempt to kill him

- *Adequate sensorimotor stimulation of infant:* Encourage mother-infant bonding. If mother is unable to provide sensori-stimulation to infant due to illness, exhaustion or sedation, another caregiver should be psychoeducated to provide same in form of massage, oil bath, singing lullabies, talking to infant, cooing, and providing a variety of colors and sounds through toys. It can ensure presence of a secure emotional attachment figure for infant.[31]
  Urgent mental health conditions: Urgent referral in case of marked agitation or suicide or infanticide at any stage of conception should be flagged as psychiatry emergency.
- *Risk assessment for infanticide and suicide in mother:* A specific enquiry must be made to assess ideas plans or any recent attempts of harm toward self, infant, or others. Structured tools for same can be used. Risk assessment and decision-making matrix are mentioned in **Table 8**.[33]

Management of Acute Agitation

Risk posed by maternal agitation for maternal and fetal safety greatly outweighs any potential risk associated with short-term exposure of psychotropics for agitation control during perinatal period. Attempt should be made for verbal de-escalation in a safe and nonstimulating environment for mild agitation. For moderate to severe agitation, antihistaminics, benzodiazepines, and antipsychotics can be used, mouth dissolving oral preparations or parenteral as per the clinical need. Details are mentioned in **Box 3**, cautious monitoring of fetal heart rate and vital monitoring of mother is needed.[34]

TABLE 8: Suicide and infanticide risk assessment.

	Suicide risk assessment		
Ask questions Suicide ideation—Plan—Lethality—Means—Previous history			
Level of risk	Low risk	Medium risk	High risk
Presentation	Fluctuating thoughts of suicide or self-injury without lethal plans or means	Thoughts and intentions of suicide without plans	Continuous thoughts of suicide, intention, plan, and means
Level of action	• Close follow-up • Adequate treatment • Involve family in treatment and monitoring	• Close follow-up • Intensive treatment • Involve family in treatment and monitoring • May offer hospitalization	• Offer inpatient treatment • Intensive treatment (Pharmacotherapy, psychotherapy, and/or ECT)

Contd...

Contd...

Infanticide risk assessment			
Ask sensitively about intrusive distressing thoughts for harming child			
Level of risk	**Low risk**	**Medium risk**	**High risk**
Presentation	• Thoughts are scary, cause anxiety, and are ego-dystonic. Mother knows harming her baby will be bad and she clearly knows she would not harm her baby • Symptoms more consistent with depression/anxiety/OCD	Thoughts are very scary, cause minimal or less anxiety. Mother is not sure if the thoughts are based on reality or whether harming baby would be a bad thing. Mother is less clear is she would not harm her baby	• Thoughts are not causing any anxiety, and ego syntonic. Mother has lack of insight, contact with reality is lost, considers these thoughts correct action to do, bizzare belief, and perceptual distortions • Symptoms are more consistent with psychosis
Intensive treatment, offer hospitalization. If mother and child are separated, regular reassessment and scheduled supervised meetings as per the Mental Healthcare Act provisions.			

(ECT: electroconvulsive therapy; OCD: obsessive-compulsive disorder)

BOX 3: Pharmacological options for management of acute agitation in perinatal population.

Antihistamine
Promethazine
Initial dosing: 25–50 mg PO, IV, or IM every 1–4 hours maximum 300 mg/day
Period of onset (PO): 15–30 minutes (IM, IV: rapid)
Side effect: Sedation and anticholinergic effects

First-generation antipsychotics
Haloperidol
Initial dosing: 5–10 mg PO, IV, or IM maximum 20 mg/day
Period of onset (PO): 2–6 hours IM, IV: 20–30 minutes
Side effect: Extrapyramidal effect, dystonia, sedation, neuroleptic malignant syndrome, and anticholinergic effects.

Second-generation antipsychotics
Olanzapine
Initial dosing: 5–10 mg PO or IM maximum 20–30 mg/day
Period of onset (PO): 15 minutes to 4 hours IM: 15–30 minutes
Side effect: Sedation, orthostatic hypotension, and extrapyramidal symptoms
Ziprasidone
Initial dosing: 20 mg IM maximum 40 mg/day
Period of onset (PO)—IM: 15–30 minutes
Side effect: Sedation, headache, nausea, and extrapyramidal symptoms

Contd...

Contd...

> **Benzodiazepines**
> **Lorazepam**
> *Initial dosing:* 0.5–2 mg PO, IV, or IM
> *Period of onset (PO):* 15–30 minutes IM and IV
> *Side effect:* Rapid sedation and respiratory depression
>
> Severe agitation may require a combination of agents. A commonly used, safe regimen—colloquially called the "B52 bomb"—is haloperidol 5 mg, lorazepam 2 mg, and promethazine 25-50 mg for prophylaxis of dystonia.

Management of Catatonia

Immobility and stuporous conditions of catatonia increase risk of deep venous thrombosis in pregnancy and pose risk of inanition which exceeds the risk of use of lorazepam for its treatment. Management can be initiated with low dose of lorazepam 3-8 mg/day in three or four divided doses. Based on response, it can be increased up to 8-16 mg/day with due monitoring of maternal and fetal vitals. Further dose may be stopped if maternal BP falls below 90/60 mm Hg or pulse <60 beats/min or fetal bradycardia, i.e., hear rate <100 beats/min. Psychotropic based on underlying dose should be started and in case of poor response to lorazepam, electroconvulsive therapy (ECT) can be given.[31]

OTHER THERAPEUTIC CHALLENGES IN PERINATAL PSYCHIATRIC DISORDERS MANAGEMENT

Long-acting Injectable Antipsychotic Usage in Perinatal Population

Level of evidence available to draw definitive conclusion about safety of long-acting injectable (LAI) in perinatal period is limited. There is no evidence to suggest that additional compounds used in making LAIs have any adverse impact on pregnancy or infant,[1] so, risk needs to be extrapolated based on evidence available from use of oral antipsychotics. Detail about LAI usage safety is mentioned in **Box 4**.[35]

Neuromodulatory Treatment Modalities Usage in Perinatal Population

Electroconvulsive Therapy

American Psychiatric Association as well as American College of Obstetricians and Gynecologists have issued statements regarding ECT as safe and effective option for treatment resistance or life-threatening conditions such as catatonia, suicidality, etc. Detail about indication and precautions for perinatal population are mentioned in **Box 5**.[40]

BOX 4: Factors governing long-acting injectable (LAI) use in perinatal period.

- *Indications:* Very effective for patients with severe mental illness or frequent episodes or with history of poor compliance
- *Benefits of LAI:* Ensure more constant plasma level of drug, reducing fetal exposure to fluctuating level of psychotropics[35] and risk of relapse to mother
- *Available level of evidence for safety:* Most evidence available is in form of case series on risperidone, paliperidone, aripiprazole, fluphenazine, zuclopenthixol LAIs, and no deleterious effect on pregnancy outcome, neonatal death, or APGAR score has been noted.[36] Isolated case reports of prematurity, small for gestation age children, and congenital anomaly have been reported though and this data has not been adjusted to other confounding factors[37]
- *Decision regarding choice of LAI:* Same parameters as for oral antipsychotic, ones with safer metabolic profile, with longer dosing interval and ones with past history of good response may be preferable[38]
- *Caution:* Dose adjustment based on pharmacokinetic changes in different stages of pregnancy may be needed, e.g., aripiprazole LAI which is metabolized by CYP2D6 whose expression in increased during pregnancy[39]
- Not advisable to initiate in cases expecting premature births

BOX 5: Electroconvulsive therapy (ECT) use principles in perinatal period.

Indications: Treatment-resistant affective and psychotic disorder, high risk of suicide or infanticide, severe depression, catatonia, psychotic agitation, marked aggression, debilitating physical condition due to poor oral intake

Pre-ECT
- Liaison with obstetrician and neonatologist if late third trimester
- To prevent risk of aspiration because of reduced gastroesophageal sphincter tone, consider following pre ECT:
  - Stop anticholinergic agents 24 hours prior
  - Strict nil per oral instructions (8 hours for solid/2 hours for liquid)
  - Prophylactic antireflux agent, e.g., proton-pump inhibitor or sodium citrate
  - To avoid precipitating factors of labor, e.g., long hours of fasting and dehydration. Consider nonglucose-containing IV fluids before and during procedure.
  - Nonstress test using tocometer in high-risk cases
  - Fetal heart rate monitoring and fetal movement monitoring
  - Adequate preoxygenation only because hyperventilation can cause fetal hypoxia because respiratory alkalosis may affect fetal oxygenation

During ECT
- Patient to be placed in the left lateral decubitus position during procedure to prevent hypotension
- Fetal heart monitoring because anesthetic induction agents and muscle relaxants cross placental barrier

Post-ECT
- Fetal movement and fetal heart rate (FHR) monitoring, if FHR reduces, oxygenate and ensure left lateral decubitus position removes the gravid uterus laterally
- Nonstress test using tocometer
- Monitor for abdominal pain and vaginal bleeding. Any uterine contractions lasting >5 minutes must be suppressed using tocolytic agents

Repeated Transcranial Magnetic Stimulation

Recommendations are not available specifically for pregnancy with regard to repeated transcranial magnetic stimulation (rTMS) but maternal safety has been confirmed in all the published case series and efficacy trials. Most published literature is for depression and patients have been in second and third trimesters. Adverse effects have similar in rTMS as well as sham stimulation group in depression. Direct stimulation of lumbar spine must be avoided and transcranial application should only be used, which is least likely to have any fetal effect because magnetic field attenuates rapidly with distance. A study examining 18 children of 18–62 months of age born to mothers who received rTMS in second or third trimester, no deleterious effect on cognitive or motor development was noticed.[40]

Other brain stimulation techniques tDCS, tACS, and VNS have been inadequately researched in perinatal period.

Management of Substance Use Disorders During Perinatal Period

With increasing prevalence of substance use disorders, it is essential to universally screen all women in perinatal period about substance use in confidential and nonjudgmental manner. Also assess for blood-borne viral infections, sexually transmitted infections, plans for pregnancy and baby, any ideas of guilt and past relapse patterns as well as determinants. Complications substance use disorder can pose for pregnancy and neonate and potential management pearls have been described in **Table 9**.[41]

TABLE 9: Substance use related complications and management issues in perinatal period.

Substance	Effect on pregnancy and infant	Management strategies
Tobacco use	Stillbirth, fetal growth restriction, decreased birth weight, prematurity, and sudden unexplained infant death	• Behavioral counseling • Varenicline, bupropion, and nicotine replacement can be considered, but lack safety data for use in pregnancy. Varenicline and bupropion have no human data to support safety during pregnancy, and animal studies show adverse and possible teratogenic effects

Contd...

Contd...

Substance	Effect on pregnancy and infant	Management strategies
Alcohol	Fetal alcohol syndrome (FAS) and congenital malformations	• Detoxification using diazepam or lorazepam taper • Relapse prevention agent naltrexone, disulfiram, and acamprosate have no human data to support safety during pregnancy, and animal studies show adverse and possible teratogenic effects
Benzodiazepine (BZD)	• "Floppy baby syndrome", (lethargy, irritability, reduced muscle tone, and respiratory depression) • Neonatal abstinence syndrome (NAS)	Psychosocial interventions and symptomatic supportive management for BZD use disorder *Management of NAS* • *Symptoms:* Irritability, hypertonia, and sleeping and feeding difficulty • *Treatment:* Supportive management suffices in most cases. Keep the baby in a quiet and dimly lit room. Ensure close, gentle interaction, and skin-to-skin contact with mother. Provide small and frequent feeds. Ensure close monitoring. In some cases, phenobarbital may be needed
Cannabis	Stillbirth, decreased birth weight, and preterm birth	Psychosocial interventions and symptomatic supportive management cannabis use disorder
Cocaine	• Maternal nasal perforation, hypertension and placental abruption, low birthweight, small for gestational age, prematurity • Infant irritability, hypertonia, and sleep disturbance	Psychosocial interventions and symptomatic supportive management for cocaine use
Amphetamine	Hypertension, preeclampsia, placental abruption, fetal demise, and neonatal death	Psychosocial interventions and symptomatic supportive management

Contd...

Contd...

Substance	Effect on pregnancy and infant	Management strategies
Opioid	• Maternal HIV/Hepatitis B/ HCV/Sexually transmitted infections • Neonatal opioid withdrawal syndrome (NOWS) • Low birthweight small for gestational age	• Maintenance regimen preferred over detoxification • Choice between methadone or buprenorphine depends on past response and availability, no rationale to switch from previously ongoing stable regimen of either of the two regimens. *Management of NOWS* • *Symptoms:* Gastrointestinal disturbances, irritability, hyperactivity, feeding, and sleeping disturbances, autonomic hyperactivity, and seizures (rare <5%) • *Monitor* within 2 hours of childbirth, thereafter every 4 hours and prefer hospitalization or close monitoring for 4–7 days. • *Treatment:* Most cases with mild symptoms only require monitoring. Severe cases can be given opioid • If withdrawal signs not adequately treated on opioid alone, consider screening for BZD, alcohol and give phenobarbitone

Breastfeeding and substance use:
- Encourage to breastfeed
- Encourage skin-to-skin contact irrespective of feeding choice
- Women on opioid maintenance treatment to be encouraged to breastfeed
- Discourage substance use while breastfeeding
- Women using alcohol intermittently to avoid breastfeeding for 2 hours after one standard drink (10 g of pure alcohol), and 4–8 hours after consuming more than one drink in a single occasion
- *Not advisable to breastfeed:* Only if currently mother is using multiple substances in large quantities, substance use is in very inconsistent manner, currently injecting drugs or using cocaine or large doses of amphetamines. It is preferable to avoid breastfeeding baby for 1–2 h after taking any street drug or medication, as this is the time of highest plasma drug concentration

Newer Promising Agent: Brexanolone

Brexanolone, i.e., allopregnanolone, is endogenous metabolite of progesterone which serves as allosteric modulator at GABA-A receptor. It is Food and Drug Administration (FDA) approved for treatment of moderate to severe postpartum depression with dosing regimen of: 30 mg/kg/h in first 4 h, followed by 60 mg/kg/h for next 20 h, then at a maximal dose of 90 mg/kg/h for next 28 h and then stepped down to 60 mg/kg/h for 4 h and 30 mg/kg/h in the last 4 h. Its administration will require hospitalization and is very expensive and not available in India currently. Its notable side effects are headache, syncope, or dizziness.[31]

CONTRACEPTIVE PLANNING FOR WOMEN WITH PERINATAL MENTAL DISORDERS ON TREATMENT

Patients should be encouraged to plan pregnancy while on psychotropics and should be psychoeducated about range of contraceptive measures available. Bidirectional impact of contraceptive use on mental illness and vice versa is discussed in **Box 6** and **Table 10** discusses potential drug interactions with different psychotropic agents.[21]

BOX 6: Bidirectional impact of contraception and psychiatric illnesses.

- *Effect of contraceptives on mental illness:* Progesterone-only pills and high-dose estrogen pills increase serotonin metabolism in brain, thereby lowering serotonin levels and predisposing to depression
- *Effect of contraceptives on psychotropics:* Synthetic estrogen stimulates protein synthesis, which may affect protein-binding of certain drugs, and inhibits some cytochrome P450 enzymes, both of which can affect blood levels of other medications
  - *Increase metabolism of psychotropics:* Oral contraceptives increase the metabolism of some benzodiazepines (lorazepam and temazepam)
  - *Decrease metabolism of psychotropics:* Oral contraceptives decrease the metabolism of some benzodiazepines (alprazolam, chlordiazepoxide, and diazepam) and tricyclic antidepressants predisposing to toxicity. It decreases metabolism of FGAs too but the effect has not been replicated in large-scale studies.
- *Effect of psychotropics on contraceptives*
- *Increases metabolism of contraceptives:* Carbamazepine, oxcarbazepine, and topiramate, mood stabilizers which induce the P450 3A4 pathway can increase the metabolism of oral contraceptives (many of which are substrates of the P450 3A4 pathway), thereby reducing their effectiveness. This effect is also seen with vaginal contraceptive rings because the hormones contained in these preparations are also metabolized by the liver

---

(FGAs: first generation antipsychotics)

TABLE 10: Psychotropics and oral contraceptives interaction.

Psychotropic class	Drug interaction and individual psychotropics			
	No interaction	Increases metabolism of oral contraceptives/ decreasing contraceptive effectiveness	Oral contraceptives increase metabolism of psychotropic/ decreasing psychotropic effectiveness	Oral contraceptives decrease metabolism of psychotropic/ predisposing to psychotropic toxicity
Antidepressant	SSRI			TCA
Antipsychotics	SGA			± FGA
Mood stabilizer	Valproate	Carbamazepine, oxcarbazepine, and topiramate	Lamotrigine	
Benzodiazepines			Lorazepam and temazepam	Alprazolam, chlordiazepoxide, and diazepam

(FGA: first generation antipsychotics; SGA: second generation antipsychotics; SSRI: selective serotonin reuptake inhibitor; TCA: tricyclic antidepressant)

Thus, patient should either change her contraceptive method or change her mood stabilizer. Contraceptive alternatives include the birth control patch (which largely avoids liver metabolism) and barrier methods can also be considered.[21]

LIASONING WITH OBSTERICIANS AND PEDIATRICIANS: SCREENING FOR COMMON MENTAL DISORDERS IN PERINATAL PERIOD

American College of Obstetrics and Gynecology recommends screening for common mental disorders at least once during perinatal period. Following easy-to-use structured clinical tools can aid in routine screening **(Table 11)**, their use should be encouraged by obstetrics and pediatric healthcare provider for screening and networking should be promoted for referral and liasoning.

INPATIENT SERVICES FOR PERINATAL MENTAL DISORDERS: CLINCIAL AND LEGAL IMPLICATIONS IN INDIA

Admission of any woman pregnant or with child <3 years of age if requires inpatient psychiatry hospitalization, Review Board must be intimated within

TABLE 11: Overview of screening tools for common mental disorders in perinatal period in reproductive child healthcare setting.

Mental disorder screened	Screening instrument	Validated for use in India
Depression	Edinburgh depression rating scale 10 items (EDPS)	Yes, in English and Hindi
	Patient health questionnaire two items and nine items (PHQ-2/PHQ-9)	Yes, in English and Hindi
	Whooley questions two items	Yes, in English
Anxiety	Generalized anxiety disorder scale two items (GAD2)	Yes, in English and Hindi
Depression and anxiety	Kessler psychological distress 10 items (K10)	Yes, in English and Hindi

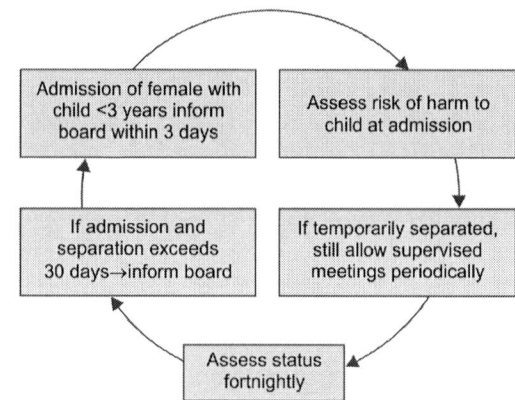

Fig. 1: Legal responsibilities as per Mental Health Care Act (MHCA) for inpatient admission in perinatal disorders.

72 hours of admission. Assessment of risk of harm to child must be done and if mother and child are separated temporarily, it is advisable to allow supervised meeting for mother-child bonding and review the decision every 15 days as detailed in **Figure 1**.[31]

Preferably such admissions must be in mother baby units (MBU), which are specific inpatient units for conjoint admission of mother and infant together under a multidisciplinary team of psychiatrist and allied health professionals. In terms of specialized perinatal service provisions and training in perinatal psychiatry, NIMHANS has been the pioneer in India. Capacity building of skilled professionals, networking with reproductive healthcare professionals, and developing such specialized services in the need of hour.[31]

CONCLUSION

Psychiatric disorders during pregnancy are common. Severe mental illnesses during pregnancy are high-risk pregnancies requiring collaboration between service users (patients and family), and all concerned healthcare providers (obstetrician, psychiatrist, and neonatologist). Regular screening for mental disorders can improve detection and following structured operational algorithms can make clinicians provide effective evidence-based uniform care. Informing the patient and family about current clinical status, course of illness, effects and side effects of medication should govern shared decision making. Concerns about effect of psychotropic safety should alone not deny due care needed for women with mental disorders. A judicious clinical decision can help to reduce burden of maternal mental disorders on mother, infant, and family.

> **KEY POINTS**
> - Perinatal period is a high risk period for mental disorders.
> - Regularly screen mothers for mental disorders in perinatal period.
> - Managing mental disorders in reproductive age group women should involve pre-emptive discussion about planning parenthood.
> - Risk benefit assessment for psychoropic use in perintal period to involve risk of discontinuation of medicine, impact of maternal illness on pregnancy and infant outcome as well as psychotropics safety.
> - Avoid sudden change in psychotropic on discovery of pregnancy.
> - Do not stop breast feeding for mothers on psychotropic.
> - Use cautious evidence based decision making of psychotropic for perinatal mental disorders.
> - Strive for collaborative care with patient, family, obstetrician and pediatrician.

REFERENCES

1. Baron EC, Hanlon C, Mall S, Honikman S, Breuer E, Kathree T, et al. Maternal mental health in primary care in five low- and middle-income countries: A situational analysis BMC Health Serv Res. 2016;16:53.
2. India State-Level Disease Burden Initiative Suicide Collaborators; Dandona R, Kumar GA, Dhaliwal RS, Naghavi M, Vos T, et al. Gender differentials and state variations in suicide deaths in India: the Global Burden of Disease Study 1990–2016. Lancet Public Health. 2018;3(10):e478-e489.
3. Campbell J, Matoff-Stepp S, Velez ML, Cox HH, Laughon K. Pregnancy-Associated Deaths from Homicide, Suicide, and Drug Overdose: Review of Research and the Intersection with Intimate Partner Violence. J Womens Health. 2021;30(2):236-44.
4. O'Hara MW, Wisner KL. Perinatal mental illness: definition, description and aetiology. Best Pract Res Clin Obstet Gynaecol. 2014;28(1):3-12.
5. World Health Organization. (2020). International Statistical Classification of Diseases and Related Health Problems, 11th edition; ICD-11. [online]

Available from https://www.who.int/standards/classifications/classification-of-diseases#:~:text=Traditional%20medicine%20conditions'.-,ICD%2D11%20enables%2C%20for%20the%20first%20time%2C%20the%20counting,and%20definitions%20nationally%20and%20internationally. [Last accessed December, 2023].

6. American Psychiatric Association. Diagnostic and Statistical Manual of Mental Disorders, 5th edition. United States: American Psychiatric Publishing; 2013.
7. Garthus-Niegel S, Radoš SN, Horsch A. Perinatal Depression and Beyond—Implications for Research Design and Clinical Management. JAMA Netw Open. 2022;5(6):e2218978.
8. Alipour Z, Kheirabadi GR, Kazemi A, Fooladi M. The most important risk factors affecting mental health during pregnancy: a systematic review. East Mediterr Health J. 2018;24(6):549-59.
9. Harsha GT, Mithun Sadashival A. Trajectory of Perinatal Mental Health in India. Indian J Soc Psychiatry. 2019;35(1):47-54.
10. Maguire J, McCormack C, Mitchell A, Monk C. Chapter 5: Neurobiology of maternal mental illness. In: Steegers EAP, Cipolla MJ, Miller EC (Eds). Handbook of Clinical Neurology. Gurugram, Haryana; Elsevier; 2020. pp. 97-116.
11. Wisner KL, Stika CS, Watson K. Pregnant women are still therapeutic orphans. World Psychiatry. 2020;19(3):329-30.
12. Kim JJ, Silver RK. Perinatal suicide associated with depression diagnosis and absence of active treatment in 15-year UK national inquiry. Evid Based Ment Health; 2016;19:122.
13. Cohen LS, Altshuler LL, Harlow BL. Relapse of major depression during pregnancy in women who maintain or discontinue antidepressant treatment. JAMA. 2006;295:499-507.
14. Epstein RA, Moore KM, Bobo WV. Treatment of bipolar disorders during pregnancy: maternal and fetal safety and challenges. Drug Healthc Patient Saf. 2014;7:7-29.
15. Dean BB, Gerner D, Gerner RH. A systematic review evaluating health-related quality of life, work impairment, and healthcare costs and utilization in bipolar disorder. Curr Med Res Opin. 2004;20:139-54.
16. Jablensky AV, Morgan V, Zubrick SR, Bower C, Yellachich LA. Pregnancy, delivery, and neonatal complications in a population cohort of women with schizophrenia and major affective disorders. Am J Psychiatry. 2005;162:79-91.
17. Glover V. Maternal depression, anxiety and stress during pregnancy and child outcome; what needs to be done. Best Pract Res Clin Obstet Gynaecol. 2014;28:25-35.
18. Creeley CE, Denton LK. Use of Prescribed Psychotropics during Pregnancy: A Systematic Review of Pregnancy, Neonatal, and Childhood Outcomes. Brain Sci. 2019;9(9):235.
19. ACOG. Clinical Management Guidelines for Obstetrician-Gynecologists Use of Psychiatric Medications During Pregnancy and Lactation. ACOG Practice Bulletin, FOCUS. 2009;7(3):385-400.
20. Hale TW. Medications in Mother's Milk, (Level III). Amaraillo (TX): Pharmasoft Publishing; 2004.
21. McAllister-Williams RH, Baldwin DS, Cantwell R, Easter A, Gilvarry E, Glover V, et al. British Association for Psychopharmacology consensus guidance on the

use of psychotropic medication preconception, in pregnancy and postpartum 2017. J Psychopharmacol. 2017;31(5):519-52.
22. Akasheh G, Sirati L, Noshad Kamran AR, Sepehrmanesh Z. Comparison of the effect of sertraline with behavioral therapy on semen parameters in men with primary premature ejaculation. Urology. 2014;83:800-4.
23. Haddad PM, Wieck A. Antipsychotic-induced hyperprolactinaemia: Mechanisms, clinical features and management. Drugs. 2004;64:2291-314.
24. Raoof NT, Pearson RM, Turner P. Lithium inhibits human sperm motility in vitro. Br J Clin Pharmacol. 1989;28:715-7.
25. Svalheim S, Sveberg L, Mochol M, Taubøll E. Interactions between antiepileptic drugs and hormones. Seizure. 2015;28:12-7.
26. Hamed SA, Moussa EM, Tohamy AM, Mohamed KO, Mohamad ME, Sherif TM, et al. Seminal fluid analysis and testicular volume in adults with epilepsy receiving valproate. J Clin Neurosci. 2015;22:508-12.
27. Austin MP, Highet N and the Expert Working Group (2017) Mental Health Care in the Perinatal Period: Australian Clinical Practice Guideline. Melbourne: Centre of Perinatal Excellence. Accessed from https://cope.org.au/wp-content/uploads/2017/10/Final-COPE-Perinatal-Mental-Health-Guideline.pdf Last accessed on 28 Dec 2023.
28. Newport DJ, Viguera AC, Beach AJ, Ritchie JC, Cohen LS, Stowe ZN. Lithium placental passage and obstetrical outcome: implications for clinical management during late pregnancy. Am J Psychiatry. 2005;162(11):2162-70.
29. Poels EMP, Bijma HH, Galbally M, Bergink V. Lithium during pregnancy and after delivery: a review. Int J Bipolar Disord. 2018;6(1):26.
30. Blake LD, Lucas DN, Aziz K, Castello-Cortes A, Robinson PN. Lithium toxicity and the parturient: case report and literature review. Int J Obstet Anesth. 2008;17(2):164-9.
31. Bharadwaj B, Endumathi R, Parial S, Chandra PS. Management of Psychiatric Disorders during the Perinatal Period. Indian J Psychiatry. 2022;64(Suppl 2):S414-28.
32. Ian B. Emotional Rejection of the Infant: Status of the Concept. Psychopathology. 2016;49:247-60.
33. Luykx JJ, Di Florio A, Bergink V. Prevention of Infanticide and Suicide in the Postpartum Period—the Importance of Emergency Care. JAMA Psychiatry. 2019;76(12):1221-2.
34. Woo MY, Gantioque R. An Obstetric and Psychiatric Emergency: Managing Acute Agitation Among Pregnant Patients in the Emergency Department. Adv Emerg Nurs J. 2023;45(4):301-10.
35. O'Sullivan DL, Byatt N, Dossett EC. Long-Acting Injectable Antipsychotic Medications in Pregnancy: A review. J Acad Consult Liaison Psychiatry. 2022;63:53-60.
36. Eleftheriou G, Butera R, Sangiovanni A, Palumbo C, Bondi E. Long-Acting Injectable Antipsychotic Treatment during Pregnancy: A Case Series. Int J Environ Res Public Health. 2023;20(4):3080.
37. Nguyen T, Frayne J, Watson S, Lebedevs T, Teoh S, Galbally M. Long-acting injectable antipsychotic treatment during pregnancy: Outcomes for women at a tertiary maternity hospital. Psychiatry Res. 2022;313:114614.

38. Kishimoto T, Hagi K, Kurokawa S, Kane JM, Correll CU. Long-acting injectable versus oral antipsychotics for the maintenance treatment of schizophrenia: a systematic review and comparative meta-analysis of randomised, cohort, and pre–post studies. Lancet Psychiatry. 2021;8(5):387-404.
39. Fernández-Abascal B, Recio-Barbero M, Sáenz-Herrero M, Segarra R. Long-acting injectable aripiprazole in pregnant women with schizophrenia: a case-series report. Ther Adv Psychopharmacol.. 2021;11:2045125321991277.
40. Goyal N, Sinha P, Kelkar R, Vidya KL. Application of Brain Stimulation Techniques during Pregnancy. Indian J Private Psychiatry. 2021;15:57-61.
41. World Health Organization. Guidelines for the Identification and Management of Substance Use and Substance Use Disorders in Pregnancy. Geneva: World Health Organization; 2014.

CHAPTER 12

Gynecological Conditions and Mental Health

Sonia Shenoy

ABSTRACT

This chapter discusses the interface between gynecology and psychiatry by including gynecological conditions such as endometriosis, hysterectomy, polycystic ovarian syndrome, infertility, gynecological cancers, white discharge per vagina, and primary ovarian insufficiency. For each of these conditions, a brief description of the condition along with the psychosocial concomitants has been discussed. The multidimensional links between the common psychiatric comorbidities such as depression, anxiety, sexual dysfunction, etc., and the maintenance of gynecological conditions have been highlighted. The common treatment approaches for comorbid psychiatric disorders have been summarized. It aims to help the readers gain insights about the importance of being aware of the psychological disturbances associated with these common gynecological conditions and the need for a multidisciplinary team to screen and manage these conditions early for better well-being and quality of life in women facing the challenges of managing these conditions.

Keywords: Gynecological disorders, mental health, endometriosis, PCOD, infertility

INTRODUCTION

The interface between gynecology and psychiatry has been a topic of discussion since ancient times and a subject of research for the past few decades.[1] Though many organ systems have symptoms overlapping with psychiatric symptoms with respect to their origins, maintenance, and exacerbations, the female reproductive system in particular has had one of the strongest associations with mental health. From physiological states such as menstrual cycle, pregnancy, lactation, and menopause to pathological conditions such as endometriosis, malignancies, and infertility, there appears to be a rich relationship between the two systems.[2]

In this chapter, gynecological conditions such as endometriosis, hysterectomy, polycystic ovarian syndrome (PCOS), infertility, and gynecological cancers, which are all known to have a significant impact on mental health in women will be discussed. Additionally, conditions such as white discharge per vagina (WDPV) and primary ovarian insufficiency (POI) will be briefly discussed.

ENDOMETRIOSIS

Endometriosis is a gynecological disorder occurring due to the presence of endometrium-like tissue outside the uterus.[3] It occurs in 5–15% of women in the reproductive age group and up to 50% in women diagnosed with infertility. The American Society for Reproductive Medicine has classified endometriosis into four stages based on factors such as quantity, depth, location, and size of the endometrium-like tissue. Stages I (minimal) and II (mild) are the initial stages, whereas stages III (moderate) and IV (severe) are the advanced stages; however, the stages do not reflect the intensity of symptoms such as pain as the initial stages can have intense pain too.[4] The exact mechanism of pathogenesis of this disorder is unclear; however theories related to it include immune dysfunction, abnormal differentiation, environmental effects, genetic factors, and epigenetic factors. The diagnosis is usually done by laparoscopic examination of the pelvis and histological assessment of the excised endometrium-like tissue. Various clinical presentations of endometriosis have been noted, for example, classification into three types namely, peritoneal endometriosis, endometriotic ovarian cysts, and deeply infiltrating endometriosis (DIE).

The common clinical symptoms and signs include chronic pelvic pain, irregular menstrual cycles, congestive dysmenorrhea, fatigue, heavy menstrual bleeding, dyspareunia, dyschezia (the inability to defecate without pain or difficulty), and infertility.[5] Around 20–25% of the patients are asymptomatic. Most women experience a delay in getting help due to the long duration (5–8.9 years) from symptom onset to diagnosis due to the nonspecific nature of symptoms as well as the invasive method of assessment.[6]

Anxiety and Depression in Endometriosis

In patients with endometriosis, anxiety and depression have been reported to occur together and also positively correlate with each other. In a study with 104 patients of endometriosis, 64.4% had moderate to severe depressive symptoms, whereas 63.5% had a high level of anxiety symptoms. The same study showed a correlation of age with depressive symptoms but not with anxiety symptoms.[7] Multiple studies have shown high levels of anxiety symptoms in patients with endometriosis, especially in women with higher scores on psychoticism, introversion, and alexithymia.[8]

Depressive symptoms were related to the presence of multiple factors such as chronic pelvic pain, dyspareunia, infertility, fatigue, delays in diagnosis, impairment in social and occupational functioning, and uncertain nature of the illness, all of which contributed to it individually or in combination.[9] A few theories have been postulated for the link between endometriosis and depression. Firstly, the psycho-neuro-immune nature of the illness wherein there is an imbalance between the production of proinflammatory [interleukin (IL)-2, IL-1β, and interferon-gamma (IFN-γ)] and anti-inflammatory(IL-4) cytokines, causing both endometriotic changes as well as shifts in mood and mental health in women, leading to depression and poorer quality of life.[10] Secondly, the "pain-focused hypothesis" implies that patients with chronic pain are vulnerable to developing depression as is seen in endometriosis.[11] A vicious cycle of endometriosis-related pain and depression has been reported wherein pain worsens depression and vice versa. A systematic review concluded that the association between endometriosis and depression is largely determined by chronic pain as women with pain during endometriosis had more depressive symptoms than those without pain symptoms without endometriosis. The review also highlighted the finding that women with endometriosis and pain did not have higher depressive symptoms in comparison to women with chronic pain without endometriosis.[9]

Other factors contributing to the development of depressive symptoms include treatment-related effects such as bloating, weight gain, and acne or greasy skin causing disturbances in self-image, infertility, and dyspareunia causing marital disharmony, absenteeism, and decrease in work productivity due to dysmenorrhea and heavy menstrual bleeding, etc.

Sexual Dysfunction and Infertility

A high percentage of women (33.5–71%) with both initial as well as advanced stages of endometriosis reported a negative impact on sexual functioning. Symptoms such as severe pelvic pain as well as dyspareunia were significant contributors to sexual dysfunction. Responses to dyspareunia included avoiding or stopping sexual intercourse in between, tolerating pain during intercourse because of a strong desire for pregnancy, or due to a need for closeness with a partner, all of which could negatively impact the sexual relationship with the partner.[6] It also caused feelings of guilt and inadequacy, thus increasing the risk of developing depression. Delays in the diagnosis of endometriosis also lead to delays in obtaining help for these symptoms. An Indian study that evaluated sexual dysfunction in patients with endometriosis found that 47.06% of the patients experienced sexual dysfunction. All the patients (100%) with severe endometriosis experienced pain and low sexual desire and 33.33% of the patients with minimal endometriosis experienced sexual dysfunction in the form of orgasm dysfunction.[12]

Treatment Options

The main goals of treatment for endometriosis are adequate pain control, prevention of recurrence, improvement of the quality of life, preservation of fertility, and reduction of anatomical damage.

The usual treatment options for endometriosis include analgesics, hormonal therapy [combined oral contraceptives, danazol, gestrinone, medroxyprogesterone acetate, and gonadotropin-releasing hormone (GnRH) agonists], minimally invasive or radical surgery, and in some cases, fertility treatment, due to high incidence of endometriosis in patients with infertility.[13] GnRH agonists can induce depressive symptoms and the patients must be ideally monitored during the course of treatment. In patients with severe depressive or anxiety symptoms, antidepressant medications such as selective serotonin reuptake inhibitors (SSRIs) and serotonin and norepinephrine reuptake inhibitors (SNRIs) can be beneficial.[8]

Psychological and mind-body interventions such as psychotherapy, mindfulness, and Yoga help in reducing stress, which in turn can alleviate the depressive symptoms as there is a link between high levels of stress and worsening of inflammatory conditions such as endometriosis. Other techniques focusing on improving coping skills, decreasing heightened vigilance toward pain, and relaxation can decrease the pain perception, which in turn can reduce depressive and anxiety symptoms and help in improving the quality of life. These interventions also improve symptoms such as fatigue, stress, sexual dysfunction, and insomnia, which are commonly seen in endometriosis. A systematic review of psychological and mind-body interventions for endometriosis reported that almost all the studies (98%) showed an improvement in pain symptoms.[14] However, better quality studies are required to substantiate the findings.

Marital therapy could benefit couples with sexual dysfunction and/or infertility due to the chronic nature of the condition and a significant strain on the quality of the marital relationship.

Improving awareness about the nature of the illness of endometriosis and its associated physical and psychological manifestations among the general population as well as healthcare professionals may help in early diagnosis of the disorder with early symptom relief, thus avoiding consequences such as infertility, marital disharmony, depression, and poor quality of life. Women diagnosed with endometriosis must also be screened for psychiatric symptoms and psychosocial difficulties.[15] A multidisciplinary approach incorporating all the different treatment options discussed above would also help in improving symptom control as well as the quality of life in patients of endometriosis.

HYSTERECTOMY

Hysterectomy is a common surgical procedure that involves the removal of the uterus to treat gynecological conditions such as fibroids, tumors, cysts, and uterine prolapse and is usually done in the perimenopausal age group.

The rate of hysterectomy in Indian women among women aged ≥45 years was 11.4% with the highest rates in women aged 45–59 years (13.8%) and lower rates in women aged ≥60 years (9.8%).[16]

Hysterectomy may be total or subtotal (cervix left intact) and may also be combined with removal of the ovaries and fallopian tubes, that is, bilateral salpingo-oophorectomy (BSO). Different types of hysterectomy include abdominal, vaginal, laparoscopic, robotic, and minilaparotomy.[17] Most of the surgeries are for elective indications to improve the quality of life in women with fibroids, cysts, abnormal uterine bleeding, endometriosis, and uterine prolapse. Only a small proportion of hysterectomies are for emergency conditions such as catastrophic bleeding or malignancies. As some gynecological conditions such as abnormal bleeding, and fibroids, get better after menopause, the decision to do a hysterectomy is made after assessing the risk-benefit ratio after comparing it with other options such as watchful waiting, medications including hormonal therapy, endometrial ablations, and myomectomy etc. However, in India, a recent survey found that the most common self-reported reason for hysterectomy procedures among women aged 15–49 years was abnormal uterine bleeding followed by cysts/fibroids.[16]

Hysterectomy and its Impact on Mental Health

Older reviews reported that 10–20% of women undergoing hysterectomy experienced depressive symptoms, sexual dysfunction, and problems with body image. In the early 1970s, the term "post-hysterectomy syndrome" was coined by Richards as a huge proportion of women (70%) had symptoms of depression along with symptoms of menopause such as hot flashes, fatigue, dizziness, and insomnia, etc.[18]

Risk factors included preoperative history of depression or other psychiatric comorbidities and sexual dysfunction, age group <40 years, uncertainty about future childbearing, fewer years of education, sensitivity to losses, inadequate knowledge about the indication and possible consequences of hysterectomy, and abnormal belief that the uterus has special psychological and sexual importance. Especially in some cultures, women hold the belief that the uterus is associated with femininity and vigor. In the older days, society perceived hysterectomized women as being desexed, neutered, shell, one-half women, and also as being promiscuous.[19] Premature loss of the uterus even in parous women not desiring more children can lead to distress due to beliefs about accelerated aging, inadequacy, and loss of femininity. Loss of menstruation is considered as missing an essential part of womanhood, losing the monthly cleansing ritual of accumulated wastes.[20] Due to these beliefs, women are prone to developing stress, anxiety, depression, and sexual dysfunction.

However, the recent reviews do not show similar rates of depression or sexual dysfunction in women who have undergone hysterectomy. Most sexual disorders improve after hysterectomy and sexual functioning remains the same or gets better.[21-23] Newer methods of hysterectomy such as laparoscopic type have a quicker recovery than the previous methods such as abdominal hysterectomy, which also left a scar symbolized as mutilation by some vulnerable patients. Rates of anxiety postoperatively were lower in women undergoing total laparoscopic hysterectomy than in those who underwent total vaginal hysterectomy.[24]

Role of the Psychiatrist

As the vulnerability in developing depression, anxiety, and sexual dysfunction posthysterectomy is more in women with known risk factors, a psychiatrist must ideally assess the mood, stressors, beliefs about sexuality and fertility, and preparedness for surgery in the vulnerable population. Special consideration must be given to premenopausal women undergoing hysterectomy along with BSO as they have to face sudden surgical menopause-related changes if estrogen therapy is not initiated immediately after surgery and if it is not maintained due to various factors such as inadequate knowledge, loss of follow-up, and logistic factors. Women who have ambivalence about future childbearing or surgery per se also have a higher risk and beliefs about these must be explored too. Postoperative assessment for emerging distress and psychiatric symptoms must be ideally done in vulnerable patients too. Antidepressants and cognitive therapy may be needed for women who experience moderate to severe depression and or anxiety symptoms.

■ POLYCYSTIC OVARIAN SYNDROME

Polycystic ovarian syndrome is a disorder characterized by a combination of factors such as hyperandrogenism, ovulatory dysfunction, and ultrasound appearance of polycystic ovaries. The manifestations are different in each individual, but the common symptoms and signs include menstrual irregularities (75-80%), infertility (75%), hirsutism (70%), acne (10-34%), sexual dysfunction (27.2-62.5%), and obesity (50%).[25] There are different types of diagnostic classifications with different criteria for diagnosis. The prevalence rate varies from 5 to 10% in the Western world, whereas the prevalence rate in India is in the range of 3.7-22.5%.[26] PCOS is associated with multiple sequelae such as insulin resistance, obesity, diabetes mellitus, endometrial cancer, and cardiovascular disorders. Mental health-related symptoms related to psychiatric disorders such as depression, anxiety, and somatization are common too.[27]

Epidemiology of Psychiatric Manifestations in Polycystic Ovarian Syndrome

In Indian women with PCOS, 54% had depressive symptoms, out of whom 72% had obesity, 70% had features of hirsutism, 61% had acne, and 56% had infertility.[28] Other Indian studies have reported rates of depression as 23.6%,[29] 25.7%,[30] and 93.5%[31] with rates of anxiety reported as 15.45%,[29] 38.6%,[30] and 100%.[31] The huge variation in the rates could be explained by various factors such as age differences, the nature of symptoms of PCOS, methods of assessment, and other contributory factors based on co-occurring medical comorbidities. Other psychiatric manifestations include suicidality (8%), obsessive-compulsive disorder (6.36%), and bipolar affective disorder (2.7%).[29] A Swedish registry of patients with PCOS (n=24,385) reported that there is a 50% increased odds of psychiatric disorders along with a 40% higher crude odds ratio for attempted suicide.[32] Women diagnosed with PCOS have three times the odds of developing depressive symptoms and four times the odds of developing anxiety symptoms.[33] The risk of postpartum depression in women with PCOS is increased by 45% compared to women without PCOS.[27]

Depression in Polycystic Ovarian Syndrome

The specific mechanisms related to higher depressive symptoms in PCOS have been attributed to an interplay of multiple factors such as imbalance of neurotransmitters [reduction in serotonin, dopamine, gamma-aminobutyric acid (GABA), and acetylcholine with increased glutamate levels], insulin resistance, obesity, hyperandrogenism, infertility, and inflammation (proinflammatory cytokines can trigger depression).

Obesity is closely related to the dysfunction of the hypothalamic-pituitary-adrenal (HPA) axis leading to depression. It can also lead to body image-related disturbances, stigma, and cognitive distortions related to one's femininity leading to depression. There is a vicious cycle between hyperandrogenism and depression, each maintaining the other. An interplay of all the factors contributes to the development of depression.

As the symptom manifestations of PCOS differ among individuals, the nature of symptoms might play a role based on the age of the patients. For example, adolescent patients might be more affected by weight gain/obesity, hirsutism, and acne causing decreased self-esteem and impaired social lives, whereas women in the reproductive age group may be impacted more by infertility-related disturbances.[34] However, the quality of life is significantly affected in each phase of life as reported in multiple studies.[30,31,33]

Sexual Dysfunction in Polycystic Ovarian Syndrome

As infertility is commonly seen in PCOS, the pressure to conceive as well as the stigma of being infertile contribute to sexual dysfunction as there is a bidirectional relationship between sexual dysfunction and infertility. Adding to this is the perceived negative self-image due to obesity and hirsutism, which is known to hamper the sexual desire in women. Hyperandrogenism and its direct impact on sexual functioning in women is unclear; however, it contributes to decreased sexual functioning due to its virilization-related disturbances. Sexual dysfunction can be manifested in various ways such as decreased sexual desire and arousal, anorgasmia, impaired lubrication, and reduced frequency of intercourse.[35]

Assessment and Management

As the rates of psychiatric disorders are high in PCOS, mandatory screening is necessary for early identification and intervention. As some of the manifestations are further worsened by the emergence of depression such as menstrual irregularities, obesity, and sexual dysfunction, it is imperative to screen for depression, anxiety, and sexual dysfunction early. Lifestyle modifications such as exercise and a healthy diet are helpful in the management of PCOS and can prevent the occurrence of psychiatric manifestations too. In patients with underlying psychiatric disorders, a thorough evaluation of treatment history specifically looking into valproate use as well as the use of antipsychotics must be noted as these medications are known to cause symptoms of PCOS such as insulin resistance and hyperandrogenism. Similarly, medications used for PCOS such as oral contraceptive pills as well as other hormonal therapy can independently induce or worsen psychiatric symptoms, so a prior screening of psychiatric symptoms is essential before starting treatment for PCOS. Nonpharmacological interventions such as Yoga, mindfulness, and cognitive behavior therapies (CBTs) for depression and anxiety help manage patients and can benefit in multiple ways by reducing stress and in turn improving blood glucose levels, blood pressure, weight, and other parameters.[34]

Increasing awareness about PCOS as well as support groups for PCOS such as LOQUS, Conquer PCOS, and HEAL PCOS may help by providing emotional support to patients with PCOS.[36] A multidisciplinary approach with early identification, earlier liaisons between gynecologists and psychiatrists, counseling, and early management can significantly help in improving the quality of life in women with PCOS.

INFERTILITY

The World Health Organization (WHO) has defined infertility as the inability to conceive after at least 1 year of regular and unprotected sexual intercourse.

Infertility has also been classified into primary infertility (for those who have not conceived previously) and secondary infertility (for those who have conceived at least once previously). As per WHO, 17.5% of the population (roughly 1 in 6 worldwide) experience infertility.[37]

The causes of infertility include one or more of these: sexual dysfunctions, dyspareunia, congenital defects, infections, chronic ill health, cervical factors, uterine factors, ovarian factors, tubal factors, and endocrinal disturbances.

Psychological Disturbances Due to Infertility

The prevalence of psychological distress among women diagnosed with infertility is 60% higher than that of the general population. It is associated with psychiatric manifestations of depression, anxiety, sexual dysfunction, adjustment disorder, and deterioration in the quality of marital life. The risks for developing anxiety and depression are 60% and 40%, respectively.[38] A cross-sectional study in India found that 78% of women with infertility had psychological problems and 45% out of these had a psychiatric disorder. The most common diagnoses were adjustment disorder, anxiety disorders, and mixed anxiety and depression disorder. However, <15% of the patients sought help from a mental health practitioner.[39] Infertility-specific stress is an umbrella term to describe the degree of emotional stress and strain associated with infertility. Risk factors include female gender, pre-existing psychiatric disorder, difficulties in marital relationships, diagnosis of primary infertility, duration of infertility, avoidant coping style, poor social support, frequent ruminations about the diagnosis with decreased acceptance or helplessness, repeated treatment failures, spontaneous abortions, as well as medical side effects.[40]

A meta-analysis reported a pooled prevalence of anxiety to be 36.17% in a sample of 5,055 women diagnosed with infertility.[41] In most cultures, giving birth to a child is closely linked to a woman's identity and femininity. The pressure from family members and society along with the stigma of being childless or "barren" induces high levels of stress and loss of self-esteem. Anxiety in the form of social anxiety and insecurity arises as there is no one to take care of them during their old age or sickness as is practiced in many cultures.[38] An Indian study done at a tertiary hospital found that 80% of women seeking help for infertility report stress and the predictive factors included the type of infertility (uterine>ovarian>tubal), coping difficulties, history of gynecological surgery, current and/or past history of psychiatric illness, the severity of premenstrual dysphoria, cycles of ovulation induction with timed sexual intercourse, and intrauterine inseminations and gynecological conditions.[42] Stress could occur at various steps ranging from difficulty in accepting a diagnosis of infertility, difficulty in dealing with the identity crisis due to the diagnostic label, difficulties in choosing and maneuvering the fertility treatment initiated, difficulty in dealing with the low success rates and possible repeated failed attempts, causing a drain emotionally, physically, and financially and lastly, difficulties in handling the unwanted effects of treatments including side effects of hormonal treatment as well as miscarriages and blood loss, etc.

Depression is one of the common presentations in women seeking help for infertility. Prevalence rates range from 31 to 51%.[43-45] Suicidality has been reported in 9.1% of the patients.[46,47] Depression is also known to further impact the chances of conception in patients undergoing in vitro fertilization. However, this has not been a consistent finding across studies.[48]

Sexual Dysfunction

Sexuality, self-identity, and fertility have multidimensional links with each other. Due to the intensive method of treatments as well as poor success rates along with a chronicity of illness, a severe impact on the well-being of couples is usually noted. Sexual dysfunction in various forms in different domains such as desire, arousal, lubrication, and orgasm have been reported.[49] Long-standing delay in conception also disturbs self-image, perceived self-attractiveness, causes decreased satisfaction, and poor marital relationship, which can all further worsen the quality of sexual relationship. Various other factors that induced sexual dysfunction included viewing conception as a goal and sex as a task, timing intercourse based on ovulation, high pressure to perform, and repeated disappointments in conception.[50] An Indian study found a prevalence of sexual difficulties in 92% of women and 86% of men after seeking help for infertility. However, a significant proportion of couples also reported sexual difficulties since the time of getting married with women (75%) reporting more than men (60%).[51]

Treatment Options

As the patients have a high prevalence of psychiatric symptoms, it is essential to screen all the patients seeking help for infertility as the success of fertility treatments also depends on the stress levels of patients acting via the psychoneuroimmunology pathway.[52] Adequate counseling, early identification, and treatment are essential to improve the quality of life. As many women are usually not keen on pharmacological treatment as they are already under treatment for fertility as well as worried about the risk of teratogenicity, caution needs to be exercised and nonpharmacological interventions can be initiated whenever it is feasible.[2] CBT and mindfulness-based interventions have been tried and have played a role in alleviating stress and anxiety in vulnerable patients.[53]

Having a practical and optimistic mindset, a better understanding of the condition as well as its treatment options, healthy communication with the doctor as well as spouse, having a strong social and peer support system, accessing help from fertility support groups as well as timely psychological interventions can help tide over the various challenges faced by women diagnosed with infertility.

GYNECOLOGIC CANCERS

Gynecologic cancer is defined as cancer of one or more of the female reproductive organs (e.g., uterine, ovarian, cervical, vaginal, vulvar, and very rarely of the fallopian tube). Approximately one out of six cases of cancer in women across the world is due to gynecologic cancers. Cervical cancers are the most common type of cancer in developing countries like India.[54]

Psychological Disturbances Due to Gynecologic Cancers

As discussed earlier in the section on hysterectomy, the uterus is considered essential for femininity and vitality by many women. Various misconceptions about cancers also are common in certain cultures, namely the possibility of being promiscuous to develop cervical cancer, the risk of spreading cancer or it being incurable, causing a lot of shame and isolation in vulnerable women. Coping skills may range from denial to minimization causing them to avoid seeking help at the right time. Cultural beliefs have a significant role in a patient's reaction to illness, help-seeking, as well as psychological responses, well-being, and quality of life.[2,55,56]

Psychological aspects of cancer differ across the developmental lifespan as it can impact areas such as childbearing, marital quality, the integrity of body image, work-related disruptions, and existential issues differently. In young adulthood (ages 19–30 years), when a woman is exploring independence, relationships, and education, cancer might indicate dependence on parents, realigning life goals, setbacks in education and college life, managing body image disturbances including alopecia due to chemotherapy, difficulty in establishing a romantic and/or sexual relationship, and the possibility of being childless due to the nature of cancer and the type of management. In mature adulthood (age 31–45 years), it would be more challenging for those who had postponed childbearing due to career or infertility. Sexual functioning-related difficulties due to vaginal stenosis, fistulas, fatigue, painful intercourse, and other factors could impact marital quality. The risk of early menopause due to oophorectomy is an added risk in this age group. Difficulties in childcare for women with young children due to the repeated trips to the hospital and treatment-related side effects could add to the women's guilt and misery about not giving enough time to her children along with the fear of leaving them motherless in the event of death due to cancer. Work-related disruptions could hamper their sense of purpose and fulfillment too. In older adulthood (age 46–65 years) and elderly (age ≥66 years), challenges could be different in the form of early retirement from work, being dependent on an aged spouse, guilt about not taking care of a spouse with health problems, and feeling dejected about spending the golden years in sickness.[2]

The common psychological disturbances reported in women with gynecologic cancer include adjustment disorder, depression, anxiety, insomnia, chronic pain, delirium, and sexual dysfunction.[57] While most women report anxiety and depressive symptoms at the time of diagnosis, around 50% develop a psychiatric disorder. Women who have poor coping skills, a history of severe psychiatric disorder, a history of suicide attempts, and poor social support are more vulnerable to developing psychological disturbances.

Depression is reported in 25% of the patients. However, Indian studies have reported rates ranging from 25 to 41.26%. The differences reported were due to the type of rating scales used and the combined assessment of anxiety and depression in one study, which reported 41.6% for anxiety/depression.[58,59] Risk factors for depression include a history of mood disorder or other psychiatric disorders, uncontrolled pain symptoms, poor prognosis of cancer, advanced stage of illness, treatments that cause disfiguring, or medications causing depressive symptoms as side effects.

Anxiety disorders are reported in 75.91% of the patients with gynecologic cancers.[60] It could occur at multiple turning points of illness such as a diagnosis, treatment failures, and recurrences. It could be secondary to pain, hospitalization, or treatment-related side effects. It is often complicated by chronic pain and nausea which is seen in many patients, especially in the advanced stages of illness. Inadequate pain relief is an unfortunate reality in many patients, which significantly impacts the quality of life and makes them vulnerable to anxiety and depression. Insomnia is also seen in up to 50% of patients, often complicated by pain.[57]

Sexual dysfunction is noted in 40–100% of the patients treated for gynecological cancer.[61] An Indian study has reported that sexual dysfunction could be of various types such as pain during intercourse, decreased interest, and decreased frequency due to vaginal stenosis. Higher dissatisfaction was reported in patients who received both surgery as well as radiotherapy and in patients in their advanced stages of illness.[62,63]

As psychiatric symptoms are so common in this population and also impact the course of illness and the quality of life, it is essential to screen and manage them as early as possible.[64,65] Multidisciplinary teams should ideally include psycho-oncologists/psychiatrists in rounds, inpatient and outpatient care for adequate screening, education, and effective management of psychiatric comorbidities.[66,67] Treatment options could include therapies such as CBT, relaxation techniques, stress management, mindfulness-based therapy, acceptance and commitment therapy, supportive psychotherapy, sleep hygiene education, spiritual care, sexual education, and counseling.[57,68] For sexual difficulties, interventions such as nerve sparing surgeries, CBT, lubricants, vaginal dilators, vaginal estrogen cream, and hormone replacement therapy can be helpful.[63] Medications such as antidepressants and benzodiazepines can be prescribed for diagnosed psychiatric comorbidities such as depression and anxiety disorders with additional benefits for pain and insomnia.[57]

WHITE DISCHARGE PER VAGINA

Vaginal discharge or WDPV is one of the most common presenting complaints in women of reproductive age group. Normal or physiological vaginal discharge is usually <4 mL per day. It is usually transparent, mucoid, colorless, or colored white, and odorless, but might be slightly malodorous. It has a pH of 4.5 and is not adherent to the vaginal wall. The nature of physiological discharge can vary throughout the different phases of the menstrual cycle and in different age groups. It is usually known to increase during the high estrogen phases such as the ovulatory phase and pregnancy. Pathological or abnormal vaginal discharge is seen in patients with infections or rarely due to foreign body, malignancy, contact dermatitis, or due to reactions to irritants.[69]

Impact on Mental Health

Though WDPV is a common presenting complaint, it is also poorly defined and misinterpreted.[70] In some cultures, women perceive white discharge as an anxiety-provoking symptom and also have associated symptoms of fatigue and pain. Various attributions ranging from food that causes "heat" within the body, disease of the internal systems in the body, consequence of tubectomy, sexual promiscuity of the husbands, family-related "tension" or stress, and effect of heavy housework have been reported by an Indian study.[71] The associated psychiatric symptoms include low mood, dysthymia, fatigue, loss of interest in work, headache, unexplained body ache, worry about health, somatization, fear about being infertile, anxiety, stigma, somatic preoccupation about hollowing of bones or weakness of eyes due to loss of nutrients via WDPV.[72] Due to the above misconception, it has been considered to be a female equivalent of Dhat syndrome, wherein men experience somatic, depressive, and anxiety symptoms along with excessive preoccupation about loss of vitality due to loss of semen as they have white discharge per urethra.[73,74] As per a study, two-thirds of the women with WDPV also considered that vitamin supplements, injections, tonics, and rest were the treatment options and even repeatedly requested the treating doctors to prescribe them.[75] Treatment options include adequate education, clearing misconceptions, psychosocial interventions, and management of clinically significant psychiatric conditions with antidepressants if required.[71]

■ PREMATURE OVARIAN INSUFFICIENCY

Premature ovarian insufficiency (POI), also called primary ovarian insufficiency, is defined as dysfunction or depletion of ovarian follicles with cessation of menstruation before the age of 40 years.[76] The incidence rates are 1 in 250 women by the age of 35 years and 1 in 100 by the age of 40 years. Usually two follicle-stimulating hormone (FSH) tests with values >25 IU/L at least 1 month apart are done to confirm the diagnosis. POI is associated with hypogonadism/hypoestrogenism and its associated features such as oligomenorrhea/amenorrhea, early menopause, vasomotor symptoms, and increased risk of osteoporosis and cardiovascular disease.[77]

Mental Health Implications of Premature Ovarian Insufficiency

As it is a life-altering irreversible condition and can impact fertility in women, it is usually associated with a high risk of developing psychiatric disorders such as depression and anxiety and a poorer quality of life. As the focus is on physical problems, up to one-third of the patients suffering from moderate to severe depression and anxiety can go undiagnosed.[78] According to a recent meta-analysis, the rates of anxiety and depression in POI were 4.89 and 3.33 times higher respectively when compared to healthy controls. The reasons for such high rates include factors related to the neuroendocrine system, common cytokines, and psychosocial factors. Low levels of estrogen and high levels of FSH and luteinizing hormone (LH) can cause dysregulation of the HPA axis, predisposing the patients to depression and anxiety. Cytokines like transforming growth factor-ß (TGF-ß) and IFN-γ are common in both POI as well as depression. Psychosocial factors include factors such as difficulty in accepting the sudden transition into the early menopause stage, stigma of illness as well as infertility, difficulties in sexual intimacy, fear about osteoporosis and cardiovascular events, and chronicity and long-term treatment of the disorder. Psychological connotations of early menopause include accelerated aging, loss of sexual life, attractiveness, and femininity early in life. The psychosocial factors related to infertility as well as early loss of menstruation have been described earlier in the chapter. Sexual dysfunction is also commonly reported due to low estrogen levels as well as low self-esteem and/or concurrent depression/anxiety. It is manifested as decreased libido, vaginal dryness causing decreased lubrication and dyspareunia, loss of vaginal elasticity, and pelvic floor hypertonicity due to persistent genitourinary symptoms.[77]

Treatment options include a multidisciplinary treatment approach with gynecologist, endocrinologist, psychiatrist, and psychologist.[79] Hormone replacement therapy, nonpharmacological treatment such as psychotherapy, lifestyle modifications in the form of exercise, and dietary modifications and medications such as SSRIs for disabling depression and anxiety are the common treatment options.[80]

> **KEY POINTS**
> - Gynecological conditions like endometriosis, polycystic ovarian syndrome, infertility, gynecological cancers, primary ovarian insufficiency, and hysterectomy are associated with psychological comorbidities.
> - Depression, anxiety, adjustment disorder and sexual dysfunction are the common psychological comorbidities.
> - Awareness, screening, and early interventions for psychological disturbances are essential to improve the well-being and quality of life.
> - Psychological therapies and/or antidepressants are helpful in managing the most common psychologic comorbidities associated with these disorders.

REFERENCES

1. Chandra PS, Ranjan S. Psychosomatic obstetrics and gynecology--a neglected field? Curr Opin Psychiatry. 2007;20(2):168-73.
2. Stotland NL, Stewart DE (Eds). Psychological Aspects of Women's Health Care: The Interface Between Psychiatry and Obstetrics and Gynecology, 2nd edition. Washington, DC, US: American Psychiatric Press; 2001.
3. Kennedy S, Bergqvist A, Chapron C, D'Hooghe T, Dunselman G, Greb R, et al. ESHRE guideline for the diagnosis and treatment of endometriosis. Hum Reprod. 2005;20(10):2698-704.
4. Lee SY, Koo YJ, Lee DH. Classification of endometriosis. Yeungnam Univ J Med. 2021;38(1):10-8.
5. Parasar P, Ozcan P, Terry KL. Endometriosis: Epidemiology, diagnosis and clinical management. Curr Obstet Gynecol Rep. 2017;6(1):34-41.
6. Culley L, Law C, Hudson N, Denny E, Mitchell H, Baumgarten M, et al. The social and psychological impact of endometriosis on women's lives: a critical narrative review. Hum Reprod Update. 2013;19(6):625-39.
7. Sepulcri R de P, do Amaral VF. Depressive symptoms, anxiety, and quality of life in women with pelvic endometriosis. Eur J Obstet Gynecol Reprod Biol. 2009;142(1):53-6.
8. Laganà AS, La Rosa VL, Rapisarda AMC, Valenti G, Sapia F, Chiofalo B, et al. Anxiety and depression in patients with endometriosis: impact and management challenges. Int J Womens Health. 2017;9:323-30.
9. Gambadauro P, Carli V, Hadlaczky G. Depressive symptoms among women with endometriosis: a systematic review and meta-analysis. Am J Obstet Gynecol. 2019;220(3):230-41.
10. Nasyrova RF, Sotnikova LS, Baystrukova NV, Krivoshchekova GV, Novitsky VV, Kupriyanova IE, et al. Psychoimmune interactions in women of reproductive age with endometriosis. Bull Exp Biol Med. 2011;152(1):93-7.

11. Lorençatto C, Petta CA, Navarro MJ, Bahamondes L, Matos A. Depression in women with endometriosis with and without chronic pelvic pain. Acta Obstet Gynecol Scand. 2006;85(1):88-92.
12. Mishra VV, Nanda S, Gandhi K, Aggarwal R, Choudhary S, Gondhali R. Female sexual dysfunction in patients with endometriosis: Indian scenario. J Hum Reprod Sci. 2016;9(4):250-3.
13. Bedaiwy MA, Allaire C, Yong P, Alfaraj S. Medical management of endometriosis in patients with chronic pelvic pain. Semin Reprod Med. 2017;35(1):38-53.
14. Evans S, Fernandez S, Olive L, Payne LA, Mikocka-Walus A. Psychological and mind-body interventions for endometriosis: A systematic review. J Psychosom Res. 2019;124:109756.
15. Pope CJ, Sharma V, Sharma S, Mazmanian D. A systematic review of the association between psychiatric disturbances and endometriosis. J Obstet Gynaecol Canada. 2015;37(11):1006-15.
16. Desai S, Singh RJ, Govil D, Nambiar D, Shukla A, Sinha HH, et al. Hysterectomy and women's health in India: evidence from a nationally representative, cross-sectional survey of older women. Womens Midlife Health. 2023;9(1):1.
17. Levenson JL (Ed). The American Psychiatric Association Publishing Textbook of Psychosomatic Medicine and Consultation-Liaison Psychiatry, 3rd edition. US: American Psychiatric Association Publishing; 2018.
18. Bachmann GA. Psychosexual aspects of hysterectomy. Womens Health Issues. 1990;1(1):41-9.
19. Drellich MG, Bieber I. The psychologic importance of the uterus and its functions; some psychoanalytic implications of hysterectomy. J Nerv Ment Dis. 1958;126(4):322-36.
20. Sloan D. The emotional and psychosexual aspects of hysterectomy. Am J Obstet Gynecol. 1978;131(6):598-605.
21. Danesh M, Hamzehgardeshi Z, Moosazadeh M, Shabani-Asrami F. The effect of hysterectomy on women's sexual function: A narrative review. Med Arch (Sarajevo, Bosnia Herzegovina). 2015;69(6):387-92.
22. Ryan MM. Hysterectomy: social and psychosexual aspects. Baillieres Clin Obstet Gynaecol. 1997;11(1):23-36.
23. Dedden SJ, van Ditshuizen MAE, Theunissen M, Maas JWM. Hysterectomy and sexual (dys)function: An analysis of sexual dysfunction after hysterectomy and a search for predictive factors. Eur J Obstet Gynecol Reprod Biol. 2020;247:80-4.
24. Bostancı Ergen E, Akpak YK, Kılıççı Ç, Abide Yayla Ç, Ayas S. Does minimally invasive surgery reduce anxiety? J Turkish Ger Gynecol Assoc. 2019;20(3):142-6.
25. ACOG Practice Bulletin No. 194: Polycystic Ovary Syndrome. Obstet Gynecol. 2018;131(6):e157-71.
26. Ganie MA, Vasudevan V, Wani IA, Baba MS, Arif T, Rashid A. Epidemiology, pathogenesis, genetics & management of polycystic ovary syndrome in India. Indian J Med Res. 2019;150(4):333-44.
27. Schoretsanitis G, Gastaldon C, Kalaitzopoulos DR, Ochsenbein-Koelble N, Barbui C, Seifritz E. Polycystic ovary syndrome and postpartum depression: A systematic review and meta-analysis of observational studies. J Affect Disord. 2022;299:463-9.
28. Sundararaman PG, Shweta, Sridhar GR. Psychosocial aspects of women with polycystic ovary syndrome from south India. J Assoc Physicians India. 2008;56:945-8.

29. Hussain A, Chandel RK, Ganie MA, Dar MA, Rather YH, Wani ZA, et al. Prevalence of psychiatric disorders in patients with a diagnosis of polycystic ovary syndrome in Kashmir. Indian J Psychol Med. 2015;37(1):66-70.
30. Chaudhari AP, Mazumdar K, Mehta PD. Anxiety, depression, and quality of life in women with polycystic ovarian syndrome. Indian J Psychol Med. 2018;40(3):239-46.
31. Prathap A, Subhalakshmi TP, Varghese PJ. A cross-sectional study on the proportion of anxiety and depression and determinants of quality of life in polycystic ovarian disease. Indian J Psychol Med. 2018;40(3):257-62.
32. Cesta CE, Månsson M, Palm C, Lichtenstein P, Iliadou AN, Landén M. Polycystic ovary syndrome and psychiatric disorders: Co-morbidity and heritability in a nationwide Swedish cohort. Psychoneuroendocrinology. 2016;73:196-203.
33. Brutocao C, Zaiem F, Alsawas M, Morrow AS, Murad MH, Javed A. Psychiatric disorders in women with polycystic ovary syndrome: a systematic review and meta-analysis. Endocrine. 2018;62(2):318-25.
34. Xing L, Xu J, Wei Y, Chen Y, Zhuang H, Tang W, et al. Depression in polycystic ovary syndrome: Focusing on pathogenesis and treatment. Front Psychiatry. 2022;13:1001484.
35. Koneru A, SP. Polycystic ovary syndrome (PCOS) and sexual dysfunctions. J Psychosexual Heal. 2019;1(2):154-8.
36. Lathia T, Joshi A, Behl A, Dhingra A, Kalra B, Dua C, et al. A practitioner's toolkit for polycystic ovary syndrome counselling. Indian J Endocrinol Metab. 2022;26(1):17-25.
37. Cox CM, Thoma ME, Tchangalova N, Mburu G, Bornstein MJ, Johnson CL, et al. Infertility prevalence and the methods of estimation from 1990 to 2021: a systematic review and meta-analysis. Hum Reprod Open. 2022;2022(4):hoac051.
38. Nik Hazlina NH, Norhayati MN, Shaiful Bahari I, Nik Muhammad Arif NA. Worldwide prevalence, risk factors and psychological impact of infertility among women: a systematic review and meta-analysis. BMJ Open. 2022;12(3):e057132.
39. Patel A, Venkata Narasimha Sharma PS, Kumar P. Psychiatric disorders in women seeking fertility treatments: A clinical investigation in India. Int J Fertil Steril. 2020;14(1):68-71.
40. Patel A, Sharma PSVN, Kumar P. "In Cycles of Dreams, Despair, and Desperation:" Research perspectives on infertility specific distress in patients undergoing fertility treatments. J Hum Reprod Sci. 2018;11(4):320-8.
41. Kiani Z, Simbar M, Hajian S, Zayeri F, Shahidi M, Saei Ghare Naz M, et al. The prevalence of anxiety symptoms in infertile women: a systematic review and meta-analysis. Fertil Res Pract. 2020;6(1):7.
42. Patel A, Sharma PSVN, Narayan P, Binu VS, Dinesh N, Pai PJ. Prevalence and predictors of infertility-specific stress in women diagnosed with primary infertility: A clinic-based study. J Hum Reprod Sci. 2016;9(1):28-34.
43. Holley SR, Pasch LA, Bleil ME, Gregorich S, Katz PK, Adler NE. Prevalence and predictors of major depressive disorder for fertility treatment patients and their partners. Fertil Steril. 2015;103(5):1332-9.
44. Sejbaek CS, Hageman I, Pinborg A, Hougaard CO, Schmidt L. Incidence of depression and influence of depression on the number of treatment cycles and births in a national cohort of 42 880 women treated with ART. Hum Reprod. 2013;28(4):1100-9.

45. Pasch LA, Holley SR, Bleil ME, Shehab D, Katz PP, Adler NE. Addressing the needs of fertility treatment patients and their partners: are they informed of and do they receive mental health services? Fertil Steril. 2016;106(1):209-15.
46. Shani C, Yelena S, Reut BK, Adrian S, Sami H. Suicidal risk among infertile women undergoing in-vitro fertilization: Incidence and risk factors. Psychiatry Res. 2016;240:53-9.
47. Rooney KL, Domar AD. The relationship between stress and infertility. Dialogues Clin Neurosci. 2018;20(1):41-7.
48. Gdańska P, Drozdowicz-Jastrzębska E, Grzechocińska B, Radziwon-Zaleska M, Węgrzyn P, Wielgoś M. Anxiety and depression in women undergoing infertility treatment. Ginekol Pol. 2017;88(2):109-12.
49. Mendonça CR de, Arruda JT, Noll M, Campoli PM de O, Amaral WN do. Sexual dysfunction in infertile women: A systematic review and meta-analysis. Eur J Obstet Gynecol Reprod Biol. 2017;215:153-63.
50. Marci R, Graziano A, Piva I, Lo Monte G, Soave I, Giugliano E, et al. Procreative sex in infertile couples: the decay of pleasure? Health Qual Life Outcomes. 2012;10(1):140.
51. Patel A, Sharma PSVN, Kumar P. "When Love Does not bear a Fruit": Patterns and Prevalence of Sexual Difficulties in Infertile Men and Women as Predictors of Emotional Distress. J Hum Reprod Sci. 2021;14(3):307-12.
52. Rao KA (Ed). The Infertility Manual. New Delhi: Jaypee Brothers Medical Publishers; 2008.
53. Patel A, Sharma PSVN, Kumar P. Application of mindfulness-based psychological interventions in infertility. J Hum Reprod Sci. 2020;13(1):3-21.
54. Sankaranarayanan R, Ferlay J. Worldwide burden of gynaecological cancer: The size of the problem. Best Pract Res Clin Obstet Gynaecol. 2006;20(2):207-25.
55. Chandrasena R, Dvoráková D, Lee SI, Loza N, Mosolov SN, Osváth P, et al. Intramuscular olanzapine vs. intramuscular short-acting antipsychotics: safety, tolerability and the switch to oral antipsychotic medication in patients with schizophrenia or acute mania. Int J Clin Pract. 2009;63(8):1249-58.
56. Chandra PS, Chaturvedi SK, Channabasavanna SM, Anantha N, Reddy BKM, Sharma S, et al. Psychological well-being among cancer patients receiving radiotherapy–a prospective study. Qual Life Res. 1998;7(6):495-500.
57. Venkataramu VN, Ghotra HK, Chaturvedi SK. Management of psychiatric disorders in patients with cancer. Indian J Psychiatry. 2022;64(Suppl 2).
58. Mendonsa RD, Appaya P. Psychiatric morbidity in outpatients of gynecological oncology clinic in a tertiary care hospital. Indian J Psychiatry. 2010;52(4):327-32.
59. Jyani G, Chauhan AS, Rai B, Ghoshal S, Srinivasan R, Prinja S. Health-related quality of life among cervical cancer patients in India. Int J Gynecol Cancer. 2020;30(12):1887-92.
60. Hu Y, Ma Z, Zhang H, Gao T, Gao J, Kong Y, et al. Prevalence of and factors related to anxiety and depression symptoms among married patients with gynecological malignancies in China. Asian J Psychiatr. 2018;37:90-5.
61. Pitcher S, Adams T, van Wijk L, Fakie N, Saidu R, Denny L, et al. Holistic sexuality post gynaecological cancer treatment: A review of recent literature. South African J Oncol. 2018;2(0):a40.
62. Shankar A, Patil J, Luther A, Mandrelle K, Chakraborty A, Dubey A, et al. Sexual Dysfunction in Carcinoma Cervix: Assessment in Post Treated Cases by LENTSOMA Scale. Asian Pac J Cancer Prev. 2020;21(2):349-54.

63. Mishra N, Singh N, Sachdeva M, Ghatage P. Sexual dysfunction in cervical cancer survivors: A scoping review. Womens Health Rep (New Rochelle). 2021;2(1):594-607.
64. D S, Chandrasekaran R, KS R, Sagar K JV. A study of psychiatric morbidity and quality of life in patients with carcinoma cervix undergoing radiotherapy. Indian J Psychol Med. 2005;26(5):78-89.
65. Rahman Z, Singh U, Qureshi S, Nisha, Srivastav K, Nishchal A. Assessment of quality of life in treated patients of cancer cervix. J Midlife Health. 2017;8(4):183-8.
66. Chaturvedi SK. Psychiatric oncology: Cancer in mind. Indian J Psychiatry. 2012;54(2):111-8.
67. Chaturvedi S. Clinical Psycho-oncology: Indian Perspectives and Research. 2021.
68. Mukherjee A, Mazumder K, Kaushal V, Ghoshal S. Effect of supportive psychotherapy on mental health status and quality of life of female cancer patients receiving chemotherapy for recurrent disease. Indian J Palliat Care. 2017;23(4):399-402.
69. Spence D, Melville C. Vaginal discharge. BMJ. 2007;335(7630):1147-51.
70. Patel V, Pednekar S, Weiss H, Rodrigues M, Barros P, Nayak B, et al. Why do women complain of vaginal discharge? A population survey of infectious and pyschosocial risk factors in a South Asian community. Int J Epidemiol. 2005;34(4):853-62.
71. Patel V, Andrew G, Pelto PJ. The psychological and social contexts of complaints of abnormal vaginal discharge: A study of illness narratives in India. J Psychosom Res. 2008;64(3):255-62.
72. Grover S, Avasthi A, Gupta S, Hazari N, Malhotra N. Do female patients with nonpathological vaginal discharge need the same evaluation as for Dhat syndrome in males? Indian J Psychiatry. 2016;58(1):61-9.
73. Chaturvedi SK, Chandra PS, Issac MK, Sudarshan CY. Somatization misattributed to non-pathological vaginal discharge. J Psychosom Res. 1993;37(6):575-9.
74. Tripathi A, Roy D, Kar SK. Distress due to nonpathological vaginal discharge: A new face of Dhat syndrome in females. J Psychosexual Heal. 2021;3(4):315-21.
75. Mehra A, Kathirvel S, Gainder S, Avasthi A, Grover S. Female Dhat syndrome in primary care setting. Ind Psychiatry J. 2021;30(2):278-84.
76. Nelson LM. Primary ovarian insufficiency. N Engl J Med. 2009;360(6):606-14.
77. Lambrinoudaki I, Paschou SA, Lumsden MA, Faubion S, Makrakis E, Kalantaridou S, et al. Premature ovarian insufficiency: A toolkit for the primary care physician. Maturitas. 2021;147:53-63.
78. Menezes C, Pravata GR, Yela DA, Benetti-Pinto CL. Women with premature ovarian failure using hormone therapy do not experience increased levels of depression, anxiety and stress compared to controls. J Affect Disord. 2020;273:562-6.
79. Słopień R. Mood disorders in women with premature ovarian insufficiency. Prz Menopauzalny. 2018;17(3):124-6.
80. Xi D, Chen B, Tao H, Xu Y, Chen G. The risk of depressive and anxiety symptoms in women with premature ovarian insufficiency: a systematic review and meta-analysis. Arch Womens Ment Health. 2023;26(1):1-10.

13 | Menarche, the Menstrual Cycle, and Menopause: Biological Cycles and Women's Mental Health

CHAPTER

Imon Paul, Anamika Das

ABSTRACT

The mental health of women is closely entwined with reproductive health and mediated by various psychobiological factors. The female reproductive period starts with the onset of menstruation or menarche, followed by cyclical hormonal changes related to ovulation, reproductive life events such as pregnancy and childbirth, and finally the cessation of menstruation or menopause. Early pubertal maturation is associated with adverse developmental outcomes in females. Hormonal changes in puberty and psychosocial factors (disparity of maturation, amplification of the disadvantaged context, and accentuation of pre-existent vulnerabilities) have been implicated as causal mechanisms. Estrogen has been implicated in the psychopathology of women, demonstrating a protective effect against psychosis and depression. Periods of estrogen-deficient states such as premenstruation and puerperium can cause symptom genesis or exacerbation. Depression and anxiety are common in perimenopausal women. Regular screening for mental health problems in vulnerable women can reduce morbidity and improve quality of life.

Keywords: Menstrual cycle, mental health, menopause, premenstrual dysphoric disorder

INTRODUCTION

The mental health of women is closely entwined with reproductive health and mediated by various psychobiological factors. The female reproductive period is heralded by the onset of menstruation or menarche, followed by cyclical hormonal changes related to ovulation, reproductive life events such as pregnancy and childbirth, and finally the cessation of menstruation or menopause. Some authors have proposed a category of reproductive-related disorders (RRDs), which include disorders with diverse phenomenology occurring at particular periods in a woman's reproductive lifespan. It is hypothesized that these disorders can occur due to genetic vulnerabilities, which are further modified by stressors and life events as well as maladaptation to the hormonal fluctuations that commonly occur in the female lifespan.[1] An understanding of the neurobiological underpinnings of the female biological cycles is required to understand the complex interplay with psychiatric disorders.

PUBERTY: A PERIOD OF CHANGES

Puberty marks the transition between childhood and young adulthood and is accompanied by myriad biological, social, psychological, and cognitive changes. Many common mental disorders such as anxiety and depression start during adolescence and often persist throughout the lifespan. An increase in psychiatric disorders in adolescents has sparked concern globally and it is particularly important in the Indian context where there is a large adolescent population. A recent meta-analysis of 41 studies from 27 countries across the globe concluded that 13.4% of children and adolescents suffered from some psychiatric disorder. Amongst these, anxiety disorders had a prevalence of 6.5%, any depressive disorder were prevalent in 2.6%, attention-deficit hyperactivity disorder in 3.4%, and any disruptive disorder was prevalent in 5.7% of the population.[2] Although mental health disorders can be seen in children, the onset is more commonly seen in adolescence. In some disorders like depression, marked preponderance in female gender emerges in puberty with girls being almost two times more likely to suffer from it compared to boys and this gender difference can persist throughout, becoming less prominent after menopause.[3] Depression and anxiety in adolescents can lead to substance use, deterioration of academic performance, reduced self-esteem, victimization by peers, and self-injurious behaviors. The adverse effects may persist throughout life causing difficulties in interpersonal relationships, poor educational and employment outcomes, and a host of mental health concerns.[4]

The emergence of psychiatric issues in puberty can be explained by:
- *Role of sex hormones:* There is an increase in the levels of sex hormones in puberty. Altered levels of these hormones can modulate neurotransmitters such as serotonin and dopamine, which can in turn influence the neural circuitry and cause disturbances in biological function, mood, and concentration, thereby increasing the risk of psychopathology.
- *Influence of psychosocial factors:* Puberty is accompanied by physical changes such as the appearance of secondary sex characteristics and changes in body morphology and voice. Adapting to the changing body and the accompanying change in societal norms and expectations can be challenging and stressful, more so if the onset of puberty is earlier or later compared to peers.

The Menstrual Cycle

Puberty in females is accompanied by the onset of menstruation. Menstruation signifies not only biological and hormonal changes but it also marks various role transitions. Menstruation in females is taken to be a sign of fecundity and it carries with it immense physiological and social responsibility.

The menstrual cycle has a basic biological underpinning in the form of hormonal fluctuations and associated changes in the reproductive organs of the female. The hormones that mainly regulate the cycle are estrogen and progesterone. The menstrual cycle starts with a menstruation phase, which may last till 7 days. At this phase, both the hormones are relatively low. This is followed by the follicular phase where there is a steady increase in estrogen and the pituitary secretes follicle-stimulating hormone (FSH) and luteinizing hormone (LH) for maturation of the eggs in the ovary. In a typical 28-day cycle, ovulation generally occurs on day 14 and the release of the egg transforms the follicle to the corpus luteum. In the subsequent luteal phase, the corpus luteum produces increasing amount of progesterone. If the egg is not fertilized then the levels of both the hormones fall and the menstrual cycle resumes with another menstruation. An understanding of these phases would help us in conceptualizing the changes in mental health over the menstrual cycle. "Premenstrual" phase is the phase just before the next menstruation and is generally referred to the mid or late luteal phase. "Perimenstrual" is used to include both the premenstrual and menstrual phase; in both these phases there is a relative low level of estrogen. The "early follicular phase" includes the menstrual and also the initial days just after the menstruation.[5] The various phases and its manifestations are tabulated in **Table 1** and the hormonal fluctuation is depicted in **Figure 1**.

Multiple mechanisms are responsible for the cyclical experiences with regard to mental health in the different phases of the menstrual cycle. They can be categorized as:[6]

- The physical discomfort causing distress and irritability, which leads to interpersonal conflicts
- The reduction in social engagement and isolation leading to psychological symptoms
- Stress related to societal stereotypes lead to negative feelings around menstruation. Women were commonly sequestered during times of menstruation across various religions and social customs and the myths and taboos regarding menstruation creates an unhealthy environment.
- The biological role of hormones

TABLE 1: Phases of menstrual cycle.

	Follicular phase	Luteal phase
Timeline	Menstruation to ovulation	Following ovulation till next menstruation
Duration	Varied in length (typically 14 days for a 28 day cycle)	Consistently 14 days
Special mention		Premenstrual phase is a part of this phase (immediately prior to menstruation).

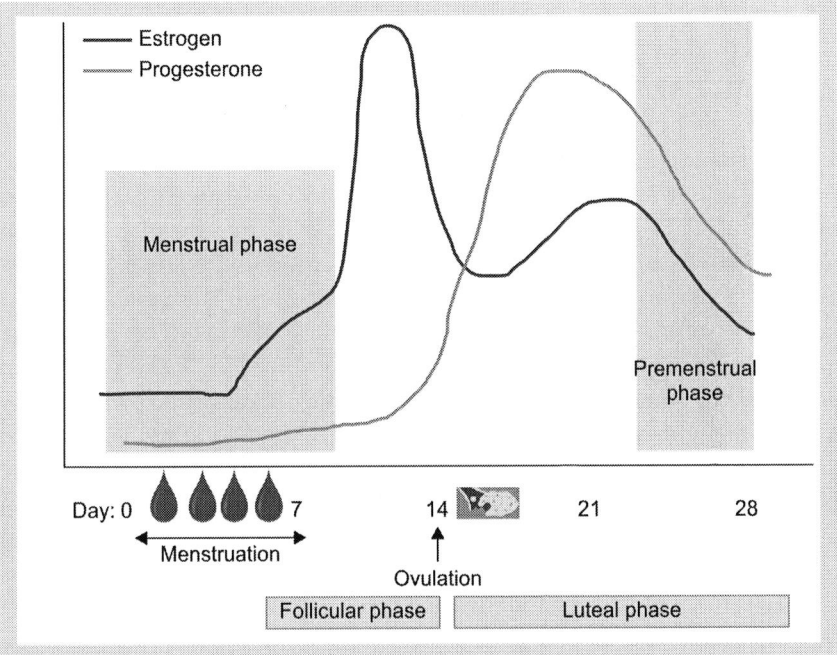

Fig. 1: Hormonal fluctuations in various phases of menstrual cycle.

The Effects of Early Pubertal Maturation

Recent research has focused on the influence of pubertal timing on mental health, particularly in females as offset pubertal timing has been associated with mental health concerns.[4,7] Early puberty can increase psychopathology by (1) an increase in level of hormones, (2) stress and adjustment problems caused due to disparity of maturation, (3) amplification of the disadvantaged context, and (4) accentuation of pre-existent vulnerabilities.[8]

■ MENARCHE AS A MARKER OF PUBERTY

Puberty is accompanied by sexual maturation including thelarche, gonadarche, pubarche, and adrenarche. Though thelarche or breast development is often the first sign of puberty in girls, it can be difficult to ascertain accurately given the variability in methods of assessment. So, while menarche or the onset of menstruation is actually a late marker of puberty, it is commonly used to determine the time of puberty as it is a significant event recollected with reasonable accuracy by most females.[9] In recent times, secular trends have noted declining menarcheal age worldwide with India being no exception.[10] Early menarche has been linked with a host of psychiatric problems including depression and anxiety disorders, externalizing disorders, and eating disorders each of which is discussed below.

Depression

Epidemiological studies reveal that major depression and dysthymia is almost twice likely to occur in females in comparison to males. This gender difference emerges in early to mid-adolescence and may be mediated by various biopsychosocial factors. In adolescent girls, the onset of menarche may trigger the pre-existent biological vulnerability to depression. The change in pubertal status accompanied by physical changes may be associated with negative affect in girls.[11] Pubertal timing or maturation relative to peers is another important factor in the genesis of depression. Early menarche has been consistently associated with depression.[12,13] Girls with an earlier age of menarche have been shown to have higher levels of depression when compared to boys or females who mature later.[13] This can be explained by the fact that girls who mature early may feel isolated and find it difficult to connect to peers who have not matured at a similar rate.[14] Females also have higher severity of symptoms, more somatic symptoms (disturbances in sleep and appetite, psychomotor retardation) and crying spells, ideas of guilt, and reduced self-esteem.[15] It is important to keep in mind that most adolescents undergo emotional changes including depressed mood at some point during the pubertal transition and these experiences are normative. The cognitive vulnerability-transactional stress model postulates that negative events give rise to negative affect and in the presence of genetic vulnerability the negative affect escalates to depression, which can in turn leads to future self-generated negative life events.[16] In females, experience of chronic strain and ruminative coping style can lead to increased vulnerability to depression.[17]

Anxiety symptoms are frequently comorbid with depression in adolescents and often precede depressive symptoms. Depression may also be co-existent with substance use disorders. Suicidal behavior is commonly seen in girls in mid adolescence with recent research focusing on the link between puberty and suicidality in girls.[11]

To summarize, latent vulnerabilities combined with biological and social transitions accompanied by stressors can lead to depressive symptoms and adverse consequences in young females.[11,14]

Anxiety Disorders

Though anxiety is frequently comorbid with depression, it is a conceptually distinct entity. The association between recency of menarche and anxiety was shown in a large cross-sectional study on Australian adolescents.[13] Among anxiety symptoms, panic attacks have been shown to be associated with pubertal stage, with increased rates of panic attacks seen in girls who are physically more mature compared to peers.[18] A review of literature of the association between puberty and anxiety concluded that advancing pubertal status is more likely to be associated with symptoms of anxiety including panic attacks in girls.[19] Studies on pubertal timing and anxiety have consistently shown that there is an increased chance of occurrence of anxiety in girls who mature early. Early maturing girls had increased lifetime prevalence of depression and anxiety in a study that investigated whether pubertal timing continued to be associated with psychopathology from mid-adolescence into young adulthood.[7]

A few studies have also examined the role of anxiety on pubertal timing with mixed results. In girls, early menarche has been correlated with family stress and mother-daughter conflict.[20] However, methodologically robust studies in this area are lacking and further research is needed to draw definitive conclusion.

Eating Disorders

Puberty is a period of risk for development of eating disorders in adolescent females. Puberty is characterized by changes in body morphology, which can cause dissatisfaction with body, concerns with weight, and reduced self-esteem in young girls. These concerns can be amplified in girls who mature early compared to their peers leading to measures such as excessive dieting and disordered eating.[14,21]

Studies on the severity and type of eating disturbance vary with some studies reporting association between bulimia and early menarche,[22,23] but not with anorexia.[23,24]

The relationship between puberty and eating disorders is also modified by life stressors and romantic relationships. The weight gain seen at the time of menarche has been implicated in causing body dissatisfaction in young girls, making them feel isolated and different from their peers and leading to eating pathologies in a bid to lose weight. In an 8-year follow-up study by Graber et al., 1994, it was noted that eating disturbances in girls who matured early was not only an episodic problem but rather a chronic problem and eating problems in adolescence can be associated with psychological disturbances, future eating disturbances, and long-term adjustment outcomes.[25]

Substance Use

Early maturation may cause young girls to be mistaken as older than their actual age. Association with older peers may expose them to substance use and risky sexual behavior. Early initiation of smoking and drinking and experimentation with marijuana and other illegal substances has been reported in girls with early puberty. Early puberty also predicts an increased risk of substance abuse in future.[14] However, some studies reported that this association between early puberty and substance use persisted only for those girls who continued to have advanced development compared to peers.[26] In another study, the same authors reported that among twin sisters with different age of menarche, the earlier developing twin was more at risk to initiate smoking and drinking at a younger age and to report a greater frequency of smoking and drinking at age 16 years than the later maturing sister,[27] thereby indicating a causal psychosocial role of early pubertal maturation.

Externalizing Behaviors

Early pubertal timing has been associated with externalizing behavior.[28] A recent Indian study found that pubertal timing but not status to be predictive for problem behaviors in Indian adolescents.[29] Like substance abuse, it can be argued that affiliation with older peers enables externalizing problem behaviors in girls who undergo early pubertal maturation. A context of risk model proposes that precocious pubertal maturation influences social surroundings, exposing girls to risk factors such as punitive parenting, and association with delinquent peers. The life history theory on the other hand takes cognizance of environmental stressors and argues that these accelerate development leading to problem behaviors.[30]

Indian Context

In India, gender plays a complex role and often girls are at a disadvantage due to their gender, which gets amplified after puberty. Girls experience unwarranted sexual advances, frequently their opportunities for educational achievement are curbed, they are burdened with more chores and responsibilities, and often are rushed into early marriages. Early marriages with consequent early pregnancies lead to increased maternal and neonatal morbidity and adverse mental health outcome. In a recent study on 13–14-year-old adolescent females of rural Karnataka, almost a third of the study population reported having little hope for the future with some having death wishes or suicidal ideation.[31] A systematic review of the effects of early menarche on sexual and reproductive health in low- and middle-income countries found that that there was dearth of methodologically robust studies in this area and existing literature revealed early menarche is associated with early sexual initiation and early marriage, early pregnancy, and sexually transmitted infections in low- and middle-income countries.[32]

THE MENSTRUAL CYCLE AND INTERFACE WITH PSYCHIATRIC MORBIDITY

Psychosis

Estrogen modulates dopamine by downregulating its transmission, thereby acting as an antipsychotic agent. Thus, estrogen confers a protective effect and individuals become vulnerable to psychosis at those stages of menstruation and reproduction (postpartum) where estrogen is low.[5]

The gender differences in schizophrenia patients can be mediated by the role of 5-hydroxytryptamine 2A (5HT2A). The lower age of onset in women, difference in symptomatology, and occurrence of a second peak, these characteristics have been explained by the protective actions of estrogen. Abnormal dopaminergic activity is held to be responsible for florid positive symptoms while abnormal 5HT functioning is linked to more refractory negative symptoms. In either cases, estrogen plays a modulatory role.[33]

The evidence of the association between estrogen and psychosis also comes from clinical studies showing fluctuation of symptoms in various phases of the menstrual cycle. There is a link between a decrease in level of estrogen and psychotic symptoms, which explains the occurrence of puerperal psychosis. Estrogen can cross the blood–brain barrier and has a role in all the major neurotransmitter systems involved in the brain. Dopamine, serotonin, and noradrenaline are various neurotransmitter systems, which play a role in mood states, and estrogen affects all of these systems.[34] Other studies have also supported this hypothesis by showing that administration of estrogen can improve puerperal psychosis. It was seen that patients having psychotic symptoms with low serum estradiol did not respond to neuroleptics, but improved after treatment with estradiol and had rebound of symptoms after discontinuation.[35] It has also been noted that there are chances of precipitation of a psychotic episode in the relatively estrogen-deficient premenstrual phase of the menstrual cycle.

Estrogen Withdrawal Associated Psychosis

Estrogen withdrawal associated psychosis (EWAP) has been conceptualized as a state where psychotic symptoms rapidly emerge subsequent to a drop in estrogen and there is recovery after normalization of estrogen levels. This hypothesis as explained by Deuchar and Brockington highlighted the role of individual predisposition as well as the effect of estrogen on central neurotransmitters. The neuroanatomical and neurobiological substrates have a complex interplay with psychosocial issues, thus producing symptomatology.[36] An interesting concept speculates on the relation of the extent of decrease of estrogen levels and psychopathology and the risk seems directly proportional to the magnitude of decrease. The association between estrogen withdrawal and nonpuerperal psychosis has also been reported in literature, the psychotic symptoms being characteristically short and reversible with recurrence occurring in cases of estrogen withdrawal.[34]

Menstrual Psychosis

Menstrual psychosis is a rare but distinct entity where psychotic symptoms present with an acute onset, short duration, usually recovering completely and occurring in sync with a woman's menstrual phases or in a circamensual

TABLE 2: Various types of menstrual psychosis according to the timing of presentation.	
Types of menstrual psychosis	Timing of symptoms
Premenstrual psychosis	Symptoms in the luteal phase with resolution at menstruation
Paramenstrual psychosis	Variable onset but always in harmony with menstrual cycle
Catamenial psychosis	Beginning at the onset of menstrual flow
Epochal menstrual psychosis	Bipolar illness with switch related to menstrual cycle
Mid cycle psychosis	Occurring at mid cycle—least in incidence

(approximately monthly and in relation to the menstrual cycle) fashion.[37] There are various types according to the timing of the presentation, which has been described in **Table 2**.[38] Multiple case reports from India have described this phenomenon in clinical cases. It has been demonstrated that there is a hormonal interplay and a link with estrogen withdrawal and level of progesterone has been postulated. The treatment strategies include use of hormones in the form of oral contraceptive pills in some cases, establishing the role of hormones in its pathophysiology. Though formal genetic studies are awaited, but the condition may run in families with case reports mentioning a positive history of menstrual psychosis in first-degree relatives.

Anxiety Disorder

There has been reports that anxiety in women is exacerbated in the premenstrual phase. Both trait and state anxiety are higher in the luteal phase as compared to the follicular phase. On the other hand, chronic anxiety increases risk for severe premenstrual symptoms. Studies have noted that sometimes there is exacerbation of anxiety in the midcycle with premenstrual improvement. There has been reports that women with generalized anxiety disorder experienced higher mental fatigue in the early follicular phase. Social anxiety and obsessive compulsive symptoms can increase in the premenstrual and menstrual phase.[5]

Substance Use Disorders

The studies of association between alcohol use and menstrual cycle show mixed results. Some studies reported increased drinking in the premenstrual phase, some reported decreased alcohol use, and others could find no relationship. The fluctuation of this drinking can be linked to progesterone to estradiol ratios. In the premenstrual phase, drinking may increase as a coping strategy to handle the negative affect mediated by low progesterone levels. On the other hand, increased drinking around ovulation was associated with social motivations and was attributed to a positive affect due to high progesterone. Craving and affective responses to tobacco was also lower in the luteal phase (where progesterone level is high) compared to the follicular phase (progesterone level is low).[5]

Depression

Estrogen has a profound effect on the mental state, mood, and memory through various neurotransmitter mechanisms. The monoamine hypothesis of mood disorders emphasizes the importance of the monoamines in the etiology of mood disorders, especially depression. The existence of premenstrual syndrome (PMS), postmenopausal depression, and postpartum depression point to an association with estrogen-deficient state, and thus the role of estrogen in the monoamine metabolism needs further discussion. Estrogen stimulates a significant increase in the serotonin (5 HT2A) binding sites in nucleus accumbens, primary olfactory cortex, anterior frontal cortex, and cingulate cortex. These areas of the brain are responsible for mediating mental processes such as cognition, behavior, emotion, and mood by pathways involving posttranslational events or classical genomic mechanisms. Thus estrogen can act as an antidepressant or can help serotonergic antidepressants in treating clinical depression.[33]

Premenstrual Symptoms

A conglomeration of emotional, behavioral, and physical symptoms manifesting in the late luteal or premenstrual phase with resolution after onset of menstrual bleeding is referred to as PMS. The symptoms generally emerge in the mid to late twenties with a chronic course if left untreated. Improvement in symptoms is noted when there are interruptions in the ovulatory cycle such as pregnancy or post ovariectomy. Presence of PMS increases risk of later depression including postpartum and perimenopausal depression.[39]

Premenstrual Dysphoric Disorder

It is a severe form of PMS with a prevalence of 3–8% and diagnosed as depressive disorder as per the Diagnostic and Statistical Manual of Mental Disorders, Fifth Edition (DSM-5; **Table 3**). It is also hypothesized that the premenstrual magnification of an existing disorder can sometimes present as premenstrual dysphoric disorder (PMDD). This diagnosis is controversial as some feel that it would pathologize normative cyclical experiences. On the other hand, it has been argued that inclusion of this diagnosis would help in further research on its symptoms and treatment, and thus would be helpful for woman experiencing this severe spectrum of PMS. The management

TABLE 3: Diagnostic criteria of PMDD as per DSM-5.[41]

Timing of symptoms	Symptoms	Severity	Consideration of other psychiatric disorders
(A) In the majority of menstrual cycles, at least 5 symptoms must be present in the final week before the onset of menses, start to improve within a few days after the onset of menses, and become minimal or absent in the week postmenses	(B) One or more of the following symptoms must be present: 1. Marked affective lability (e.g., mood swings, feeling suddenly sad or tearful, or increased sensitivity to rejection) 2. Marked irritability or anger or increased interpersonal conflicts 3. Markedly depressed mood, feelings of hopelessness, or self-deprecating thoughts 4. Marked anxiety, tension, and/or feelings of being keyed up or on edge	(D) The symptoms are associated with clinically significant distress or interference with work, school, usual social activities, or relationships with others	(E) The disturbance is not merely an exacerbation of the symptoms of another disorder, such as major depressive disorder, panic disorder, persistent depressive disorder (dysthymia) or a personality disorder (although it may co-occur with any of these disorders)

Contd...

Contd...

Timing of symptoms	Symptoms	Severity	Consideration of other psychiatric disorders
(F) Criterion A should be confirmed by prospective daily ratings during at least 2 symptomatic cycles (although a provisional diagnosis may be made prior to this confirmation)	**(C)** One (or more) of the following symptoms must additionally be present to reach a total of 5 symptoms when combined with symptoms from criterion B above: • Decreased interest in usual activities • Subjective difficulty in concentration • Lethargy, easy fatigability, or marked lack of energy • Marked change in appetite; overeating or specific food cravings • Hypersomnia or insomnia • A sense of being overwhelmed or out of control • Physical symptoms such as breast tenderness or swelling; joint or muscle pain, a sensation of "bloating" or weight gain		**(G)** The symptoms are not attributable to the physiological effects of a substance (e.g., drug abuse, medication, or other treatment) or another medical condition (e.g., hyperthyroidism)

(DSM-5: Diagnostic and Statistical Manual of Mental Disorders, Fifth Edition; PMDD: premenstrual dysphoric disorder) consists of selective serotonin reuptake inhibitors (SSRIs), anxiolytics, and ovulation suppressing agents such as oral contraceptive pills.[40]

Suicide

In a meta-analysis on the effects of menstrual cycle on mental health outcomes, it was found that the chances of suicide increased in the menstrual phase. This outcome is likely due to both the psychological and physiological impacts of menstruation. Physical pain and dysmenorrhea, psychological symptoms such as lower self-esteem, dysphoria, and higher levels of anxiety can play a role. When completed suicides were considered, the menstrual phase posed the highest risk. Psychiatric admissions increased both during the premenstrual and menstrual phase. The overall risk of poor mental health outcomes was also increased in these phases.[6] Histopathological reports of completed suicides showed higher incidence during the menstrual phase. Women with existing mental health disorders are about five times more likely to attempt suicide in the menstrual phase.[5]

Sleep

Multiple central nervous system areas such as basal forebrain, dorsal raphe nucleus, coeruleus, hypothalamus are involved in sleep regulation and both estrogen and progesterone receptors are widely present in these areas. Although the mechanism is not fully explainable, it has been seen that ovarian steroids can influence circadian rhythms through effects on the master pacemaker suprachiasmatic nucleus.[42]

Various aspects of sleep have been studied vis-à-vis menstrual cycle. They are described as follows:

- *Sleep quality (subjective/self-reported):* Sleep disturbances are commonly reported during the first few days of menstrual bleeding phase (early follicular) and the last few premenstrual days (late luteal) phase. Changes in the progesterone and estrogen levels rather than absolute values in the premenstrual phase may be responsible for altered sleep quality. Other factors such as anxiety, depression, cramps, headaches, and breast tenderness during the menstrual phase may also be responsible for the altered sleep quality.
- *Sleep quality (objective):* This was studied by polysomnography (PSG) and actigraphy. The sleep efficiency (SE) and total sleep time (TST) were decreased in the week just prior to menstruation. The other confounding factors were smoking, obesity, or financial stressors. PSG studies showed that there was a decline in the rapid eye movement (REM) sleep in the luteal phase. Electroencephalography (EEG) studies have found that

upper frequency range sleep spindles were increased in the luteal phase. This may occur due to modulation of gamma-aminobutyric acid (GABA) receptors by progesterone metabolites.
- *Circadian rhythms:* Blunted amplitude of body temperature rhythm was present in the luteal phase primarily due to progesterone. The heart rate was raised in this phase.
- *Sleep duration:* Short sleep duration was associated with altered menstrual cycles both in adolescents and adulthood. Women with sleep <6 hours reported variance in the menstrual cycle duration (either long or short). This can impact reproductive function in turn.

Sleep Disturbances in Premenstrual Syndrome and Premenstrual Dysphoric Disorder

Sleep disturbance is present in many cases of PMS and is one of the specified five symptoms for diagnosis of PMDD as per DSM-5. Frequent sleep disturbances are experienced by women with severe PMS. It includes effects on sleep quality, fatigue, daytime sleepiness, disturbing dreams, and insomnia.[43] Women with PMS/PMDD had poor sleep quality when assessed with sleep rating tools.[44] This disruption in sleep quality can be both a state and trait factor. The menstrual state can be a cause as well as a precipitant of sleep disturbance in females with preexistent sleep problems.

Various studies have found a link between PMS and daytime sleepiness. Women with PMS were less alert and more sleepy with increased fatigue in the late luteal phase as compared to the follicular phase. There were more prone to psychomotor slowing and slower reaction times in this phase.[45]

There are studies that found a link between menstrual cycle phases and melatonin levels and rhythm suggesting circadian rhythm dysfunction in patients with PMDD. There is evidence of decreased melatonin amplitude in the luteal phase. Less responsiveness to bright light shift in melatonin secretion in the luteal phase as compared to the follicular phase has been noted.[46,47]

Sleep and Dysmenorrhea

Painful menstrual cramps of the uterine origin, either primary or secondary, are referred to as dysmenorrhea. There is an integral connection of pain and sleep. Due to the increased pain sensitization, both quality and quantity of sleep was affected in patients with dysmenorrhea. Adequate analgesia with control of heavy bleeding by hormonal methods not only improves dysmenorrhea but also improves the related sleep disturbances.[48]

MENOPAUSE AND ITS EFFECT ON MENTAL HEALTH OF WOMEN

Menopause is said to occur after one year of last menstrual bleeding. It is a transitional state experienced by women in late forties or early fifties. The quality of life is impacted at this stage due to various biological, psychological, and social constructs. Multiple studies have been done to show the impact of this transitional stage on mental health. Depression is the most common psychiatric disorder, which is corelated with perimenopausal and menopausal stage.

The Study of Women's Health across the National Mental Health Study (SWAN MHS) was a longitudinal, community-based, multicentric study over 8 years, involving 3,302 participants. It consisted of an annual follow-up of pre and perimenopausal women with questionnaires about their health, lifestyle, psychosocial factors, anthropometry, and a fasting blood sample in the early follicular phase. Depression was assessed annually using the Center for Epidemiological Studies Depression (CES-D) scale, with a score of ≥16 showing potential depression. The important findings of the study are as follows:[49]

- It showed that there is an increase in depression risk in late perimenopausal or postmenopausal period compared to pre or early perimenopausal period ($p<0.001$). Premenopausal was defined as having regular menses in past 3 months, early perimenopausal with irregular menses in last 3 months, late perimenopausal as no menses in last 3 months but some bleeding in last 12 months, and postmenopausal as no bleeding occurring in last 12 months.[50]
- Higher testosterone levels and an increase in testosterone levels from baseline correlated with high CES-D scores. Testosterone is aromatized to estradiol and it also increases serotonin receptors in the brain and the relative androgenicity in the menopausal transition may disrupt mood. The annual estimation of the levels in the study may have been unable to detect the variability of the hormonal patterns, which seems to be the recent understanding in the concept of menopausal depression.
- Depressive symptoms were increased in women with frequent vasomotor symptoms, stressful life events, and low social support.[50]
- In a meta-analysis of prevalence of sleep disorders during menopause, it was found that about 51.6% of the women in postmenopausal group had sleep disorders with the most common being restless legs syndrome.[51]

A biopsychosocial approach has been summarized in **Table 4**.[49,50]

It has been seen that history of depression and use of antidepressants increased the risk of early perimenopausal transition by about three times as compared to nondepressed individuals. They also showed lower levels of estradiol and high levels of FSH and LH.[52]

TABLE 4: Biopsychosocial approach and its risk factors.

Construct	Risk factors (aggravating risk)
Biological	• Decreased reproductive hormonal level (estrogen deficiency and fluctuations) • Fluctuating and irregular pattern of FSH release • Long premenopausal period • Severe menopausal symptoms including long-term vasomotor symptoms (directly aggravate depression or precipitate an episode) • Sleep abnormalities due to the problematic hot flushes • Type of menopause—surgical • Premature menopause • Chronic medical diseases/physical disorders • History of premenstrual syndrome
Psychological	• History of depressive disorder or any other mood disorder • Negative attitude toward menopause and aging • Family history of psychiatric disorder • History of postpartum depression or postpartum blues • Perceived loss OF femininity and attractiveness • Loss of reproductive capacity • Physical problems of dry vagina and memory issues • Dissatisfaction with relationships • Sense of loss of control over menopausal symptoms
Social	• Empty nest syndrome (breakage in family structure due to children leaving home for education or job or getting married) • Additional responsibilities of care giving or loss of role of a mother • Associated change in work place and functioning • Retirement of self or spouse • Shift in roles and responsibilities

Older age at menopause leading to longer exposure to endogenous estrogens and thus longer reproductive period can lead to a protective action for depression in later life.[53]

Management of Depression Associated with Menopause

As with other depressive episodes, antidepressants remain the mainstay of treatment. Some patients may remain unresponsive or partially responsive for whom transdermal estrogen patches can be helpful. Treatment with venlafaxine, duloxetine, or escitalopram has shown promise by reducing both the depressive symptoms and the vasomotor symptoms.[54] The Canadian Network for Mood and Anxiety Treatments (CANMAT) guidelines identify desvenlafaxine and cognitive behavioral therapy as first line for depression among perimenopausal women. Second-line agents include transdermal estradiol, duloxetine, mirtazapine, escitalopram, and venlafaxine extended release preparation.[55] A treatment approach that takes into consideration the biopsychosocial factors has been found to be of maximum benefit.

Menopause and Bipolar Illness

Bipolar disorder in women differ from men in having more burden of depression, higher frequency of episodes, rapid cycling, and mixed features. The frequency of symptom-free euthymic intervals decreases gradually with increasing age. This may be explained by episodic accumulation due to sensitization or kindling. The variation in hormonal levels with age has also been implicated. Bipolar illness exacerbation has an association with female reproductive stages. Women transitioning to menopause have more depression. The highest risk remains at the juncture of early post menopause when gonadal hormones go through a marked fluctuation. Euthymia and mood elevation was found to decrease with progress in the reproductive age phase. Hormonal fluctuation is thought to be responsible in the perimenopausal and postmenopausal group.[56] Estrogen and progesterone both modulate intracellular signaling pathways used by mood stabilizers. Oxidative stress and brain-derived neurotrophic factor are neurobiological factors implicated in the neurobiology of bipolar disorders and also affected by these hormones. Factors such as inflammation, diet, and structural changes to the brain can also have causal role.[57,58]

Menopause and Psychosis

The possible protective action of estrogen on psychosis has been discussed earlier. This leads to the assumption that menopause may result in exacerbation of psychotic symptoms. Menopause being a period of profound hormonal changes has an impact on the disease trajectory. The altered pharmacokinetic and pharmacodynamics of antipsychotics also has its impact. It has indeed been seen that there is a late life rise in psychotic episode in women. It has also been shown that there is a need of dose escalation of antipsychotics in women post menopause. Data obtained from a large cohort of 61,889 Finnish patients with schizophrenia-spectrum disorders [International Classification of Diseases, 10th Revision (ICD-10) diagnosis of F20 and F25) showed that antipsychotic effectiveness decreased after the age of 45 and the chances of relapse also increased. This is majorly due to the pharmacokinetics regulation of antipsychotics by estrogen. Estrogen is a potent inhibitor of CYP1A2 responsible for metabolism of various antipsychotics (majorly olanzapine and clozapine) and inducer of CYP3A4, which metabolizes quetiapine. Estrogen also increases the sensitivity of dopamine receptors (D2). Thus, in premenopausal state the antipsychotic levels remain higher and also the D2 receptor occupancy of antipsychotics is more, thus exerting the protective role of estrogen in patients with schizophrenia spectrum disorders. The loss of these roles of estrogen leads to lowered effectiveness of antipsychotics in postmenopausal period, thus leading to more relapses and increased hospital admission.[59] Even in premenopausal women, dose adjustments are recommended by some during menstruation phase. It is recommended that side effect profile needs to be monitored after menopause due to higher chances of QTc prolongation, hyperprolactinemia, and tardive dyskinesia. Some studies have shown that use of selective estrogen receptor modulator (raloxifene) with antipsychotics proved beneficial in menopausal women.[60] Hormone replacement therapy (HRT) can also be used in perimenopausal women with schizophrenia. They are indeed helpful for the physical symptoms associated with menopause. As far as psychotic symptoms are concerned, it has been seen that addition of HRT or raloxifene at a dosage of 120 mg/day in postmenopausal women decreased positive symptoms without any added adverse effects. There is also less extrapyramidal side effects and a protection against tardive dyskinesia in patients with HRT. Improvement in various aspects of cognition such as attention and processing speed improved with HRT. The safest time to institute HRT is during the postmenopausal women under age of 60 or within 10 years of menopause. Caution should be taken about breast and cardiovascular complications. There is also evidence that changes should be done in the antipsychotic regimen of postmenopausal women. This is because of the changed metabolism and need for increased dosage, which gradually increases with the increased duration from the time of menopause and other ancillary factors such as treatment of comorbid disorder. Antipsychotics causing hyperprolactinemia should be avoided. Drugs causing weight gain may provide some benefit by increasing estrogen but pose other health hazards, and thus preferably should be avoided. It has also been seen that intramuscular administration is more effective than oral formulation. Thus, during menopause clinicians should regularly monitor for side effects and also periodically review the need for modification of type, dose, and mode of antipsychotic medications.[61]

▌ INDIAN STUDIES

Indian studies have reported occurrence of depression, anxiety, mood swings, irritability, and sleep disturbances in perimenopausal women.[62-64] The COVID-19 pandemic may have led to an exacerbation of depression, anxiety, and stress in this age group.[65] A recent review noted that factors such as reduced Vitamin D and estrogen levels and increased stress can contribute to depression and anxiety in postmenopausal women. Psychological distress is often ignored and under-reported by these women due to reduced awareness and associated stigma.[66] Routine screening for mental health problems in vulnerable women can reduce morbidity and improve quality of life.

> **KEY POINTS**
> - Menstrual cycle is an integrated part of female physiology and its various phases have different psychological underpinnings and variation in psychopathology due to the widespread hormonal fluctuations and psychosocial impact.
> - Early pubertal maturation is associated with adverse developmental outcomes in females such as depression (which may persist through adolescence and adulthood), anxiety, substance abuse, eating disturbances, body dissatisfaction, and externalizing behaviors. Implicated causal mechanisms include hormonal changes and various psychosocial factors.
> - Estrogen is the major hormone that plays a major role in modulating psychopathology. It has a protective action against both psychosis and depression.
> - Periods of low estrogen levels such as premenstruation, pregnancy, puerperium, and postmenopause are vulnerable periods for both psychosis and depression.
> - PMS and PMDD are conditions that should be kept in mind when evaluating such patients.
> - Perimenopausal period is a major transition phase in females with various biopsychosocial changes. Psychiatric symptoms arising at this time should be handled with sensitivity and consideration.
> - Patients with schizophrenia attaining menopause can be offered HRT with due caution and the dose, mode, and type of antipsychotics should be modified if warranted.

REFERENCES

1. Halbreich U. Women's reproductive related disorders (RRDs). J Affect Disord. 2010;122(1-2):10-3.
2. Polanczyk GV, Salum GA, Sugaya LS, Caye A, Rohde LA. Annual research review: A meta-analysis of the worldwide prevalence of mental disorders in children and adolescents. J Child Psychol Psychiatry. 2015;56(3):345-65.
3. Steiner M, Dunn E, Born L. Hormones and mood: from menarche to menopause and beyond. J Affect Disord. 2003;74(1):67-83.
4. Richburg AG, Kelly DP, Davis-Kean PE, Richburg A. Depression, anxiety, and pubertal timing: Current research and future directions. University of Michigan Undergraduate Research Journal. 2021;15.
5. Handy AB, Greenfield SF, Yonkers KA, Payne LA. Psychiatric symptoms across the menstrual cycle in adult women: a comprehensive review. Harv Rev Psychiatry. 2022;30(2):100-17.
6. Jang D, Elfenbein HA. Menstrual cycle effects on mental health outcomes: a meta-analysis. Arch Suicide Res. 2019;23(2):312-32.
7. Graber JA, Seeley JR, Brooks-Gunn J, Lewinsohn PM. Is pubertal timing associated with psychopathology in young adulthood? J Am Acad Child Adolesc Psychiatry. 2004;43(6):718-26.
8. Ge X, Natsuaki MN. In search of explanations for early pubertal timing effects on developmental psychopathology. Curr Dir Psychol Sci. 2009;18(6):327-31.

9. Lee Y, Styne D. Influences on the onset and tempo of puberty in human beings and implications for adolescent psychological development. Horm Behav. 2013;64(2):250-61.
10. Pathak PK, Tripathi N, Subramanian SV. Secular trends in menarcheal age in India-evidence from the Indian human development survey. PLoS One. 2014;9(11):e111027.
11. Born L, Shea A, Steiner M. The roots of depression in adolescent girls: is menarche the key? Curr Psychiatry Rep. 2002;4(6):449-60.
12. Stice E, Presnell K, Bearman SK. Relation of early menarche to depression, eating disorders, substance abuse, and comorbid psychopathology among adolescent girls. Dev Psychol. 2001;37(5):608-19.
13. Patton GC, Hibbert ME, Carlin J, Shao Q, Rosier M, Caust J, et al. Menarche and the onset of depression and anxiety in Victoria, Australia. J Epidemiol Community Health. 1996;50(6):661-6.
14. Mendle J, Turkheimer E, Emery RE. Detrimental psychological outcomes associated with early pubertal timing in adolescent girls. Dev Review. 2007;27(2):151-71.
15. Rao U, Chen LA. Characteristics, correlates, and outcomes of childhood and adolescent depressive disorders. Dialogues Clin Neurosci. 2009;11(1):45-62.
16. Hankin BL, Abramson LY. Development of gender differences in depression: An elaborated cognitive vulnerability–transactional stress theory. Psychol Bull. 2001;127(6):773.
17. Nolen-Hoeksema S, Larson J, Grayson C. Explaining the gender difference in depressive symptoms. J Pers Soc Psychol. 1999;77(5):1061.
18. Hayward C, Killen JD, Hammer LD, Litt IF, Wilson DM, Simmonds B, et al. Pubertal stage and panic attack history in sixth-and seventh-grade girls. Am J Psychiatry. 1992;149(9):1239-43.
19. Reardon LE, Leen-Feldner EW, Hayward C. A critical review of the empirical literature on the relation between anxiety and puberty. Clin Psychol Rev. 2009;29(1):1-23.
20. Kim K, Smith PK. Childhood stress, behavioural symptoms and mother–daughter pubertal development. J Adolesc. 1998;21(3):231-40.
21. Klump KL. Puberty as a critical risk period for eating disorders: A review of human and animal studies. Horm Behav. 2013;64(2):399-410.
22. Kaltiala-Heino R, Rimpel M, Rissanen A, Rantanen P. Early puberty and early sexual activity are associated with bulimic-type eating pathology in middle adolescence. J Adolesc Health. 2001;28(4):346-52.
23. Ruuska J, Kaltiala-Heino R, Koivisto AM, Rantanen P. Puberty, sexual development and eating disorders in adolescent outpatients. Eur Child Adolesc Psychiatry. 2003;12(5):214-20.
24. Fairburn CG, Cooper Z, Doll HA, Welch SL. Risk factors for anorexia nervosa: three integrated case-control comparisons. Arch Gen Psychiatry. 1999;56(5):468-76.
25. Graber JA, Brooks-Gunn J, Paikoff RL, Warren MP. Prediction of eating problems: An 8-year study of adolescent girls. Dev Psychol. 1994;30(6):823.
26. Dick DM, Rose RJ, Viken RJ, Kaprio J. Pubertal timing and substance use: associations between and within families across late adolescence. Dev Psychol. 2000;36(2):180.

27. Dick DM, Rose RJ, Pulkkinen L, Kaprio J. Measuring puberty and understanding its impact: A longitudinal study of adolescent twins. J Youth Adolesc. 2001;30(4):385-99.
28. Dimler LM, Natsuaki MN. The effects of pubertal timing on externalizing behaviors in adolescence and early adulthood: A meta-analytic review. J Adolesc. 2015;45:160-70.
29. Kanwar P. Pubertal development and problem behaviours in Indian adolescents. Int J Adolesc Youth. 2020;25(1):753-64.
30. Klopack ET, Simons RL, Simons LG. Puberty and girls' delinquency: a test of competing models explaining the relationship between pubertal development and delinquent behavior. Justice Q. 2020;37(1):25-52.
31. Beattie TS, Prakash R, Mazzuca A, Kelly L, Javalkar P, Raghavendra T, et al. Prevalence and correlates of psychological distress among 13–14 years old adolescent girls in North Karnataka, South India: a cross-sectional study. BMC Public Health. 2019;19(1):1-2.
32. Ibitoye M, Choi C, Tai H, Lee G, Sommer M. Early menarche: A systematic review of its effect on sexual and reproductive health in low-and middle-income countries. PloS One. 2017;12(6):e0178884.
33. Fink G, Sumner BE, Rosie R, Grace O, Quinn JP. Estrogen control of central neurotransmission: effect on mood, mental state, and memory. Cell Molecular Neurobiol. 1996;16(3):325-44.
34. Mahé V, Dumaine A. Oestrogen withdrawal associated psychoses. Acta Psychiatr Scand. 2001;104(5):323-31.
35. Ahokas A, Aito M. Role of estradiol in puerperal psychosis. Psychopharmacology. 1999;147:108-10.
36. Deuchar N, Brockington I. Puerperal and menstrual psychoses: the proposal of a unitary etiological hypothesis. J Psychosom Obstet Gynaecol. 1998;19(2):104-10.
37. Ray R, Paul I. Menstrual psychosis: A not so forgotten reality. Indian J Psychiatry. 2020;62(5):585.
38. Brockington I. Menstrual psychosis. World Psychiatry. 2005;4(1):9-17.
39. Ramachandran VS (Ed). Encyclopedia of human behavior, 2nd edition. US: Academic Press; 2012.
40. Chrisler JC. Teaching taboo topics: Menstruation, menopause, and the psychology of women. Psychol Women Q. 2013;37(1):128-32.
41. Freeman EW. Premenstrual syndrome and premenstrual dysphoric disorder: definitions and diagnosis. Psychoneuroendocrinology. 2003;28:25-37.
42. Baker FC, Lee KA. Menstrual cycle effects on sleep. Sleep Med Clin. 2022;17(2):283-94.
43. Baker FC, Lamarche LJ, Iacovides S, Colrain IM. Sleep and menstrual-related disorders. Sleep Med Clin. 2008;3(1):25-35.
44. Khazaie H, Ghadami MR, Khaledi-Paveh B, Chehri A, Nasouri M. Sleep quality in university students with premenstrual dysphoric disorder. Shanghai Arch Psychiatry. 2016;28(3):131-8.
45. Baker FC, Colrain IM. Daytime sleepiness, psychomotor performance, waking EEG spectra and evoked potentials in women with severe premenstrual syndrome. J Sleep Res. 2010;19(1p2):214-27.
46. Parry BL, Martínez LF, Maurer EL, López AM, Sorenson D, Meliska CJ. Sleep, rhythms and women's mood. Part I. Menstrual cycle, pregnancy and postpartum. Sleep Med Rev. 2006;10(2):129-44.

47. Parry BL, Meliska CJ, Sorenson DL, Martínez LF, López AM, Elliott JA, et al. Reduced phase-advance of plasma melatonin after bright morning light in the luteal, but not follicular, menstrual cycle phase in premenstrual dysphoric disorder: an extended study. Chronobiology international. 2011;28(5):415-24.
48. Baker FC, Driver HS, Rogers GG, Paiker J, Mitchell D. High nocturnal body temperatures and disturbed sleep in women with primary dysmenorrhea. Am J Physiol. 1999;277(6):E1013-21.
49. Bromberger JT, Schott LL, Kravitz HM, Sowers M, Avis NE, Gold EB, et al. Longitudinal change in reproductive hormones and depressive symptoms across the menopausal transition: results from the Study of Women's Health Across the Nation (SWAN). Arch Gen Psychiatry. 2010;67(6):598-607.
50. Bromberger JT, Matthews KA, Schott LL, Brockwell S, Avis NE, Kravitz HM, et al. Depressive symptoms during the menopausal transition: the Study of Women's Health Across the Nation (SWAN). J Affect Disord. 2007;103(1-3):267-72.
51. Salari N, Hasheminezhad R, Hosseinian-Far A, Rasoulpoor S, Assefi M, Nankali S, et al. Global prevalence of sleep disorders during menopause: a meta-analysis. Sleep and Breath. 2023:1-5.
52. Azizi M, Fooladi E, Abdollahi F, Elyasi F. Biopsychosocial risk factors of depression in the menopausal transition: a narrative review. Iran J Psychiatry Behav Sci. 2018;12(4):e12928.
53. Georgakis MK, Thomopoulos TP, Diamantaras AA, Kalogirou EI, Skalkidou A, Daskalopoulou SS, et al. Association of age at menopause and duration of reproductive period with depression after menopause: a systematic review and meta-analysis. JAMA Psychiatry. 2016;73(2):139-49.
54. Friedman SH, Prakash C, Moller-Olsen C. Psychiatric considerations in menopause. Curr Psychiatr. 2018;17(10):11-6.
55. Murray G. Adjunctive psychosocial interventions for bipolar disorder: Some psychotherapeutic context for the Canadian Network for Mood and Anxiety Treatments (CANMAT) & International Society for Bipolar Disorders (ISBD) guidelines. Bipolar Disord. 2018;20(5):494-5.
56. Marsh WK, Ketter TA, Crawford SL, Johnson JV, Kroll-Desrosiers AR, Rothschild AJ. Progression of female reproductive stages associated with bipolar illness exacerbation. Bipolar Disord. 2012;14(5):515-26.
57. Hu LY, Shen CC, Hung JH, Chen PM, Wen CH, Chiang YY, et al. Risk of psychiatric disorders following symptomatic menopausal transition: a nationwide population-based retrospective cohort study. Medicine. 2016;95(6):e2800.
58. Musial N, Ali Z, Grbevski J, Veerakumar A, Sharma P. Perimenopause and first-onset mood disorders: A closer look. Focus. 2021;19(3):330-7.
59. Sommer IE, Brand BA, Gangadin S, Tanskanen A, Tiihonen J, Taipale H. Women with schizophrenia-spectrum disorders after menopause: a vulnerable group for relapse. Schizophr Bull. 2023;49(1):136-43.
60. González-Rodríguez A, Guàrdia A, Monreal JA. Peri-and post-menopausal women with schizophrenia and related disorders are a population with specific needs: a narrative review of current theories. J Pers Med. 2021;11(9):849.
61. Brzezinski A, Brzezinski-Sinai NA, Seeman MV. Treating schizophrenia during menopause. Menopause. 2017;24(5):582-8.

62. Kumar V, Singh V, Kumar A. Mental health issues in menopause. Indian J Clin Psychiatry. 2023;3(1):18-26.
63. Jagtap BL, Prasad BS, Chaudhury S. Psychiatric morbidity in perimenopausal women. Ind Psychiatry J. 2016;25(1):86-92.
64. Yadav V, Jain A, Dabar D, Goel AD, Sood A, Joshi A, et al. A meta-analysis on the prevalence of depression in perimenopausal and postmenopausal women in India. Asian J Psychiatr. 2021;57:102581.
65. Khatak S, Gupta M, Grover S, Aggarwal N. Depression among peri- and post-menopausal women during COVID-19 pandemic in Chandigarh, North India: A Study from Community. J Midlife Health. 2022;13(3):233-40.
66. Madaan S, Acharya N, Jaiswal A, Dewani D, Kotdawala K. Anxiety and depression in post-menopausal women: A short review. Ann Geriatr Educ Med Sci. 2021;8(2):38-41.

SECTION 3

Gender-based Violence and Vulnerable Groups

- **Intimate Partner Violence: Impact on Mental Health and Evidence-based Interventions**
  Madhuri H Nanjundaswamy, Rini Joseph
- **Rights of Women with Mental Illness**
  Shivanee Kumari, Sai Chaitanya Reddy B, Suresh Bada Math
- **Mental Health Issues among Women in Sexual Minority Groups**
  Debadutta Mohapatra, Aruna Yadiyal, Amrit Pattojoshi
- **Sexual Violence: Mental Health Consequences and Interventions**
  Arunashree B, Abhilasha Das, Veena A Satyanarayana

CHAPTER 14

Intimate Partner Violence: Impact on Mental Health and Evidence-based Interventions

Madhuri H Nanjundaswamy, Rini Joseph

ABSTRACT

Intimate partner violence (IPV) is a global problem with severe implications for women's mental health. It includes physical, sexual, emotional, coercive control, and economic abuse, affecting women from diverse backgrounds. The relationship between IPV and mental health is bidirectional. Exposure to IPV increases the risk of mental health problems, such as depression, anxiety, posttraumatic stress disorder (PTSD), substance abuse, and suicidal thoughts. Concurrently, individuals with preexisting mental health issues are more vulnerable to experiencing IPV.

Perinatal IPV poses a particular risk, leading to mental health issues and adverse obstetric outcomes. Children exposed to IPV, especially during pregnancy, face a higher risk of developing mental health issues.

Evidence-based interventions, including the LIVES (Listen, Inquire, Validate, Enhance safety, and support) approach and cognitive behavioral therapy (CBT), are effective in addressing the mental health consequences of IPV. Screening for IPV during perinatal care is crucial for early detection and referral to mental health treatment. Addressing the mental health impact of IPV is critical to supporting women's well-being. Introducing a trauma- and violence-informed, equity-oriented approach to interventions addressing IPV at all stages of prevention signifies a significant transformation in IPV research, practice, and policy.

Keywords: Mental health, trauma, intimate partner violence, trauma-informed care, counselling, women's mental health, domestic abuse

INTRODUCTION

Violence against women is a widespread global problem with severe implications for human rights and public health.[1] Worldwide, almost one-third (30%) of all women who have been in a relationship have experienced physical and/or sexual violence by their intimate partner.[2] The profound and detrimental impact of abuse on women hinders their capacity for happiness and productivity, encompassing various forms such as physical, sexual, emotional, and economic violence across diverse backgrounds and cultures.[3] In the last few years, the relationship between intimate partner violence (IPV) and mental health problems has become more apparent, and there is now much more recognition of the link. Mental health problems are more commonly observed than physical health problems. Experiencing more than one form of IPV can increase the severity of outcomes.[4] The link between IPV and mental health is complex. Being exposed to IPV, whether in childhood or adulthood, increases the likelihood of developing a range of mental health problems, including thoughts of suicide and suicide attempts. Additionally, individuals with preexisting mental health issues are more vulnerable to experiencing IPV. This relationship is bidirectional, meaning that IPV can serve as both a predictor of future mental health problems and a potential consequence of preexisting mental health challenges.[5-7]

Mental health issues are associated with various types of IPV and can have significant implications for the mental well-being of those who face violence, especially women.[8,9] IPV carries a multitude of mental health consequences for women. These consequences include depression, anxiety, posttraumatic stress disorder (PTSD), substance abuse, personality disorders, eating disorders, psychosis, and suicidal thoughts.[5,10] Even cyber victimization is known to impact mental health.[11]

Women are indeed more likely to experience IPV than men, and research has consistently shown that a larger proportion of women experience mental health problems related to IPV. However, it is important to emphasize that anyone, regardless of gender, can experience IPV, and the impact is not limited to one gender.[12,13] Recognizing the distinct trauma of IPV survivors is essential for tailoring effective therapeutic interventions. The COVID-19 pandemic worsened violence against women, causing a notable surge in cases, including severe outcomes such as homicides and suicides in some instances.

Types of IPV include the following:
- *Physical violence:* Pushing, slapping, hitting, kicking, and beating.
- *Sexual violence:* Forced sexual intercourse and other forms of sexual coercion, sexual assault, and harassment.
- *Emotional (psychological) violence:* Insults, belittling (putting down), constant humiliation, intimidation (e.g, destroying things), threats of harm, threats to take away children, and excessive jealousy.
- *Controlling behaviors:* Including isolating a person from family and friends; monitoring their movements; and restricting access to financial resources, employment, education or medical care.
- *Financial (economic) violence:* Limiting access to money, excessive control in spending, and financial dependence.

MENTAL HEALTH IMPACT OF INTIMATE PARTNER VIOLENCE

Experiencing IPV can result in profound psychological challenges. They may grapple with diminished self-esteem, guilt, and shame, internalizing their abusers' criticisms and feeling unworthy of love and respect. Some employ emotional numbness and detachment as coping mechanisms. Ongoing fear of abuse can lead to anxiety and hyper-vigilance. Severe or prolonged IPV can trigger depression and PTSD, with symptoms such as flashbacks and nightmares. These psychological effects can have a lasting impact, hindering their ability to form new relationships and trust others.

COMMON MENTAL HEALTH DISORDERS

Depression, anxiety, PTSD, and substance misuse have been the most assessed mental health outcomes in both observational and interventional studies, often relying on self-reported measures.

A comprehensive review and meta-analysis revealed significant associations between domestic violence and mental health disorders among women. The findings indicated a threefold rise in the probability of experiencing depressive disorders, a fourfold increase in the likelihood of anxiety disorders, and a staggering sevenfold increase in the possibility of PTSD among women who have experienced domestic violence and abuse.[5,6]

Depression

Depression exhibits a strong correlation with IPV, with the intensity and persistence of the violence closely tied to the severity of depressive symptoms.[12] In a US-based prospective study on women with a history of IPV, it was revealed that, even after 5 years, they had significantly higher levels of depressive symptoms, functional impairment, lower self-esteem, and reduced life satisfaction, highlighting the enduring mental health risks faced by women who have experienced IPV.[14] The disease burden with mental health disorders and IPV is very high.[15] Various types of violence, including controlling behavior, have demonstrated a causal relationship with symptoms of depression.[16]

Anxiety

There is a significant association between a positive history of IPV and elevated anxiety levels in women, with an adjusted incidence rate ratio of 1.99. This association remained even after controlling for variables such as income, education, age, comorbidity of depression, and the severity of anxiety symptoms. Furthermore, it was noted that the severity of state anxiety was notably higher in women who exhibited more severe depressive symptoms. The findings imply that the presence of anxiety symptoms in abused women is closely linked to the severity and frequency of the abuse they have endured.[12,17]

Posttraumatic Stress Disorder

Several studies related to PTSD in women who have experienced IPV unanimously indicated a positive association between a history of IPV and an increased incidence of PTSD symptoms. A study estimated that women with a history of IPV were 2.3 times more likely to develop PTSD compared to women who had never been abused.[18] The prevalence rates of PTSD varied widely across studies but consistently indicated a higher risk among women with a history of IPV. The severity and sustained experience of abuse were found to be linked to higher levels of PTSD symptoms, with women who had experienced multiple forms of abuse showing more significant symptomatology.[19] The presence of depression and the type of abuse experienced were also associated with the risk of developing PTSD.[12] A study revealed a high prevalence of complex posttraumatic stress disorder (CPTSD) among women who had a history of IPV. Fear of the perpetrator, low resilience, and emotional suppression were found to increase the risk of CPTSD.[20]

Substance Use

Studies report high prevalence rates of substance use coexisting with IPV. For many who have experienced IPV, substance use acts to cope with the physical and emotional pain due to IPV, while others may be coerced into using substances by their abusive partner. When compared to the general population, people who experience IPV are almost twice as likely to use alcohol. The relationship between IPV and substance use is bidirectional, as shown in **Figure 1**.

There exists a potentially cyclical relationship between exposure to IPV, substance misuse, and mental health issues, increasing the vulnerability to revictimization.[21]

Women facing IPV who also struggle with substance use encounter significant obstacles in seeking help and support. Some of these barriers include stigma, the risk of their testimony being dismissed, and legal

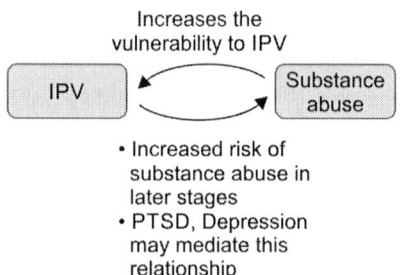

Fig. 1: Bidirectional relationship between IPV and substance use. (IPV: intimate partner violence; PTSD: posttraumatic stress disorder)

complexities like the potential loss of child custody. Moreover, abusive partners may intensify these challenges by isolating those who face IPV, pressuring them to continue substance use, exploiting societal stigma to discredit them, falsely accusing them, or manipulating their dependency to exert control.[22]

Suicidal Thoughts and Self-Harm

Individuals in abusive relationships may contemplate suicide as a way out. Even after a suicide attempt, discussing violence is often challenging for those who face violence due to shame or lack of awareness about the connection. It is crucial to approach them empathetically, understanding the complexity of their situations and offering support. In a comprehensive World Health Organization (WHO) multicountry study on women's health and domestic violence,[23] pooled data from 15 sites across 10 countries revealed alarming statistics. Women who had encountered physical or sexual violence, or both, were three times more prone to suicidal ideation and nearly four times more likely to have attempted suicide compared to women who had never experienced partner violence. People facing violence frequently turn to substance abuse, and drug overdoses can contribute to an elevated risk of self-harm and suicide.

After controlling for likely common mental health disorders, the most consistent risk factors for suicide attempts were childhood sexual abuse, having a mother who had experienced IPV, nonpartner physical violence, and having ever been divorced, separated, or widowed.[10] Inquiring about IPV is essential when someone seeks help for suicidal despair or after self-harm. Individuals who are at risk of self-harm and suicide may benefit from interventions aimed at lowering the frequency and duration of IPV.[24]

Personality Disorders

Specific aspects related to anger and impulsivity in borderline personality disorder (BPD) were independently linked to various violent outcomes, including severity, repetition, and injury.[25] However, it is essential to emphasize that those who face domestic violence are never at fault, and full accountability for these actions rests with the perpetrators. Environmental factors contributing to early BPD include familial maltreatment, such as abuse and neglect and conflicted parent-child relationships. Early trauma is believed to disrupt the development of cognition, affectivity, and emotional awareness, leading to posttraumatic reactions, dissociation, and alexithymia. Maltreated children may internalize negative perceptions of themselves, others, and relationships, fostering BPD through insecure attachment. Recurring trauma from caregivers or partners heightens psychiatric risks. CPTSD, akin to BPD, emerges from prolonged early traumas, influencing relationships and self-harming behaviors.[26] Individuals diagnosed with BPD are more likely to report experiences of childhood adversity compared to those with different clinical diagnoses.[27]

Sexual violence can lead to adverse consequences for women, including sexually transmitted infections and a heightened risk of human immunodeficiency virus (HIV). These experiences may result in sexual dysfunction, characterized by decreased interest, arousal difficulties, and painful intercourse. The presence of such dysfunction can further escalate violence when a woman resists sexual intimacy.

Severe Mental Disorders

Individuals diagnosed with severe mental health issues face significantly high rates of IPV in the preceding 1-3 years, with women reporting approximately double the rates compared to men. About 60% of women with severe mental illness (SMI) were likely to be exposed to IPV.[6,7] This elevated risk might stem from abusive partners exploiting moments when individuals with mental health problems, such as during certain states of psychosis involving disinhibition or preoccupation with one's thoughts, make them less capable of protecting themselves.

The most frequently reported forms of violence were emotional and controlling behaviors, followed by physical violence, with sexual violence being the least commonly reported.[28] Patients with SMI face a significantly higher risk of domestic and sexual violence compared to the general population, particularly with a greater prevalence of family violence.[29] Even men with severe mental illness had an increased risk of IPV. Alternatively, prolonged exposure to IPV is associated with severe mental health issues.[12]

MENTAL HEALTH PROBLEMS AS A RISK FACTOR FOR PERPETRATING INTIMATE PARTNER VIOLENCE

Individuals with mental health problems, such as depression and anxiety, have a higher risk of perpetrating IPV. Alcohol and drug use problems are strong risk factors for IPV perpetration.

While most individuals with mental health problems are not violent, some may be at an increased risk of committing IPV, possibly due to psychological traits and substance misuse. Further research is needed to understand the mechanisms behind this increased risk, including the role of familial factors and detection rates. Individuals who both experience and commit violence are at the greatest risk of developing mental health disorders.[7] When Ross and Babcock (2009) examined the male perpetrators for their patterns of violence and its relationship to personality, they found that proactive violence was associated with antisocial personality disorder, whereas reactive violence was associated with borderline personality disorder.[30]

Mental Health Impact of Perinatal Intimate Partner Violence

Exposure to IPV over a lifetime, as well as experiencing IPV during pregnancy and the postpartum period, significantly increases the risk for women to develop PTSD, depression, contemplate suicide, and engage in substance abuse during the perinatal periods.[31-34] The impact on the fetus can be a miscarriage, stillbirth, or low birth weight. The impact on mothers' obstetric health—high blood pressure, vaginal bleeding, urinary tract infection, placental abruption, and premature rupture of membranes. In a study done among 462 women in South India, domestic violence predicted suicidal ideation in the current pregnancy.[35] Perinatal IPV may have long-term consequences on the child, such as executive and cognitive functioning difficulties, insecure and disorganized attachment, and exposure to additional traumatic events.[36]

In a systematic review, the prevalence of antenatal and postnatal depression showed wide variation, ranging from 15 to 65% during the antenatal period and 5 to 35% postnatally. Suicidal thoughts were reported by 5-11% during pregnancy and 2-22% postpartum. Notably, individuals facing IPV during pregnancy had a significantly increased risk of antenatal and postnatal depression, influenced by factors such as the study's location and the nature and severity of the violence. In all cases, those experiencing IPV had a substantially higher risk of perinatal depression compared to those who did not.[37]

It is crucial to look for IPV during perinatal healthcare visits to identify women who may be vulnerable to adverse obstetric health outcomes. This process helps in several key ways: early detection, risk assessment, safety planning, and referral to mental health treatment.[36]

Impact of Intimate Partner Violence on Children

Individuals who have face violence were more likely to have experienced childhood abuse or witnessed IPV during their childhood, in contrast to who have not faced violence.[4]

Children born to mothers who faced IPV during pregnancy face a higher risk of anxiety, depression, attention-deficit hyperactivity disorder (ADHD), and conduct disorder compared to those born to mothers who did not experience IPV during pregnancy. A meta-analysis exploring the long-term consequences of children's exposure to IPV unveiled a prospective connection between such exposure and various adjustment difficulties, encompassing externalizing, internalizing, and overall adjustment issues. Interestingly, this association appeared to intensify over time.[38]

Perpetrators of Intimate Partner Violence

Intimate partner violence perpetrators may have experienced childhood violence, societal influences, anger and control issues, personality disorders, substance or mental health problems, or cognitive impairments contributing to their behavior. These factors do not excuse their actions but emphasize the importance of interventions addressing root causes to ensure safety for both perpetrators and those who experience violence. Efforts to reduce IPV should focus on addressing the abusive behaviors of perpetrators. Mental healthcare providers need support in identifying and responding to IPV perpetration. Inquiries about IPV should be persistent, as perpetrators often deny or minimize their actions. Disclosure acknowledgment and conveying that abusive behavior is unacceptable should be part of the response. Providers should work with perpetrators, emphasize possible change, and use motivational interviewing techniques. Clinical responses should target modifiable risk factors in perpetrators with mental health issues without excusing violent behavior. This may involve therapies, antipsychotic medication, and interventions for substance or alcohol misuse.[7]

Intimate Partner Violence in Women in the LGBTQIA+ Group

The prevalence of IPV in lesbian, gay, and bisexual (LGB) couples is reportedly higher than that in heterosexual couples, with lesbian women facing a particularly elevated risk and more complex outcomes. Conventional IPV services encounter challenges in addressing the unique aspects of LGB relationships, necessitating adapted assessments. Healthcare providers play a crucial role and must recognize, empathize, ensure safety, and aid survivors in distancing from difficult situations. Standard screening methods may fall short in effectively addressing LGB cases, requiring a nuanced approach that involves openly inquiring about sexual orientation using inclusive language to avoid perpetuating homophobic attitudes.

Accurate assessment serves an educational purpose, shedding light on the often-invisible nature of LGB IPV. Public and specialized education is recommended to mitigate incidence rates and fortify support systems, encouraging early help-seeking. Essential measures include specific training for LGB IPV assessment, education on homophobia, and the development of tailored response protocols for law enforcement.[39,40]

Barriers to Help-seeking and Help Provision

Service users, especially women seeking help in mental health settings, face several barriers to disclosing domestic violence to professionals. These obstacles include fears of negative consequences such as involving child protection services, doubts about being believed, concerns that disclosure could trigger more abuse, the hidden nature of the violence, re-victimization of the actions of the abuser, and feelings of shame.

Moreover, women fear not being taken seriously when sharing their abuse experiences, as they anticipate mental health professionals concentrating solely on their symptoms. The stigma attached to mental illness further hinders their willingness to disclose. Additionally, a lack of privacy is a substantial obstacle when discussing abuse in the presence of their abusive partners, increasing the risk of further harm.

Mental health professionals sometimes refrain from discussing IPV due to several barriers. These obstacles include personal discomfort, therapeutic nihilism, concerns about causing retraumatization, and time limitations. Residents, in particular, encounter difficulties in addressing IPV, driven by inadequate knowledge, unease, safety concerns, and worries about legal matters. Notably, the study found that around 71% of the residents highlighted the absence of formal training as a significant hindrance to effectively addressing IPV-related issues.[41,42]

TRAINING MENTAL HEALTH PROFESSIONALS IN ADDRESSING THE MENTAL HEALTH IMPACT OF INTIMATE PARTNER VIOLENCE

The WHO recommends training programs addressing IPV for healthcare staff to improve their attitudes, incorporate safety planning, enhance communication skills, and provide guidance on referring those who experience violence to specialized community resources. Additionally, there is a crucial requirement for culturally sensitive IPV resource materials tailored for healthcare professionals to address IPV within clinical settings effectively. This approach ensures that healthcare providers are well-equipped to support and respond to IPV cases in a culturally sensitive and effective manner.

Feminist Principles Regarding Intimate Partner Violence

Feminist intervention principles include the following:
- *Critical awareness:* Acknowledging that a woman's difficulties arise within a sociopolitical framework influenced by patriarchy and gender inequality, feminist analysis underscores how conventional gender norms and prevailing ideals of masculinity, termed "hegemonic masculinities", play a role in shaping gender hierarchies. These norms prescribe certain characteristics such as dominance, aggression, emotional restraint, and success as the ideal for men. Societal approval of these norms can perpetuate gender disparities by prioritizing and legitimizing the authority and advantages of specific men while marginalizing those who deviate from these expectations. Ultimately, these norms are closely

tied to endorsing the use of violence by men against women.[43] In this context, men are predominantly viewed as the primary perpetrators, while women are primarily cast as victims.[44] Women's experiences of violence can be different based on things such as their race, social class, and sexual orientation. These factors all intersect and affect how women may experience and deal with violence in their lives, known as the intersectionality principle.

- *Advocacy for social change:* There is a need to challenge traditional gender roles and societal expectations that fuel unequal power dynamics and educate about the importance of seeking consent. Feminists advocate for legal and policy reforms by improving access to resources and strengthening consequences for perpetrators. Community engagement and activism are prioritized to cultivate a culture that rejects violence, encourages healthy relationships, and supports survivors within a broader social context.[45]

It is important to avoid simple either/or ideas when we aim to render socially just treatments. Understanding the history of violence and cultural influences on a specific couple is crucial. The treatment should recognize and adapt to changing power dynamics, and it should always maintain a stance against oppression and emphasize that nonviolence is central to treatment.[46]

- *Egalitarian counseling relationship:* Building a counseling dynamic founded on authenticity, mutual respect, and equality is vital.
- *Strength-based approach:* Reframing trauma symptoms as survival strategies and coping mechanisms, avoiding victim-blaming. This aligns with the principles of trauma-informed care.

INTIMATE PARTNER VIOLENCE AND MENTAL HEALTH IN THE INDIAN CONTEXT

Research in the Indian context reveals an alarming correlation between spousal violence and poor mental health in women, highlighting the impact on depression, suicidal tendencies, and other disorders. In this chapter, we tend to highlight few studies from the Indian context. A study exploring the contributing factors to IPV highlights poverty, low education, alcohol use, and childhood exposure to violence. Social support emerges as a protective factor, emphasizing the enduring impact of childhood experiences on mental health.[47,48] In Delhi, a study found that around 25.3% of women experienced poor mental health and suicidal thoughts compared to those who had not faced violence.[49,50] Women subjected to IPV exhibited elevated PTSD and depression scores, with a positive correlation between the severity of violence and sexual coercion with PTSD.[51] A study (n = 100) from a tertiary care psychiatric hospital revealed a majority of the women were facing moderate IPV, contributing to mental illness post-marriage and childhood exposure and alcohol use heightened IPV.[52]

A study delved into the prevalence of IPV and its associated factors among 100 women with severe mental illness in a psychiatric hospital. The results disclosed that 22% of the participants had encountered IPV, and this was connected to detrimental consequences such as suicidal behavior, depression, compromised physical health, and somatic symptoms.[28] A cross-sectional study in pregnant women from South India reported DV predicted suicidality in current pregnancy.[35] Additionally, a survey from Mumbai studied that economic abuse independently correlated with increased risks of moderate-severe depression, anxiety, and suicidal ideation.[53] A very high prevalence of violence (32.5%, n = 412) was noted during the pandemic.[54]

ETHICAL ISSUES IN PROVIDING CARE

In addressing IPV, it is vital to uphold principles of confidentiality to protect women's privacy, prioritize women's safety, respect their autonomy in decision-making, and work to minimize the risk of further violence. Providing awareness of their rights and available resources, acting in their best interest (beneficence), and seeking justice to hold perpetrators accountable and address systemic issues are integral to a compassionate and comprehensive approach to supporting those who face IPV while working to prevent future violence.

ASSESSMENT OF INTIMATE PARTNER VIOLENCE

In a recent survey conducted among psychiatry residents in India, both the spontaneous disclosure of IPV and routine clinical assessment of IPV among women seeking mental health services were found to be low. Residents cited challenges such as lack of knowledge, comfort, safety concerns, and medicolegal issues. Nearly 71% of the residents lack formal training, and current IPV training in clinical rotations varies, depending on individual consultants' emphasis on gender issues rather than a standardized curriculum.[41]

While there is insufficient evidence to justify universal screening for IPV, considering the high prevalence in mental health settings (30%), case finding and a trauma-informed model of care for all is essential.[55,56]

The process of case finding for IPV involves being vigilant for signs and symptoms of various mental health disorders. This also includes inquiring about past or ongoing IPV and recognizing potential barriers to disclosure, such as fear, shame, or economic dependence. Cultural competence is essential, and a female interviewer may sometimes be needed to facilitate disclosure without increasing the patient's risk.[56] Engaging the woman in the assessment process can have a therapeutic effect.

When dealing with someone who has experienced IPV, as a care provider, the following should be kept in mind:
- Recognize connections of symptoms with trauma
- Pay attention to safety concerns
- Use context, clinical judgment, and training rather than relying on tools alone
- Create a private, secure, and supportive environment
- Clarify confidentiality boundaries and ensure privacy when discussing IPV
- Do not use family members as translators
- Know local legislation and services
- Refer appropriately to other services
- Document carefully
- Consider other comorbidities
- Recognize difficulties with trust
- Do not push her to leave
- Couple therapy is not safe in severe abuse
- Pay attention to countertransference

Whenever IPV is disclosed, remember to use the following communication skills and be mindful of what NOT to do:
- Validation ("Anyone in your situation would have felt the same way")
- Affirmation ("Violence is unacceptable—you deserve to feel safe at home.")
- Support ("There are things we can discuss that can help.")
- Ask about safety and plan as needed!
- No critical remarks ("Why don't you just leave?")
- Respect the individual's concerns and decisions

Signs of possible IPV are as follows:
- Unexplained injuries (or unlikely explanations)
- Unexplained fear (especially of partner)
- Social withdrawal from friends or family
- Restricted access to family finances
- Sudden absences or changes in plans.

Some examples of questions that can be asked during routine clinical interviews are given in the **Box 1**.

When providing first-line support to a woman who has been subjected to violence, the following needs require attention:
- Immediate emotional/psychological health needs
- Immediate physical health needs
- Ongoing safety needs
- Ongoing support and mental health needs

Let us discuss each of these components in detail.

> **BOX 1:** Some disclosure questions.
> - "It's important for me to understand my patient's safety in close relationships."
> - "Sometimes partners or ex-partners use physical force-Is this happening to you?"
> - "Have you felt humiliated or emotionally harmed by your partner or ex-partner?"
> - "Do you feel safe in your current or previous relationships?"
> - "Have you ever been physically threatened or harmed by your partner or ex-partner?"
> - "Have you ever been forced to have any kind of sexual activity by your partner or ex-partner?"
> - "Do you feel your partner over-controls you in your relationships with family, friends or in financial matters?"

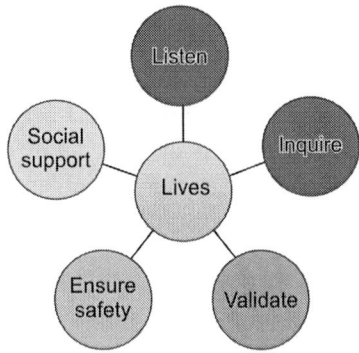

Fig. 2: WHO LIVES (Listen, Inquire, Validate, Enhance safety, and Support) model.

Immediate Psychological Management

Supportive psychological first aid should be given using the WHO LIVES model **(Fig. 2)**. LIVES is an acronym that stands for:

- *Listen* to their concerns in an empathic and non-judgmental manner
- *Inquire* about their needs and concerns (emotional, physical, social, and practical)
- *Validate* their emotions and show you believe and understand them. Reassure the woman that her reaction is understandable. Reassure this is a safe, confidential environment.
- *Enhance* safety by initiating discussion on how to protect against further harm. Ask if it is safe to return home today and assist with referrals to appropriate services locally.
- *Support* by connecting them to medicolegal services and social support.

Do a current mental status examination to assess mood and cognition. Demonstrate stress reduction exercises (breathing, muscle relaxation) to them and encourage them to practice with you.

Use grounding techniques if needed and focus on the present. These include simple strategies to detach from severe emotional pain (flashbacks and anxiety). It aims to create a safe place to regain control over overwhelming

> **BOX 2:** Grounding technique.
> - Touch the chair you are in and describe it
> - Make them repeat a safe statement "I am safe here"
> - Think about a soothing scene
> - Tap feet on the floor
> - Ask them to "name five things you can see, four things you can hear, three things you can touch, two things you can smell, and 1 thing you can taste

emotions or "numbing". Distract the person by focusing on the external world rather than inward. **Box 2** provides statements that can be used in this technique.

If psychological supports do not work, short-term benzodiazepines can be used for severe anxiety. There is no evidence for the use of propranolol, escitalopram, temazepam, or gabapentin to prevent PTSD. Interventions depend on the patient, the severity and frequency of abuse, relationship dynamics, readiness for change, resilience, and culture.

Educate them on the effects of trauma, such as anxiety, hyperarousal, irritability, sleep disturbances, and re-experiencing trauma.

Ongoing Support and Mental Health Needs

An IPV assessment should encompass aspects such as the nature of the violence, its duration, frequency, and severity, and protective and risk factors. This comprehensive approach empowers women by presenting various options for them to consider and plan their next steps.

Schedule a follow-up visit for further assessments and management.

Immediate Physical Health Needs

Treat the physical injuries. Do a pregnancy test and provide emergency contraception measures if required. Assess and treat (including prophylaxis) for sexually transmitted infections (STIs), including HIV. Refer for a forensic examination/specimen collection. Document all injuries and management carefully.

Ongoing Safety Needs

Refer the person experiencing IPV to social and legal services. Inform them that perpetrators are often more violent during times of separation, increasing their risk for harm, including severe and life-threatening injury.

It is vital to make an emergency safety plan as described follows:
- *If staying at home:*
    - *Identify support:* Identify people and places for help (police, places of worship, hospital, school, friends, and neighbors). Inform neighbors to contact the police if they hear signs of violence.

> **BOX 3:** Emergency kit for exit plan.
> - Identification documents like Adhaar, ration card, passport
> - Keys for house/car
> - Bank book, cheque book, ATM card, money
> - Important documents of yourself and children: Birth Certificates, Driver's license, children's school, and vaccination records
> - A set of clothes

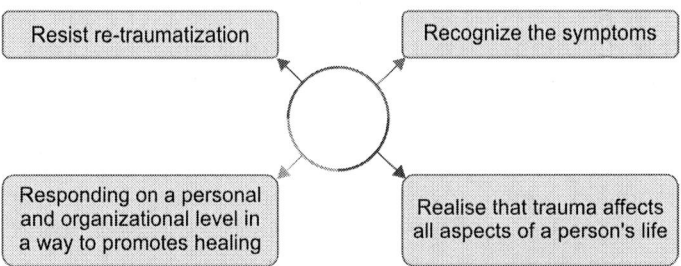

Fig. 3: Trauma-informed model of care framework (4 R's).

- *Assess children's safety:* Teach them emergency contacts, memorize phone numbers, and make them aware of safety measures. Teach children what to do, that is, contact the number of family members. Make them remember important telephone numbers.
- *Emergency numbers on the phone:* Program your phone with essential numbers (police, neighbors, family, and friends).
- *If you plan to leave home:*
  - Emergency kit **(Box 3)**.
  - *Practice safe exit:* Plan safe escape routes, including stairs, elevators, doors, and fire escapes.
  - *Safe destinations:* List safe places to go (Shelter homes, family or friends willing to help during periods of crisis).

TRAUMA-INFORMED MODEL OF CARE (FIG. 3)

Trauma-informed model of care (TIC) is a holistic approach aimed at evaluating the effects of trauma on those who experience violence, taking steps to address trauma, and empowering them to experience a sense of security and recovery. The service providers must consider the patient's present and past condition to provide care with a healing touch.

Key principles include safety, trustworthiness, transparency, peer support, collaboration, mutuality, empowerment, voice, choice, cultural, historical, and gender issues.[57]

Trauma-informed care shifts the focus from "What's wrong with you?" to "What happened to you?" This approach helps to alleviate the isolation, shame, and self-blame of the woman.

EVIDENCE-BASED INTERVENTIONS

Numerous psychological and pharmacological treatments have substantial supporting evidence of at least moderate strength of efficacy, including exposure therapy, cognitive processing therapy (CPT), cognitive therapy (CT), mixed therapies involving cognitive behavioral therapy (CBT), eye movement desensitization and reprocessing (EMDR), narrative exposure therapy, fluoxetine, paroxetine, sertraline, topiramate, and venlafaxine.[58]

Cognitive Behavioral Therapy-Informed Interventions

Randomized control studies have applied CBT principles to those who have experienced domestic violence, leading to significant reductions in depressive and PTSD symptoms.[59] CPT has proven effective, helping them recognize and challenge cognitive distortions related to their traumatic experiences and reducing PTSD, anxiety, and depression symptoms. It involves psychoeducation about PTSD, assisting individuals to understand their condition and its impact, and equips them with the tools to confront and reframe these negative thought patterns.[60-62] The Psychological Advocacy Towards Healing (PATH) intervention, consisting of eight one-hour sessions, is a CBT-informed psychological intervention delivered by specialist psychological advocates. It demonstrated clinically significant improvements in mental health outcomes compared to standard advocacy care.[63] In a review encompassing 70 studies with 4,761 participants, individual trauma-focused cognitive behavioral therapy (TFCBT) and EMDR were found to be more effective than waitlist or usual care in reducing the severity of PTSD symptoms.[64]

Mind-body Interventions

Mind-body interventions recognize the connection between the mind and body. In one randomized controlled trial (RCT) by Franzblau et al. in 2008, a yogic breathing intervention was found to significantly reduce depressive symptoms in 40 women who had experienced violence.[65] Two RCTs adapted mindfulness-based stress reduction (MBSR) programs for women with interpersonal violence experiences, addressing their specific needs.[66,67] Another RCT focused on counseling, dietary habits, exercise, and stress management to reduce stress, depression, and anxiety, improving the quality of life for women with a history of IPV.[68]

Group Interventions

Group psychotherapy can be a valuable therapeutic approach for certain participants, particularly when it comes to addressing symptoms related to dissociation and self-esteem.[69]

Other Interventions

Two studies, "iSAFE"[70] and "I-DECIDE"[71], explored the effectiveness of online safety decision aids in enhancing the mental health of women experiencing IPV over a year. These interventions involved online decision aids assessing relationship priorities and generating tailored action plans to address IPV-related circumstances.

Advocacy-based Interventions

These interventions had a dual focus—enhancing outcomes for those facing violence by addressing violence factors and improving clinicians' preparedness to address domestic violence. Training clinicians in domestic violence and connecting those who face violence with advocacy services can improve responses to psychiatric services.[72] It mainly includes facilitation for shelters, emergency housing, ongoing support, and legal and financial services.

> **KEY POINTS**
> - IPV is a pervasive global issue, affecting women from diverse backgrounds. It encompasses various forms of abuse, and its consequences extend beyond physical harm to profound mental health implications.
> - The link between IPV and mental health is complex and bidirectional. Those who experience violence are at an increased risk of developing mental health problems, while individuals with preexisting mental health issues are more vulnerable to experiencing IPV.
> - IPV during pregnancy and the postpartum period significantly increases the risk of mental health issues in women, with potential consequences for both mothers and their children.
> - It is important for the service providers to identify violence and use LIVES approach by the WHO as a first-line response.
> - Various evidence-based interventions, including trauma-focused CBT, EMDR, mind-body approaches, and group therapy, have been developed to address the mental health consequences of IPV.
> - For women facing violence, a trauma-informed care offers the opportunity to engage more fully in their health care, develop a trusting relationship with their provider, and improve long-term health outcomes.
> - Addressing the mental health impact of IPV is essential for the overall well-being of women.

■ REFERENCES

1. Garcia-Moreno C, Jansen HAFM, Ellsberg M, Heise L, Watts CH; WHO Multi-country Study on Women's Health and Domestic Violence against Women Study Team. Prevalence of intimate partner violence: findings from the WHO multi-country study on women's health and domestic violence. Lancet Lond Engl. 2006;368(9543):1260-9.

2. World Health Organization. (2013). Global and regional estimates of violence against women. [online] Available from: https://www.who.int/publications-detail-redirect/9789241564625 [Last accessed December, 2023].
3. Kilpatrick DG. What is violence against women: defining and measuring the problem. J Interpers Violence. 2004;19(11):1209-34.
4. Lagdon S, Armour C, Stringer M. Adult experience of mental health outcomes as a result of intimate partner violence victimisation: a systematic review. Eur J Psychotraumatology. 2014;5(1):24794.
5. Trevillion K, Oram S, Feder G, Howard LM. Experiences of domestic violence and mental disorders: a systematic review and meta-analysis. PloS One. 2012;7(12):e51740.
6. Oram S, Khalifeh H, Howard LM. Violence against women and mental health. Lancet Psychiatry. 2017;4(2):159-70.
7. Oram S, Fisher HL, Minnis H, Seedat S, Walby S, Hegarty K, et al. The Lancet Psychiatry Commission on intimate partner violence and mental health: advancing mental health services, research, and policy. Lancet Psychiatry. 2022;9(6):487-524.
8. Carbone-López K, Kruttschnitt C, Macmillan R. Patterns of intimate partner violence and their associations with physical health, psychological distress, and substance use. Public Health Rep Wash DC 1974. 2006;121(4):382-92.
9. Ludermir AB, Schraiber LB, D'Oliveira AFPL, França-Junior I, Jansen HA. Violence against women by their intimate partner and common mental disorders. Soc Sci Med 1982. 2008;66(4):1008-18.
10. Devries K, Watts C, Yoshihama M, Kiss L, Schraiber LB, Deyessa N, et al. Violence against women is strongly associated with suicide attempts: evidence from the WHO multi-country study on women's health and domestic violence against women. Soc Sci Med 1982. 2011;73(1):79-86.
11. Cantu JI, Charak R. Unique, additive, and interactive effects of types of intimate partner cybervictimization on depression in Hispanic emerging adults. J Interpers Violence. 2022;37(1-2):NP375-99.
12. Dillon G, Hussain R, Loxton D, Rahman S. Mental and physical health and intimate partner violence against women: a review of the literature. Int J Fam Med. 2013;2013:313909.
13. Coker AL, Davis KE, Arias I, Desai S, Sanderson M, Brandt HM, et al. Physical and mental health effects of intimate partner violence for men and women. Am J Prev Med. 2002;23(4):260-8.
14. Zlotnick C, Johnson DM, Kohn R. Intimate partner violence and long-term psychosocial functioning in a national sample of American women. J Interpers Violence. 2006;21(2):262-75.
15. Vos T, Astbury J, Piers LS, Magnus A, Heenan M, Stanley L, et al. Measuring the impact of intimate partner violence on the health of women in Victoria, Australia. Bull World Health Organ. 2006;84(9):739-44.
16. Lövestad S, Löve J, Vaez M, Krantz G. Prevalence of intimate partner violence and its association with symptoms of depression; a cross-sectional study based on a female population sample in Sweden. BMC Public Health. 2017;17(1):335.
17. Chandan JS, Thomas T, Bradbury-Jones C, Russell R, Bandyopadhyay S, Nirantharakumar K, et al. Female survivors of intimate partner violence and

risk of depression, anxiety and serious mental illness. Br J Psychiatry J Ment Sci. 2020;217(4):562-7.
18. O'Campo P, Kub J, Woods A, Garza M, Jones AS, Gielen AC, et al. Depression, PTSD, and co-morbidity related to intimate partner violence in civilian and military women. Brief Treat Crisis Interv. 2006;6(2):99.
19. Houry D, Kemball R, Rhodes KV, Kaslow NJ. Intimate partner violence and mental health symptoms in African American female ED patients. Am J Emerg Med. 2006;24(4):444-50.
20. Fernández-Fillol C, Pitsiakou C, Perez-Garcia M, Teva I, Ruzzante NH. Complex PTSD in survivors of intimate partner violence: risk factors related to symptoms and diagnoses. Eur J Psychotraumatology. 2021;12(1):2003616.
21. Mehr JB, Bennett ER, Price JL, de Souza NL, Buckman JF, Wilde EA, et al. Intimate partner violence, substance use, and health co-morbidities among women: a narrative review. Front Psychol. 2022;13:1028375.
22. National Center on Domestic Violence, Trauma, and Mental Health. (2015). The relationship between intimate partner violence and substance use: An applied research paper. [online] Available from: https://ncdvtmh.org/resource/the-relationship-between-intimate-partner-violence-and-substance-use-an-applied-research-paper-2015/ [Last accessed December, 2023].
23. Ellsberg M, Emmelin M. Intimate partner violence and mental health. Glob Health Action. 2014;7:25658.
24. McManus S, Walby S, Barbosa EC, Appleby L, Brugha T, Bebbington PE, et al. Intimate partner violence, suicidality, and self-harm: a probability sample survey of the general population in England. Lancet Psychiatry. 2022;9(7):574-83.
25. González RA, Igoumenou A, Kallis C, Coid JW. Borderline personality disorder and violence in the UK population: categorical and dimensional trait assessment. BMC Psychiatry. 2016;16(1):180.
26. Bozzatello P, Rocca P, Baldassarri L, Bosia M, Bellino S. The role of trauma in early onset borderline personality disorder: A biopsychosocial perspective. Front Psychiatry. 2021;12:721361.
27. Porter C, Palmier-Claus J, Branitsky A, Mansell W, Warwick H, Varese F. Childhood adversity and borderline personality disorder: a meta-analysis. Acta Psychiatr Scand. 2020;141(1):6-20.
28. Nair S, A Satyanarayana V, Desai G. Prevalence and clinical correlates of intimate partner violence (IPV) in women with severe mental illness (SMI). Asian J Psychiatry. 2020;52:102131.
29. Khalifeh H, Moran P, Borschmann R, Dean K, Hart C, Hogg J, et al. Domestic and sexual violence against patients with severe mental illness. Psychol Med. 2015;45(4):875-86.
30. Ross JM, Babcock JC. Proactive and reactive violence among intimate partner violent men diagnosed with antisocial and borderline personality disorder. J Fam Violence. 2009;24(8):607-17.
31. Cheng D, Salimi S, Terplan M, Chisolm MS. Intimate partner violence and maternal cigarette smoking before and during pregnancy. Obstet Gynecol. 2015;125(2):356-62.
32. Rodriguez MA, Heilemann MV, Fielder E, Ang A, Nevarez F, Mangione CM. Intimate partner violence, depression, and PTSD among pregnant Latina women. Ann Fam Med. 2008;6(1):44-52.

33. Varma D, Chandra PS, Thomas T, Carey MP. Intimate partner violence and sexual coercion among pregnant women in India: Relationship with depression and posttraumatic stress disorder. J Affect Disord. 2007;102(1):227-35.
34. Howard LM, Oram S, Galley H, Trevillion K, Feder G. Domestic violence and perinatal mental disorders: a systematic review and meta-analysis. PLoS Med. 2013;10(5):e1001452.
35. Ananthanpillai S, Kandavel T, Satyanarayana V, Thomas S, Desai G, Jangam K, et al. Suicidality in early pregnancy among antepartum mothers in urban India. Arch Womens Ment Health. 2016;19.
36. Hahn CK, Gilmore AK, Aguayo RO, Rheingold AA. Perinatal intimate partner violence. Obstet Gynecol Clin North Am. 2018;45(3):535-47.
37. Halim N, Beard J, Mesic A, Patel A, Henderson D, Hibberd P. Intimate partner violence during pregnancy and perinatal mental disorders in low and lower middle income countries: A systematic review of literature, 1990-2017. Clin Psychol Rev. 2018;66:117-35.
38. Vu NL, Jouriles EN, McDonald R, Rosenfield D. Children's exposure to intimate partner violence: A meta-analysis of longitudinal associations with child adjustment problems. Clin Psychol Rev. 2016;46:25-33.
39. Messinger AM. Invisible victims: same-sex IPV in the National Violence Against Women Survey. J Interpers Violence. 2011;26(11):2228-43.
40. Rollè L, Giardina G, Caldarera AM, Gerino E, Brustia P. When intimate partner violence meets same sex couples: A review of same sex intimate partner violence. Front Psychol. 2018;9:1506.
41. Mathur P, Sharma LP, H Nanjundaswamy M, S Chandra P. Training needs of psychiatry residents in handling Intimate Partner Violence (IPV) in clinical situations—A survey. Asian J Psychiatry. 2020;53:102379.
42. Rose D, Trevillion K, Woodall A, Morgan C, Feder G, Howard L. Barriers and facilitators of disclosures of domestic violence by mental health service users: qualitative study. Br J Psychiatry. 2011;198(3):189-94.
43. Namy S, Carlson C, O'Hara K, Nakuti J, Bukuluki P, Lwanyaaga J, et al. Towards a feminist understanding of intersecting violence against women and children in the family. Soc Sci Med 1982. 2017;184:40-8.
44. Dobash RE, Dobash R. (1979). Violence against wives - a case against the patriarchy. [online] Available from: https://www.ojp.gov/ncjrs/virtual-library/abstracts/violence-against-wives-case-against-patriarchy [Last accessed December, 2023].
45. McPhail BA, Busch NB, Kulkarni S, Rice G. An integrative feminist model: the evolving feminist perspective on intimate partner violence. Violence Women. 2007;13(8):817-41.
46. George J, Stith SM. An updated feminist view of intimate partner violence. Fam Process. 2014;53(2):179-93.
47. Kumar S, Jeyaseelan L, Suresh S, Ahuja RC. Domestic violence and its mental health correlates in Indian women. Br J Psychiatry. 2005;187(1):62-7.
48. Kamimura A, Ganta V, Myers K, Thomas T. Intimate partner violence and physical and mental health among women utilizing community health services in Gujarat, India. BMC Womens Health. 2014;14(1):127.

49. Sharma KK, Vatsa M, Kalaivani M, Bhardwaj D. Mental health effects of domestic violence against women in Delhi: A community-based study. J Fam Med Prim Care. 2019;8(7):2522-7.
50. Vachher AS, Sharma A. Domestic violence against women and their mental health status in a colony in delhi. Indian J Community Med Off Publ Indian Assoc Prev Soc Med. 2010;35(3):403-5.
51. Chandra PS, Satyanarayana VA, Carey MP. Women reporting intimate partner violence in India: Associations with PTSD and depressive symptoms. Arch Womens Ment Health. 2009;12(4):203-9.
52. Narasimha Vranda M, Naveen Kumar C, Muralidhar D, Janardhana N, Thangaraju Sivakumar P. Intimate partner violence, lifetime victimization, and sociodemographic and clinical profile of women with psychiatric illness at a tertiary care psychiatric hospital in India. Indian J Psychol Med. 2021;43(6):525-30.
53. Kanougiya S, Daruwalla N, Gram L, Gupta AD, Sivakami M, Osrin D. Economic abuse and its associations with symptoms of common mental disorders among women in a cross-sectional survey in informal settlements in Mumbai, India. BMC Public Health. 2021;21(1):842.
54. Kamath A, Yadav A, Baghel J, Mundle S. Locked down: Experiences of domestic violence in Central India. Glob Health Sci Pract. 2022;10(4).
55. O'Doherty L, Hegarty K, Ramsay J, Davidson LL, Feder G, Taft A. Screening women for intimate partner violence in healthcare settings. Cochrane Database Syst Rev. 2015;2015(7):CD007007.
56. Stewart DE, Chandra PS. WPA International competency-based curriculum for mental health providers on intimate partner violence and sexual violence against women. World Psychiatry. 2017;16(2):223-4.
57. SAMHSA's Trauma and Justice Strategic Initiative. (2014). SAMHSA's Concept of Trauma and Guidance for a Trauma-Informed Approach. [online] Available from https://ncsacw.acf.hhs.gov/userfiles/files/SAMHSA_Trauma.pdf [Last accessed December, 2023].
58. Jonas DE, Cusack K, Forneris CA, Wilkins TM, Sonis J, Middleton JC, et al. Psychological and pharmacological treatments for adults with posttraumatic stress disorder (PTSD) [Internet]. Rockville (MD): Agency for Healthcare Research and Quality (US); 2013.
59. Johnson DM, Johnson NL, Perez SK, Palmieri PA, Zlotnick C. Comparison of adding treatment of PTSD during and after shelter stay to standard care in residents of battered women's shelters: Results of a randomized clinical trial. J Trauma Stress. 2016;29(4):365-73.
60. Resick PA, Galovski TE, Uhlmansiek MO, Scher CD, Clum GA, Young-Xu Y. A randomized clinical trial to dismantle components of cognitive processing therapy for posttraumatic stress disorder in female victims of interpersonal violence. J Consult Clin Psychol. 2008;76(2):243-58.
61. Iverson KM, Gradus JL, Resick PA, Suvak MK, Smith KF, Monson CM. Cognitive-behavioral therapy for PTSD and depression symptoms reduces risk for future intimate partner violence among interpersonal trauma survivors. J Consult Clin Psychol. 2011;79(2):193-202.

62. Iverson KM, Resick PA, Suvak MK, Walling S, Taft CT. Intimate partner violence exposure predicts PTSD treatment engagement and outcome in cognitive processing therapy. Behav Ther. 2011;42(2):236-48.
63. Ferrari G, Feder G, Agnew-Davies R, Bailey JE, Hollinghurst S, Howard L, et al. Psychological advocacy towards healing (PATH): A randomized controlled trial of a psychological intervention in a domestic violence service setting. PLoS ONE. 2018;13(11):e0205485.
64. Bisson JI, Roberts NP, Andrew M, Cooper R, Lewis C. Psychological therapies for chronic posttraumatic stress disorder (PTSD) in adults. Cochrane Database Syst Rev. 2013;2013(12):CD003388.
65. Franzblau SH, Echevarria S, Smith M, Van Cantfort TE. A preliminary investigation of the effects of giving testimony and learning yogic breathing techniques on battered women's feelings of depression. J Interpers Violence. 2008;23(12):1800-8.
66. Kelly A, Garland EL. Trauma-informed mindfulness-based stress reduction for female survivors of interpersonal violence: Results from a stage I RCT. J Clin Psychol. 2016;72(4):311-28.
67. Dutton MA, Bermudez D, Matas A, Majid H, Myers NL. Mindfulness-based stress reduction for low-income, predominantly African American women with PTSD and a history of intimate partner violence. Cogn Behav Pract. 2013;20(1):23-32.
68. Kokka A, Mikelatou M, Fouka G, Varvogli L, Chrousos GP, Darviri C. Stress management and health promotion in a sample of women with intimate partner violence: a randomized controlled trial. J Interpers Violence. 2019;34(10):2034-55.
69. Karatzias T, Ferguson S, Gullone A, Cosgrove K. Group psychotherapy for female adult survivors of interpersonal psychological trauma: a preliminary study in Scotland. J Ment Health Abingdon Engl. 2016;25(6):512-9.
70. Koziol-McLain J, Vandal AC, Wilson D, Nada-Raja S, Dobbs T, McLean C, et al. Efficacy of a web-based safety decision aid for women experiencing intimate partner violence: Randomized controlled trial. J Med Internet Res. 2018;19(12):e426.
71. Hegarty K, Tarzia L, Valpied J, Murray E, Humphreys C, Taft A, et al. An online healthy relationship tool and safety decision aid for women experiencing intimate partner violence (I-DECIDE): a randomised controlled trial. Lancet Public Health. 2019;4(6):e301-10.
72. Trevillion K, Byford S, Cary M, Rose D, Oram S, Feder G, et al. Linking abuse and recovery through advocacy: an observational study. Epidemiol Psychiatr Sci. 2014;23(1):99-113.
73. World Health Organization. (2019). Caring for women subjected to violence: a WHO curriculum for training health-care providers. [online] Available from: https://www.who.int/publications/i/item/9789241517102 [Last accessed December, 2023].

SUGGESTED READING

1. Ministry of Women & Child Development, Government of India. NIMHANS STREE MANORAKSHA PROJECT. Training in psychosocial issues and mental

health care to support women facing gender-based violence. [online] Available from: http://nimhansstreemanoraksha.in/project-stree-manoraksha/ [Last accessed December, 2023].
2. Stewart DE, Chandra PS. WPA International Competency-Based Curriculum for Mental Health Providers on Intimate Partner Violence and Sexual Violence Against Women. World Psychiatry. 2017;16(2):223-4.
3. World Health Organization. (2013). Responding to intimate partner violence and sexual violence against women – Summary. [online] Available from: https://www.who.int/publications/i/item/WHO-RHR-13.10 [Last accessed December, 2023].
4. World Health Organization. (2019). RESPECT women, Preventing violence against women [online] Available from: https://www.who.int/publications/i/item/WHO-RHR-18.19 [Last accessed December, 2023].

CHAPTER 15

Rights of Women with Mental Illness

Shivanee Kumari, Sai Chaitanya Reddy B, Suresh Bada Math

▌ ABSTRACT

Women's mental health is influenced by various social, cultural, and biological factors. Mental illness itself inflicts great suffering upon an individual, and being a woman often puts them at a double disadvantage, and at risk for violation of their rights.

Studies from India have shown that more women (54.26%) than men (45.74%) have been confined to mental hospitals. These women face upheavals in their family life, divorce, abandonment, and homelessness. Research on psychiatric long-stay institutions has reported confinement, physical and sexual abuse, inhumane or degrading treatment, violation of reproductive rights, and lack of proper maintenance of hygiene and sanitation for women.

The Mental Healthcare Act 2017 sheds light on the rights of women suffering from mental illness in various sections, especially *Sections 20-21*, where women are given the right to dignity, privacy, and equality. The National Commission for Women and the National Institute for Mental Health and Neurosciences have also made efforts and recommendations for the protection of the rights of women with mental illness.

Keywords: Human rights, women, mental illness, legal rights

▌ INTRODUCTION

The Mental Health Care Act (MHCA) 2017[1] defines mental illness as a substantial disorder of thinking, mood, perception, orientation, or memory that grossly impairs judgment, behavior, capacity to recognize reality or ability to meet the ordinary demands of life, and mental conditions triggered by the abuse of alcohol and drugs. However, intellectual disability, which is a condition of arrested or incomplete development of the mind of a person specially characterized by subnormality of intelligence, does not fall within the Act's ambit. Women's mental health is influenced by various social, cultural, and biological factors. Mental illness itself inflicts great suffering upon an individual, and being a woman often puts them at a double disadvantage, and at risk for violation of their rights.[2-4] In this chapter, we are focusing on the human rights, disadvantages of women with mental illness, violation of their rights, studies, cases, and laws pertaining to their human rights, and recommendations to prevent the violation of rights.

HUMAN RIGHTS AND MENTAL ILLNESS

Contrary to the constitutional provision, a quality review of the status of human rights in 36 psychiatric institutions across India by the National Human Rights Commission (NHRC) in 1997 found that infrastructure, manpower, and services were not adequate; water supply systems had outlived their utility; there was lack of rehabilitation facilities and support system; confinement in closed environments was common; there were deficiencies in disability certification and specialized services for children and elderly. The situation is particularly graver for women due to the denial of economic resources, education, legal and health services, lack of physical and mental nurturance, and sexual or other forms of physical and mental abuse.[5] Research from a tertiary care center in India shows that the majority of economically disadvantaged women suffering from mental illness have a lack of basic facilities like food and water, adequate access to toilets and sanitary facilities, and were found to be in pitiable living conditions.[6]

DISADVANTAGES FOR WOMEN WITH MENTAL ILLNESS IN THE COMMUNITY

The Hans Study 2019 was conducted across 43 psychiatric facilities in 24 states of India. It found that more women (54.26%) than men (45.74%) have been confined to mental hospitals. In addition, women form a larger proportion of such people who live in long-stay psychiatric homes. The proportion of disabled women is also more than that of men in such institutions. Such women suffering from disabling mental illnesses encounter several difficulties while living in society. They face upheavals in their family and marital life that lead to irreconcilable relationship conflicts, separation, divorce, and even abandonment by the partner and family. Narratives from different women reveal that they are often left without a home because their families consider them a "burden" if they cannot carry out household chores. Many report that their opinions are not considered while making household decisions and that they are not considered capable. Most homeless women suffering from psychiatric illness are from disadvantaged castes, with poor educational backgrounds. Some women are also left to fend for their children alone, without any financial support.[7,8] In India, women from disadvantaged castes with mental illness are more likely to face penury as compared to men due to a higher degree of stigma. The condition of stark poverty makes survival even more difficult for them.[9] Such double disadvantages make women more vulnerable to the violation of their basic human rights.

VIOLATION OF RIGHTS OF WOMEN WITH MENTAL ILLNESS

Violence

The lifetime prevalence rate of violence against women ranges from 16 to 50%.[10] A study from India reported the prevalence of violence against mentally ill women to be 80%. It also found that violence predisposed women to mental illness, which in turn, led to the perpetration of further violence upon them by family members for purposes of behavioral control and, thus leading to the creation of a vicious cause-effect circle.[4]

Sexual Coercion

At least one in five women are reported to be subjected to rape or attempted rape in their lifetime.[10] Homelessness further makes them vulnerable to sexual abuse.[4] A study from our country reported the prevalence of sexual coercion to be 34% among 146 women with severe mental illness (SMI), mostly inflicted upon them by their spouses.[11]

Childhood Sexual Abuse

Several research studies have found high rates of sexual abuse in childhood among women with SMI.[12,13] In a study done among women with SMI in our country, 18 out of 50 respondents reported a history of childhood sexual abuse (CSA).[11]

Reproductive Rights

Over the years, issues of violation of reproductive rights have also been raised after reports of illegally carrying out abortions on mentally ill women without their consent.[14] Coerced sterilization, hysterectomies, and tubal ligations on nonconsenting women with SMI, lack of proper sanitation provisions during menstruation, and forced separation from children are also sensitive issues that need to be tackled. Women with psychiatric disorders are also susceptible to incest and sexually transmitted diseases (STDs).[15,16]

Healthcare and Community Living

Women in mental health establishments (MHEs) are often abandoned by their families even after they achieve remission of their illnesses. Due to poverty and stigma, these women hesitate to leave the MHE and are unable to integrate with the community.[17]

STUDIES ON VIOLATION OF RIGHTS OF WOMEN WITH MENTAL ILLNESS IN PSYCHIATRIC INSTITUTIONS AND HOMES IN INDIA

Human Rights Watch 2014

Human Rights Watch 2014 reported that instances of violence against women with mental disabilities including confinement, physical and sexual abuse, inhumane or degrading treatment, and excessive electroshock therapy were high in residential care facilities for psychiatric patients. These facilities lacked adequate monitoring and supervision. Within the family and community, women with disabilities were also subjected to violence. They also faced violations of their reproductive rights in the form of involuntary sterilization.[18]

NIMHANS and National Commission for Women 2016

A study was conducted by the National Institute of Mental Health and Neurosciences (NIMHANS) in collaboration with the National Commission for Women in 2016, where 245 women with mental illness were interviewed and visits were done to 10 mental hospitals and residential care facilities in different cities of the nation. Onsite evaluation by a multidisciplinary team of mental health professionals found that the wards were dimly lit in some institutes, overcrowded, there was a hot water shortage, bathrooms were poorly maintained and slippery and some patients were defecating in the open. There were a number of women who were shunned and abandoned by their families, staff shortages in the institutes, poor surveillance, lack of legal aid, and a dearth of safe and supportive community-based rehabilitation services.

The study further showed that informed consent was not taken from women for treatment. They were neither allowed to go out of the wards nor given access to communication with their family members, that is to say, they were kept in restraint for most of the day without the opportunities for participation in any group, cultural, or spiritual activities. The majority of these women were not aware of their rights. No forms of extra care were provided to those who were pregnant or breastfeeding. The research also highlighted the dearth of female staff in psychiatric institutions dedicated to the task of ministering to the needs of these women.[19]

National Commission for Women 2019

The National Commission for Women 2019 conducted a study by reviewing the status of 27 institutions and 19 Psychiatric Homes in the country. The study revealed that women often had to overstay due to the refusal of family members to take them back, stigma, remarriage of the spouse to another, and denial of property rights. Family members were not allowed to visit the patients, therefore limiting their participation in the care and treatment of the women with mental illness. In many of the institutions, women often stayed for a period of >5 years due to desertion by family members.

The study also highlighted overcrowding, lack of nutritious food, and deficiencies in sanitation and hygiene requirements of women, including inadequate personal toiletries, sanitary napkins, inner garments, and clothes. They were not provided privacy during bathing or changing clothes; tonsuring was done without consent and recreational facilities were also lacking. Confidentiality was not maintained regarding the treatment of these women. They would be at risk of sexual abuse from institutional authorities, but there was no functioning internal committee in the mental hospitals for the prevention of sexual harassment. The study also showed that women with mental illness had less access to mental health care services, and utilization of the female beds was low compared to the male beds.

In addition, the study showed that staff was deficient across all categories, especially nurses and medical attendants, who provided day-to-day support. Separate wards for women were not available in some institutes, and entry into the same was also not regulated. Many of these institutes were not associated with any nongovernmental organizations (NGOs) or Civil Societies that helped in the rehabilitation of these women.[20]

■ WOMEN WITH MENTAL ILLNESS IN PRISONS

Prisoners needing treatment for mental diseases should be kept in the psychiatric wing of the prison hospital or MHE, instead of prison. However, women suffering from mental illnesses are often housed in prisons due to a lack of other appropriate facilities, thereby hindering their right to access basic healthcare.[21] A study done in India found that lack of personal contacts and fading familial communications were major sources of mental health issues in incarcerated women.[22] Research on prisons has shown that there is a lack of separate sections for women, female staff, basic facilities, sanitation amenities, recreation, necessary services needed for childcare, and legal aid in the prisons. Asian Centre for Human Rights (ACHR) also stated that custodial rape remains one of the worst forms of torture perpetrated on women by law enforcement personnel and many custodial rapes of women take place at regular intervals.[23,24] The Bangalore Prison Study 2011 revealed that one in four women were undernourished, had poor knowledge about legal aid, did not have access to rehabilitation services, and that women with mental illness felt that they were discriminated against.[25]

WOMEN WITH MENTAL ILLNESS DURING CONFLICT AND HUMANITARIAN CRISIS

Reports from Cooperative or Assistance and Relief Everywhere (CARE) International suggest humanitarian crises have a worse impact on women, especially if they are disabled.[26] A recent study from India showed that women with mental illness have a higher risk of relapse during disasters. They have less help-seeking behavior, cannot protect themselves and their support system is also poor, making them more vulnerable to abuse and violence in disaster situations. The study highlighted the need for relief agencies to come up with mechanisms to protect women with mental illness during disasters.[27] Research by the Women's Refugee Commission (WRC) showed that women experienced violence in all contexts, including sexual violence, and that those with intellectual or mental disabilities were at the most risk. In addition, such women were not aware of menstrual hygiene, had poor access to reproductive health services, and also had a lack of livelihood opportunities. In Handicap International's Survey, disabled women reported that they did not have adequate access to basic assistance such as water, shelter, food, and health, which is a gross violation of their basic rights.[28]

MENTAL HEALTHCARE ACT, 2017 AND RIGHTS OF MENTALLY ILL WOMEN

The United Nations Convention on the Rights of Persons with Disabilities (UNCRPD) recognized that women with disabilities were at higher risk for violence, injury or abuse, neglect, maltreatment, and exploitation. Acknowledging this, the convention directed for ensuring the full development, advancement, and empowerment of women, for the purpose of guaranteeing them the exercise and enjoyment of human rights and fundamental freedoms. It also ensured their access to social protection and poverty reduction programs.[29]

India passed the MHCA 2017 after ratifying the UNCRPD in 2007. The Act gives utmost importance to the informed choice, rights, and autonomy of persons with mental illness (PMI). It emphasizes on the assessment of the mental capacity to consent.[30] The rights of PMI have been elaborately described in Sections 18–28 of Chapter 5 of MHCA 2017. In addition, the Act sheds light on the rights of women suffering from mental illness in various sections.[1]

Section 18

Right to access mental healthcare and treatment from mental health services without discrimination on the basis of gender, sex, or sexual orientation.

Section 20

Right to live with dignity *(protection from cruel, inhuman, and degrading treatment, provision of sanitary conditions and hygienic environment, privacy, recreational facilities, prohibition of shaving head, and protection from abuse)*
- *Subsection 2* instructs for adequate addressal of women's personal hygiene by providing access to items that may be required during menstruation.

Section 21

Right to equal treatment with physical illness in the provision of all healthcare (including no discrimination based on gender).
- *Subsection 2* also stresses that a child under 3 years of age shall not be separated from the mother who is receiving care at an MHE. Provided that the treating psychiatrist feels there is a risk to the child, temporary separation may be allowed, but the decision needs to be reviewed every 15 days, and the mother shall continue to have access to her child under the supervision of the staff or family. Permission from the authority will be required if the separation exceeds 30 days.

Information regarding the admission of women in the MHE needs to be intimated to the Mental Health Review Board (MHRB) within 3 days of admission under *Sections 86, 89, and 90*. According to *Section 87*, when a minor girl is admitted, a female attendant shall be appointed by the nominated representative if he is a male and, under all circumstances, she shall stay with the minor girl in the MHE for the entire duration of her admission.

Section 95

It emphasizes that sterilization is prohibited when it is intended as a treatment for mental illness. Women who have valid gynecological indications may undergo hysterectomy.

Apart from these, some gender-neutral rights have been provided by MHCA 2017 under *Sections 19 and 22-28*.

THE SCHEDULE FOR MINIMUM STANDARDS OF MENTAL HEALTH ESTABLISHMENTS[31]

It has specified regulations specifically to cater to the needs of women in MHEs, which are enumerated below:
- *Special diet:* Must be given to women who are elderly, pregnant, lactating, or have recently undergone abortion or miscarriage based on distinct nutritional requirements.

- *Physical examination and treatment:* Shall be in the presence of a female attendant or female nursing staff.
- *Privacy:* Separate wards, toilets, and bathrooms need to be provided for male and female inpatients.
- *Hygiene and sanitation:* Disposal facilities for sanitary napkins are mandatory.

Some landmark judgments in the context of women with mental illness are enumerated in **Table 1**.[5,32,33]

TABLE 1: Landmark judgments for women with mental illness.

Case	Description	Violation of rights	Court verdict
Suchita Srivastava and Another versus Chandigarh Administration (Although this is a case of mental retardation, the court has upheld a woman's right to dignity and privacy. The verdict is broad and by the argument proposed, an extension may be considered for women with mental illness)	The Chandigarh Administration approached the Punjab and Haryana High Court to seek permission to medically terminate the pregnancy of a mentally retarded girl	• Sexual assault (rape) • Cruel and inhumane treatment • Reproductive choices • Dignity	*Supreme Court:* A Woman's right to privacy, dignity, and bodily integrity should be respected including reproductive choice to continue with the pregnancy
Mansi versus the State of Punjab and others	Detention of a 2-year-old child of a mentally ill mother at the hands of her husband and in-laws	Right to equal treatment and no discrimination on the basis of gender	*Punjab and Haryana High Court:* In the case of a mother, especially where the custody concerns a child <5 years old, she ought to be granted custody unless she is so mentally or physically incapacitated that handing over custody to her would be physically or mentally detrimental to the health of the child

Contd...

Contd...

Case	Description	Violation of rights	Court verdict
Sheela Barse versus Union of India and others	Sheela Barse, a female journalist, wrote a letter to the Supreme Court addressing the issue related to custodial violence and lack of proper legal assistance to women prisoners in Bombay Central jail	• Cruel and inhumane treatment • Right to legal aid	*Supreme Court:* Legal assistance to be provided to the prisoners, 4–5 lockups with all the facilities available for the women prisoners in a good locality and guarded by female constables to be allotted, interrogation to be done in the presence of a female constable
Binoo Sen versus State of West Bengal through the Principal Secretary, Department of Social Welfare, and others	Remanding mentally ill persons to Rehabilitation Homes that are not equipped for treatment	Access to mental health care	*Calcutta High Court:* Need to send a person for a medical check-up at a hospital that is well-equipped to conduct such a test and provide mental healthcare to him/her before sending to a Rehabilitation Home

EFFORTS MADE TO EMPOWER WOMEN WITH MENTAL ILLNESS

Apart from the above judgments, the authors feel it is significant to mention regarding a commendable effort from the society, which helped unite a mentally ill mother with her child. In 2019, a woman with behavioral abnormalities was spotted with her newborn child at a railway station and was admitted to a rehabilitation center while her child was sent to a foster family by the Child Welfare Committee (CWC). Over the course of time, her mental illness improved and she wished to be reunited with her child. Though the foster family resisted, considering the mother's mental and physical fitness and her right to motherhood, the CWC ordered the foster family to hand over the child to the biological mother.[34]

Boxes 1 and 2[35] below highlight attempts and initiatives by several organizations (Banyan and Anjali) to ensure the restoration of the rights of women with mental illness.

> **BOX 1:** Anjali—An NGO based in West Bengal.
>
> An NGO based in West Bengal called "Anjali" aspires to translate the aims of the MHCA 2017 into reality. One of their initiatives was helping women in Berhampore Mental Hospital and Calcutta Pavlov Hospital achieve their basic individual right to vote. Dhobi Ghar is an initiative by Anjali, which was launched in May 2016 where the participants worked in shifts to wash the linen of the Calcutta Pavlov Hospital. The organization attempts to provide vocational experience to expedite re-integration into the community. One example of this is providing work at a tea stall within the campus of the hospital. During the COVID pandemic, the organization conducted workshops on trauma counseling.

> **BOX 2:** Banyan—An NGO based in South India.
>
> The Banyan is an NGO established in 1993 in South India, which has worked to create alternative institutional care and rehabilitation for independent community living. Their initiative to rehabilitate led to the starting of Adaikalam, Clustered Group Homes (CGH), and Home Again. These initiatives strive to provide a long-term safe space and rented accommodations in the community for women with mental illnesses. One of the key priorities is re-integration with family and continuity of care to prevent abandonment and homelessness.

Along with the above efforts, NIMHANS has also made some efforts to empower women with mental illness. The institution initiated the process of getting voter cards and Aadhar cards to help the women in long-stay wards.[36] In addition, a halfway home is run by the Institute, which is known as Sakalwara Community Mental Health Centre, where all measures for community rehabilitation and restoration of the dignity of women with mental illness are taken into account.[20]

■ RECOMMENDATIONS

Considering the extensive violation of the rights of women with mental illness, the authors have summarized recommendations for psychiatric institutions for the protection of the rights of women with mental illness,[19,20,35] which are enumerated as follows:
- *Gender-sensitive treatment facilities:* One of the vital steps to prevent rights violations is establishing gender-sensitive mental healthcare. Separate special treatment environments are needed for women to feel safe and provide them with peer support. They should have life-stage focused care, trauma-informed care, access to maternity and child care, as well as protection from violence and sexual abuse.
- *Adequate human resources including female staff:* Each psychiatric home should have an adequate number of psychiatrists/specialists and at least one should be a woman amongst them. Female nurses in accordance

with the number of women admitted and high representation of female attendants is mandatory.

- *Gender-sensitive toiletries, undergarments, and sanitary napkins in psychiatric homes:* All the items of personal toiletries should be issued to individual female patients admitted in inpatient departments. These items should be issued on a regular basis.
- *Recreational and educational facilities:* An organization of adequate recreational programs in the form of conventional indoor and outdoor games should take place. They should be participative in nature, such as group dance, musical evenings, singing, and devotional songs (bhajan sessions).
- *Foster ways to increase acceptance by family, community, and society:* The family members of the women admitted to the inpatient department should have free access to visitation, and also be fully involved in the treatment process by giving all the relevant information regarding medication, care practices, likely duration of the treatment, need for continued stay in the psychiatric home, etc. The family members of the patient also need to be made aware about the benefits, such as free/subsidized treatment, disability benefits, and travel benefits available to mentally ill patients. All psychiatric homes need to have a midway/halfway home of their own for the women with mental illness, who have been treated and are in a near normal mental state and require transfer to family/community.
- *Adequate skill training to discourage long-stay homes:* Psychiatric homes should arrange for continuous skill training of patients in accordance with their abilities and interests. Skills that help the patient to become self-reliant may be given preference while choosing the skills training programs. All institutions should develop associations with NGOs/Civil Societies for various purposes, such as counseling, recreational activities, skill development/vocational training, and rehabilitation.
- *Legal aid and provisions for child care (without separation):* Legal aid services should be made available to admitted women with mental illness through the NGO/District Level Services Authority (DLSA). Also, the woman should not separate from a growing infant for the mere presence of a mental illness unless she poses a threat to the infant.
- *Community-level facilities like vocational or rehabilitation centers:* Women's respite/halfway home facilities/rehabilitation centers need to be set up, including treatment for addiction-related problems. Shelters, daycare facilities, self-help groups, and link-ups with vocational centers also need to be provided.
- *Identification of women with mental illness by other agencies like NGOs and bringing them for treatment:* Detection of a woman with mental illness need to be ensured from other settings, such as Beggar's Home,

Prisons, Juvenile Homes for adolescent girls, Old Age Homes for women, and Private Residential facilities by NGOs and they should be given proper access to treatment facilities.

For a detailed report of the recommendations, refer to "Addressing Concerns of Women Admitted to Psychiatric Institutions in India: An In-depth Analysis," 2016, and "Review of Psychiatric Homes/Mental Hospitals of Government Sector in India with Special Reference to Female Patients in IPD," 2019 by NCW.[19,20] Apart from the aforementioned, the authors would like to make some additional recommendations as follows:

- Gender-sensitive training for all staff working in mental health including students, law enforcement personnel and members of MHRBs, etc.
- Women and child units can be established in all MHEs
- Women with mental illness with children to be given priority in outpatient departments (OPDs)
- MHCA 2017 needs to be amended to make provisions for PMI more gender-sensitive.

The status of women, especially of those suffering from mental illness, is abject. Along with mental illness, they face a number of different problems, such as poor understanding of illness, lack of access to health care services, stigma, abandonment, sexual abuse, and loss of reproductive rights. In spite of various efforts over the years, the situation has improved only minimally. The rights, decisions, and autonomy of women with mental illnesses, continue to be compromised at various levels. In light of the new MHCA 2017, there is hope that further steps will be taken in the direction of protection of the rights of persons with mental illness and access to treatment, which may indirectly help safeguard the rights of women with mental illness. Still, considering research from recent studies, we still have a long way to go before we can say that women's rights have been fully ensured in our country.

KEY POINTS

- Women's mental health is influenced by various social, cultural. and biological factors.
- National studies have shown that more women (54.26%) than men (45.74%) have been confined to mental hospitals.
- Research on psychiatric long-stay institutions have reported confinement, physical and sexual abuse, inhumane or degrading treatment, violation of reproductive rights, lack of proper maintenance of hygiene and sanitation for women.
- The Mental Healthcare Act 2017 sheds light on the rights of women suffering from mental illness in various sections, especially *Sections 20–21*, where women are given the right to dignity, privacy, and equality.
- NIMHANS, and NGOs such as Anjali and Banyan have taken initiatives to empower women with mental illness and protect their rights.

REFERENCES

1. Mental Healthcare Act. 2017. [online]. Available from http://www.prsindia.org/uploads/media/Mental%20Health/Mental%20Healthcare%20Act,%202017.pdf [Last accessed December, 2023].
2. Nambi S. Marriage, mental health and the Indian legislation. Indian J Psychiatry. 2005;47(1):3-14.
3. Rao TS, Tandon A. Women and mental health: Bridging the gap. Indian J Psychiatry. 2015;57:S199-200.
4. Vijayalakshmi P, Gandhi S, Sai Nikhil Reddy S, Palaniappan M, Badamath S. Violence against women with mental illness and social norms and beliefs: nursing professional perspective. Community Ment Health J. 2021;57(2):212-8.
5. Nagaraja D, Murthy P. Mental health care and human rights. New Delhi: National Human Rights Commission; 2008.
6. Poreddi V, Thimmaiah R, Math SB. Human rights violations among economically disadvantaged women with mental illness: An Indian perspective. Indian J Psychiatry. 2015;57(2):174-80.
7. The Hans Foundation. (2019). National Strategy for Inclusive and Community Based Living for Persons with Mental Health Issues. [online]. Available from https://thehansfoundation.org/wp-content/uploads/2020/07/THF-National-Mental-Health-Report-Final.pdf [Last accessed December, 2023].
8. Vijayalakshmi P, Reddemma K. Does a woman with mental illness have human rights? Indian J Psy Nsg. 2013;5:47-52.
9. Trani JF, Bakhshi P, Kuhlberg J, Narayanan SS, Venkataraman H, Mishra NN, et al. Mental Illness, Poverty and Stigma in India: A Case-Control Study. BMJ Open. 2015;5(2):e006355.
10. World Health Organization. Gender and women's mental health. Gender disparities and mental health: The Facts. Geneva: World Health Organization; 2001.
11. Chandra PS, Deepthivarma S, Carey MP, Carey KB, Shalinianant MP. A cry from the darkness: women with severe mental illness in India reveal their experiences with sexual coercion. Psychiatry. 2003;66(4):323-34.
12. Chandra PS. Hidden but not forgotten: The trauma experience among women with severe mental illness and our role as mental health professionals. J Psychosoc Rehab Ment Health. 2019;6:5-8.
13. Read J, Harper D, Tucker I, Kennedy A. Do adult mental health services identify child abuse and neglect? a systematic review. Int J Mental Health Nurs. 2017;27(1):7-19.
14. James S. Abortion in India: Issues & Concerns. InHealth Laws in India 2022(pp. 196-224). Routledge.
15. Pradhan M, Dileep K, Nair A, Al Sawafi KM. Forced Surgeries in the Mentally Challenged Females: Ethical Consideration and a Narrative Review of Literature. Cureus. 2022;14(7):e26935.
16. Agoramoorthy G. Are women with mental illness & the mentally challenged adequately protected in India?. Indian J Med Res. 2011;133(5):552-4.
17. Kaur K. Implications of the Mental Healthcare Act, 2017 on the Rights of Women with Mental Illnesses in India. J Int Women's Stud. 2018;19(4):13.

18. Human Rights Watch. Treated Worse than Animals. Human Rights Watch. Available from https://www.hrw.org/report/2014/12/03/treated-worse-animals/abuses-against-women-and-girls-psychosocial-or-intellectual [Last accessed December, 2023].
19. Math SB. Addressing Concerns of Women Admitted to Psychiatric Institutions in India: An In-depth Analysis. New Delhi: National Institute of Mental Health & Neurosciences, Bangalore and National commission for Women; 2016.
20. National Women Commission. (2019). Review of Psychiatric Homes and Mental hospitals of Government Sector in India with Special Reference to the Female Patients in IPD. Available from http://ncw.nic.in/sites/default/files/Psychiatric%20Home%20Report%202019_0.pdf [Last accessed December, 2023].
21. Ministry of Women and Child Development, Government of India. (2018). Women in Prisons—India. 2018. [online]. Available from https://wcd.nic.in/sites/default/files/Prison%20Report%20Compiled.pdf [Last accessed December, 2023].
22. Kaur N, Roy S. Mental Health Status of Incarcerated Women in India: A Perspective from a Social Worker. Indian J Gend Stud. 2022;29:113-30.
23. www.indiacode.nic.in. Prisons Act. 1894. [online]. Available from https://www.indiacode.nic.in/bitstream/123456789/18475/1/prisons_act_1894.pdf [Last accessed December, 2023].
24. Kasera P. Rights of Women Prisoners in India. Available from https://ssrn.com/abstract=3621467 or http://dx.doi.org/10.2139/ssrn.3621467 [Last accessed December, 2023].
25. Math SB, Murthy P, Parthasarathy R, Kumar CN, Madhusudhan S. Mental health and substance use problems in prisons. Bangalore: NIMHANS; 2011.
26. CARE International. Women more worried about food security, mental health during humanitarian crises. Available from https://www.care-international.org/news/women-more-worried-about-food-security-mental-health-during-humanitarian-crises [Last accessed December, 2023].
27. Nanjundaswamy MH, Kumar CN, Chandra PS, Badamath S. Need for perinatal services and support during and after disasters - A viewpoint. Asian J Psychiatr. 2023;88:103731.
28. Rohwerder B. (2006). Women and girls with disabilities in conflict and crises. https://assets.publishing.service.gov.uk/media/5b9a458540f0b67866ffbd56/032-Women_and_girls_with_disabilities_in_crisis_and_conflict.pdf [Last accessed December, 2023].
29. United Nations. (2006). Convention on the Rights of Persons with Disabilities. [online]. Available from https://www.ohchr.org/en/instruments-mechanisms/instruments/convention-rights-persons-disabilities [Last accessed December, 2023].
30. Math SB, Basavaraju V, Harihara SN, Gowda GS, Manjunatha N, Kumar CN, et al. Mental Healthcare Act 2017 – Aspiration to action. Indian J Psychiatry. 2019;61(Suppl 4):S660-6.
31. Central Mental Health Authority. (2020). Mental Healthcare (Central Mental Health Authority) Regulations. [online] Available from: Mental Healthcare (Central Mental Health Authority) Regulations, 2020..pdf [Last accessed December, 2023].

32. Kaur K. Gender, Human Rights and Law: Women with mental illness in India: A healthcare and legal analysis. In: Thomas SE (Ed). Gender, Human Rights and Law. Bengaluru: National Law School of India University; 2021. pp. 95-112.
33. indiankanoon.org. Mansi vs State of Punjab and others. 2022 [online] Available from https://indiankanoon.org/doc/36958415/ [Last accessed December, 2023].
34. Menon VK. (2020). Mumbai: Woman beats mental illness to win baby back from fosterage. [online] Available from https://www.mid-day.com/mumbai/mumbai-news/article/Mumai--Woman-beats-mental-illness-to-win-baby-back-from-fosterage-23143216 [Last accessed December, 2023].
35. Chandra PS, Vinod P. Women Mental Health. India: National Human Rights Commission. 2023; pp. 9-10.
36. Sivakumar T, James J. Facilitating Aadhaar and Voting for Long-Stay Patients: Experience from a Tertiary Care Center. Indian J Psychol Med. 2019;41(5):472-5.

CHAPTER 16

Mental Health Issues among Women in Sexual Minority Groups

Debadutta Mohapatra, Aruna Yadiyal, Amrit Pattojoshi

ABSTRACT

People belonging to sexual minority groups have been shown to be suffering from significant mental health issues, which seem to be much more accentuated in the women in this group. The problem appears to be much more augmented in the milieu of poor social support, prevalent stigma and discrimination, and disparity in access to mental healthcare services. Even as research in this area is limited, this chapter tries to bring into focus the specific mental health disorders studied in this group which includes mood and anxiety disorders, psychotic disorders, sleep and sexual disorders, somatization, and suicides. Along with this, a discussion on the risk factors and protective factors, assessment and treatment considerations in this specifically vulnerable group will help in furthering our understanding on the said topic. A note at the end of the chapter tries to throw light on the Indian context of the scenario as well.

Keywords: Sexual minority, women, mental health

INTRODUCTION

The term "sexual minority" refers to a group of people whose sexual orientation, sexual identity, and/or practices diverge from mainstream of the society. This term is often used to describe individuals who are Lesbian, Gay, Bisexual, Transgender, Queer and Intersex. Though there have been definite changes in the social acceptance of LGBTQI people after the landmark judgment by honorable Supreme Court of India, mental health concerns of this group are yet to be addressed adequately. Further, factors such as poor societal support, lack of proper sexuality education, high-risk sexual behaviors, and negative psychosocial behaviors such as bullying, violence, and sexual harassment tend to augment the mental health issues. Historical trends show that increase in societal acceptance corresponds to a decrease in the age of coming out.[1] As a result, people now usually come out during a developmental period characterized by peer influence, opinion along with strong social and interpersonal regulation of gender, sexuality, and even homophobia.[2] The binary male-female dichotomy prevalent in the heteronormative societies tends to pathologize the "nonconformity" of these sexual minority groups, thus, creating immense psychological distress and "minority stress". This minority stress is a conceptual model which describes stressors embedded in the social position of individuals belonging to sexually minority groups.

MENTAL HEALTH OF THE GROUP

Lesbian, gay, bisexual, and transgender (LGBT) individuals have historically faced societal marginalization, leading to health disparities, particularly in mental health. Meyer's minority stress model explores the connection between prejudice, discrimination, and the resulting distress experienced by LGBT individuals. The model identifies unique stressors, including discrimination, concealment of sexual orientation, expectations of rejection, and internalized homophobia, as important contributors of negative mental health outcomes. The importance of coping strategies and social support within the LGBT community in mitigating these negative effects has been emphasized in studies. Additionally, Hatzenbuehler's framework integrates general psychological processes and group-specific stressors to explain the link between stigma-related stress and adverse mental health outcomes. Recent studies mention the historical context of depathologizing homosexuality but note that negative attitudes persist among some mental health professionals too. Several mental health organizations and societies have strongly opposed unethical practices like interventions to change sexual orientation or gender identity. There is also increasing importance of studying and addressing the mental health of LGBT populations through awareness, knowledge expansion, and policy interventions.[3] The concept of "double discrimination" experienced by specific subpopulations, such as bisexual individuals, ethnic minority LGB individuals, older homosexuals and transgender adults, is noteworthy. It is important to study the minority stress model in diverse cultural contexts, addressing the limitation of predominantly white/Caucasian samples in many studies, which hinders exploration of potential confounding factors related to ethnicity and sexual minority status. Additionally, the prevalence of cross-sectional designs in most studies limits the ability to infer causality.

Use of LGBTQ-inclusive policies can positively impact the mental health outcome in sexual minority populations. Long-term mental health improvements are expected in the areas where such policies are implemented. Meanwhile, individual along with community-based interventions focusing on greater LGBTQ inclusion, promoting resilience, and addressing minority stress can contribute to narrowing the gap in mental health disparities in the short- and mid-term.

Risk Factors

Universal risk factors like family conflict and substance use are found at a greater prevalence in this population along with some LGBT specific risk factors such as stigma and discrimination too.[1] Stigma and minority stress exist at individual, interpersonal, and structural levels. Individual forms of stigma include internalized homophobia/transphobia, rejection sensitivity, and concealment. Interpersonal stigma includes interactions characterized by abuse, discrimination, and rejection. Structural stigma includes state policies and institutional practices.[4] LGBT women were more likely to report harassment and feeling unwelcome and unsafe than non-LGBT women. Some LGBT women also reported of delayed or missed care with lack of interaction with other veterans. These findings point toward interventions that could help LGBT women to feel more safe and welcome at care facilities, thereby, reducing the barriers to access needed care.[5]

There are various psychosocial and psychophysiological mechanisms underlying stigma and minority stress that impairs LGBT mental health.

- *Vigilance:* Experiences with stigma make individuals more vigilant in anticipating and avoiding stigmatizing situations. Perceptual vigilance, linked to cardiovascular effects in the general population, is heightened in sexual minority individuals, impacting mental health, particularly leading to depressive symptoms.
- *Rumination:* Repeated encounters with stigma and stressors can lead to rumination, a maladaptive emotion regulation strategy. Sexual minority individuals, especially adolescents and adults, tend to ruminate more than their heterosexual counterparts and this is associated with psychological distress in them.
- *Loneliness:* Stigma and minority stressors may increase feelings of loneliness, affecting interpersonal relationships and they may experience heightened loneliness, introversion, psychological distress, and social anxiety.
- *Internalized homophobia:* Internalized homophobia refers to the negative feelings and beliefs that the persons who identify as LGBTQ+ may have about themselves, their identity, and their place in society because of societal attitudes and discrimination. The constant struggle to reconcile one's sexual orientation with societal expectations can lead to chronic stress and emotional distress. It can lead to feelings of shame, guilt, and self-hatred. This internal conflict can manifest in various mental health issues such as depression, anxiety, low self-esteem, and even suicidal thoughts. The association between internalized homophobia and depression emphasizes the need to address the internalized homophobia while treating or preventing depression.[6]

A systematic review of qualitative studies found 5 core themes in relation to challenges of mental health faced by sexual and gender minority (GM) youth including (1). isolation, rejection, phobia, and need for support, (2) Depression, self-harm, and suicidality, (3) Marginalization, (4) Connectedness, (5) Policy and environment.[7]

Physiologic Mechanisms Related to Stress Response

Stigma along with existing minority stress impacts the hypothalamic-pituitary-adrenal (HPA) axis, affecting cortisol regulation. Chronic stress leads to HPA axis dysregulation and which in turn is associated with the negative health outcomes like cardiovascular disease and diabetes. Structural stigma during adolescence may result in a blunted cortisol response to stressors in adulthood among sexual minority individuals.

In summary, stigma and minority stress influence cognitive processes, emotional regulation, loneliness, and physiologic mechanisms, all of which contribute to the overall adverse health outcomes in LGBT individuals.

Protective Factors

The journey of LGBT youth into adulthood is also marked by resilience and positive development, although research has primarily focused on risks rather than protective factors. This discussion highlights various contextual elements that affirm the identities of LGBT youths, encompassing aspects such as school policies, family acceptance, dating experiences, and the process of coming out.

Studies consistently emphasize the positive impact of supportive school environments on the mental health of LGBT youth. States with comprehensive antibullying laws that include sexual orientation and gender identity witness significantly lower rates of homophobic victimization. Additionally, Gay-Straight alliances (GSAs) in schools play a crucial role in fostering a sense of safety, reducing depressive symptoms, substance use, and suicidal thoughts among LGBT students. Beyond school policies inclusive curriculums that incorporate LGBT-related content have been associated with improved psychological adjustment in LGBT students. Training for teachers, staff, and administrators on LGBT issues also contributes to a more supportive school environment.

Interpersonal relationships, both within families and peer groups, significantly influence the well-being of LGBT youth. Support from parents, friends, and communities, especially in acknowledging and affirming one's sexual orientation and gender identity, is linked to positive mental health outcomes.[8]

Despite societal challenges, romantic relationships are recognized as important developmental experiences for LGBT adolescents. Overcoming social barriers related to dating same-sex partners is crucial for their well-being, as studies show that such relationships are associated with improved mental health and lower substance use.

The process of coming out, while potentially exposing youth to harassment and the loss of friends, has positive long-term effects. Those who come out in high school, despite facing higher risks of victimization, report lower levels of depression and greater overall well-being in young adulthood.

In summary, a combination of supportive school environment, inclusive curriculums, interpersonal support, healthy dating experiences, and the process of coming out contribute to the positive development in this population.

SPECIFIC DISORDERS IN LESBIAN, GAY, BISEXUAL, AND TRANSGENDER GROUP

Depression and Anxiety Disorder

Depression is a significant issue in the LGBTQIA+ community affecting individuals at higher rates than general population.[3] The risk of depression is twice as high for lesbian, gay, and bisexual women than rest of the population. The risk was found to be four times higher for trans people. A study by Stonewall found that half of LGBTIQ+ people had experienced depression, and three in five had experienced anxiety. LGBTQIA++ youth had 1.75 times more anxiety and depression as those of the rest of society, while transgender community is more vulnerable as they suffer 2.4 times higher anxiety and depression.[2] Studies have shown that 30-60% of LGBT women deal with anxiety and depression at some point during their lives. It is around 1.5-2.5 times higher than that of their gender-conforming counterparts. The high levels of anxiety in the LGBT community can be attributed to the experience of being a minority group facing discrimination and prejudice daily. The continual threats to housing and job security, need for hiding one's own identity, leading an unwanted double life, lack of social and emotional support from families, the long-term effects of bullying, violence, and gradual reduction in self-esteem contribute to intensified levels of anxiety in LGBT. Prevalence of lifetime mental health disorder is likely to be more than twice in LGBTQ individuals as compared to the heterosexual women with 2.5 times more likelihood of depression, anxiety, and substance misuse compared with heterosexual individuals.[9-11]

Psychotic Disorders

The recently conducted GROUP study concluded that there is an elevated rate of "psychotic disorders" particularly nonaffective psychotic disorders (NAPD).[12] Chakraborty et al. (2011) found elevated rates of psychotic disorders in nonheterosexual individuals (3.75 unadjusted odds ratio).[12] Gevonden et al. (2014) in Netherlands found elevated rates of psychotic symptoms in the LGB population compared with heterosexuals during two consecutive periods (NEMESIS-1 and NEMESIS-2).[13] Chakraborty et al. (2011) found elevated rates of psychotic disorders in nonheterosexual individuals (3.75 unadjusted odds ratio).[14]

Sleep Disorders

There is paucity of well-established body of literature specifically addressing sleep disorders in sexual minorities. Sleep disorders in this particular group can be explained though from the interconnected nature of ongoing chronic stress, mental health conditions and its impact on sleep, where disruptions in one domain can adversely affect the other,[15] and the understanding of this relationship could be just evolving.

Sexual Disorders

According to the report by National Institute of Medicine in 2011, individuals in the LGBT community face elevated hate crimes, risks of violence, and sexually transmitted infections (STIs). Sexual and reproductive health (SRH) disparities among LGBT individuals are often discussed in relation to their sexual orientation, emphasizing the unique SRH healthcare needs of each subgroup.[16] Lesbian and bisexual (LB) women frequently experience challenges within the healthcare system, with their SRH needs often inadequately addressed compared to those of heterosexual women.[17] Research suggests that LB women face higher risks of STIs, unwanted pregnancies, sexual violence, and partner violence than heterosexual women. They are also more likely to use emergency contraceptives and pregnancy prevention methods and receive SRH services.[18-21] Bisexual women may face additional risks, such as having multiple partners and engaging in intercourse with partners who use drugs.[22] LB women are also reported to undergo screenings for colon, breast, and cervical cancers less frequently than their heterosexual counterparts, often due to fears of inadequate health services.[20,21,23]

Transgender individuals, even after completing gender transition, may carry health risks associated with their assigned gender at birth. For instance, transgender women with a history of prostate cancer in their family are at risk and require prostate examinations. Similarly, transgender men, despite undergoing breast reduction surgery, may still have residual breast tissue and need mammography screening for breast cancer. Most transgender men also have a cervix and should be screened for cervical cancer.[24]

The role of healthcare professionals is crucial in addressing the unique SRH needs of LGBT individuals. Unfortunately, studies indicate that homophobic or transphobic attitudes among healthcare providers, along with discomfort in serving LGBT individuals, and a lack of knowledge and clinical experience in addressing SRH problems specific to this population, hinder the provision of adequate healthcare services.[20] The predominant focus of SRH services on heterosexual individuals may further contribute to the oversight of the distinct healthcare needs of LGBT individuals, despite evidence that these needs differ significantly from those of heterosexual individuals.

Suicide

Research links underlying mental disorders like depression and bipolar disorder to an increased risk of suicide attempts and thoughts of suicide among sexual minority (SM) populations.[16,25-27] A cohort study found that the reported likelihood of suicide attempts among trans-women was five times greater than that of heterosexuals, with a 19 times greater probability compared to completed suicides.[28] Inclusion issues in research and the frequent incorrect use of the term SM further complicate accessing relevant information.[29] Further, there is a compelling need for multidirectional studies and evidence-based research, which focused on suicide ideation and attempts in sexual minorities to produce high levels of evidence to help effective interventions in this area.[30,31] Analyzing an unpublished National Epidemiologic Survey on Alcohol and Related Conditions (NESARC) analysis by Haas et al., after adjusting for psychiatric disorders, suicide attempt rates among SM individuals were generally two to three times higher than those of heterosexual participants.[31] This could be attributed to these populations facing discrimination, stigmatization, violence, and rejection, resulting in elevated stress levels.[30,32] Many SM individuals report encountering homophobic abuse, violence, or discrimination, and research indicates that LGBT youth often experience minority-related stress in schools.[33] Those who routinely face discrimination due to their gender identity and perceive their identity as under attack are more prone to suicidal thoughts and behaviors. Another health-related challenge is that many SM individuals fear discrimination, and believe that they cannot access the psychiatric help they need, thus leading to dissatisfaction with available services.[34]

Somatization Disorder

We could find some research, scattered across time and ethnicities, which specifically mentioned somatization, which included somatic complaints, body-related distress, various pains including migraine and headache, and decreased functionality and physical health which affected the quality of life of the sexually minority groups in a negative way. Fibromyalgia and related somatic symptoms such as physical pain, fatigue, and impaired general health were found to be highly prevalent in this group.[35] Significantly, higher levels of somatization were found along with depression and anxiety in a group of young transgender women who were also survivors of intimate partner violence. Around 27.5% of the transgender population samples in the USA in an online survey done in 2013 had somatization, along with depression (44.1%) and anxiety (33.2%).[36,37] A systemic review, done in 2020, on 26 studies provided substantial evidence supporting the relationship between minority stress in SMs and biological outcomes which included overall physical health, immune responses, human immunodeficiency virus

(HIV)-specific, cancer-related and hormonal outcomes, all of which can present with somatic complaints.[38] A study done on Latinos showed positive correlation between minority stress and somatization, anxiety, and hostility.[39] In a sample of 477 SM women who had posttraumatic stress disorder (PTSD), social support, and SM status were interactive and the association was significant for somatic complaints and functional impairment.[40] A recent study done on 2,104 bisexual women showed that micro-aggressions of any type were associated with same-day increase in somatic complaints and negative affect.[41] Data from a national health interview survey done in the USA from 2013 to 2018, showed prevalence of migraines and headache to be the highest in bisexual women (36.8%) followed by lesbians (24.7%), bisexual women (22.8%), and gay men (14.8%) when compared to their heterosexual counter parts (9.8-19.7%).[42] Data from a Midlife in US Study (MIDUS) showed that individuals belonging to SM groups had increased levels of C-reactive protein and interleukin-6, both biological markers of inflammation, when compared to heterosexuals after controlling for age, race, gender, and education and these differences were partially explained by perceptions of discrimination.[43] A higher prevalence of migraine and more worse physical health outcomes were noted in adults belonging to sexual minority groups in a year-long study done on national representative sample of the US adults.[44] A 13-year-old review study done on 332 male-to-female transgenders undergoing gender reassignment surgery in Brazil showed a great number of surgical adverse events such as meatal stenosis, vaginal strictures, and healing disorders (3-40%), with preserved functionality, which could explain the occurrence of somatic complaints in them.[45] One-third of the 232 patients who underwent male-to-female sex reassignment surgery, in a study, reported of urinary stream problems and were least satisfied with vaginal lubrication, touch and erotic sensation, which could manifest as somato-sexual complaints.[46] Statistically significant dose-response relationship was present between daily and lifetime perceived discrimination, psychological distress, and chronic pain in those discriminated for their sexual orientation and gender nonconformation.[47] Pelvic pain was found to be a common condition in female to male transgender persons at any point in the transition process which could be multifactorial according to a recent study.[48] A recently reported case report published in 2021 revealed somatic symptoms of arthralgia, myalgia, headache, and fatigue to be veiling gender dysphoria in an adolescent.[49]

■ FACTORS CONTRIBUTING TO MENTAL HEALTH CONCERNS

Psychosocial Factors

Studies revealed that childhood trauma, bullying in adolescence, and lifetime discrimination were factors mediating the association between LBG status and affective or psychotic disorders. The indirect effects of these factors were significant with bullying showing a smaller effect compared to childhood trauma and discrimination. LBG individuals may also experience increased psychological strain due to social adversity leading to the formation of biased cognitive schemas exacerbated by having an "outsider status".

Neurodevelopmental and Biological Mechanisms

Exposure to social stressors during critical periods of brain development is hypothesized to lead to sensitization, resulting in a permanent excess of basal presynaptic transmission of dopamine, potentially increasing the risk for psychosis and thereby secondary disturbed emotional states.

Importance of Sexual Identity Disclosure

Sexual identity disclosure has been shown to improve the overall mental health of LBG individuals, and those who have disclosed their sexual preference may experience lower cortisol levels and fewer psychiatric symptoms.

Challenges in Establishing a Steadfast Sense of Self

Difficulties in establishing a steadfast sense of self have also been reported, and the study suggests that LBG individuals who face victimization as children may be deprived of the developmental conditions needed for healthy identity and body-image formation.

■ ASSESSMENT OF PSYCHIATRIC DISORDERS

Assessing mental health disorders within the sexual minority group involves careful consideration of unique stressors, experiences, and vulnerabilities that may contribute to psychological challenges. The process requires a culturally competent and inclusive approach that recognizes the impact of societal attitudes, discrimination, and stigma specific to sexual orientation. Here are key aspects to consider in the assessment of mental health disorders within the sexual minority group:

Cultural Competence

Mental health professionals should be culturally competent and knowledgeable about the diverse experiences within the sexual minority community. Understanding the terminology, identities, and unique stressors is essential for effective assessment. Being aware of the impact of intersectionality—how various identities such as race, gender, and socioeconomic status intersect with sexual orientation—helps in understanding the complexity of individuals' experiences.

Creating a Safe and Affirming Environment

Establishing a safe and affirming therapeutic environment is crucial. Creating a space where individuals feel comfortable disclosing their sexual orientation fosters trust and openness during the assessment process. Avoiding assumptions about heteronormativity and using inclusive language helps to validate diverse identities within the sexual minority community.

Understanding Minority Stress

Recognizing the impact of minority stress on mental health is essential. This includes stressors related to stigma, discrimination, and prejudice specific to sexual orientation. Understanding the concept of internalized homophobia—negative beliefs and attitudes directed inward based on societal stigma—helps in assessing the internal struggles individuals may face.

Assessment Tools and Measures

Utilizing assessment tools that are inclusive and sensitive to sexual minority experiences is important. General mental health measures may be complemented by instruments designed to capture the unique stressors faced by this population. Assessment tools may cover a range of mental health domains, including anxiety, depression, substance use, and suicidal ideation. It is beneficial to use instruments validated for diverse sexual orientations.

Intersectionality in Assessment

Considering the intersectionality of identities is critical. For example, experiences of discrimination may vary based on both sexual orientation and racial or ethnic identity. Intersectional approaches acknowledge the complexity of individuals' lives and contribute to a more nuanced understanding of mental health challenges within the sexual minority group.

Counselor Sensitivity and Training

Mental health professionals should undergo training to enhance their sensitivity and competence in working with sexual minority clients. This includes staying informed about current research, policy changes, and best practices in LGBTQ+ mental health. Continuing education on sexual orientation-related issues is essential for mental health professionals to provide effective and affirming care.

Assessing Resilience and Coping Mechanisms

Evaluating individuals' resilience and coping mechanisms are crucial. Some sexual minorities may develop strong coping strategies and support networks that contribute to their mental well-being. Understanding the role of community connections, chosen families, and other sources of support helps in assessing protective factors.

Regular Monitoring and Follow-up

Mental health assessments should not be one-time events. Regular monitoring and follow-up are essential to track changes in mental health status and to adjust interventions accordingly. Creating an ongoing dialogue with clients helps in addressing emerging mental health concerns and adapting treatment plans as needed.

In summary, a comprehensive assessment of mental health disorders in the sexual minority group requires a holistic and culturally competent approach. By considering the unique stressors, strengths, and diverse identities within this community, mental health professionals can contribute to more effective and affirmative mental health care for sexual minority individuals.[50,51]

■ TREATMENT CONSIDERATIONS

In 2011, the Institute of Medicine (IOM) highlighted the health disparities faced by sexual minorities, and Healthy People 2020 emphasized the need to address sexual orientation-based health disparities. Interventions are necessary at different levels.

Intraindividual Level (Heterosexual Individuals)

Here the emphasis is on reducing prejudice and enhancing allyship among heterosexual individuals to address experiences of stigma and their impact on mental health. Strategies include intergroup contact, perspective-taking, and empathy.

Interpersonal Level (Organizations and Communities)

Facilitating education and positive intergroup dynamics in organizations, particularly in educational settings, is recommended at this level. Creating safe spaces like GSAs can contribute to better psychological functioning among sexual minority youth. Additionally, fostering community connectedness and protecting local LGBTQ resources are crucial.

Institutional Level (Academic and Legal Structures)

At this level, it is encouraged to enhance research attention to diversify the representation of sexual minorities in disparities research and to redefine measures of prejudice to capture modern manifestations. Also, legal protections, including the expansion of civil rights, inclusive family policies, and religious freedom bills that promote equality help in effective interventions.

The effectiveness of an intervention, proud and empowered, in addressing minority stress and improving mental health among SM and GM adolescents was found in a randomized controlled trial conducted in four high schools reported significant reductions in minority stress, anxiety, and depressive symptoms compared to the control group. The intervention is a 10-session therapy, each of 45 minutes addressing various issues. Furthermore, the intervention moderated the relationship between minority stress and symptoms of PTSD, depression, and suicidality, indicating that it helped to mitigate the negative impact of stress on mental health outcomes.[52] In another study it was seen that in a contact intervention, led by LGBT educators, involving discussion, personal stories, and interaction activities resulted in significant reduction in modern LGBT negativity immediately postintervention and at follow-up. However, it had limited impact on old-fashioned prejudice, attitudes toward public displays of affection, and gender nonconformity.[53] However, there is a need for social action to address sexual stigma and health disparities, with a focus on well-intentioned individuals, organizations, communities, researchers, and policymakers taking directed steps to bring about positive change. Healthcare professionals also lack adequate knowledge about this and which in turn adds to the stigma and discrimination and peer healthcare deliveries to these groups. Proper training of the healthcare providers and development of treatment guidelines are thus the need of the hour.[50]

■ INDIAN CONTEXT

LGBTQ+ youth in the Indian subcontinent face various mental health issues. Some of the challenges they encounter include a discord between gender identity and societal expectations, poor self and social acceptance of their sexual orientation, verbal, physical, and sexual abuse from friends, family, and peers, discrimination, loneliness, fear of law enforcement, and a lack of coping mechanisms. Adverse childhood events, such as experiences of sexual violence, also contribute to their mental health struggles. However, the lack of standardized statistics and research on LGBTQ+ health status in India hinders a comprehensive understanding of their specific mental health needs.[54] A content review from 2009 to 2019 reveals that LGBTQIA+ individuals showed high rates of mental health concerns. The adapted minority stress model may explain and stand out as a crucial pathway for the above. Factors related to mental well-being, one's lived experiences, and societal attitudes have also a strong impact. Relatively lesser interventional studies and less representation of certain groups of LGBT women in the research are also some contributors.[55,56]

Women belonging to sexual minority groups form a special vulnerable cohort who tend to experience "minority stress" which predisposes them to intense psychological pressures, both from within and from external sources. The heteronormative societies, in which these women have to live, tend to pathologize the "nonconformity" of these sexual minority groups, thus creating an unfavorable milieu of poor support, stigma, discrimination, and disparity toward mental healthcare access. Various psychosocial and psychophysiological mechanisms underlying stigma and minority stress such as vigilance, ruminations, loneliness, and internalized homophobia tend to impair LGBT mental health, leading to increased prevalence of depression, anxiety, psychotic disorders, sleep and sexual disorders, somatization disorders, and finally may end fatally in suicides. Many psychosocial factors and neurodevelopmental and biological mechanisms lie behind these adverse mental health outcomes, necessitating a comprehensive assessment and a holistic and culturally competent approach toward this group. Interventions at intraindividual level of both heterosexuals and homosexuals, interpersonal level of organizations and communities, and institutional level of academic and legal structures are necessary to counter the unique stressors, strengths, and diverse identities within this community, through which, mental health professionals can contribute to more effective and affirmative mental healthcare for women in this minority group.

> **KEY POINTS**
> - Women in sexual minority group used to face a lot of challenges like poor social support, stigma discrimination, and disparity in getting mental healthcare.
> - Although there is less availability of research, studies are suggestive of higher prevalence of mental health conditions in this group.
> - Adequate planning of policy and development of guideline is a key step.
> - Training of healthcare providers is the need of the hour.
> - Awareness in the society and inclusion in the society are two welcome steps.

REFERENCES

1. Russell ST, Fish JN. Mental health in lesbian, gay, bisexual, and transgender (LGBT) youth. Ann rev clin psychol. 2016;12:465-87.
2. Yarns BC, Abrams JM, Meeks TW, Sewell DD. The Mental Health of Older LGBT Adults. Curr Psychiatry Rep. 2016;18(6):60.
3. Wilson C, Cariola LA. LGBTQI+ Youth and Mental Health: A Systematic Review of Qualitative Research. Adolescent Res Rev. 2020;5:187-211.
4. Akré ER, Anderson A, Stojanovski K, Chung KW, Van Kim NA, Chae DH. Depression, Anxiety, and Alcohol Use Among LGBTQ+ People During the COVID-19 Pandemic. Am J Public Health. 2021;111(9):1610-9.

5. Shipherd JC, Darling JE, Klap RS, Rose D, Yano EM. Experiences in the Veterans Health Administration and Impact on Healthcare Utilization: Comparisons Between LGBT and Non-LGBT Women Veterans. LGBT Health. 2018;5(5):303-11.
6. Yolaç E, Meriç M. Internalized homophobia and depression levels in LGBT individuals. Perspect Psychiatr Care. 2021;57(1):304-10.
7. Johnson B, Leibowitz S, Chavez A, Herbert SE. Risk Versus Resiliency: Addressing Depression in Lesbian, Gay, Bisexual, and Transgender Youth. Child Adolesc Psychiatr Clin N Am. 2019;28(3):509-21.
8. Ryan C, Russell ST, Huebner D, Diaz R, Sanchez J. Family acceptance in adolescence and the health of LGBT young adults. J Child Adolesc Psychiatr Nurs. 2010;23(4):205-13.
9. Killen M, Hitti A, Mulvey KL. Social development and intergroup relations. In: Mikulincer M, Shaver PR, Dovidio JF, Simpson JA (Eds). APA Handbook of Personality and Social Psychology, Vol. 2. Group processes. United States: American Psychological Association. 2015. pp. 177-201.
10. Hatzenbuehler ML, Pachankis JE. Stigma and minority stress as social determinants of health among lesbian, gay, bisexual, and transgender youth: Research evidence and clinical implications. Pediatr Clin. 2016;63(6):985-97.
11. Mongelli F, Perrone D, Balducci J, Sacchetti A, Ferrari S, Mattei G, et al. Minority stress and mental health among LGBT populations: An update on the evidence. Minerva Psichiatrica. 2019;60(1):27-50.
12. Post D, Veling W. Sexual minority status, social adversity and risk for psychotic disorders-results from the GROUP study. Psychol med. 2021;51(5):770-6.
13. Gevonden MJ., Selten JP, Myin-Germeys I, de Graaf R, ten Have M, van Dorsselaer S, et al. Sexual minority status and psychotic symptoms: Findings from the Netherlands mental health survey and incidence studies (NEMESIS). Psychol Med. 2014; 44(2):421-33.
14. Chakraborty A, McManus S, Brugha TS, Bebbington P, King M. Mental health of the non-heterosexual population of England. Br J Psychiatry. 2011;198(2):143-8.
15. Patterson CJ, Potter EC. Sexual orientation and sleep difficulties: a review of research. Sleep Health. 2019;5(3):227-35.
16. Taşkın L, Erenel AŞ, Sözbir ŞY, Gönenç İM, Yücel Ç, Dikmen HA, et al. Sexual health/reproductive health-related problems of lesbian, gay, bisexual and transgender people in Turkey and their health-care needs. Florence Nightingale J Nurs. 2020;28(1):97.
17. Munson S, Cook C. Lesbian and bisexual women's sexual healthcare experiences. J Clin Nurs. 2016;25(23-24):3497-510.
18. Agénor M, Krieger N, Austin SB, Haneuse S, Gottlieb BR. At the intersection of sexual orientation, race/ethnicity, and cervical cancer screening: assessing Pap test use disparities by sex of sexual partners among black, Latina, and white US women. Soc Sci Med. 2014;116:110-8.
19. Mc Lafferty M, Ross J, Waterhouse-Bradley B, Armour C. Childhood adversities and psychopathology among military veterans in the US: the mediating role of social networks. J Anxiety Disord. 2019;65:47-55.
20. Marrazzo JM, Stine K. Reproductive health history of lesbians: implications for care. Am J Obstet Gynecol. 2004;190(5):1298-304.

21. Ward BW, Dahlhamer JM, Galinsky AM, Joestl SS. Sexual orientation and health among U.S. adults: national health interview survey, 2013. Natl Health Stat Report. 2014;(77):1-10.
22. Estrich CG, Gratzer B, Hotton AL. Differences in sexual health, risk behaviors, and substance use among women by sexual identity: Chicago, 2009-2011. Sex Transm Dis. 2014;41(3):194-9.
23. Blosnich JR, Mays VM, Cochran SD. Suicidality among veterans: implications of sexual minority status. Am J Public Health. 2014;104(Suppl 4):S535-7.
24. Cahill S, Makadon H. Sexual Orientation and Gender Identity Data Collection in Clinical Settings and in Electronic Health Records: A Key to Ending LGBT Health Disparities. LGBT Health. 2014;1(1):34-41.
25. Pepping CA, Lyons A, McNair R, Kirby JN, Petrocchi N, Gilbert P. A tailored compassion-focused therapy program for sexual minority young adults with depressive symotomatology: study protocol for a randomized controlled trial. BMC Psychol. 2017;5:5.
26. Cochran SD, Mays VM, Sullivan JG. Prevalence of mental disorders, psychological distress, and mental health services use among lesbian, gay, and bisexual adults in the United States. J Consult Clin Psychol. 2003;71(1):53-61.
27. Schneeberger AR, Dietl MF, Muenzenmaier KH, Huber CG, Lang UE. Stressful childhood experiences and health outcomes in sexual minority populations: a systematic review. Soc Psychiatry Psychiatr Epidemiol. 2014;49(9):1427-45.
28. Dhejne C, Lichtenstein P, Boman M, Johansson AL, Långström N, Landén M. Long-term follow-up of transsexual persons undergoing sex reassignment surgery: cohort study in Sweden. PLoS One. 2011;6(2):e16885.
29. Muller A, Hughes TL. Making the invisible visible: a systematic review of sexual minority women's health in Southern Africa. BMC Pub Health. 2016;16:307.
30. Barboza GE, Dominguez S, Chance E. Physical victimization, gender identity and suicide risk among transgender men and women. Prev Med Rep. 2016;4:385-90.
31. Haas AP, Eliason M, Mays VM, Mathy RM, Cochran SD, D'Augelli AR, et al. Suicide and suicide risk in lesbian, gay, bisexual, and transgender populations: review and recommendations. J Homosex. 2011;58(1):10-51.
32. Nuttbrock L, Hwahng S, Bockting W, Rosenblum A, Mason M, Macri M, et al. Psychiatric impact of gender-related abuse across the life course of male-to-female transgender persons. J Sex Res. 2010;47(1):12-23.
33. Greytak EA, Kosciw JG, Diaz EM. Harsh Realities: The Experiences of Transgender Youth in Our Nation's Schools. New York: Gay, Lesbian and Straight Education Network (GLSEN); 2009.
34. Zimmer-Gembeck MJ, Webb HJ, Pepping CA, Swan K, Merlo O, Skinner EA, et al. Review: Is Parent–Child Attachment a Correlate of Children's Emotion Regulation and Coping? Int J Behav Develop. 2017;41(1):74-93.
35. Levit D, Yaish I, Shtrozberg S, Aloush V, Greenman Y, Ablin JN. Pain and transition: Evaluating fibromyalgia in TG individual. Clin Exp Rheumatol. 2021;39-130(3):27-32.
36. Garthe RC, Hidalgo MA, Goffnett J, Hereth J, Garofalo R, Reisner SL, et al. Young transgender women survivors of IPV: A latent class analysis of protective processers. Psychol Sexual Orient Gender divers. 2020;7(4):386.

37. Bockting WO, Miner MH, Swinburne Romine RE, Hamilton A, Coleman E. Stigma, Mental health and resilience in an online sample of US TG Population. Am J Public Health. 2013;103(5):943-51.
38. Flentje A, Heck NC, Brennan JM, Meyer IH. The relationship between Minority stress and biological outcomes: A systematic review. J Beh Med. 2020;43(5):673-94.
39. Alamilla SG, Kim BSK, Lam NA. Acculturation, Enculturation, perceived racism, minority status stress and psychological symptomatology among Latinos. Hispanic J Beh sciences. 2010;32(1):55-76.
40. Weiss BJ, Garvert DW, Cloitre M. PTSD and Trauma related difficulties in SM women: The impact of perceived social support. J Traumatic stress. 2015;28(6):563-71.
41. Smith AU, Bostwick WB, Burke L, Hequembourg A, Santuzzi A, Hughes T, et al. How deep is the cut? The interaction of daily micro aggressions on bisexual women's health. Psychol Sex Orient Gender Divers. Advance online publication. 2022.
42. Heslin KC. Explaining disparities in severe headache and migraine among sexual minority adults in the US, 2013-2018. J Nerv Mental dis. 2020;208(11):876.
43. Wardecker BM, Graham-Engeland JE, Almeida DM. Perceived discrimination predicts elevated biological markers of inflammation among sexual minority adults. J Beh Med. 2021;44(1):53-6.
44. Nagata JM, Ganson KT, Tabler J, Blashill AJ, Murray SB. Disparities across sexual orientation in Migraine, among US adults. JAMA Neurol. 2021;78(1):117-8.
45. Neto RR, Hintz F, Krege S, Rubben H, VanDorp F. Gender reassignment surgery: A 13-year review of surgical outcomes. Int Braz J Urol. 2012;38(1):97-107.
46. Lawrence AA. Patient reported complications and functional outcomes of male to female sex reassignment surgery. Arch sex Beh. 2006;35(6):717-27.
47. Brown TT, Partanen J, Chuong L, Villaverde V, Chantal Griffin A, Mendelson A. Discrimination hurts: The effect of discrimination as development of chronic pain. Soc sci Med. 2018;204:1-8.
48. Moulder JK, Carillo J, Carey ET. Pelvic pain in the transgender man. Curr Obstet Gynaecol Rep. 2020;9:138-45.
49. Morabito G, Cosentini D, Tornese G, Gortani G, Pastore S, Genovese MRL, et al. Case report: Somatic symptoms veiling gender dysphoria in an adolescent. Front Pediatr. 2021;28(9):679004.
50. Santos GM, Ikeda J, Coffin P, Walker J, Matheson T, Ali A, et al. Targeted Oral Naltrexone for Mild to Moderate Alcohol Use Disorder Among Sexual and Gender Minority Men: A Randomized Trial. Am J Psychiatry. 2022;179(12):915-26.
51. Matthews AK, Steffen AD, Kuhns LM, Ruiz RA, Ross NA, Burke LA, et al. Evaluation of a Randomized Clinical Trial Comparing the Effectiveness of a Culturally Targeted and Nontargeted Smoking Cessation Intervention for Lesbian, Gay, Bisexual, and Transgender Smokers. Nicotine Tob Res. 2019;21(11):1506-16.
52. Cramwinckel FM, Scheepers DT, Wilderjans TF, de Rooij RB. Assessing the Effects of a Real-Life Contact Intervention on Prejudice Toward LGBT People. Arch Sex Behav. 2021;50(7):3035-51.

53. Vargas SM, Wennerstrom A, Alfaro N, Belin T, Griffith K, Haywood C, et al. Resilience Against Depression Disparities (RADD): a protocol for a randomised comparative effectiveness trial for depression among predominantly low-income, racial/ethnic, sexual and gender minorities. BMJ Open. 2019;9(10):e031099.
54. Gaur PS, Saha S, Goel A, Ovseiko P, Aggarwal S, Agarwal V, et al. Mental healthcare for young and adolescent LGBTQ+ individuals in the Indian subcontinent. Front Psychol. 2023;14:1060543.
55. Wandrekar JR, Nigudkar AS. What Do We Know About LGBTQIA+ Mental Health in India? A Review of Research From 2009 to 2019. J Psychosexual Health. 2020;2(1):26-36.
56. Pai NM, Naik SS, Kumar CN, Badamath S (Eds). Manual on Mental health care of Transgender persons in India. NIMHANS publication no: 205. Bengaluru: National Institute of Mental Health and Neurosciences; 2021.

CHAPTER 17: Sexual Violence: Mental Health Consequences and Interventions

Arunashree B, Abhilasha Das, Veena A Satyanarayana

ABSTRACT

Sexual violence (SV) is a serious violation of human rights, and it can occur across all age groups, resulting in both physical and mental scars. This chapter provides a holistic understanding of the prevalence, mental health consequences, and interventions for sexual violence. When interviewing survivors, it is important to broaden the assessment with the understanding of contextual factors, including protective factors that influence recovery. Further, our approach to intervention needs to be more comprehensive to incorporate medical and legal services along with enhancing community/social support. The chapter also discusses specialized interventions for psychological recovery from a trauma-informed perspective.

Keywords: Sexual violence, mental health outcomes, psychological interventions

INTRODUCTION

Violence against women is identified as a public mental health problem,[1] with a bidirectional association between violence against women and mental disorders, such as depression, substance use, post-traumatic stress, and suicidal behavior.[2] While violence can be a predisposing or triggering factor for the onset of mental illness, and ongoing violence a maintaining factor of mental illness, women with preexisting psychiatric illnesses are also at an increased risk of violence victimization.

Sexual violence (SV) can be defined through a public health lens as well as from a legal standpoint since it is a punishable offense.[3,4] In the Indian Penal Code, laws related to sexual violence use the terminologies of rape (Sections 376, 376A, 376B, 376C, and 376D), sexual harassment (Section 354A), domestic violence which includes sexual violence by partner (Section 398A), and assault to outrage one's modesty (Section 354 and 354B).[5]

PREVALENCE OF SEXUAL VIOLENCE

Sexual violence is one of the most common types of violence against women. Globally, 27% of ever-partnered women aged 15–49 years are estimated to have experienced physical or sexual, or both types of intimate partner violence (IPV) in their lifetime, with 13% experiencing it in the past year.[6]

In India, the National Family Health Survey 5 (2019–2021) reported that 6% of women aged between 18 and 49 years have experienced sexual violence in their lifetime. Among married survivors of sexual violence, 83% report the perpetrator to be the current husband, and 13% report a former husband.[7] 20% of women with severe mental illness reported experiencing IPV, including emotional, physical, and sexual violence, in the past year.[8]

Two meta-analyses showed the global prevalence rate of sexual violence victimization, including digital sexual violence, among higher education students to be ranging between 7.2 and 17.4%.[9,10] A study in New Zealand[11] found that among people with disabilities (physical, intellectual, or psychological), 11.1% experienced lifetime nonpartner sexual violence. The pooled sexual violence rate against female children was found to be 0.24 [95% confidence interval (CI): 0.20-0.27] in the meta-analysis by Qu et al. 2022.[12]

Characteristics of Sexual Violence

Although the legal definitions of sexual violence vary according to the laws of the country, most legal codes recognize that the use of physical force, intimidation, and lack of consent constitutes a crime.[13] It is essential to understand its patterns and characteristics to provide appropriate care for recovery, as this information should aid our clinical assessments and judgment about the known and unknown impact of such violations over one's overall well-being in a sensitive manner.

Type of Sexual Contact

Any sexual act, oral, vaginal or anal penetration, and nonpenetrative acts, inflicted without the consent of an individual are categorized as sex crimes worldwide. However, other acts that get subtly discarded as nonserious offenses such as stalking, sexual remarks, and harassment can also leave a victim with lasting psychological distress and fear of safety. As mental health professionals (MHPs) we must broaden our assessment to include contextual factors, like the setting where violence occurred, the relationship with the perpetrator, and the type of coercion in order to have a nuanced understanding of this complex phenomenon.

■ CONTEXTUAL FACTORS

Setting

Few studies in this area showed that assault occurring in a private setting (e.g., at home) were associated with lower perceptions of postassault safety and found that socioenvironmental contexts such as assault setting (intimate spaces) and intoxication at the time of the assault have a higher contribution to the current psychological distress. This throws light on the maintaining factors for psychological distress from such traumatic experiences which highly rely on the context in which the offense took place, and associated cues rather than the characteristics of the assault alone.[14,15]

Relationship with Perpetrator

Studies have found that assault by strangers was associated with greater postassault fear, anxiety, and post-traumatic stress disorder (PTSD). Whereas, a known perpetrator significantly increases the risk of postassault psychological impact, in terms of interpersonal relationships and self-concept due to the complexities of betrayal and trust. Prior sexual experiences with a perpetrator have been found to have varied impacts on distress based on past and present reports.[13,15]

TYPES OF COERCION

Coercion here could range from verbal threats to forcing on an individual who is not in the state of giving consent, such as an intoxicated state. Studies have revealed that actively forced sex either through physical force, ignoring direct refusals, or physical force by threatening, suffered the most with negative thoughts about self and societal blame compared to other coercion tactic groups, such as incapacitated and situations coercion.[16] Physical violence involved in rape can pose a severe threat to life. As much as rape victims reported that the incident affected their social life and relationships, they were also more likely to disclose and seek mental health intervention. Studies have also shown that incapacitated rape had similar impacts of long-term psychological consequences as those of coercion, which is considered more traumatic. However, the perceived responsibility of assault on the perpetrator was seen to be higher for both the groups-active force and incapacitated rape victims when compared to verbal coercion victims.[17] Clinical perspective must thus focus on the narration of subjective experiences and their internal processes about the act too.

SEXUAL INTIMATE PARTNER VIOLENCE

Sexual victimization within intimate relationships takes many forms, including unwanted but consensual sex, coerced sex, rape, or attempted rape. Disclosure or seeking help is complicated here due to the social stigma, self-blame, and shame which may be unique because of the relationship dynamics.[18] Spousal sexual violence has high consequences on reproductive health outcomes in women leading to high-risk fertility behaviors, such as unintended pregnancy, limited access to contraception, terminated pregnancy, infant mortality, and short-delivery intervals.[19,20]

Therefore, apart from psychological aid, appropriate referrals for medical and social support also become paramount to overcome the adverse consequences which most individuals become aware of after a period of probable denial or confusion.

■ MENTAL HEALTH CONSEQUENCES

Sexual violence severely impacts the mental health of its survivors.[21] During or in the event's immediate aftermath, it can elicit strong emotions, such as fear, numbness, helplessness, and shame.[22] Survivors of sexual violence often also have to address physical and reproductive health complications such as sexually transmitted infections and unwanted pregnancies following the abuse, which adds to their distress.[2]

In the long term, sexual violence victimization can also play an important role in mental illness among the survivors. Sexual violence and mental illness share various types of association—violence can predispose, precipitate, or maintain the illness. Mental illness can also coexist with violence or can increase vulnerability to violence.[23] Mental illnesses that are commonly implicated in this context include anxiety,[24] depression, and post-traumatic stress disorder.[25] Complex post-traumatic disorder characterized by disturbances in self-organization has also been found among women exposed to IPV.[26] Additionally, studies have found that survivors of sexual IPV experience insomnia, somatic symptoms, dissociative experiences, and suicidality.[25]

An Indian study found somatic symptoms, depressive symptoms, and PTSD symptoms to be more severe in women survivors of sexual coercion during pregnancy.[27] The severity of sexual violence was seen to be related to more severe psychiatric symptomatology. College students faced with dating apps facilitated sexual violence reported a decrease in perceived control, higher loneliness, and lower self-esteem.[28]

Sexual violence was found to independently predict PTSD and dissociative experiences.[25] Resilience was found to be a partial mediator between perceived stress and depressive symptoms, while the link between perceived stress and PTSD symptoms was partially mediated by social support.[29]

Personality vulnerabilities among women, especially borderline personality features, have also been found to be significantly associated with a history of sexual abuse victimization. Childhood sexual abuse, in particular, is a risk factor for borderline personality disorder and predicts greater severity of symptoms and poorer prognosis.[30]

The bidirectional relationship between sexual abuse and mental illness can be understood partly through the substance use pathway too. Women with a history of abuse are more vulnerable to harmful use of substances

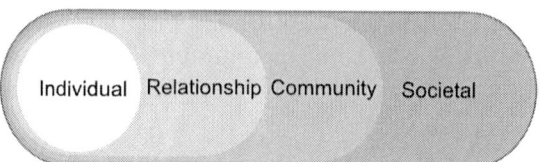

Fig. 1: Social-ecological model for risk of sexual violence.
Source: Centers for Disease Control and Prevention. (2022). The Social-Ecological Model: A Framework for Prevention. [online] Available from: https://www.cdc.gov/violenceprevention/images/theSocialEcologicalModel.PNG?_=23860 [Last accessed December, 2023].

such as alcohol, which puts them at greater risk of further sexual violence victimization.[31]

Furthermore, it is essential to acknowledge that survivors of sexual violence often have to face stigma and discrimination from their families, communities, and workplaces.[32] This can take the form of being blamed for the violence, rejection, being prevented from marrying, and being excluded from groups at work. Institutions where women seek help after sexual violence, such as medical and legal facilities, also sometimes do not practice sensitivity in their interactions with the women, for example, forcing them to recount details of the incident repeatedly. All these sociocultural factors have been found to contribute significantly to the mental health consequences of sexual violence.[33]

Factors that put women at risk for sexual violence can be understood using the social-ecological model.[34] According to the model, not only do individual factors such as age, education level, and history of abuse but also relationship, community, and societal factors including peer norms, neighborhood environment, and gender norms have an influence on experiences of violence. The interactions among the various factors are significant as each level has an impact on the others (as illustrated by overlapping rings in **Figure 1**). The model thus suggests that efforts to prevent violence and address the impact of violence on survivors need to be made keeping in mind all the various factors.

PROTECTIVE FACTORS THAT BUFFER AGAINST SEXUAL VIOLENCE IMPACT
Social Support

The role of social support has always been a crucial factor in recovery from acute and long-term impact of sexual violence and this enables better help-seeking behavior and motivation to get treatment. Studies have identified two kinds of social support—informal such as friends, family, and significant others; and formal such as nurses, police, attorneys, and therapists. Survivors' disclosure about the assault and the extent of these support systems largely impacts their recovery and willingness to fight for justice.[35-37] This is significant in the context of reports of negative disclosure experiences with either kind of support system, which can have huge negative consequences. Studies showed that the survivors received "*insensitive reactions*" and "*inappropriate support*" for the assault. These survivors were blamed for putting themselves in vulnerable positions and were frequently told that they should have known better.[23,24] This can further increase PTSD symptoms and their vulnerability to retraumatization due to hostile or nonsupportive reactions. Thus, multilevel, and interdisciplinary measures must be implemented for interventions focusing on survivors of sexual violence.

■ INTERVENTION

Women who experience sexual violence need attention for various medical conditions, psychological impact, guidance on legal issues, social support, advice on the prevention of unwanted pregnancy, and prophylaxis against STDs.[13,38] Models of intervention need to be interdisciplinary and must be comprehensive for overall well-being. Social stigma, victim blame, and shame associated with disclosure of such assault need to be eradicated at grassroots levels and not just in therapy rooms. Sensitization to acute distress and the long-term impact of sexual assault should be carried out in other sectors of support—medical, social, and legal systems, along with medical and psychological interventions.

Medical Services

Sexual violence is strongly associated with poor sexual and reproductive health of victims, such as unwanted pregnancy, sexually transmitted infections (STIs), human immunodeficiency virus (HIV)/acquired immunodeficiency syndrome (AIDS), hepatitis B, recurrent urinary tract infection, pelvic pain, and pelvic inflammatory disease as well as genital injury and trauma.[13] Irrespective of the disclosure of sexual violence in the first place, medical services that cater to various health-related impacts must also be sensitive and holistically evaluated. A trauma-informed approach and care, as advocated by Caswell R J et al., (2020) is needed, which not only broadens the awareness of the need for psychological safety during consultation and examination but also empowers patients with an agency of choice and also access to wider avenues of care services.[39]

In case of sexual IPV incidences, since the reproductive health care unit is sometimes the only contact to the health care system for several women in India, these clinics should be involved in unveiling and reporting sexual IPV. Providing counseling programs on partner violence at these units could also contribute to reducing domestic violence and protecting a potential victim[20] This should especially be implemented in countries like ours where marital rape is decriminalized. The way forward requires educating healthcare providers to have a holistic approach while being sensitive to a survivor's safety needs and empowerment by referring them to appropriate contacts.[40]

Legal Services

A police station would probably be the first place of redressal for sexual offenses. Legal proceedings like filing a First Information Report (FIR), producing evidence through various forensic examinations, and seeking counseling and compensation, all involve multiple stops at different hierarchical levels within the legal system which can be overwhelming. Sexual offenses are not just a matter of legal concern but also involve sensitive and emotional aspects, and therefore officers who provide legal aid should ideally address survivors more empathetically.[41] Police personnel's sensitivity to acute psychological distress when victims first disclose the assault can prevent revictimization, disengagement, and noncooperation for further investigation.[37]

Within Indian legal systems, multiple amendments have been made to address the increasing rates of sexual violence, such as involvement of women officers as a first point of contact, recording statements at the victim's residence or place of her choice, online portal for registration, victim's consent for medical examination, and free treatment. The One Stop Centers that came up through the Nirbhaya fund have proved to be of great significance in India which provides integrated services, such as medical aid, police assistance, legal counseling, court case management, psychosocial counseling, and temporary shelter to women affected by violence. It adopts a victim-centric approach that involves a systematic focus on the needs and concerns of a victim, to ensure compassionate and sensitive delivery of services in a nonjudgmental manner. It seeks to minimize retraumatization associated with the criminal justice process by providing support from advocates and counselors while empowering survivors to engage in the process of receiving care and justice.

Although there are strong legal protections for victims of sexual offenses, barriers to accessing justice often also happen due to failure to enforce the existing laws. Examples include refusal or delay in FIR registration, discrimination toward minority groups, such as Dalit survivors, corruption within legal systems, and lack of safety concerns. To overcome these barriers, States must also adopt an integrated approach of preventive, punitive, rehabilitative, and a compensatory method, along with a change in the attitude of counselors involved in the implementation of these laws.[41]

Psychological Interventions

India has adopted, in 2013, the guidelines published by the World Health Organization (WHO), for medicolegal care for victims of sexual violence.[42] These guidelines aim at providing a holistic understanding about the impact of sexual violence, the needs and rights of survivors/victims, and highlight the medical and forensic responsibilities of health professionals. Along with creating immediate access to healthcare services postassault, it also recognizes the need to create a sensitive environment that reduces self-blame and enhances healing opportunities for survivors. Singh et al., have also published clinical practice guidelines for assessment and management in psychiatric emergencies, with emphasis on the clinician's role in recovery through empathic listening and promoting emotional recovery, discharge, and follow-up treatment plans for ongoing support. They also provide guidelines for special populations, such as children and adolescents, the elderly, persons with disabilities, and queer community.[38] In a nutshell, these guidelines take cognizance of physical, emotional, and behavioral consequences of sexual violence and indicate physical and psychological safety as fundamental to recovery. They not only provide means for redressal of violation but also promote empowerment for future challenges of seeking justice, be it legally or psychologically.

In 2020, WHO[43] came up with guidelines for the clinical management of rape and IPV survivors by any qualified healthcare provider (medical doctors, clinical officers, midwives, and nurses) working in humanitarian settings. It adopts a survivor-centered approach that prioritizes the survivors' rights, needs, and wishes. It is implemented through developing a workable protocol, staff training, pooling available resources, and referral systems to tackle violence. The LIVES model that is used for such training is enumerated in **Box 1**.

This protocol aims to increase access to services while providing the initial psychological aid with minimal training to different healthcare providers, which can act as a buffer for accessing MHPs for further in-depth psychological interventions. Within mental health settings, intensive care should focus on pharmacological and/or psychotherapeutic interventions as needed. The complexities of sexual abuse can engulf one's identity and internal coping resources. Therefore, psychological interventions must adopt trauma-informed and trauma-focused techniques to increase healthy coping.

Therapeutic interventions that are strength-based and trauma-informed in approach can significantly promote a healthy recovery journey. Intervention components include:
- Access to resources and services
- Enhancing safety, control, and support

> **BOX 1:** LIVES model.
> - *Listening:* Listen with empathy and without judgment
> - *Inquiring* about needs and concerns: Assess and address various needs and concerns—emotional, physical, social, and practical (e.g., childcare)
> - *Validating:* Ensuring that the varied emotional experiences, one may go through are valid and reducing self-blame
> - *Enhancing safety:* To mutually plan an action to protect from further harm if violence occurs again.
> - *Supporting:* By helping to access information, services, and social support

- Increasing knowledge about trauma responses and postassault reactions
- Alterations to affective states and cognitions
- Increased skills to cope and improve self-management
- Improved family and/or social relations was found to be most effective for survivors of sexual violence.[44]

Interventions designed specifically for PTSD[45] can also be considered effective treatment protocols for sexual violence survivors. These include:

- *Cognitive behavioral therapy (CBT):* CBT with a trauma focus uses standard CBT principles together with trauma processing which may include relaxation training, psychoeducation, therapeutic exposure, or cognitive restructuring. [See adult prevention and early treatment for PTSD by the International Society for Traumatic Stress Studies (ISTSS)]
- *Cognitive processing therapy (CPT):* It is also a specific type of CBT that helps patients learn how to restructure unhelpful beliefs related to the trauma and helps create a new understanding of the traumatic event so that it reduces its ongoing negative effects on current life.
- *Prolonged exposure:* It is again a type of CBT that teaches individuals to gradually approach trauma-related memories, feelings, and situations. Eventually, survivors learn that memories and cues are not threatening and need not be avoided.
- *Eye movement desensitization and reprocessing therapy (EMDR):* It is a structured therapy that encourages the patient to briefly focus on the trauma memory while simultaneously experiencing bilateral stimulation (typically eye movements), which is associated with a reduction in the vividness and emotion related-to the trauma memories. EMDR is a conditional suggestion for PTSD that requires detailed clinical assessment and clinician training in delivering.
- *Narrative exposure therapy (NET):* It is most recent in its effectiveness helps in establishing a coherent life narration that conceptualizes traumatic experiences while reprocessing its meaning and restoring survivor's rights.

In most clinical situations, an integrated form of therapy approach that incorporates theory and techniques that best suit the client's needs is often adopted. An integrated therapy that provides such a phasic approach to treatment can be most helpful in reprocessing and reintegration of traumatic elements. The phases may include—stabilization (safety enhancement and skill building), trauma processing, and future generalization and prevention that is tailor-made to suit the individual's pace and need.

In a broader context, service-providing systems (e.g., child and/family welfare, education, criminal and juvenile justice, primary health care, etc.) must also engage from a trauma-informed perspective to sustain not just survivors' recovery but also families and the community at large. Substance Abuse and Mental Health Services Administration (SAMHSA)[46] prescribed six key principles that are fundamental for developing trauma-informed care within the system's culture. They include:

- *Safety:* The organization understands the importance of safety in trauma survivors and promotes a sense of safety—physical and psychological for every individual involved within a system.
- *Trustworthiness and transparency:* The organization takes effective steps to conduct operations and decisions with transparency as a way to build and maintain trust among everyone involved in the organization; staff and client alike.
- *Peer support:* Trauma survivors come together to provide peer support through their lived experiences and stories to promote recovery and healing. It is one of the key principles for enhancing trust, hope, and collaboration.
- *Collaboration and Mutuality:* Importance is placed on leveling power differences among service providers, staff, and clients to demonstrate that healing happens within interpersonal relationships and meaningful sharing of decision-making power. It is based on the premise that everyone in the organization has a role to play in trauma recovery.
- *Empowerment, voice, and choice:* Building capacities and resilience is at the core of a trauma-informed approach to recovery. The organization aims to cultivate self-advocacy skills and support clients with shared decision-making, choice, and goal-setting for moving forward.
- *Cultural, historical, and gender issues:* The organization actively works on being sensitive to various cultural differences and gender issues when promoting recovery. It offers access to gender-responsive services, healing values of cultural connections, and addressing historical trauma.

Additionally, practitioners could also integrate theories like feminist theory with a trauma-informed approach when working with women survivors for better conceptualization of violence impact and healing. As per Pemberton and Loeb (2020),[14] feminist theories' key hallmarks are incorporated within the six principles, for example, enhancing safety is of the highest priority as violence leads to hypervigilance and anxiety of various forms and ingrained negative cognitions like self-blaming, can hinder the understanding of trauma experiences. To enhance trust, trauma-informed feminist practitioners could calculatedly use self-disclosure to build an alliance and transparency to achieve a more egalitarian relationship. Peer support systems could also enhance better understanding through the sharing of mutual experiences of trauma from a larger contextual perspective. Feminist theory highlights the need for sensitivity to intersectionality such as culture, gender, race, and identity when working with survivors due to the obvious disproportionality in violence toward vulnerable groups.[47]

> **KEY POINTS**
> - Sexual violence is one of the most common types of violence against women and is a public health issue. Characteristics of the assault, relationship with the perpetrator, and context of the violence are important dimensions to assess while working with survivors of sexual violence.
> - Sexual violence and mental health share a bidirectional relationship. Sexual violence survivors are at a higher risk of developing mental illnesses, such as depression, anxiety, and post-traumatic stress disorder. Women suffering from mental illness are in turn at higher risk of experiencing sexual violence.
> - A multipronged approach is required to support survivors of sexual violence. Stakeholders from medical, legal, and mental health institutions need to adopt trauma-informed practices and work in collaboration with each other to prevent retraumatization. Reducing stigma and discriminatory acts from the community at large is also imperative.
> - World Health Organization's LIVES framework is useful for providing first-response care for survivors. Specialized interventions for addressing mental health consequences of sexual violence include CBT formats and NET.

REFERENCES

1. Oram S, Khalifeh H, Howard LM. Violence against women and mental health. Lancet Psychiatry. 2017;4(2):159-70.
2. Grose RG, Roof KA, Semeza DC, Leroux X, Yount KM. Mental health, empowerment, and violence against young women in lower-income countries: A review of reviews. Aggress Violent Behav. 2019;46:25-36.
3. World Health Organization. (2021). Violence against women—intimate partner and sexual violence against women. [online] Available from: https://www.who.int/news-room/fact-sheets/detail/violence-against-women [Last accessed December, 2023].
4. Basile KC, Smith SG, Breiding MJ, Black MC, Mahendra R. Sexual Violence Surveillance: Uniform Definitions and Recommended Data Elements, Version 2.0. Atlanta (GA); Centers for Disease Control and Prevention, National Center for Injury Prevention and Control; 2014.
5. Indian Penal Code. Indian Penal Code, 1860. [online] Available from: https://www.indiacode.nic.in/bitstream/123456789/4219/1/THE-INDIAN-PENAL-CODE-1860.pdf [Last accessed December, 2023].

6. Sardinha L, Maheu-Giroux M, Stöckl H, Meyer SR, García-Moreno C. Global, regional, and national prevalence estimates of physical or sexual, or both, intimate partner violence against women in 2018. Lancet. 2022;399(10327):803-13.
7. International Institute for Population Sciences. National Family Health Survey 5 (2019-2021). India; 2021. [online] Available from: https://dhsprogram.com/pubs/pdf/FR375/FR375.pdf [Last accessed December, 2023].
8. Nair S, A Satyanarayana V, Desai G. Prevalence and clinical correlates of intimate partner violence (IPV) in women with severe mental illness (SMI). Asian J Psychiatr. 2020;52:102131.
9. Steele B, DPhil N, Mphil M, Sciarra A, Degli M, DPhil E, et al. Global prevalence and nature of sexual violence among higher education institution students: a systematic review and meta-analysis. 2021;398(S16):1.
10. Patel U, Roesch R. The Prevalence of Technology-Facilitated Sexual Violence: A Meta-Analysis and Systematic Review. Trauma Violence Abuse. 2022;23(2):428-43.
11. Malihi ZA, Fanslow JL, Hashemi L, Gulliver PJ, McIntosh TKD. Prevalence of Nonpartner Physical and Sexual Violence Against People With Disabilities. Am J Prev Med. 2021;61(3):329-37.
12. Qu X, Shen X, Xia R, Wu J, Lao Y, Chen M, Gan Y, Jiang C. The prevalence of sexual violence against female children: A systematic review and meta-analysis. Child Abuse Negl. 2022;131:105764.
13. Blake M de T, Drezett J, Vertamatti MA, Adami F, Valenti VE, Paiva AC, et al. Characteristics of sexual violence against adolescent girls and adult women. BMC Womens Health. 2014;14:15.
14. Culbertson KA, Vik PW, Kooiman BJ. The Impact of Sexual Assault, Sexual Assault Perpetrator Type, and Location of Sexual Assault on Ratings of Perceived Safety. Violence Against Women. 2001;7(8):858-75.
15. Blayney JA, Read JP. Sexual Assault Characteristics and Perceptions of Event-Related Distress. J Interpers Violence. 2018;33(7):1147-68.
16. Kern SG, Peterson ZD. From Freewill to Force: Examining Types of Coercion and Psychological Outcomes in Unwanted Sex. J Sex Res. 2020;57(5):570-84.
17. Brown AL, Testa M, Messman-Moore TL. Psychological consequences of sexual victimization resulting from force, incapacitation, or verbal coercion. Violence Against Women. 2009;15(8):898-919.
18. Kennedy AC, Meier E, Saba J. Sexual violence within intimate relationships. Routledge Int Handb Domest Violence Abus. 2021;:203-19.
19. Bramhankar M, Reshmi RS. Spousal violence against women and its consequences on pregnancy outcomes and reproductive health of women in India. BMC Womens Health. 2021;21(1):382.
20. Das M, Tóth CG, Shri N, Singh M, Hossain B. Does sexual Intimate Partner Violence (IPV) increase risk of multiple high-risk fertility behaviours in India: evidence from National Family Health Survey 2015-16. BMC Public Health. 2022;22(1):2081.
21. In: Chandra P, Herrman H, Fisher J, Riecher-Rössler A (Eds). Mental Health and Illness of Women. Berlin: Springer; 2020.
22. Chandra PS, Deepthivarma S, Carey MP, Carey KB, Shalinianant MP, Garey KB. A Cry from the Darkness: Women with Severe Mental Illness in India Reveal Their Experiences with Sexual Coercion. Psychiatry. 2003 Winter;66(4):323-34.

23. Rai R, Rai AK. Sexual violence and poor mental health of women: an exploratory study of Uttar Pradesh, India. Clin Epidemiol Glob Heal. 2020;8(1):194-8.
24. Tarzia L, Maxwell S, Valpied J, Novy K, Quake R, Hegarty K. Sexual violence associated with poor mental health in women attending Australian general practices. Aust N Z J Public Health. 2017;41(5):518-23.
25. Honda T, Wynter K, Yokota J, Tran T, Ujiie Y, Niwa M, et al. Sexual violence as a key contributor to poor mental health among Japanese women subjected to intimate partner violence. J Women's Heal. 2018;27(5):716-23.
26. Fernández-Fillol C, Pitsiakou C, Perez-Garcia M, Teva I, Hidalgo-Ruzzante N. Complex PTSD in survivors of intimate partner violence: risk factors related to symptoms and diagnoses. Eur J Psychotraumatol. 2021;12(1):2003616.
27. Varma D, Chandra PS, Thomas T, Carey MP. Intimate partner violence and sexual coercion among pregnant women in India: Relationship with depression and post-traumatic stress disorder. J Affect Disord. 2007;102(1-3):227-35.
28. Echevarria SG, Peterson R, Woerner J. College Students' Experiences of Dating App Facilitated Sexual Violence and Associations with Mental Health Symptoms and Well-Being. J Sex Res. 2023;60(8):1193-205.
29. Catabay CJ, Stockman JK, Campbell JC, Tsuyuki K. Perceived stress and mental health: The mediating roles of social support and resilience among black women exposed to sexual violence. J Affect Disord. 2019;259:143-9.
30. de Aquino Ferreira LF, Queiroz Pereira FH, Neri Benevides AML, Aguiar Melo MC. Borderline personality disorder and sexual abuse: a systematic review. Psychiatry Res. 2018;262:70-7.
31. Pitpitan E V, Kalichman SC, Eaton LA, Sikkema KJ, Watt MH, Skinner D. Gender-based violence and HIV sexual risk behavior: alcohol use and mental health problems as mediators among women in drinking venues, Cape Town. Soc Sci Med. 2012;75(8):1417-25.
32. Josse E. "They came with two guns": The consequences of sexual violence for the mental health of women in armed conflicts. Int Rev Red Cross. 2010;92(877):177-95.
33. Dworkin ER, Weaver TL. The Impact of Sociocultural Contexts on Mental Health Following Sexual Violence: A Conceptual Model. Psychol Violence. 2021;11(5):476-87.
34. Bronfenbrenner U. Ecology of the family as a context for human development: Research perspectives. Dev Psychol. 1986;22(6):723-42.
35. Ullman SE. Correlates of Social Reactions to Victims' Disclosures of Sexual Assault and Intimate Partner Violence: A Systematic Review. Trauma, Violence, Abus. 2023;24(1):29-43.
36. Peter-hagene LC, Ullman SE. Sexual assault-characteristis effects of PTSD and psychosocial mediators: a cluster-analysis approach to sexual assault types: Correction to Peter-Hagene and Ullman (2014). Psychol Trauma Theory Res Pract Policy. 2015;7(2):170.
37. Hansen NB, Hansen M, Nielsen LH, Bramsen RH, Elklit A, Campbell R. Rape Crimes: Are Victims' Acute Psychological Distress and Perceived Social Support Associated With Police Case Decision and Victim Willingness to Participate in the Investigation? Violence Against Women. 2018;24(6):684-96.

38. Singh O, Sarkar S, Singh V. Clinical practice guidelines for assessment and management of psychiatric emergencies in victims of sexual violence. Indian J Psychiatry. 2023;65(2):175-80.
39. Caswell RJ, Maidment I, Ross JDC, Bradbury-Jones C. How, why, for whom and in what context, do sexual health clinics provide an environment for safe and supported disclosure of sexual violence: Protocol for a realist review. BMJ Open. 2020;10(6):e037599.
40. Chattopadhyay S. The Responses of Health Systems to Marital Sexual Violence–A Perspective from Southern India. J Aggress Maltreatment Trauma. 2019;28(1):47-67.
41. Nagarathna A. Investigation of Sexual Offenses against Women in India – A Review of Legal Procedural Mandates and Directives. Natl Law Sch J. 2019;15:173-91.
42. Ministry of Health and Family Welfare. Guidelines & protocols - Medico-legal care for survivors/victims of sexual violence. [online] Available from: https://main.mohfw.gov.in/sites/default/files/953522324.pdf [Last accessed December, 2023].
43. World Health Organization, United Nations Population Fund (UNFPA), United Nations High Commissioner for Refugees (UNHCR). Clinical management of rape and intimate partner violence survivors: Developing protocols for use in humanitarian settings. [online] Available from: https://www.un.org/sexualviolenceinconflict/wp-content/uploads/2020/04/9789240001411-eng.pdf [Last accessed December, 2023].
44. Paphitis SA, Bentley A, Asher L, Osrin D, Oram S. Improving the mental health of women intimate partner violence survivors: Findings from a realist review of psychosocial interventions. PLoS One. 2022;17(3):e0264845.
45. American Psychological Association. (2017). Clinical practice guideline for the treatment of PTSD in adults American Psychological Association Guideline development panel for the treatment of PTSD in adults. [online] Available from: https://www.apa.org/ptsd-guideline/ptsd.pdf [Last accessed December, 2023].
46. Substance Abuse and Mental Health Services Administration. (2014). SAMHSA's Concept of Trauma and Guidance for a Trauma-Informed Approach. HHS Publication No. (SMA) 14-4884. [online] Available from: https://ncsacw.acf.hhs.gov/userfiles/files/SAMHSA_Trauma.pdf [Last accessed December, 2023].
47. Pemberton JV, Loeb TB. Impact of Sexual and Interpersonal Violence and Trauma on Women: Trauma-Informed Practice and Feminist Theory. J Fem Fam Ther. 2020;32(1-2):115-31.

SECTION 4

Interventions and Services

- **Cultural Formulation in Women's Mental Health**
  Sai Spoorthy Mamidipalli, Sucharita Mandal, Sai Krishna Tikka

- **Gender-sensitive Mental Health Services and Ethical Issues in Care**
  Sunita Simon Kurpad

- **Measurement and Assessment Tools for Women's Mental Health**
  Gunja Sengupta, Sundarnag Ganjekar

- **Neuromodulation in Women**
  Nishant Goyal, Shobit Garg

- **General Principles of Psychopharmacology in Women**
  Vikas Menon, Chandrima Naskar

CHAPTER 18

Cultural Formulation in Women's Mental Health

Sai Spoorthy Mamidipalli, Sucharita Mandal, Sai Krishna Tikka

ABSTRACT

Culture influences the thought process, emotions, understanding of illness, assessment/formulation/diagnostic process, and treatment decisions. Gender is a critical determinant of mental health and mental illnesses. Several mental disorders, such as depression, anxiety disorders, and somatization disorders are more common in women compared to men. Gender influences the way individuals communicate, and express their emotions and feelings and is also influenced by their sociocultural background/culture-devised gender roles. Culture hence plays an important role. The Diagnostic and Statistical Manual (DSM)-5 in fact has proposed a brief semistructured interview for systematically assessing cultural factors in assessment termed the Cultural Formulation Interview (CFI).

In the South Asian region, causal attributions of mental illness in women are highly influenced by their cultural beliefs as well as customs and rituals followed. Mostly, supernatural causes, moral reasons such as bad character and past life sins are believed to be the cause for the illness and women often seek religious strategies for treatment. Depending upon the country of origin and degree of social support various cultural theories have been put forward regarding the etiology of disorders, such as depression, dissociation, and postpartum psychiatric disorders. Certain factors such as migration and interpersonal violence frequently seen in women from low- and middle-income (LAMI) countries were found to be causal factors for several common mental disorders. Barriers affecting past and current help-seeking among women with psychiatric disorders include stigma, unawareness, affordability, lack of human resources who are gender-sensitive, caregiving role, somatoform expression of distress, and explanatory models of illness.

In this chapter, we start by giving an outline of women's mental health and its relationship to culture and then move on to describe cultural formulation in the context of women's mental health. Here, we elaborate on the various domains of CFI. The cultural definition of the problem, cultural perception of the cause, context and support, cultural factors affecting self-coping, and past help-seeking, and cultural factors affecting current help-seeking. We lay special emphasis on cultural aspects of mental health issues related to gender-based violence, suicide, self-harm, and perinatal mental health.

Keywords: Culture, women, mental health, explanatory models, help seeking.

INTRODUCTION

Culture refers to the meanings, values, and behavioral norms that are learned and transmitted in the dominant society and within its social groups. It powerfully influences cognition, feelings, and self-concept as well as the assessment/formulation/diagnostic process and treatment decisions **(Fig. 1)**.

The Diagnostic and Statistical Manual (DSM)-5[1] defines culture as:
- The values, knowledge, and practices that individuals derive from membership in diverse social groups (such as ethnic, faith, and occupational groups).
- Aspects of an individual's background, developmental experiences, and current social context(s) that influence their perspectives (such as geographical origin, religion, sexual orientation, and ethnicity)
- Influences from family, friends, and other community members on the individual's experience of mental illness. Most individuals and groups are exposed to multiple cultures, which they use to fashion their own identities and make sense of experiences.

The six important components of culture are—it is learned, passed on from one generation to the next, a "set of meanings" in which words, behaviors, events, and symbols have meanings—agreed upon by the cultural group, *acts as a template to "shape and orient" future behaviors and perspectives within and in between generations*, culture exists in a *constant state of change*, culture includes patterns of both *subjective and objective components* of human behavior. In general, the relationship between culture and psychiatric illness is understood as below:[2]
- Culture shapes how and what psychiatric symptoms are expressed
- Culture influences the meanings that are given to symptoms
- Culture also impacts the interaction between the patient and the healthcare system
- Psychiatrists can be influenced by their own culture or by the culture/race of the patients
- Can lead to a biased diagnosis.

WOMEN'S MENTAL HEALTH AND CULTURE

Gender is a crucial determinant of mental health and mental illnesses. There is a gross difference in the prevalence of several mental disorders such as depression, affective disorders, anxiety disorders, schizophrenia, and somatization disorder with *females* outnumbering males as per data from large-scale community studies.[3] Other differences in females are with respect to the age of presentation of different psychiatric disorders, the clinical presentation (predominantly somatic nature), frequency of psychotic symptoms, treatment response, tolerability of psychotropics, unique pharmacokinetic and pharmacodynamic changes, and dose adjustments of drugs during perinatal period, course, social adjustment, and overall prognosis.

There is an obvious difference between females and males with respect to their "psychological makeup." Women's brains are "wired" differently than men when it comes to information processing and reactions to external events.[4] The way women communicate, and express their emotions and feelings is colored by their sociocultural background/culture-devised gender roles. Mental illnesses form a major contributor to ill health among women in the reproductive age group. This burden is comparatively much higher in low- and middle-income countries (LAMI) like India.[5]

Culture influences when, where, how, and to whom patients narrate their subjective experiences and associated distress. The pattern and predominant symptoms of patients at presentation (particularly women), the development of symptoms/syndrome, patient's perceptions about causes of illness and acceptable treatment strategies, course of illness, and clinician's understanding of symptoms and diagnoses are all heavily influenced by culture.[4,6]

Mental health practitioners wanting to use structured questions as part of the assessment can use the Cultural Formulation Interview (CFI). The CFI is a brief semistructured interview for systematically assessing cultural factors in assessment (detailed description given in upcoming section). Here in the next sections, we try to summarize how culture shapes women's mental health and how the cultural formulation of DSM-5 can be understood in the perspective of women's mental health.

CULTURAL FORMULATION AND WOMEN'S MENTAL HEALTH

Based on the description given in the previous section, it is clear that culture affects almost every clinician-patient interaction and it is not restricted to a subgroup of patients. The inclusion of evaluation about a patient's culture forms the basis for any comprehensive assessment in psychiatry.

The first step toward the incorporation of culture into the classificatory systems started with the DSM-IV. It is definitely an achievement in the history of classificatory systems and a milestone for cultural psychiatry as the relevance of culture to psychiatric diagnoses gained attention. This inclusion was carried out under three categories:

1. The inclusion of how cultural factors can influence the expression, assessment, and prevalence of specific disorders
2. An outline of a cultural formulation of clinical diagnosis to complement the multiaxial assessment
3. A glossary of relevant cultural-bound syndromes from around the world.

The "Outline for Cultural Formulation" was "meant to supplement the multiaxial diagnostic assessment and to address difficulties that may be encountered in applying DSM-IV criteria in a multicultural environment." Despite this, only a proportion of the content proposed by the task force for DSM-IV was retained in the final version. It presents a short list of questions with minimal introduction and no illustrated case vignettes. Also, the 'culture-bound syndromes were added in the appendix section leading to under recognition of the same.

The next milestone which occurred in the same decade was the preparation of the World Mental Health Report. This was a compilation of literature available throughout the world to find out the range of mental health and behavioral problems with a specific focus on low-income countries in Africa, Latin America, Asia, and the Pacific. One important observation by this report was with respect to the social causes/roots of poor mental health among women from these countries. Hunger, labor-intensive dangerous work settings/unstable employment, cultural shock (in migrants) and domestic violence are predominant factors specific to these LAMI countries that contribute to psychiatric illnesses in women.[7]

Despite the widespread knowledge across the world about the DSM-IV outline for cultural formulation for the next two decades, the implementation rates by clinicians were limited. Reasons for limited use/barriers for wide use include lack of clarity on when, where, and how it should be used, that is, for which patients, for what purposes, by which staff members, and at which point in the course of clinical care.[7]

So, the American Psychiatric Association and DSM-5 cross-cultural issues subgroup revised the existing tool to prepare a more feasible, acceptable, and clinically useful tool with clear indications. This was called the "Cultural Formulation Interview,"[8] which helps in performing client-centered cultural assessments aiding in diagnosis and treatment planning. This tool can be used in all clinical encounters by *all clinicians* and for *all patients* and its use is not restricted to cultural minorities or cultural discrepancy between patients and clinicians. This is because all of us bring our own cultures, values, and expectations to the clinical encounter, including often invisible influences on how we approach specific aspects of care.

The cultural formulation of psychiatric disorders has been deemed important in many different ways, including:
- The prevention of misdiagnoses
- Obtaining crucial clinical information/helps clinicians in understanding the patient's illness as a whole
- Improving the therapeutic relationship
- Improving adherence to treatment
- Improving therapeutic effectiveness and
- Serving as a guide to clinical studies and cultural epidemiological studies on psychiatric disorders.

Although recommended for all clinical encounters by DSM-5, there are five main clinical situations with respect to clinical care where it is a "must use"[9] (**Fig. 1**).

The evolution of the CFI made the OCF more operational. There are two forms in the CFI, one which has to be filled by the patient and the other form meant for the caregivers/informants. The evaluation in these two forms is carried out under four different domains[10] (**Flowchart 1**):
- The cultural definition of the problem items.[1-3]
- The cultural perception of the cause, context, and support items.[4-10]

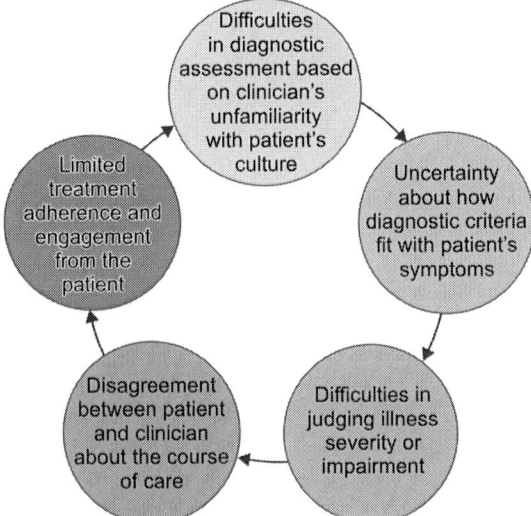

Fig. 1: Main clinical situations in which Cultural Formulation Interview (CFI) is a "must-use."

Flowchart 1: Domains of Cultural Formulation Interview.

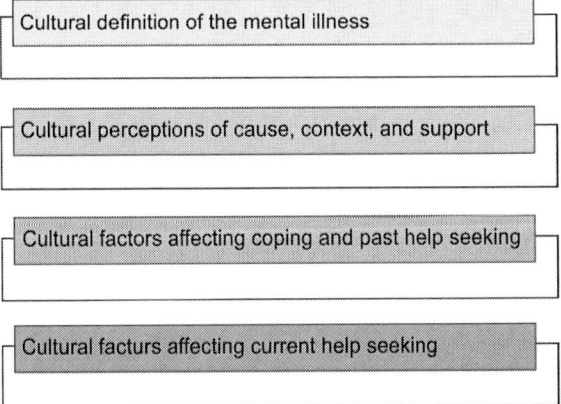

- The cultural factors affecting self-coping, and past help-seeking items.[11-13]
- The cultural factors affecting current help-seeking items.[14-16]

Cultural Definition of the Mental Illness in Women

Gender plays a major role in cultural perceptions and the likelihood of diagnosis/definition of the problem in mental illness. For women, there is often a "double jeopardy" at play. First, many psychiatric disorders are more common in women as discussed; second, women are predominantly the caregivers across cultures, adding further difficulty and demand to their lives.[2]

In South Asian region, causal attributions of mental illness are highly influenced by their cultural beliefs, customs, and rituals followed. Mostly, supernatural causes, moral reasons such as bad character and past life sins are believed to be the cause for the illness (more so in psychotic illness/postpartum psychosis/trans and possession) and women sought religious strategies for treatment more often.

Similarly, culture has different effects while shaping the psychopathology in women with psychiatric disorders. Though the mechanisms are similar in both genders, the clinical conditions or signs produced or the underlying factors responsible for these effects are heavily influenced by the female gender **(Table 1)**.[12-14]

Cultural Perceptions of Cause, Context, and Support

Hysteria

It was once considered an exclusively female disease. Two different theories of causation were put forward—magicodemonological and scientific views. At that time, it was perceived that women were not only vulnerable to mental disorders, but were weak and easily influenced (by supernatural powers or by organic degeneration). From the 13th century till the end of the 19th

TABLE 1: Cultural definition of mental illness in women.

Effect of culture	Clinical condition/signs/factors	Mechanism
Pathoplastic effect	• Somatic symptoms • Persecutory delusions • Religious delusions • Infanticidal thoughts • Dissociation (trance and possession) • Self-guilt, unworthiness, and suicidal conduct ("Western" depression)	a, b, c. Represent "culture-specific expression" of psychological distress d. Culture shaping themes e, f. "Culturally acceptable" way

Contd...

Contd...

Effect of culture	Clinical condition/signs/factors	Mechanism
Pathogenic influence (culture-bound syndromes)	• Susto • Toas • Lom pid duan • Aire • Caida de mollera • Sanni/Janni/Janni Ekkendi/Sanni Patam • Latah • Dhat syndrome (Females) • Ataque de nervios • Pibloktoq • Falling out/blacking out • Sati (culture-bound suicide)	• A condition that is "understood only in certain cultural context" and is labeled based on "the specific ways in which each cultural group understands distress, tension, illness and health" • Culture is the *direct causative factor* in forming or "generating" psychopathology
Pathoelaborating effects	• Gender preference at birth • *Modern cultural contexts*: Family structure, workplace, and maternity leave • Poor control over contraception due to lack of agency or religious beliefs	Culture elaborates on the clinical manifestation
Pathofacilitatory effect	• Poor social support • Low self-esteem • Stressful life events • Multiparity • Domestic violence • Immigration • Female baby	Culture promoting the frequency of occurrence
Pathoreactive effect	• *Faith healing practices* in India • People attribute illness as a result of *"black magic" and react to it by offering rituals* • Mental illness due to "not getting married"	• Culture shaping folk responses to the clinical condition • The role of culture is *interpretation and reaction to illness*

century most of the theories centered around "hysteria" still considered it as a "symbol" of feminity. Given below in the table are different cultural perceptions of the cause of this illness across different countries and different time frames[14] **(Table 2)**.

In a recent study conducted in North India among women with conversion disorder, using the CFI authors have tried to assess the perceived causes of illness and contextual stressors.

TABLE 2: Cultural perceptions of causes of hysteria.

Country/time period	Cultural explanation of the cause of "hysteria"
Egyptian theories (first and second century BC) (Eber Papyrus and Kahun Papyrus)	• Movement of the uterus upward or downward causes hysteria • Therapeutic measures include placing of malodorous and acrid substances near the mouth or nostrils if it has moved upward, and scented substances near the vagina and vice versa in case of downward movement
Greek theories (fifth century BC) (Melampus, Plato, Hippocrates, Trotula, Aristotle, and St Thomas Aquinas)	• Related to the lack of normal sexual life • Due to abnormal movements of the uterus in the body due to an inadequate sexual life (bad uterus) • "Woman is a failed man" • Treatment is living an adequate sexual life
Rome (Cornelius Celsus, Claudius Galen, and Soranus) (first century BC, second century AD)	• The term "hysteria" was given, the effect on the uterus causes symptoms in the rest of the system • Hysterical disorders among women arise from the toils of procreation; their recovery is encouraged by sexual abstinence and perpetual virginity
Middle ages Europe (13–14th century)	• Manifestations of mental illness are seen as obscene bonds between women and the devil or due to sorcery • Mental illness is due to "sins" • "Hysterical" women are subjected to exorcism—considered a cure but not a punishment
Modern age (16–18th century) (Thomas Willis, Thomas Sydenham, Pierre Roussel, Franz Anton Mesmer, and Jean-Martin Charcot)	• The disease is explained by the nonfulfillment of natural desire • Not related to the uterus but related to the brain and nervous system • Symptoms may simulate almost all forms of organic diseases • Suggestion as a method of treatment (mesmerism); hypnosis as a method of treatment

Contd...

Contd...

Country/time period	Cultural explanation of the cause of "hysteria"
Contemporary age France (Pierre Janet and Sigmund Freud)	• Hysteria is a pathology in which dissociation appears autonomously for neurotic reasons; reason is the idée fixe (subconscious) • Janet studied five hysteria symptoms—anesthesia, amnesia, abulia, motor control diseases, and modification of character • Caused by a lack of libidinal evolution (setting the stage of the Oedipal conflict) and the failure of conception is the result not the cause of the disease • Concept of "secondary advantage"
Late 19 and 20th centuries	• Evolution of the concept of "Briquet's syndrome" • Deletion of hysterical neurosis from DSM-III
Late 20th centuries (observations from World War I and II)	• Hysteria, as one of the somatic ways of expressing emotional distress • Importance of transcultural psychiatry • The role of environmental factors in modifying psychopathology was emphasized

As per the results, biological, traditional cultural, psychological, and social factors are found to be causes of conversion disorder (given here).[15]

- *Biological:*
  - Physical illnesses/weakness
  - "Body heat"
  - Neurological causes
- *Traditional-cultural:*
  - External evil forces
- *Psychological:*
  - Emotional dysregulation
  - Inability to express emotions
  - Cognitive causes
- *Social:*
  - Domestic violence
  - Stigma
  - Perceived lack of social support
  - Interpersonal stress
  - Excessive stimulation
  - Occupational stressors

Depression

Women are more likely to have winter depression, atypical depression, and depression due to underlying thyroid disorder, and depression during different phases of the reproductive cycle (menstruation, pregnancy, postpartum, and menopause).

South Asian women's social isolation, powerlessness/being overly controlled by their families, additional home and work responsibilities, abuse, low self-esteem/autonomy, low support, and poor literacy are the cultural factors that have also been identified as potential contributors to increased risk of depression. It is regarded that the phenomena of "turning in on oneself" leads to the causation of depression in women from South Asian regions. Apart from the increased prevalence, and predominance of somatic symptoms in the presentation of the disorder, the "somatic veil of depression" particularly in those belonging to LAMI countries reflects the underlying cultural aspects.[16]

In south India, in the region of Kerala, the literacy rate is over 98% among women, yet suicide rates are the highest in the Indian nation. This phenomenon has been linked to discrepancies between the achievement and aspirations of highly educated women, many of whom find it difficult to find work or come under social pressure not to work after marriage. Low rates of diagnosis in particular ethnic groups might reflect the diagnostic bias or clinicians' deeply held views about mental illness in that particular subgroup.[2]

Somatization

Similar to depression, somatization is found more frequently in women compared to men. In these individuals "body" acts as a metaphor for events of "personal" and "social" meaning. "Bodily themes" are perceived as acceptable ways of expressing distress and getting help in a less stigmatic way in the majority of women and ethnic minorities. This type of expression is seen in women from developing countries compared to the developed countries. Western women consider "somatization" as an inferior way of dealing with emotions and intrapsychic conflicts as they rely on independence and autonomy.[17]

Gender-based Violence

Intimate personal violence (IPV) though much underreported, is pretty common among women from South Asian countries. The lifetime prevalence rates of physical or sexual violence as per a 10-country study by the World Health Organization (WHO) were found to be between 15 and 71%. Though research in this area is still emerging some of the correlates like forced and arranged marriages, social isolation (especially when coupled with language barriers), and low socioeconomic and educational status, which make women more vulnerable to being controlled by men, are likely to be among crucial factors for interpersonal violence.

Most South Asian countries follow collectivist cultures and patriarchal ideology which emphasizes the dominant role of male members in the family and imposes subordination of views and needs of women in favor of family relations. These values make the women more tolerant to several forms of IPV and also make them reluctant to disclose about the same in fear of stigma.

According to a UN report, around two-thirds of the married women in India are victims of domestic violence. The common forms of violence against Indian women are female feticide, domestic violence, dowry death or harassment, mental and physical torture, sexual trafficking, and public humiliation. Their expected role of bearing children, the consequences of infertility, and the failure to beget a male child have been linked to wife-battering and suicide.[4]

A type of IPV, female genital mutilation might predispose women to an increasing number of perinatal mental illnesses and post-traumatic stress disorder (PTSD) as per anecdotal evidence. It reflects the social attitudes to sex and female sexuality among some cultures.

Though in-depth evaluation is lacking factors such as trafficking, forced prostitution, sexual abuse, and being rendered stateless can all increase the vulnerability of women to a range of issues such as depression, PTSD, anxiety disorders, increased risk of suicide, and somatic conditions including disabling physical pain and dysfunction.[2]

Migration

Most migrant women have poor support (practical and emotional) compared to their country of origin and the absence of close relationships. Staying away from their native place can also take the form of "cultural bereavement"— including grief for the loss of home and shared cultural identity. These trigger several common mental disorders, such as anxiety, depression, and perinatal depression in particular.[18]

A study was conducted among Hmong people (originally from the hills of Laos in South Asia) residing in the United States. It was found that despite their "immigrant" status strict adherence to their postpartum practice of 30-day rest after birth combined with support from family reduced the vulnerability to postpartum depression.[19]

Pregnancy and Infertility

Though pregnancy was once considered a protective period for the development of psychiatric disorders, it has been proved that the antenatal period increases the development of various mental disorders. Several factors such as past personal history of sexual, physical, or emotional abuse, current exposure to intimate partner violence or coercion, current social adversity, and coincidental adverse life events have led to increased incidence of psychiatric disorders in pregnancy. Additional culture-specific causative factors from developing countries include poverty, gender disadvantage, marital disharmony, poor social support, and restricted access to the health care system. Certain protective factors, such as good social support and self-confidence were also identified.[20] Moreover, with changing gender roles, especially in women's employment, work-life balance along with lack of sufficient maternity leaves tends to have an adverse effect on women's mental health during pregnancy.

Pressure to begetting children is common in several countries. The importance attached to parenthood portrays infertility as undesirable and is stigmatized. Though males and females are discriminated against, males have the option of opting out of marriage or remarriage. Hence, infertility in women tends to cause depression, low self-esteem, and other psychiatric disorders.[21]

In LAMI countries, belief in evil spirits and supernatural powers as causes of infertility is still prevalent leading to treatment delays. In a study from India, it was found that in both men and women, low spousal support, financial constraints, and social coercion in the early years of marriage predict infertility distress.[22] Introduction of various assisted reproductive procedures for the treatment of infertility has resulted in hope as well as psychological turmoil before and during pregnancy. However, most women seek alternative treatment and assisted techniques take a secondary preference. In those who seek assisted conception, it has been shown to cause various adverse psychiatric problems.[20,23]

Postpartum Psychiatric Disorders

Postpartum depression and postpartum psychosis are serious disorders that affect women across the world. The *causation* of these illnesses is linked to a range of cultural factors/aspects that occur in and around the period of pregnancy along with biological, psychological, familial, and social factors. The prevalence of postpartum depression in Asian countries varies between 1 and 20%. The lower prevalence of the disorder in certain cultural groups is due to the alleviating effect of the culture. It is believed that in cultures that have *strong social support* for new mothers, women tend to have lower rates of postpartum disorders.

A study done in India found that several causative explanatory models of postpartum psychosis were held among patients and caregivers. Respondents most often held more than one explanatory model of illness (EMI).

Biomedical or physical EMI, supernatural causation, spiritual and religious causes, stressors unique to "childbirth," and marital stress were among the EMI. Nonbiomedical models are common among these women with postpartum psychosis.[24]

Cultural traditions like "doing the month" (the traditional practice of women being relieved from work for a month after giving birth) and "peiyue" were found to be protective against the development of postpartum depression in Chinese and Taiwanese cultures. The ritual of "Satogaeri bunben" followed in Japan was not found to make a difference in the occurrence of postpartum depression in women.[25-28]

On the other hand, lack of cultural traditions or presence of some cultural traditions (staying together with the husband's parents or interfering role of parents or perceived unmet needs) during the postpartum period served as a deteriorating factor for postpartum depression.

Studies done in India have shown that *cultural beliefs* about "preference for male child/sadness about female gender" served as a significant risk factor for the development of postpartum depression and marital violence. On the other hand, giving birth to a "male child" was found to be protective of depression and interpersonal relationship issues.[19,29,30]

Substance Use Disorders

Women tend to face unique issues with respect to substance use. Though the prevalence is less in women compared to men the duration needed from use to dependence level is comparatively shorter. The differences are affected by biological basis (female sex itself) and gender roles (based on cultural definitions). It rarely comes in isolation and is influenced by social personal and economic factors. Women who are victims of domestic violence or sexual assault or survivors of abuse are at increased risk of substance use. Divorce, loss of child custody, or the death of a partner or child can trigger the initiation of substance use in them. Other reasons/factors responsible for substance use are as a means of controlling weight, overcoming exhaustion, pain relief, and attempts to self-medicate for mental health issues.[31]

Self-medication (illicit drugs, prescription drugs, and alcohol) is the means of initiation of substance use in women contrary to men who start using substances due to peer pressure. Underlying causes for self-medication include comorbid psychiatric disorders (anxiety, depression, grief, PTSD, and bipolar disorder), trauma, loneliness, and major lifestyle changes. Trauma, as a cause of self-meditation is of special mention as drugs/alcohol, may transiently reduce the impact but may actually worsen mental health issues.[32]

In some Indian subcultures, consumption of alcohol and tobacco chewing are culturally sanctioned and are therefore vulnerable to developing severe forms of substance use disorders (SUDs).

Suicide

Suicide attempts, far more frequent in female teenagers, are too often felt as the only solution for girls to advocate some freedom. Besides, the ultraconservative upbringing of many females paves the way to the development of morbid fear of sexual intercourse and even to nonconsummation of marriage.

Certain forms of suicide like "*Sati*"/"*Suttee*"—the death of women after the demise of their husbands were culturally accepted and followed by societies till the late 18th century. The prevalence rates of suicide attempts were found to be significantly higher in South Asian women compared to their Western counterparts. Several social and cultural factors are responsible for these higher rates:[33,34]

- Female gender itself
- Gender-role expectations
- Family or interpersonal conflicts
- Domestic violence
- Cultural conflict (among migrants)
- Poor self esteem
- Alcohol use in the family

Studies conducted in India have shown that rates of attempted suicides were as high as 0.8%. The strongest predictors of suicide were found to be common mental disorders, violence, and hunger. Other factors responsible include failures in life, difficulties in interpersonal relationships, and dowry-related harassment. The precipitants for suicide among women are as follows: Dowry disputes, love affairs, illegitimate pregnancies, and quarrels with spouses or parents-in-law. Spousal violence has been found to be specifically associated as an independent risk factor.[4]

Specific factors influencing the cultural perceptions of cause, context, and support among women in South Asian regions have been summarized in **Figure 2**.

Cultural Factors Affecting Coping and Past Help-Seeking/Current Help-Seeking in Women

General-Coping and Past Help-Seeking[5,35]

Women with mental illness do not receive the same amount of treatment and suffer from worse clinical and social outcomes. In LAMI countries, the proportion of women receiving psychiatric emergency services/in-patient services was around one-third of the total patients seeking care. The reasons depicted by most studies are delays in treatment-seeking and poor compliance. The other reasons for this gross disproportion of mental health care gap are:

- Burden of *cultural taboos and stigma* of mental disorders/their treatment—prevents women from seeking help—as this can increase of their risk of not getting married/getting divorced or separated; and increase their risk of being sexually/physically abused.
- *The dual curse* of being a "woman" and "mentally ill"—being ostracized and discriminated leading to poor service-seeking
- *The experiences* of self-worth, competence, autonomy, and economic independence, as well as physical, sexual, and emotional safety and security, are systematically denied to most women simply due to gender—this contributes to the growing burden of mental health issues in women.
- Though *effective preventive and treatment* strategies exist, these services remain *unavailable* to most women in LAMI countries.
    - Quality of *evidence and implementation* for integration of these evidence-based interventions into nonspecialized health care settings

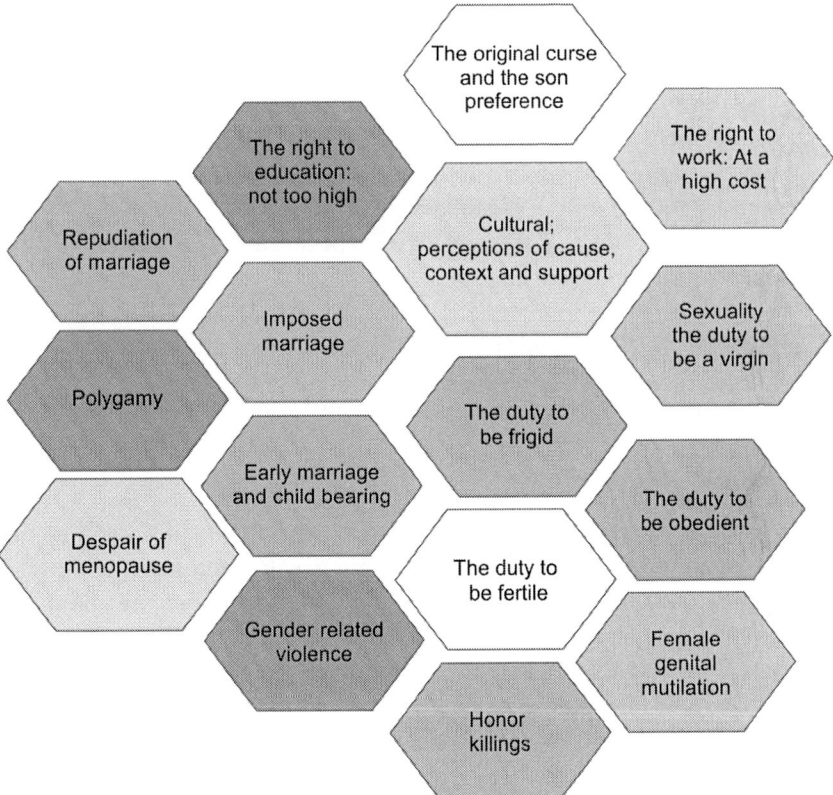

Fig. 2: Factors influencing the cultural perception of cause, context, and support.
Source: Douki S, Zineb SB, Nacef F, Halbreich U. Women's mental health in the Muslim world: cultural, religious, and social issues. J Affect Disord. 2007;102(1-3):177-89.

(primary care, maternal and child health care, and community care) seems to be *lacking*.
- The creation of mental health *goals* based on the systems from high-income countries (HICs) lacks the locally felt *priorities* and *sociocultural* context of LAMIs.

Current Help-Seeking—South Asian Region (Particular Reference to India)[36-38]

- Lack of awareness and acknowledgment of mental health issues are the important barriers to help-seeking
- Inadequate human resources and limited access to mental health care resources
- Affordability of mental health care services
- Stigma and discrimination
- *The caregiving role* for most if not all family members (children, elderly with/without chronic physical illnesses)—makes their own mental health issues a *low priority* compared to the expectations of the role they play.
- Women are *less aggressive and dangerous* during the acute episode—enhances family tolerance and causes further delay in help-seeking
- "*Somatoform expression*" of the underlying psychological distress misdirects the pathway to help-seeking toward physicians/general practitioners rather than psychiatrists
- Perceptions about the illness or explanatory models of illness (supernatural models of illness)
- Women's rights are frequently violated by major stakeholders, including mental health professionals
- Inadequate management of existing resources
- Help-seeking process itself

Depression and Self Harm

Apart from the general factors, the following specific factors/barriers are responsible for help-seeking behavior in women with depression.
- Language acquisition for migrant groups increases women's likelihood of seeking help and receiving a diagnosis.
- *Barriers to access:* Confidentiality concern
- Unawareness of available services
- *Inadequate service response:* Lack of cultural understanding

Somatization/Medicalizing Symptoms and Dissociative Disorder

As discussed earlier, a lack of distinction between physical and psychological symptoms and beliefs in supernatural causes/variable illness beliefs are commonly seen in women from South Asian regions. Thin in turn leads to delay in help-seeking as they land up with medical specialists/superspecialists or with faith healers for the treatment.[11,39]

"Somatization" was found to be the common "idiom of distress" for help-seeking in Havik Brahmin women from South India. Factors such as weak social support and limited opportunities to ventilate and seek help from others were found to be responsible for this transformation.[40,41]

A number of barriers such as social barriers (stigma and lack of caregiver), resource constraints (finance, time, and lack of awareness), and illness-related (impairing symptoms and anticipation of treatment/outcome), and institutional barriers were found to be the reasons for delayed help-seeking in women with dissociative disorder.[15]

In a recent study conducted in North India, it was shown that women with conversion disorder tend to use emotion-focused coping strategies (recreational activity, occupational activity, meditation and relaxation, and behavioral disengagement) more often compared to problem-focused coping strategies (resolution of conflicts and use of psychological therapies). Other coping strategies, such as alternative healing methods, religious coping, and ventilation are also sought by patients.[15]

Gender-based Violence

Most South Asian countries follow collectivist cultures and patriarchal ideology which emphasizes the dominant role of male members in the family and imposes subordination of views and needs of women in favor of family relations. These values make the women more tolerant to several forms of IPV and also make them reluctant to disclose about the same in fear of stigma.[2]

Migration

Minority women, who might have less choice in the decision to migrate because of the patriarchal nature of their countries of origin, might experience migration as a form of trauma, thus making them vulnerable to mental health problems, depression, and anxiety in particular. Women who become refugees or asylum seekers face additional stresses as a result of their migration status (or lack thereof), which means they have limited or no access to the services, rights, and legal protections afforded to members of the majority population or settled migrants. Language barriers and lack of awareness of the cultural customs and norms of the countries to which they have migrated contribute to social isolation, increased vulnerability to mental health problems, and challenges in accessing services.[42]

Additionally, women's central role in maintaining family and kinship networks, including pressure to send money home and to sponsor others to join them, whilst raising their children without access to the support of extended families can be extremely stressful. Women report that these stresses negatively impact their marital relationships, especially where there are financial worries and/or women become the chief or only sources of family income, which generates tensions from the reversal of gender-based roles within their culture. The possibility of divorce and family breakdown represents further stressors for women with pressure to remain in situations that are detrimental to their mental health for fear this would bring shame, stigma, and potential financial ruin to their families.[42]

Substance Use Disorders

It is important to note that treatment for SUDs in women may progress differently than for men. Treatment response is different in women compared to men. However, for all persons with SUD, there will be a definite delay and several barriers for help-seeking. Women in particular may be afraid to get help during or after pregnancy or otherwise due to possible legal or social fears and lack of child care while in treatment. Women in treatment often need support for handling the burdens of work, home care, child care, and other family responsibilities. Services such as child care, parenting classes, supportive therapies, family engagement, and job training should be included as a part of treating women with SUDs.[31]

Measures were suggested by Substance Abuse and Mental Health Services Administration (SAMHSA), 2021 advisory in treating Asian women with SUDs to overcome barriers to treatment.[43] These include:
- Incorporation of drug and alcohol education to reduce the stigma attached to substance use and SUD.
- Approach treatment from the vantage point of promoting overall health rather than focusing solely on substance use; include a holistic connection between body, mind, and spirit.
- Provide a nurturing environment that does not encourage cultural and gender-related tendencies toward self-blame.

Pregnancy-related Psychiatric Disorders

A systematic review was conducted from the synthesis of studies addressing barriers to help-seeking among ethnic minorities (Bangladeshi, Pakistani, Indian, South Asian, Asian, Mixed Asian/British, Pathan, Black, Black African, Nigerian, Ghanaian, Black Caribbean, Portuguese, White American, and White Australian) in Europe. The factors responsible for help-seeking among these women were categorized into themes. They include unawareness and beliefs about mental health, the influence of culture (key finding), symptoms and coping strategies, emotional isolation and seeking support, accessing mental health services, experiences of mental health services, and what women want. Unawareness about the services and avoidance of existing services due to bad past experiences or assumptions due to cross-cultural mismatch also hampers help-seeking.[44]

Postpartum Disorders

Appropriate psychiatric treatment during postpartum period is affected by multiple barriers like nonreporting of symptoms to a health care professional, inability to express feelings to family members, poor satisfaction about the initial contact with health professionals, acceptance of myths, stigma, lack of time, and child care issues, limited evidence on feasible detection and treatment strategies for maternal mental disorders, lack of mental health specialists in the public health sector, lack of prescribing guidelines for pregnant and breastfeeding women, and stigmatizing attitudes among primary health care staff and the community.[45]

A recent study conducted in South India assessed the help-seeking patterns in women with postpartum disorders. It has been found that about 47 % of women with postpartum disorders first visited general practitioners/faith healers for help-seeking. Among 52% who first contacted the Psychiatrist, a past history of psychiatric illness was significantly higher. This suggests that lack of awareness and resources are the main barriers for help-seeking in this group.[46]

■ CONCLUSION

Women's mental health cannot be understood in a comprehensive manner without the sociocultural underpinnings. Hence, to achieve the goal of addressing women's mental health needs health policies should also target the social and cultural factors. Such an emphasis calls for Governments' policies that invest in education, economic empowerment, violence reduction, legal, and political mechanisms that enhance women's status.[35] In addition, research is called for to examine the social factors that influence women's health in specific cultural contexts and to identify effective community-based interventions in improving women's health status.[7]

KEY POINTS

- Various aspects of psychiatric disorders such as definition, symptom presentation, psychopathology, help-seeking, diagnosis, and treatment adherence in women are influenced by cultural background and traditions.
- Cultural formulation interview from DSM-5 can be used while eliciting a history from a female with a mental illness.
- Culture-specific risk factors such as interpersonal violence, poor socioeconomic status, subordinate position, burden of caregiving, and migration can lead to psychiatric disorders in women from LAMI countries.

- Predominant barriers for help-seeking include stigma, unawareness, explanatory models of illness, scarce resources, and improper implementation of healthcare policies and programs.
- Comprehensive assessment with a special focus on domains of cultural formulation needs to be carried out while evaluation of women for mental health disorders.

REFERENCES

1. American Psychiatric Association. Diagnostic and statistical manual of mental disorders. [online] Available from https://www.psychiatry.org/psychiatrists/practice/dsm [Last accessed December, 2023].
2. Edge D, Bhugra D. Ethnic and cultural effects on mental health care for women. In: Castle DJ, Abel KM (Eds). Comprehensive Women's mental health. Cambridge: Cambridge University Press; 2016. pp. 14-27.
3. Chandra PS, Saraf G, Bajaj A, Satyanarayana VA. The current status of gender-sensitive mental health services for women-findings from a global survey of experts. Arch Womens Ment Health. 2019;22(6):759-70.
4. Malhotra S, Shah R. Women and mental health in India: An overview. Indian J Psychiatry. 2015;57(Suppl 2):S205-11.
5. Tol WA, Ebrecht B, Aiyo R, Murray SM, Nguyen AJ, Kohrt BA, et al. Maternal mental health priorities, help-seeking behaviors, and resources in post-conflict settings: a qualitative study in eastern Uganda. BMC Psychiatry. 2018;18(1):39.
6. Niaz U, Hassan S. Culture and mental health of women in South-East Asia. World Psychiatry. 2006;5(2):118-120.
7. López SR, Guarnaccia PJ. Cultural psychopathology: uncovering the social world of mental illness. Annu Rev Psychol. 2000;51:571-98.
8. www.psych.org. (2013). Cultural formulation Interview. available at http://www.psych.org/practice/dsm/dsm5/online-assessment-measures [Last accessed December, 2023].
9. Lewis-Fernández R, Aggarwal NK, Bäärnhielm S, Rohlof H, Kirmayer LJ, et al. Culture and psychiatric evaluation: operationalizing cultural formulation for DSM-5. Psychiatry. 2014;77(2):130-54.
10. DeSilva R, Aggarwal NK, Lewis-Fernandez R. The DSM-5 cultural formulation interview and the evolution of cultural assessment in psychiatry. Psychiatric Times. 2015;32(6):10.
11. Birtel MD, Mitchell BL. Cross-cultural differences in depression between White British and South Asians: Causal attributions, stigma by association, discriminatory potential. Psychol Psychother. 2023;96(1):101-16.
12. Tikka SK, Thippeswamy H, Chandra PS. The Influence of culture on perinatal mental health. Key Topics in Perinatal Mental Health. 2022;18:287-302.
13. Kapoor A, Juneja R, Singh DC. Cultural specific syndromes in India – an overview. Int J Cur Res Rev. 2018;10(11): 2-6.
14. Tasca C, Rapetti M, Carta MG, Fadda B. Women and hysteria in the history of mental health. Clin Pract Epidemiol Ment Health. 2012;8:110-9.
15. Lakhani S, Sharma V, Desai NG. Qualitative content analysis of cultural formulations of clients suffering from conversion disorder in North India. Indian J Psychiatry. 2022;64(1):73-9.

16. Bohra N, Srivastava S, Bhatia MS. Depression in women in Indian context. Indian J Psychiatry. 2015;57(Suppl 2):S239-45.
17. Moldavsky D. The implication of transcultural psychiatry for clinical practice. Isr J Psychiatry Relat Sci. 2003;40(1):47-56.
18. In: James C, Este D, Thomas WB, Benjamin A, Lloyd B, Turner T (Eds). Race and well-being: The Lives, Hopes and Activism of African Canadians. Fernwood Publishing Co Ltd; 2010.
19. Bina R. The impact of cultural factors upon postpartum depression: a literature review. Health Care Women Int. 2008;29(6):568-92.
20. Satyanarayana VA, Lukose A, Srinivasan K. Maternal mental health in pregnancy and child behavior. Indian J Psychiatry. 2011;53(4):351-61.
21. Kuug AK, James S, Sihaam JB. Exploring the cultural perspectives and implications of infertility among couples in the Talensi and Nabdam Districts of the upper east region of Ghana. Contracept Reprod Med. 2023;8(1):28.
22. Patel A, Sharma PSVN, Kumar P, Binu VS. Sociocultural Determinants of Infertility Stress in Patients Undergoing Fertility Treatments. J Hum Reprod Sci. 2018;11(2):172-9.
23. Ali S, Sophie R, Imam AM, Khan FI, Ali SF, Shaikh AY, et al. Knowledge, perceptions and myths regarding infertility among selected adult population in Pakistan: a cross-sectional study. BMC Public Health. 2011;11:760.
24. Thippeswamy H, Dahale A, Desai G, Chandra PS. What is in a name? Causative explanatory models of postpartum psychosis among patients and caregivers in India. Int J Soc Psychiatry. 2015;61(8):818-23.
25. Huang YC, Mathers N. Postnatal depression -- biological or cultural? A comparative study of postnatal women in the UK and Taiwan. J Adv Nurs. 2001;33(3):279-87.
26. Kirmayer LJ. Cultural variations in the response to psychiatric disorders and emotional distress. Soc Sci Med. 1989;29(3):327-39.
27. Heh SS, Coombes L, Bartlett H. The association between depressive symptoms and social support in Taiwanese women during the month. Int J Nurs Stud. 2004;41(5):573-9.
28. Yoshida K, Yamashita H, Ueda M, Tashiro N. Postnatal depression in Japanese mothers and the reconsideration of 'Satogaeri bunben'. Pediatr Int. 2001;43(2):189-93.
29. Patel V, Rodrigues M, DeSouza N. Gender, poverty, and postnatal depression: a study of mothers in Goa, India. Am J Psychiatry. 2002;159(1):43-7.
30. Rodrigues M, Patel V, Jaswal S, de Souza N. Listening to mothers: qualitative studies on motherhood and depression from Goa, India. Soc Sci Med. 2003;57(10):1797-806.
31. National Institute on Drug Abuse. (2020). Substance Use in Women Research Report. [online] Available from https://nida.nih.gov/publications/research-reports/substance-use-in-women/summary [Last accessed December, 2023].
32. Robinson L, Smith M. (2021). Self-medicating depression, anxiety, and stress. [online] Available from https://www.helpguide.org/articles/addictions/self-medicating.htm [Last accessed December, 2023].
33. Bhugra D, Desai M. Attempted suicide in South Asian women. Advances in Psychiatric treatment. 2002;8(6):418-23.

34. Özen-Dursun B, Kaptan SK, Giles S, Husain N, Panagioti M. Understanding self-harm and suicidal behaviours in South Asian communities in the UK: systematic review and meta-synthesis. BJPsych Open. 2023;9(3):e82.
35. Douki S, Zineb SB, Nacef F, Halbreich U. Women's mental health in the Muslim world: cultural, religious, and social issues. J Affect Disord. 2007;102(1-3):177-89.
36. Sen G, Ostlin P. Gender inequity in health: Why it exists and how we can change it. Glob Public Health. 2008;3(Suppl 1):1-12.
37. Chandra PS, Satyanarayana VA. Gender disadvantage and common mental disorders in women. Int Rev Psychiatry. 2010;22(5):513-24.
38. Amarasinghe GS, Agampodi SB. Help-seeking intention for depression and suicidal ideation during pregnancy and postpartum in rural Sri Lanka, a cross-sectional study. Rural Remote Health. 2022;22(3):7273.
39. Karasz A, Patel V, Kabita M, Shimu P. "Tension" in South Asian women: developing a measure of common mental disorder using participatory methods. Prog Community Health Partnersh. 2013;7(4):429-41.
40. Nichter M. Idioms of distress: alternatives in the expression of psychosocial distress: a case study from South India. Cult Med Psychiatry. 1981;5(4):379-408.
41. Desai G, Chaturvedi SK. Idioms of distress. J Neurosci Rural Pract. 2017;8(Suppl 1):S94-97.
42. Delara M. Social Determinants of Immigrant Women's Mental Health. Advances in Public Health. 2016;1-11.
43. Substance Abuse and Mental Health Services Administration. (2021). Addressing the Specific Needs of Women for Treatment of Substance Use Disorders. [online] Available from https://store.samhsa.gov/sites/default/files/pep20-06-04-002.pdf [Last accessed December, 2023].
44. Watson H, Harrop D, Walton E, Young A, Soltani H. A systematic review of ethnic minority women's experiences of perinatal mental health conditions and services in Europe. PLoS ONE. 2019;14(1):e0210587.
45. Baron EC, Hanlon C, Mall S, Honikman S, Breuer E, Kathree T, et al. Maternal mental health in primary care in five low- and middle-income countries: a situational analysis. BMC Health Serv Res. 2016;16:53.
46. Thippeswamy H, Desai G, Chandra P. Help-seeking patterns in women with postpartum severe mental illness: a report from southern India. Arch Womens Ment Health. 2018;21(5):573-8.

CHAPTER 19

Gender-sensitive Mental Health Services and Ethical Issues in Care

Sunita Simon Kurpad

■ ABSTRACT

This chapter discusses the impact of gender on the mental health of women. Relevant terminology in this field is explained. Awareness of the role of gender in the experience of mental illness and its management is important for effective care. The resources that are available to sensitize health professionals are cited. Gender equity is recognized as important in research. Gender-responsive mental health care is discussed, in the context of ground realities in India with the need to audit such services. Handling ethical dilemmas safely needs an understanding of the practical implications of our interventions. Some problems can be handled by the sensitivity and expertise of mental health professionals, while others may reflect more deep-rooted social problems that need community involvement to make effective changes. Various ethical issues in care are discussed. While the focus of this chapter is women, gender-sensitive mental health care services will help all genders.

Keywords: Gender, mental health, psychiatric services, women, mental illness, trauma-informed

■ INTRODUCTION

Gender is an important social determinant of health.[1] Both higher-income and lower-income countries face challenges in their effort to handle this issue in health care. This chapter will focus on some key areas in an effort to sensitize all trainees on the issue of gender in the mental health of women.

A person's biological sex is determined by chromosomes, sexual organs, and hormones and is generally assigned at birth. However, one's gender is a social, cultural, behavioral, and psychological construct and comprises of one's identity as well as gender norms held by the society one lives in. It also includes the social roles one is expected to fulfill and even the activities one can participate in and the opportunities available. If one's gender is different from one's biological sex, if one's gender expression is at variance with one's biological sex, or if sexual orientation is not accepted by a heteronormative society, then there is a high risk of facing discrimination and even violence.[2] While the focus is on women's mental health in this chapter—persons identifying as lesbian, gay, bisexual, transgender, intersex, queer/questioning, and asexual (LGBTQiA) and even some men too may face specific challenges due to gender roles and bias in our society.[3,4]

No one culture is representative of India and while some women in India may enjoy the benefits of education, work, financial independence, leisure, supportive relationships, and the agency to make decisions on issues ranging from health care to finance, there are many women who are dependent on others (usually men) to even visit the doctor, let alone taking decisions about own health care. All of this points to the importance for doctors, especially psychiatrists and other mental health professionals to be sensitive to these issues.

SOME RELEVANT TERMINOLOGIES

Intersectionality

Intersectionality was a term originally coined by law Professor Kimberle Crenshaw in 1989, in the context of race and gender discrimination. She pointed out that it was important to recognize that black women faced discrimination on both counts (i.e., being a person of color and being a woman) and these "intersected or overlapped" with each other and with issues of class and individual characteristics.[5] The World Health Organization (WHO) refers to "intersectionality" in health in that gender does cause inequalities that intersect with other social and economic discriminations such as socioeconomic status, ethnicity, geographic location, disability, and age among others and this leads to further discrimination.[1]

Trauma-informed Care

Women may face multiple traumas. An experience of sexual abuse and/or domestic violence impacts mental illness and its treatment. Due to multiple common vulnerabilities, vulnerable women face a "lifetime spiral of gender violence"—from the risk of female feticide, less nutritious food as a baby, less education opportunities for a girl child, violence as a teen/young adult/married woman or elder.[6] Trauma-informed care is being mindful of the trauma a person can experience over their lifetime and offering services that reflect this understanding.[7] It involves engaging effectively with the victim survivor, empathetic communication, and being sensitive to possible triggers of reexperiencing trauma. Being sensitive to cultural, historical, and gender issues is one of six integral guiding principles of a trauma-informed approach to care (the others being "safety, trustworthiness and transparency, peer support, collaboration, and mutuality and empowerment and choice").[8] Gender-responsive trauma-informed care will be discussed further a little later in this chapter.

Patient

While many doctors feel it is appropriate to call patients as clients- in this chapter the word patient will be used, in recognition to the intrinsic vulnerability of the patient in the doctor-patient dynamic.[9] This chapter refers to women but does not mean that gender is a binary concept.

Domestic Violence/Intimate Partner Violence

Domestic violence is the broader term as it includes violence experienced at home—with perpetrators being spouses/in-laws/children/partners. Intimate partner violence (IPV) is in the context of people experiencing violence, psychological aggression, or stalking with the current or former partner involved in an intimate relationship.[10]

Victim/Survivor

In the context of violence, victim is generally a term used by the police or in court. 'Victim' is also used to describe a person in the immediate aftermath of the violence, while "survivor" implies that the person identifies with a degree of recovery and resilience. It is suggested that sometimes it can be premature to use the term survivor, and it is best to respectfully ask the person whether they prefer to be called victim or survivor.[11] In India, particular sensitivity is required with different languages and dialects—not least when a translator is being used.

■ SENSITIVE USE OF LANGUAGE

There is a need to be sensitive/take care about the language we use to describe people/issues as it may risk gender stereotyping or being perceived as gender stereotyping. A recently released handbook released by the Supreme Court of India for the legal fraternity on gender-sensitive language for speaking and writing is a useful read.[12] Some words that people may use without thought (that being considered acceptable many years ago would no longer be considered acceptable today) have better alternatives, for example, affair—relationship outside of marriage, housewife—homemaker, spinster—unmarried woman, and unwed mother—mother.

■ GENDER AND MENTAL ILLNESS

Gender inequality affects women and girls in a far higher proportion than men and boys.[1] The link between mental illness and gender is complex due to the issues of intersectionality and the spiral of gender violence. However, listed below are some issues that have already been known about gender and mental health. Any gender-sensitive mental health service should ensure the health professionals working with them are aware of these issues. The well-known adage in the practice of medicine that the "eye will not see, what the mind does not know," would hold true in this area too.

Nature of Mental Illness

Depression, Anxiety, and Bipolar Disorders

Both depression and anxiety have consistently shown to be commoner in women than men across countries over the last several decades. However, in countries where women have better gender equality, this gender gap is closing, attributed to changing gender roles for women which allows for more access to protective factors like employment.[13] While bipolar disorder was traditionally considered to have equal prevalence in men and women, some recent clinical studies (not epidemiological)—seem to suggest that bipolar 2 is increasingly being recognized in women. Dell'Osso pointed out that rapid cycling, suicide attempts, and depression are more common in women with bipolar affective disorder (BPAD), and possibly women with BPAD are more likely to be misdiagnosed as major depressive disorder—perhaps as the first episode is often depression.[14]

Substance Use

The intrinsic biological differences between men and women make it more likely for women to absorb alcohol quickly, metabolize it less efficiently, and be more prone to complications of alcohol use earlier. The risk of liver cirrhosis, cardiac muscle damage, brain atrophy, cognitive decline, and cancer of the mouth, throat, colon, and liver, and not just breast cancer have been flagged as particular concerns of excessive alcohol use as a risk in women's health.[15]

Women with alcohol and other substance use often have other medical and mental health comorbidity, and doctors can miss this history of substance use unless they routinely try to elicit this information sensitively.[16] This is important as women may find it more difficult to report and access care for substance dependence. The occurrence of medical comorbidity may in reality present a useful opportunity to intervene.

The association between alcohol and sexual violence is complex. The cognitive and motor effects of alcohol use may make women less able to protect themselves. One should not compound the self-blame victim's experience if they have been drinking. In some men—alcohol use compounds the risk of them assaulting women. One way to reduce this risk of violence is not just educating women about the risks of alcohol, but educating men too, especially as some men make assumptions about a woman's willingness to have a sexual activity with them just because she has consumed alcohol.[17] Some women too get aggressive under the influence of alcohol.

Schizophrenia and Other Psychoses

Chandra has discussed the importance of psychiatrists being alert to the experience of trauma in women with schizophrenia. This can present as dissociative symptoms, something which is not traditionally recognized/accepted as a comorbidity in schizophrenia.[18]

Post-traumatic Stress Disorder

Post-traumatic stress disorder (PTSD) is three times more common in women than in men. While it is never acceptable to gender stereotype, there is a body of recent evidence which suggests sex and gender-specific factors which could account for the differences in symptom profile and even outcome. These have been linked to sex-specific epigenetic factors and neuroendocrine responses to stress, for example, the oxytocin response in women versus the vasopressin response in men. The kind of trauma experienced by men and women may be different, with women often experiencing trauma at an earlier age when they are even more neurobiologically vulnerable. Women tend to present more often with depression, anxiety, and dissociative symptoms. It has been suggested that they tend to cope with stress using the "tend and befriend" mechanism (tending to young ones and befriending each other), which can be why lack of social support is a particular risk factor in women. Women tend to do better with therapy and are less likely to drop out. The use and abuse of substances is a way that all genders use to cope with PTSD.[19,20]

Deliberate Self-harm and Suicide

In India, the suicide rates in women are higher than in men and even higher than the global average.[21] Unlike in the West, women here are as likely as men to die by violent methods like hanging. Social issues such as economic hardship, problems with in-laws, domestic violence, and alcohol use in spouses seem to contribute more to deliberate self-harm attempts than diagnosable mental illness.[22] Recognizing and treating depression is important, but addressing relevant social issues is also necessary. However, there is limited research evidence on gender-specific risk and protective factors.[23]

Life Stage and Mental Illness

Women can face particular risks to mental health depending on the life cycle stage they are abused when young, issues related to pregnancy/delivery in the reproductive age group to elder abuse, and dementia when older.[24] The stressors and needs of the older woman need to be looked at from both the life stage and gender lens. Women are more likely to be caregivers. Inadequate services like daycare for persons with dementia add significantly to the burden of having to care for children, sick, and other elderly in the family which can lead to her compromising on her own health.

PREGNANCY, CHILDBIRTH, AND LACTATION

Pregnancy and breastfeeding of children affect treatment choices regarding pharmacotherapy.[25] Substance Abuse and Mental Health Administration (SAMHSA) in their recent document titled "Addressing the specific need of women for treatment of substance use disorders" have discussed the additional challenge of treatment during pregnancy. They recommend that buprenorphine is safer than naltrexone and methadone in the treatment of pregnant women with opioid dependence. Regarding alcohol use in pregnancy, there is no safe limit.[26]

In India, antenatal care may occur in one place with the actual delivery in another. The availability of extended family support would intuitively seem to be a protective factor. Equally, the lack of support from family would be a concern. India has tried to address the gaps in maternal and perinatal health care with better coverage of the District Mental Health Programme. The Mental Health Care Act 2017 mandates mother and child care done simultaneously when a mother is admitted for mental illness.[27]

Biological Vulnerabilities of Women on Psychotropic Medication

Women are more likely to have dose-dependent higher prolactin levels when exposed to certain psychotropics. The effects of lowering estrogen have been linked to premature aging. There is a likelihood of a more severe metabolic syndrome in women.[28]

Culture, Somatic Complaints, and Somatization

Cross-cultural studies seem to suggest that the earlier belief that it is non-Western cultures tend to "somatize" as a way to express psychological distress, may not be true. It seems to be a cross-cultural phenomenon. Some women with depression do present to doctors with physical complaints, and others even with medically unexplained/inadequately explained symptoms. Interestingly not only have patient-related factors been reported, but that of doctors and health care settings. Patients seem more likely to report somatic symptoms in a "walk-in" clinic, rather than one which offers a more personalized primary care.[29] In India it has been reported that being a woman and poor are important correlates of somatization disorder.[30]

GENDER AND PHYSICAL HEALTH

There is a complex interplay between sex, gender, and health. While it is relevant for many illnesses- two conditions of particular relevance for psychiatrists are discussed here:

Cardiovascular Health

Gender has been recognized to have an impact on outcomes in cardiovascular disease. The excess mortality in women is reportedly not just due to clinical factors such as atypical and delayed presentations, but actual gender bias with factors ranging from misdiagnosis (wrongly attributing symptoms to anxiety) to women being more likely to be undertreated. On one hand, some women seem more likely to somatize, yet ironically others are more likely to die of cardiac complaints as they do not seek help for physical symptoms. For women who are obese, weight stigma (which includes self-stigma and is not gender-specific) may lead to avoidance of health screenings which further compounds the risk. Both women and clinicians need to be sensitized to these issues.[31] Psychiatrists are also physicians and patients coming for mental health treatment should also have simple checks such as weight and blood pressure, and appropriate physical review when indicated.

Human Immunodeficiency Virus Infection

Here biological factors related to mucosal tears and gender related issues like being less empowered to demand condom use by partners can make women especially vulnerable. Both sex workers and married women within a relationship can be at risk. Sexual violence compounds human immunodeficiency virus (HIV) risk. Health education can play a significant role in reducing risk by creating awareness. The National Aids Control Organization (NACO) and the Ministry of Health and Family Welfare (MoHFW) in India have created useful documents which are freely available online to sensitize health workers at the grass root level to the gender issues in HIV and acquired immunodeficiency syndrome (AIDS).[32]

■ CLINICAL PRACTICE, EDUCATION, AND RESEARCH

After developing an understanding about how gender (and sex) impacts mental and physical health, translating that understanding into clinical practice for the benefit of patients and caregivers, education of health personnel, and research in this constantly evolving field is important.

Clinical Practice

Awareness about the role of gender in medicine should translate into practice. This starts with sensitive history taking and physical examination. It should go beyond diagnosis and immediate management to planning follow-up care. As gender is a well-known determinant of access to health care- this should be explored in the context of the individual woman patient in front of us. Many women in India are dependent on others often men, to bring them to hospital. Factors such as transportation, difficulty in traveling back late, the male attendant being away from work for a day to bring the patient to the hospital, and the option of some teleconsultation sessions have to be factored in when planning follow-up care.

Education

Medical students, doctors, and other health personnel need to be sensitized to issues of sex and gender in medicine[33] and to trauma-informed care. Some factors relating to gender are more easily modifiable like the differential use of diagnostics and therapeutics. Others like empowering women in a predominantly patriarchal society will need community involvement and the help of advocacy groups.

The particular challenge would be to ensure that the "older" health professional is also sensitized. Continuing medical education programs are a useful forum to focus on these particular issues.

The World Psychiatry Association has released a competency-based curriculum to train health workers on violence against women.[34] Using the LIVES acronym by WHO is a useful reminder "Listen, Inquire, Validate, Enhance (safety), and Support (connect to services and social support)."[35]

Research

Gender Equity

In recognition of the absence of gender equity in research, the US now has a policy on sex as a biological variable. They suggest 4 Cs to address this issue—"consider (design studies to take this into account/or explain why not), collect and tabulate sex-based data, characterize (analyze sex-based data), and communicate (report and publish sex-based data)."[36]

There are challenges and opportunities for research in this area. Greaves and Ritz point out that when research merely looks at the sex binary of male females or the gender binary of men and women, there is potentially already a loss in useful information, as findings cannot be generalized. Understanding the role of sex and gender better is an intrinsic component of evidence-based precision medicine.[37]

Need to Study Impact of Gender on Health

The issues around women and mental health have been raised in India.[24] There has been pioneering work in the field of perinatal mental health.[38] Aspects of gender sensitivity in mental health care have also been highlighted recently.[39] There is a need to create a body of evidence-based literature looking at sex and gender on various aspects of mental health and illness, including service utilization and outcomes. Issues of intersectionality with other issues such as caste and religion, both extremely sensitive topics in India, need to be studied safely.[40,41] As these issues are linked to historical (multigenerational) trauma, they need to be handled with particular sensitivity.

GENDER AND MENTAL HEALTH SERVICES

Once awareness of sex and gender issues in mental health is created, then it is easier for mental health professionals to ensure that mental health services do reflect that sensitivity. Listed below are some of the issues which would be relevant.

Gender-responsive Care

While being gender-sensitive implies that one is sensitive to the issues around gender, gender-responsiveness is the higher ideal that aspires to modify one's behavior to address gender inequality. Gender-responsive care was described in the context of care of women prisoners in the US.[42] Gender-responsiveness has been described to have five components:[43]

1. *Relationship-based*—acknowledging the importance of social connections and relationships for women.
2. *Strengths-based*—focusing on the patient's strengths, seeing negative behaviors as sometimes starting as adaptive strategies and then teaching new skills.
3. *Trauma informed*—as discussed earlier in this chapter.
4. *Culturally competent*—ensures practitioners are capable of valuing diversity and working cross-culturally.
5. *Holistic*—acknowledges the larger context of the lives of women, their feelings, and decision-making.

Involving Women Stakeholders

In the document "Addressing the unmet needs of women's mental health," Abel and Newbigging from the UK pointed out the importance of involving women stakeholders in policies regarding mental health care in the spirit of collaborative care and shared decision-making effort.[28] A landmark document from India, where the authors visited several mental health institutions and spoke to the women patients- gives a powerful voice to these women patients. Satisfaction with physical facilities was noted in several centers. However, the document lists several concerns for women in terms of human rights and ethics, which will be discussed later in this chapter.[44]

Structural and Logistic Issues

Adequate Beds and Spaces for Women

While on one hand there is an underutilization of psychiatric services by women in India (partly attributed to stigma), there is a need for adequate beds for women in acute psychiatric services.[24] In many countries, the importance of having separate wards and toilets for women has been highlighted,[39] but in India traditionally these have always been separated for men and women. While one understands the need for privacy, the use of lockable doors is considered to be a risk for self-harm in many acute care centers. In India, patients need to have attenders with them in order to be admitted into the hospital (family, friends, or paid workers). This creates its own challenges but generally affords a degree of safety in a psychiatric ward.

Handling Violent Women

Inpatient and outpatient facilities should have adequate facilities to deal with aggressive or violent women sensitively, yet safely. While appropriate use of restraints has been discussed in the Mental Health Care Act of India 2017, attention to deescalation and protecting the human rights of patients is necessary.[45,46] Steps like explaining to the woman what is going to be done and why, taken. If a brief physical holding of the aggressive woman is warranted to get the situation under control, it is best to use trained female staff, nursing aides, or even security. When planning the service, one needs to ensure adequate numbers of female personnel who can handle violence are available round the clock. To expect male personnel to even briefly hold an agitated women patient can make it extremely traumatic for the woman if she has been a victim of violence in the past and also placing male personnel in an inappropriate situation.

Workplace Policies

The law in India does protect the rights of working women by ensuring much-needed policies like maternity (and paternity) leave. Audits may be required to ensure that women are not discriminated against while hiring personnel. One cannot expect a workforce to deliver effective gender-responsive service if the needs of women employed by them are not addressed effectively.

Implications for Forensic Psychiatry

Research in the West has shown that there is a disproportionate number of women with a history of trauma and mental illness in conflict with the law. In the US, the idea of "therapeutic jurisprudence" has gained support with the establishment of mental health courts. While the focus is on persons of any gender with a history of mental illness and nonviolent crime, there is some evidence to suggest that women are more likely to be referred to these programs and a trauma-informed approach focusing on building resilience seems to reduce recidivism.[47,48]

Audit of Services

It is important to audit how gender-sensitive services are on the ground. Chandra et al. surveyed how satisfied mental health professionals across the globe were about gender sensitivity in their mental health services. The seven domains they evaluated in themselves are a useful checklist. The domains are gender-sensitive structural arrangements, creating an atmosphere of safety and respect, having choices and meaningful access to care including advance directives, gender-specific training of mental health professionals, information (including on grievance redressal and legal aid), and gendered data analysis.[39] Developing and improving on existing quality checks for accreditation purposes could mandate some changes.

▪ ETHICAL ISSUES IN CARE

Listed below are some of the common ethical issues which may be relevant when discussing gender and mental health.

Ethical Decision-making in Clinical Care

Context is important in ethical decision-making. The well-known known ethical principles form a useful ethical framework to make decisions in clinical care.[49] In the context of gender an example would be the issue of domestic violence in India. How should one handle it if the patient confides in the doctor that she is a victim of physical abuse from her spouse, but is unwilling for the doctor to raise it with the spouse. Let us assume for the sake of discussion that this information was elicited while evaluating her depression. Let us see how the principles play out.

Autonomy

In situations where the woman has the capacity to make decisions, one has to respect her autonomy. Going against her wishes will make her lose trust in the doctor. While the role of family is important in Asian cultures, the choice to involve her parents or sibling should still rest with the patient.

Beneficence

The doctor may well feel that talking to the husband about his aggression toward his spouse may deter him from hitting her again. In reality, the patient's reluctance may be due to her fear that this would put her at greater risk of aggression. What may benefit her is empowering her over several sessions to deal with this issue, trying to therapeutically engage with the spouse himself, and working with the couple. If she has clinical depression, that needs to be treated effectively too.

If there is an ongoing risk and the husband is unlikely to change his behavior, then arranging for additional support would be helpful. Involving the police may be beneficial, especially as there are now laws to protect women from domestic violence and dowry harassment. Many women may initially feel this is not a feasible option as they are dependent on their spouse.[50]

Nonmaleficence

Do no harm is often stated as the most important ethical principle. Understanding the woman's concerns about discussing the violence with her spouse is imperative. While well-intentioned, the health professional confronting the husband risks him getting even more violent with her when she gets home. If she has no other option but to go back to her spouse and is also dependent on him to bring her back to the hospital, it is vital to ensure one's interaction with her spouse will not deter him from bringing her back to the hospital.

Justice

Traditionally this is described in the context to being fair and just in the context of allocation of scarce resources. But here we will focus on the important role mental health professionals have in advocating for patients and their rights. In this situation, it is important to educate the woman on her legal rights and put her in touch with services that could help her. Documenting all relevant information properly in the medical notes is necessary.

Confidentiality, Informed Consent, and Protection of Human Rights

It is important to protect the confidentiality of the health professional-patient interaction, unless mandated by the law (for example as in child sexual abuse in India). Privacy of the documents—paper or digital, should also be maintained, and there should not be any disclosure of patient details unless there is a request from a court of law. If feasible, if the mental health professional is unsure what should be done, it is useful to contact a legal expert or a senior colleague. Even if disclosure is mandated, the proper process should be followed, and always advisable to tell the patient why disclosure is necessary and what exactly will and will not be disclosed.[45,51]

Women patients in India have reported some specific concerns about the care in some mental health institutions such as "not being educated about illness, not allowed to make health care decisions, not being informed of rights, no informed consent taken for treatment, and confidentiality not being maintained by staff and even hair cut without consent."[44]

In India, the law does protect the reproductive rights of women. Handling unplanned pregnancies, especially in the context of sexual violence can be traumatic for the patient. Health professionals need to be aware of the law regarding the Medical Termination of Pregnancy in India. People who practice different religions in India may have differing opinions on the sensitive issue of abortion, depending on when they believe life begins in the womb. Health professional should not impose their own values upon the patient, but if they feel their own opinion on the matter prevents them from handling the patient in a professional manner, it is best to hand over their care to another professional in a sensitive manner.[52]

Protecting Everyone's Rights

Sometimes family courts adjudicate on custody issues and as doctors, we advocate for justice for our patients with mental illness. Persons with mental illness, when stable on regular management of mental illness can make excellent parents. However, in the rare situation when the woman with severe mental illness is poorly adherent to medication and her mental illness prevents her from safely looking after children questions need to be answered truthfully in court, in order to protect the child and to be fair to husbands too. It is always good to prepare the patient for the fact that as a doctor you have to state the truth and its likely outcomes.

Research Ethics

Research on the issues of gender, intersectionality, and mental health is the need of the hour. Women in India are designated as a vulnerable group in research by the Indian Council for Medical Research.[53] Special care should be taken in groups with additional vulnerabilities like prisoners. A detailed discussion on the ethical issues in research in persons with mental illness is outside the scope of this chapter, but literature is available.[54] Existing national guidelines should be followed when planning and conducting research.[53]

Other Issues

As with any ethical practice, there is a need to ensure supervision and a safe space to discuss challenging work. Self-reflection is a must. Professional boundaries should be respected. Sometimes unethical things can happen in clinical work and in research and there is a need for safe whistleblowing.[55-57] It is important to be aware of current ethical guidelines and the law.

■ CONCLUSION

This chapter has outlined some of the key issues around gender, mental health services, and related ethical issues. This is a constantly evolving area.

While much is already known about the problems that exist, there is a need for further research to understand the complex interplay of factors involved in gender and mental health, mental illness, and its outcome in the context of mental health services and their utilization and efficacy.

> **KEY POINTS**
> - Gender is an important social determinant of mental health.
> - Gender can affect the experience of mental illness and its treatment, thereby influencing outcome.
> - Gender-responsive mental health services aim to deliver gender-responsive care in an effort to rectify the fact that gender inequality in women adversely impacts their mental and physical health.
> - Handling the ethical issues that arise in the care of patients and ethical decision-making needs a practical understanding of what can be achieved by a mental health professional's expertise and what needs community involvement to effect a change.

■ REFERENCES

1. World Health Organization. (2021). Gender and health. [online] Available from https://www.who.int/news-room/questions-and-answers/item/gender-and-health [Last accessed December, 2023].
2. Council of Europe. (2023). What is gender-based violence? [online] Available from https://www.coe.int/en/web/gender-matters/what-is-gender-based-violence [Last accessed December, 2023].
3. United Nations. LGBTQI+ Free and equal, not criminalized. [online] Available from https://www.un.org/en/fight-racism/vulnerable-groups/lgbtqi-plus [Last accessed December, 2023].
4. Centre for Disease control and Prevention. (2023). LGBTQ+ Youth: addressing health disparities with a school-based approach. [online] Available from https://www.cdc.gov/lgbthealth/youth.htm [Last accessed December, 2023].
5. Crenshaw K. Demarginalizing the Intersection of Race and Sex: A Black Feminist Critique of Antidiscrimination Doctrine, Feminist Theory and Antiracist Politics. University of Chicago Legal Forum. 1989;8(1).
6. Asian Pacific Institute on Gender-Based Violence. (2002). Lifetime Spiral of Gender Violence. [online] Available from https://www.api-gbv.org/about-gbv/our-analysis/lifetime-spiral/ [Last accessed December, 2023].
7. Jayasundara D, El-Jarrah H, Dabby C, Ahmed D. From the Roots of Trauma to the Flowering of Trauma-Informed Care. Plano, Texas: Texas Muslim Women's Foundation and Asian Pacific Institute on Gender-Based Violence; 2020.
8. Office of Readiness and Response (CDC) and National Centre for Trauma informed care (SAMSHA). (2020). Infographic: 6 guiding principles to a trauma-informed approach. [online] Available from https://www.cdc.gov/orr/infographics/6_principles_trauma_info.htm [Last accessed December, 2023].
9. Kurpad SS, Machado T, Galgali RB, Daniel S. All about elephants in rooms and dogs that do not bark in the night: Boundary violations and the health professional in India. Indian J Psychiatry. 2012;54(1):81-7.

10. Centre for Disease control and Prevention. (2022). Fast Facts: Preventing intimate partner violence. Centers for disease control and prevention. [online] Available from https://www.cdc.gov/violenceprevention/intimatepartnerviolence/fastfact.html#:~:text=Intimate%20partner%20violence%20(IPV)%20is,and%20how%20severe%20it%20is. [Last accessed December, 2023].
11. Women against abuse. The language we use. [online] Available from https://www.womenagainstabuse.org/education-resources/the-language-we-use [Last accessed December, 2023].
12. Supreme Court of India. Handbook on combating gender stereotypes. [online] Available from https://main.sci.gov.in/pdf/LU/04092023_070741.pdf [Last accessed December, 2023].
13. Seedat S, Scott KM, Angermeyer MC, Berglund P, Bromet EJ, Brugha TS, et al. Cross-National Associations Between Gender and Mental Disorders in the World Health Organization World Mental Health Surveys. Arch Gen Psychiatry. 2009;66(7):785-95.
14. Dell'Osso B, Cafaro R, Ketter TA. Has Bipolar Disorder become a predominantly female gender related condition? Analysis of recently published large sample studies. Int J Bipolar Disord. 2021;9:3.
15. Center for Disease Control and Prevention. (2022). Excessive alcohol use is a risk factor for women's health. [online] Available from https://www.cdc.gov/alcohol/fact-sheets/womens-health.htm [Last accessed December, 2023].
16. McCaul ME, Roach D, Hasin DS, Weisner C, Chang G, Sinha R. Alcohol and Women: A Brief Overview. Alcohol Clin Exp Res. 2019;43(5):774-9.
17. Queensland Centre for Domestic and Family Violence Research QCDFVR. (2018). Insights from Literature. Alcohol use and violence against women. [online] Available from https://noviolence.org.au/wp-content/uploads/2018/10/Alcohol-Use-and-Violence-Against-Women.pdf [Last accessed December, 2023].
18. Chandra PC. Hidden but not forgotten: the trauma experience among women with severe mental illness and our role as mental health professionals. J Psychosoc Rehabil. Ment Health. 2019;6(7):5-8.
19. Olff M. Sex and gender differences in post-traumatic stress disorder: an update. Eur J Psychotraumatol. 2017;8(suppl 4):1351204.
20. Hiscox LV, Sharp T, Olff M, Seedat S, Halligan SL. Sex-Based Contributors to and Consequences of Post-traumatic Stress Disorder. Curr Psychiatry Rep. 2023;25(5):233-45.
21. World Health Organization. (2021). Suicide worldwide in 2019. [online] Available from https://www.who.int/publications/i/item/suicide-in-the-world [Last accessed December, 2023].
22. Parkar SR, Dawani V, Weiss MG. Gender, Suicide, and the Sociocultural Context of Deliberate Self-Harm in an Urban General Hospital in Mumbai, India. Cult Med Psychiatry. 2008;32(4):492-515.
23. Ramesh P, Taylor PJ, McPhillips R, Raman R, Robinson C. A Scoping Review of Gender Differences in Suicide in India. Front Psychiatry. 2022;13:884657.
24. Malhotra S, Shah R. Women and mental health in India: An overview. Indian J Psychiatry. 2015;57(Suppl 2):S205-11.
25. National Institute for Health and Care Excellence. (2020). Antenatal and postnatal mental health: clinical management and service guideline. [online]

Available from https://www.nice.org.uk/guidance/cg192/resources/antenatal-and-postnatal-mental-health-clinical-management-and-service-guidance-pdf-35109869806789 [Last accessed December, 2023].
26. Substance Abuse and Mental Health Services Administration. (2021). Addressing the Specific Needs of Women for Treatment of Substance Use Disorders. [online] Available from https://store.samhsa.gov/sites/default/files/pep20-06-04-002.pdf [Last accessed December, 2023].
27. Ganjekar S, Thekkethayyil AV, Chandra PS. Perinatal mental health around the world: priorities for research and service development in India. BJ Psych Int. 2020;17(1):2-5.
28. Abel KM, Newbigging K. (2018). Addressing the unmet needs of women's mental health. British Medical association. [online] Available from https://www.bma.org.uk/media/2115/bma-womens-mental-health-report-aug-2018.pdf [Last accessed December, 2023].
29. Simon GE, VonKorff M, Piccinelli M, Fullerton C, Ormel J. An international study of the relation between somatic symptoms and depression. N Engl J Med. 1999;341(18):1329-35.
30. Chander KR, Manjunatha N, Binukumar B, Kumar CN, Bada Math S, Janardhan Reddy YC. The prevalence and its correlates of somatization disorder at a quaternary mental health centre. Asian J Psychiatr. 2019;42:24-7.
31. Bosomwoth J, Khan Z. Analysis of Gender-Based Inequality in Cardiovascular Health: An Umbrella Review. Cureus. 2023;15(8):e43482.
32. National AIDS Control Organisation. Shaping our lives: learning to live safe and healthy, free from HIV/Syphilis & other STIs. [online] Available from https://naco.gov.in/sites/default/files/Shaping%20Our%20Lives%20-%20version%202.pdf [Last accessed December, 2023].
33. Mauvais-Jarvis F, Bairey Merz N, Barnes PJ, Brinton RD, Carrero JJ, DeMeo DL, et al. Sex and gender: modifiers of health, disease, and medicine. Lancet. 2020;396(10250):565-82.
34. Stewart DE, Chandra PS. WPA International Competency-Based Curriculum for Mental Health Providers on Intimate Partner Violence and Sexual Violence Against Women. World Psychiatry. 2017;16(2):223-4.
35. World Health Organization. (2021). Caring for women subjected to violence: a WHO curriculum for training health-care providers, revised edition, 2021. [online] Available from https://www.who.int/publications/i/item/9789240039803 [Last accessed December, 2023].
36. National Institutes of Health. NIH policy on sex as a biological variable. [online] Available from https://orwh.od.nih.gov/sex-gender/nih-policy-sex-biological-variable [Last accessed December, 2023].
37. Greaves L, Ritz SA. Sex, Gender and Health: Mapping the Landscape of Research and Policy. Int J Environ Res Public Health. 2022;19(5):2563.
38. Chandra PS, Desai G, Reddy D, Thippeswamy H, Saraf G. The establishment of a mother-baby inpatient psychiatry unit in India: Adaptation of a Western model to meet local cultural and resource needs. Indian J Psychiatry. 2015;57(3):290-4.
39. Chandra PS, Saraf G, Bajaj A, Satyanarayana VA. The current status of gender-sensitive mental health services for women-findings from a global survey of experts. Arch Womens Ment Health. 2019;22(6):759-70.

CHAPTER 19: Gender-sensitive Mental Health Services and Ethical Issues in Care

40. Gupta A, Coffey D. Caste, Religion, and Mental Health in India. Popul Res Policy Rev. 2020;39(6):1119-41.
41. Johri A, Anand PV. Life Satisfaction and Well-Being at the Intersections of Caste and Gender in India. Psychological Studies. 2022;67:317-31.
42. Benedict A, Ney B, Ramirez R. (2015). Gender responsive Discipline and Sanctions Policy Guide for women's facilities. National resource Centre for Justice Involved Women. [online] Available from https://cjinvolvedwomen.org/wp-content/uploads/2018/04/Combined-Discipline-Guide-031518.pdf [Last accessed December, 2023].
43. Benedict A. The office CORE Practice areas of gender responsiveness. Copyright Core associates. [online] Available at https://demoiselle2femme.org/wp-content/uploads/Five-Core-Practice-Areas-of-Gender-Responsiveness.pdf [Last accessed December, 2023].
44. Murthy P, Naveen KC, Chandra PS, Bharat S, Math SB, Bhola P, et al. (2016). Addressing Concerns of Women Admitted to Psychiatric Institutions in India: An In-depth Analysis. New Delhi: National Institute of Mental Health & Neurosciences, Bangalore and National Commission for Women. [online] Available from http://ncw.nic.in/ncw-reports/addressing-concerns-women-admitted-psychiatric-institutions-india-depth-analysis [Last accessed December, 2023].
45. The Mental Health Care Act 2017. (2017). The Gazette of India. Ministry of Law and Justice. [online] Available from http://www.prsindia.org/uploads/media/Mental%20Health/Mental%20Healthcare%20Act,%202017.pdf [Last accessed December, 2023].
46. Raveesh BN, Lepping P. Restraint guidelines for mental health services in India. Indian J Psychiatry. 2019;61(Suppl 4):S698-705.
47. Bureau of Justice assistance, US Department of Justice. (2012). Mental Health Courts Program. [online] Available from https://bja.ojp.gov/program/mental-health-courts-program/overview [Last accessed December, 2023].
48. Honegger L, Dewald S. Making a Case for Gender-Responsive, Trauma-Informed Mental Health Courts: An Exploration of Participant Trauma Histories. J Forensic Soc Work. 2023;7(1):72-90.
49. Beuchamp TL, Childress JF. Principles of biomedical ethics, 5th edition. Oxford: Oxford University Press; 2001.
50. Sabri B, Rai A, Rameshkumar A. Violence Against Women in India: An Analysis of Correlates of Domestic Violence and Barriers and Facilitators of Access to Resources for Support. J Evid Based Soc Work (2019). 2022;19(6):700-29.
51. National Medical Commission; Ethics and registration Board. National Medical Commission Registered Medical practitioner (Professional Conduct), Regulations August 2023. [online] Available from https://www.nmc.org.in/MCIRest/open/getDocument?path=/Documents/Public/Portal/LatestNews/NMC%20RMP%20Conduct%20Regulations%202023.pdf [Last accessed December, 2023].
52. Kurpad SS. High Risk Sexual behavior. In: David Cooper (Ed). Ethics in Mental health Substance Use. United Kingdom: CRC Press Taylor and Francis Group; 2017.

53. Indian Council Of Medical Research. (2018). Handbook on National Ethical Guidelines for Biomedical and Health Research involving human participants. [online] Available from https://ethics.ncdirindia.org/asset/pdf/ICMR_National_Ethical_Guidelines.pdf [Last accessed December, 2023].
54. Kurpad S. Research Ethics in Participants with mental Illness. In: Mathur R, Muthuswamy V, Kumar NK (Eds). Biomedical Ethics Perspectives in the Indian Context by ICMR and NCDIR. New Delhi: Jaypee Brothers Medical Publishers (P) Ltd; 2022. pp. 42-51.
55. Kurpad SS, Ethics in psychosocial interventions. Indian J Psychiatry. 2018;60(Suppl 4):S571-4.
56. Indianjpsychiatry.org. IPS Task Force on Boundary Guidelines. Guidelines for doctors on sexual boundaries in the doctor patient relationship. Version 3.4. Guidelines for doctors on Sexual boundaries Version 3.4 IPS. [online] Available from https://www.nmc.org.in/MCIRest/open/getDocument?path=/Documents/Public/Portal/LatestNews/Guidelines%20for%20doctors%20on%20Sexual%20Boundaries-03.04.2019.pdf [Last accessed December, 2023].
57. Kurpad SS, Bhide A. Sexual boundaries in the doctor–patient relationship: Guidelines for doctors. Indian J Psychiatry. 2017;59(1):14-6.

CHAPTER 20

Measurement and Assessment Tools for Women's Mental Health

Gunja Sengupta, Sundarnag Ganjekar

ABSTRACT

Women's health is influenced by physiological, psychological, and social processes that evolve throughout the lifespan of a woman. Mental health is an interplay of "biopsychosocial" paradigms and gender is one of the important determinants that affect all of them. While there is no substitute for a good clinical history and evaluation, research in the area requires tools that are developed and validated to understand the unique dimensions of the life of women to screen, classify, and quantify determinants of women's mental health. This chapter has reviewed some of the important measures and though by no means complete, tries to describe measures that are commonly sought after. Some tools are also culture-specific and address the position of women in India and South Asia. The measures reviewed address psychosocial vulnerabilities and a reproductive life course approach. Wherever available, literature published in India with regard to these measures has been highlighted.

Keywords: Women's mental health, scales, tools, assessment

INTRODUCTION

The experience of being a woman is a complex phenomenon with biological, psychological, and social underpinnings. Women, by virtue of their gender, maybe more vulnerable to several psychological and psychosocial adversities. Physiological processes such as menarche, pregnancy, postpartum, and menopause may also predispose women to develop specific psychiatric disorders. The literature around the world has documented differences in the onset, course, and prognosis of both common mental disorders (CMDs) and severe mental illnesses (SMIs) between men and women. This includes the higher lifetime risk of anxiety disorders as well as major depression and dysthymic disorder in women.[1] Depression in women is more common as well as more persistent.[2] Approximately one-fifth of women who are pregnant and one-sixth of postpartum women in low- and middle-income countries (LMICs) experience common perinatal mental disorders (CPMD).[3] One in three women in India experience physical or sexual abuse in their lives, usually at the hands of an intimate partner.[4] The mental health experiences that are encountered during the life course of a woman and during a vulnerable period warrant specific assessment tools to evaluate the vulnerabilities, strengths, symptom domains, severity of the problem, and overall impact on her functioning. This chapter has made an attempt to discuss available assessment tools for women's mental health.

■ BRIEF OUTLINE

Since the concept of gender encompasses dimensions beyond biological, this chapter will discuss tools under two headings related to psychosocial issues and also the reproductive life course.

Scales for assessing patriarchy, gender discrimination, gender-based violence (GBV), intimate partner violence (IPV), and their mental health outcomes are addressed in the first section and those for disorders and experiences related to the reproductive life cycle in the next section. This will cover menstruation, sexual functioning, pregnancy, and postpartum, and menopause.

Part 1: The Psychological, Social, and Cultural Dimension

Gender plays a major role in mental health which includes the effects of different social roles that are imparted to women, attitudes towards women, and traumatic events like violence of different kinds which are more commonly found in women than men. It has been seen that women may face more chronic and daily stress than men.[5] It can be said that women are exposed to certain kinds of unique stressors because of their gender and gender-based roles.[6] This part of the chapter will classify the instruments based on these gender-specific psychosocial entities.

- *Violence Against Women:* Violence against women is defined by the United Nations as "any act of GBV that results in, or is likely to result in, physical, sexual, or mental harm or suffering to women, including threats of such acts, coercion or arbitrary deprivation of liberty, whether occurring in public or in private life." There are different forms of such violence, as delineated below.
  - *Intimate Partner Violence:* IPV refers to actions within an intimate relationship by a current or former intimate partner that may harm the victim physically, sexually, or psychologically. Examples include physical violence, sexual coercion, psychological abuse, and controlling behavior. It is one of the most common forms of violence against women. Nearly a third (27%) of women aged 15–49 worldwide who have been in a relationship have reported to being subjected to IPV. Numerous reports and studies have extensively documented that violence inflicted upon women by their partners and sexual violence are significant factors contributing to women's mental health issues, specifically depression and suicidality as well as

sexual and reproductive health problems, injuries, and other chronic health ailments. The adverse health and social consequences of such violence can persist for extended periods. Moreover, IPV against women also adversely affects their offspring, manifesting in low birth weight, child health, and development issues.[7] The following scales are available to evaluate IPV:

- *Composite Abuse Scale (CAS):*[8] The CAS is a 30-item scale developed by Hegarty et al. which is multi-dimensional. The final scale has four dimensions, namely, *severe combined abuse, emotional abuse, physical abuse,* and *harassment.* The target population for this scale is women with present or past intimate partners for longer than a month. The four factors presented good internal reliability, as evidenced by Cronbach's alpha exceeding 0.85. Moreover, the corrected item total correlations displayed high levels of correlation, exceeding 0.5. The Composite Abuse Scale (CAS) has demonstrated validity across multiple domains, including face, content, criterion, and construct. A validation study for adaptation of the CAS in Kannada and Dakhani Urdu is currently underway (according to an email from Ms. A. Banu, PhD scholar, NIMHANS (banu17khadirnavar@gmail.com) on November 30, 2023).

- *Composite Abuse Scale (Revised)-Short Form (CASR-SF):*[9] This CASR-SF is a 15-item revised version of the CAS. It retained 12 items of the original scale and three new items were added based on literature and expert consultations. The items encompass three distinct domains of abuse: physical, sexual, and psychological. These domains are evaluated through inquiries that aim to gauge lifetime, recent, and current exposure, in addition to frequency of abuse. The internal consistency of the CASR-SF has been found to be 0.942, indicating high reliability in measurement. Moderate correlation has been found with measures of depression, coercive control, and post-traumatic stress disorder (PTSD), establishing concurrent validity. The reliability and validity profiles have been studied to be comparable to those of the original CAS.

- *Revised Conflict Tactics Scales (CTS-2):*[10] The CTS-2 is composed of 78 items which aim to evaluate both the occurrences of victimization and perpetration. Among these items, the victimization scale is comprised of 39 items, which are further divided into five subscales. These subscales are responsible for measuring the frequency of physical assault, psychological aggression, sexual coercion, negotiation, and injury between partners. Notably, the subscale dedicated to physical assault consists of 12 items, which may be categorized into minor and severe forms.

The CTS-2 can be applied to those in cohabitating, marital as well as dating relationships. The CTS-2 has evidence for internal consistency, convergent, discriminant, and factorial validity.

- *Questionnaires Used in Research Settings:* There have been large community prevalence studies on national and international levels for estimation of IPV that have used questionnaires formulated for the target populations.
  - *WHO Multi-country Study on Women's Health and Domestic Violence:*[11] This instrument is extensively utilized in countries with low- and middle-income populations. Primarily intended for prevalence surveys, although also employed in clinical research, it includes the assessment of physical, sexual, and psychological abuse as well as the evaluation of the frequency and duration of abuse occurring within the previous 12 months and throughout adulthood. In addition, it assesses certain repercussions of IPV, such as injuries, living in a state of fear, and the impact on mental well-being. The women's questionnaire is comprised of an individual consent form and 12 distinct sections designed to elicit comprehensive information regarding the respondent and her community, encompassing aspects of general and reproductive health, financial autonomy, children, partner dynamics, encounters with both partner and non-partner violence, and the consequences of violence on her overall life. It has been culturally adapted and translated during the original study.
  - *National Family Health Survey (NFHS):*[4] The questionnaire used by NFHS 5 includes questions to ever-married women about their experience with physical spousal violence, emotional spousal violence, and sexual spousal violence by current or former husband. It also includes assessing current or past experience with violence by anyone on both married and unmarried women and physical violence during pregnancy.
  - *Indian Council of Medical Research (ICMR) Task Force Study on Domestic and Partner Violence:*[12] The instrument consisted of 18 forms of abusive behavior which were classified into psychological abuse (such as the use of abusive language, making threats, and neglecting), physical abuse (such as hitting, scalding, and burning), and sexual abuse (including coercion, denial, and causing sexual injury) from a spouse and/or other members of the family. The presence of violence was indicated if the participants answered affirmatively to any abusive behavior within the three categories. A multiphase approach was employed to create these questionnaires in order to ensure their cultural and linguistic appropriateness. Initially, the questionnaire was prepared in English and then translated and back-translated to guarantee both semantic and content validity.

Other scales and perspectives on measurement of IPV have been delineated in the article by the Lancet Psychiatry Commission on IPV and mental health.[13]

- *Domestic Violence (DV):* While IPV is a phenomenon noted worldwide; another term widely used in India is DV. The Protection of Women from Domestic Violence Act was passed in 2005 to safeguard women from DV. According to this act, DV includes any harm, injury, harassment, or threats to a woman in a domestic relationship. It includes the categories of physical abuse, sexual abuse, verbal and emotional abuse and financial abuse. It also has within its purview abuse or threats for demand of dowry.[14] The core difference in concept from IPV is that it includes relationships beyond an intimate partner, to everyone who is sharing or has shared a household, including members of a joint family. According to NFHS 5, a significant proportion of married women in India, constituting 29.3%, between the ages of 18 and 49 have been subjected to domestic and/or sexual violence. Additionally, a notable 3.1% of pregnant women aged 18–49 have encountered physical violence during their pregnancy.[4]
- *Indian Family Violence and Control Scale (IFVCS):*[15] The IFVCS is a 63-item questionnaire which was developed and validated in India by a mixed-methods study. It has two subscales: control and violence. Concurrent validity has been established in comparison to CTS-2. Construct validity was examined by the association between established correlates of DV from existing literature and the control and violence subscales of the IFVCS, as well as the abbreviated version of the CTS-2. All variables that exhibited a correlation with the NFHS-3 CTS-2 also displayed a significant correlation with the IFVCS. Internal consistency was established with item response theory analysis where 56 out of 63 items had statistically significant factor loading. It has been developed in English, Hindi, and Marathi.
- *Domestic Violence Questionnaire:*[16] This is a 20-item questionnaire validated for married women from 18 to 55 years of age to identify DV over the past 1 year. It has 7 items for measuring physical violence and 13 items for measuring psychological violence. The internal consistency reliability of the questionnaire is 0.92, indicating a high level of internal consistency and coherence among the items. With a cutoff score of 5, the measure has a sensitivity of 89.5% and a specificity of 87.2%.
- *Sexual Violence:* The classification of violence against women by the United Nations includes IPV and sexual violence, defined "as any sexual act, attempt to obtain a sexual act, or other act directed against a person's sexuality using coercion, by any person regardless of their relationship to the victim, in any setting." It encompasses

rape, attempted rape, and unwanted sexual touching. It also includes noncontact forms of sexual violence.[17] According to the 2021 annual report issued by the National Crime Records Bureau (NCRB), the number of rape cases registered throughout the nation totaled 31,677, with an average of 86 cases per day.[18] It has been seen to predispose, precipitate, and perpetuate mental disorders.[19]

- *Sexual Experiences Survey (SES):* The SES is a self-report questionnaire developed to measure sexual aggression and sexual victimization. It was developed based on responses from university students in 1986. It is a 10-item questionnaire with answers in yes–no format. Internal consistency was 0.74 for women and 0.89 for men. In test–retest reliability, the mean item agreement was 93%.[20] Construct validity was further verified in a multicenter study in 1997.[21]

- *Sexual Experiences Survey–Short Forms Victimization and Perpetration:* Based on the pitfalls noted, the authors of SES updated the survey instrument in 2007. Changes were made in the heterosexist language, language was also updated in terms of existing legal statutes, and redundant terms were eliminated. The scale was changed to a format of two parallel scales of victimization and perpetration. There is a long and short version of each scale.[20] The in-person and internet versions were validated in a separate study. The internal consistency is 0.92 and 0.98, respectively, for victimization and perpetration scales. Rates of disclosure are noted to be comparable to the original scale. Both subscales have been seen to have good predictive validity, to trauma symptomatology and to hypermasculinity and hyper-gender ideology. The study also showed comparative results for in-person and computer-based data collection.[22]

- *Other Scales for GBV:* Social norms and beliefs about GBV Scale
  This social norms and belief about GBV Scale has 30 items that measure beliefs about GBV. It has three subscales, "Response to Sexual Violence," "Husband's Right to Use Violence", and "Protecting Family Honor". It has two domains, namely, personal beliefs and injunctive norms. The scale was validated in South Sudan and Somalia. Notably, the injunctive norms domain has Cronbach alphas varying from 0.69 to 0.75, while the personal beliefs domain has Cronbach alphas ranging from 0.71 to 0.77. The scale is also seen to demonstrate good construct validity.[23]

- *Severity of Violence Against Women Scales (SVAWS):*[24] SVAWS are two versions of a 10-point scale measuring male violence against women based on 46 possible acts. The results are classified into actual mild, moderate, and severe violence and threats of mild, moderate, and severe violence. However, psychometric properties have not been well studied for this scale.

- *Interpersonal Trauma:* It has been seen that men and women differ in the types of trauma they face. Women may be more prone to experience earlier onset and high impact trauma. Women also have twice to thrice the risk of PTSD as compared to men.[25] Traumatic experiences have cultural underpinnings. What constitutes a traumatic event may be different in different cultures.[24]
    - *Childhood Trauma Questionnaire (CTQ):*[26] The CTQ serves as a retrospective assessment tool for childhood trauma that has undergone psychometric evaluation in various populations. It comprises five subscales, namely emotional abuse, physical abuse, sexual abuse, emotional neglect, and physical neglect. The initial validation of the CTQ involved psychiatric and community samples with interrater reliability kappa ranging from 0.9 to 1.0. Subsequent validation studies of the CTQ have been conducted in both community and clinical samples, with findings consistently supporting the measure's validity. It has also been correlated with prospective assessment of violence with three of the five subscales show significant correlation.[27]
    - *Indian Interpersonal Trauma Interview:*[28] Indian Interpersonal Trauma Interview comprises 49 questions pertaining to instances of trauma, which are organized according to different stages of life: 0–5 years, 6–18 years, and 18+ years; e.g., separation from parental caregivers and loss of a parent in the 0–5 years age group, and body shaming, bullying, and different kinds of abuse at 6–18 years. In adulthood (18 years and above), individuals encounter culture-specific traumatic events, such as dowry harassment, the repeated rejection by potential partners in an arranged marriage setting, distressing relationships with one's spouse and in-laws, infertility, and trauma experienced during pregnancy and childbirth. It was devised as a holistic interview for traumatic experiences in Indian women. Validation studies are awaited.
- *Patriarchy:* Patriarchy is a concept of a social system that encompasses dominance by men in terms of authority and power and gives a disadvantaged and subordinate position to women. It has been shown to have implications on the mental health of women through GBV, oppression, lack of opportunities, and ostracization of nonconformists.[29]
    - *India Patriarchy Index:*[30] Indian Patriarchy Index was developed to quantify the societal and ideological concept of patriarchy utilizing empirical evidence pertaining to familial organization and gender roles. It built on the original Patriarchy Index developed by Gruber and Szołtysek in Europe. By utilizing data derived from the NFHS 1, 3, and 4, India Patriarchy Index was devised to effectively assess the gendered social standing within households, taking into account

factors such as sex and age distribution, patrilocality, sex ratio disparity among offspring, and gender-specific economic roles. Favorable internal consistency (Cronbach's alpha 0.77) and construct validity has been demonstrated on validation, with validity being evidenced by its correlation with three gender equality measures utilized in India [United Nations (GDI) Gender Development Index, WEI (Women's Empowerment Index), and GVI (Gender Vulnerability Index)]. Additionally, spatial and temporal analyses have highlighted substantial variation in India Patriarchy Index scores at the state level as well as its gradual evolution over time.

- *The Patriarchal Beliefs Scale (PBS):*[31] The PBS has 35 items with three factors: Institutional Power of Men (F1, 12 items), Inherent Inferiority of Women (F2, 12 items) and Gendered Domestic Roles (F3, 11 items). The PBS has demonstrated construct validity and reliability (Crohnbach's alphas are 0.97, 0.97, 0.95, and 0.96 for the total scale, F1, F2 and F3 respectively).

- *Gender-based Roles:* The manner in which men and women exhibit their psychological distress may be influenced by sociocultural factors that act through socially imposed roles and patterns of behavior. Differences in social stress may have implications on women's mental health being poorer on certain domains. Gender-related factors have been determined to have a significant impact in determining the extent to which women receive psychological care. Specifically, research has shown that a higher degree of adherence to traditional gender roles correlates with a greater likelihood of women seeking psychological care.[6]
  - *Feminine Gender Role Stress (FGRS) Scale:*[32] The FGRS is a 39-item scale. There were five factors identified during validation of the FGRS scale that reflect categories of female gender role stressors: fear of unemotional relationships, fear of physical unattractiveness, fear of victimization, fear of behaving assertively, and fear of not being nurturant. The FGRS scale has demonstrated internal consistency (Cronbach's alphas 0.73–0.83 through all the factors), and test–retest reliability ($r = 0.82$).
  - *Gender Role Attitudes Scale (GRAS):*[33] The GRAS has 20-items, developed in Spain, measuring attitudes and beliefs about gender roles, with responses scored on a Likert scale of five possible responses to each item (totally agree to totally disagree). It has been found to be highly reliable (Cronbach's alpha 0.99). However, construct validity has not been established.

Other Scales: Conformity to Feminine Norms Inventory (CFNI), Conformity to Masculine Norms Inventory (CMNI)[6]

- *Gender Disadvantage/Discrimination:* Gender disadvantage has been defined by Blumberg as "the extent to which societal members are unequal in their access to the scarce values of their society, on the basis of their membership in a certain gender category".[34] This includes restriction in choices, lesser access to adequate nutrition, lesser school education, unequal pay, obstacles in reaching leadership positions, workplace harassment and poverty. The terms gender disadvantage, gender discrimination, gender disparities and gender inequalities are synonymous. The interplay of these factors with specific situations like migration, disasters, food insecurity may increase the vulnerability of women to mental disorders.[35] The World Health Organization (WHO) has acknowledged inequity in health outcomes as well. Perceived gender discrimination often leads to mental health problems. A cohort study on child-bearing women revealed that 10.7% had perceived gender discrimination, and that group had more depressive symptoms through the course of time.[36] There was a study exploring tools used in assessing gender discrimination. They found 57 such studies with questionnaires mainly developed by individual research teams, most with no validation data.[37] For gender disadvantage, CAGED has been developed and validated in India (see below).
  - *The Checklist for Assessment of Gender Disadvantage (CAGED):*[38] The CAGED covers four domains **(Table 1)** with 15 items. It has been culturally validated in India. The scale has established internal consistency (Cronbach's alpha 0.74) and test–retest reliability (0.84). It has been used to measure gender disadvantage in adolescent girls in India during the COVID pandemic.
  - *The Schedule of Sexist Events (SSE):*[39] The SSE scale has 20-items, measuring recent and lifetime sexist discrimination in the lives of women. It identified four factors: sexist degradation, sexism in distant relationships, sexism in close relationships, and sexist discrimination

TABLE 1: Domains of Checklist for Assessment of Gender Disadvantage (CAGED).

Domain	Evaluates	Items
Gender discrimination	Male preference/criticism from others	3
Violence and sexual harassment	Physical/sexual violence within and outside of the family	5
Barriers to personal growth related to gender	Barriers to privacy, personal goals, education	4
Emotional distress related to gender disadvantage (impact subscale)	Suicide/self-harm, sadness	3

in the workplace. The internal-consistency and split-half reliability of the SSE-Lifetime and SSE-Recent scales have been found to be high, with values of 0.92 and 0.90 as well as 0.87 and 0.83, respectively. The SSE scale also has established convergent validity.

- *Perceived Gender Discrimination Scale (PGDS):*[40] The PGDS is a 45-item tool developed in Pakistan that quantifies the inequitable disparity that arises from the identification of an unjust imbalance between the circumstances faced by women across eight vital domains, namely, education (6 items), employment/career (9 items), familial matters (8 items), financial matters (5 items), general social rights (6 items), appreciation and encouragement (5 items), abuse and violence (6 items), and gender-based stereotyping (6 items), as compared to their male counterparts. Each item scored on a 5-point Likert scale, with total scores ranging from 56 to 280. The scale has established factorial validity and internal consistency (Cronbach's alpha 0.84).

Part 2: Reproductive Life Cycle Approach

Women are at an increased vulnerability to acquiring psychiatric disorders during certain intervals, namely, menarche, pregnancy, postpartum, and menopause. Psychiatric disorders that affect only women include premenstrual dysphoric disorder (PMDD), antenatal/postpartum depression, postpartum psychosis, and perimenopausal disorders.[41] In addition, there is a notable difference between the sexual functioning of males and females. This section describes assessment tools used to evaluate disorders associated with specific biological periods among women.

- *Menstruation:* The female menstrual cycle is accompanied by a series of alterations that may manifest in the psychological realm as somatic symptoms or behavioral modifications. In 1931, Frank was the first to document premenstrual syndrome (PMS).[42] PMS exhibiting more severe symptoms was designated as late luteal phase dysphoric disorder (LLPDD) by the DSM-IIIR (Diagnostic and Statistical Manual of Mental Disorders, Third Edition, Revised). Subsequently, it was categorized as PMDD and incorporated within the Depressive Disorder Not Otherwise Specified in the DSM-IV-TR. Furthermore, PMS is identified as the "associated feature" of PMDD in the appendix of the DSM-IV. The DSM-V proceeded to position the diagnosis of PMDD under depressive disorders. PMDD necessitates the presence of at least one psychological symptom, such as affective lability, irritability, sad mood, or anxiety, in conjunction with at least four psychological, somatic, or behavioral manifestations. The estimated prevalence of PMDD varies within a range of 2%–4% based on symptom evaluation. The diagnosis of PMDD is dependent on the prospective ratings obtained over two consecutive cycles.[43] There are both retrospective and prospective rating scales that are accessible for evaluating PMDD.

- *Menstrual Distress Questionnaire (MDQ):*[44] The MDQ was developed by Moos, wherein a list of 47 symptoms with eight predominant factors was examined. These factors pertained to pain, focus, water retention, behavioral change, autonomic responses, negative affect, arousal, and control. The symptoms were graded according to their severity, ranging from nonexistent to moderately incapacitating. Assessment and symptom ratings were generated for the premenstrual, menstrual, and intermenstrual experiences.

  The MDQ has been subjected to a lot of criticism because of the conspicuous insufficiency of substantial research conducted on the MDQs reliability, accompanied by issues concerning the normative sample and indeterminate validity. Specifically, the MDQ has been shown to gauge constructs that have no correlation with the menstrual cycle and inaccurately define PMS. Furthermore, the factor structure of this tool may be prone to instability.[45]

  The revised version of the MDQ was constructed utilizing a 4-point rating scale in order to mitigate the complexity associated with the original MDQ. This modified MDQ comprises 35 items that center on the premenstrual phase without any reference to other phases of the menstrual cycle.[46] The internal reliability remains uncertain in terms of content validity, as it is grounded in the original MDQ and, thus, warrants scrutiny.[47]

- *Premenstrual Assessment Form (PAF):*[48] The PAF questionnaire accommodates subcategories of premenstrual alterations, including bipolar continua, unipolar summary scales, and typological categories. It encompasses an assortment of behavioral, psychological, and somatic modifications. An evaluation of symptoms from the preceding three menstrual cycles is conducted. The lengthiness of the PAF impeded its routine employment and posed challenges in its administration. Abbreviated versions of this scale have been developed and evince substantial internal consistency and dependability.[49]

  The PAF represented an advancement over preceding tools that tended to amalgamate varying dysphoric moods such as depression, anxiety, and irritability. The respondent also had the capacity to elaborate on and provide a duration for her premenstrual phase. This tool augmented specificity by facilitating the differentiation between non-premenstrual states and other chronic psychiatric ailments. Furthermore, this form was shown to be an improvement over the MDQ in terms of validity and reliability.[47]

- *Premenstrual Symptom Screening Tool (PSST):* The initial PSST was designed to translate DSM-IV category fields into a quantitative rating scale framework, complete with severity grading. This 4-point rating scale is brief and practical, serving as an effective screening tool. Subsequent to this screening, it is incumbent upon the psychiatrist to eliminate the possibility of other psychiatric afflictions. In the event of any uncertainty, it may be useful to employ prospective charting.[50] The tool has been translated into the Gujarati language through the use of forward and backward translation methods. Both the English and Gujarati versions of the PSST have been utilized in this study among medical and nursing/arts/commerce students, respectively. However, the study does not address the validation of the Gujarati version of the PSST.[51]
- *Daily Rating Form (DRF):*[52] The DRF evaluates symptoms throughout the menstrual cycle by utilizing a 20-item measure and a severity Likert scale ranging from 1 (absent) to 6 (extremely severe). Emphasis is placed on the pre- and postmenstrual periods, specifically the 5-day window. The rater is granted some flexibility, and trends may be compared across cycles. The DRF has provided evidence supporting the concept of premenstrual alterations. While internal reliability testing has yet to be conducted, content validity has been established.
- *Calendar of Premenstrual Experiences (COPE):*[53] The COPE questionnaire comprises 10 physical and 12 behavioral questions. These items were developed based on the daily symptom reports of women seeking treatment for PMS. The scale measures symptoms on a 4-point range from 0 (no symptoms) to 3 (severe or painful symptoms). A diagnosis of PMS requires a follicular phase value of under 40 and a luteal phase score above 42. Test–retest reliability was found to be high when the COPE was administered during the same phase of two consecutive menstrual cycles. In terms of construct validity, COPE has been tested with the Beck Depression Inventory (BDI) and the Profile of Mood State (POMS) assessments. COPE is a valuable tool for both research and therapeutic purposes, as it has the potential to differentiate between individuals experiencing various illnesses.
- *Daily Record of Severity of Problem (DRSP):*[54] The DRSP form has undergone development to aid medical practitioners in evaluating and diagnosing PMDD through the implementation of DSM-IV criteria. The form comprises 24 distinct elements that are meticulously assessed on a 6-point severity scale. As evidenced by various studies, both individual DRSP elements and summary scores exhibit

remarkable test-retest reliability and demonstrate a high degree of sensitivity to therapeutic interventions. Moreover, summary scores exhibit high levels of internal consistency.
- *Carolina Premenstrual Assessment Scale (C-PASS):*[55] The utilization of the C-PASS, a standardized rating system, along with the DRSP provides a systematic approach to diagnosing PMDD, as outlined in the DSM-V. This rating system is made accessible through various mediums, such as a worksheet, Excel macro, and SAS macro, and has enabled researchers to accurately interpret PMDD across diverse samples, individuals, and menstrual cycles.

The details of scales used for PMS/PMDD such as timing of assessment, number of items, psychometric properties, drawbacks and resources has been summarized in **Table 2**.

- *Sexual Functioning:* Female sexual dysfunction (FSD) is a widespread debilitating ailment that results in a suboptimal quality of life. Despite the fact that nearly 40% of women experience sexual dysfunction, only a small proportion seek therapeutic intervention.[56] Vaginal lubrication, soreness, discomfort during intercourse, reduced excitement sensation, and challenges in achieving orgasm are the most common symptoms associated with FSD. We present a number of objective tools employed in the assessment of FSD.
  - *Female Sexual Functioning Index (FSFI):*[57] The self-reported scale is comprised of 19 items and is organized into six domains, namely arousal, sexual desire, lubrication, orgasm, satisfaction, and pain. The cutoff score for this scale is set at 26. It is worth noting that the scale has demonstrated good discriminant validity, thereby making it a viable screening and diagnostic tool. However, it is important to acknowledge that the assessment is limited to the preceding 4 weeks, and as such, the classification of different sexual disorders cannot be solely based on this particular scale.
  - *Arizona Sexual Experience Scale (ASEX):*[58] ASEX is a concise questionnaire consisting of 5 items that can be administered either self-rated or clinician-administered utilizing a Likert scale, ranging from 1 to 6. This instrument assesses various factors such as drive, arousal, penile erection/vaginal lubrication, capacity for orgasm, and orgasmic satisfaction, which are commonly affected by sexual disorders. Furthermore, the scale exhibits high levels of validity, sensitivity, and reliability. It is noteworthy that there are two variations of this scale available for both men and women.
  - *Female Sexual Distress Scale (FSDS)—Revised:*[59] The self-administered scale consisting of 12 items has undergone validation. The items in the scale are designed to assess sexual distress experienced by women

TABLE 2: Scales for premenstrual syndrome.

S. No.	Name of scale	Type	Time of assessment	No. of items and scale structure	Psychometric properties	Critique	Resource
1.	Menstrual Distress Questionnaire (MDQ)	R	All stages	47 Form C (cycle) Form T (today)	Internal reliability unclear. Test-retest reliability of the MDQ was conducted on 15 cases	• User acceptability poses a threat to the face validity, owing to the intricacy of the rating system • Overlapping symptoms	*Manual is available:* Moos, RH. (1977). Menstrual distress questionnaire manual. Stanford University, Department of Psychiatry and Behavioral Sciences https://journals.lww.com/psychosomaticmedicine/Abstract/1968/11000/The_Development_of_a_Menstrual_Distress.6.aspx
2.	Modified MDQ	R	Only premenstrual phase	35	The internal reliability is unclear regarding content validity	Psychometric properties are underpinned by the original MDQ and hence questionable	
3.	Premenstrual Assessment Form (PAF)	R	Last three menstrual cycles measured	97	High internal consistency and reliability of original scale and shortened versions	Lengthy, hence shortened versions created	A shortened 10 item version is available. https://onlinelibrary.wiley.com/doi/abs/10.1111/j.1600-0447.1982.tb00820.x?sid=nlm%3Apubmed

Contd...

S. No.	Name of scale	Type	Time of assessment	No. of items and scale structure	Psychometric properties	Critique	Resource
4.	Premenstrual Symptom Screening Tool (PSST)	R	–	4-point screening tool	Several translations validated across the world	Gujrati version available but psychometric properties of the version unclear	Researchers can mail to asranis@mcmaster.ca https://link.springer.com/article/10.1007/s00737-003-0018-4 Gujarati: https://journals.lww.com/indianjpsychiatry/pages/default.aspx
5.	Daily Rating Form (DRF)	P	5 days of the pre- and postmenstrual periods.	20 items severity scale (not at all) to 6 (extreme)	Internal reliability testing has not been done, though content validity has been demonstrated	• The rater has flexibility of scoring • Comparisons of patterns over the periods is possible	https://www.sciencedirect.com/science/article/abs/pii/0165032786900352?via%3Dihub
6.	Calendar of Premenstrual Experiences (COPE)	P	Follicular and luteal phase	22 items 4-point scale from 0 (no symptoms) to 3 (severe or painful symptoms)	Test-retest reliability in two consecutive cycles; construct validity established	Beneficial in both research as well as clinical settings	https://obgyn.onlinelibrary.wiley.com/doi/abs/10.1016/0020-7292%2891%2990644-K

Contd...

S. No.	Name of scale	Type	Time of assessment	No. of items and scale structure	Psychometric properties	Critique	Resource
7.	Daily Record of Severity of Problem (DRSP)	P	DSM-IV criteria	24 items 6-point severity scale	Test-retest reliability and internal consistency established	Responsive to change during treatment	https://link.springer.com/article/10.1007/s00737-005-0103-y https://psychscenehub.com/wp-content/uploads/2020/10/Daily-Record-of-Severity-of-Problems-PMDD.pdf
8.	Carolina Premenstrual Assessment Scoring System (C-PASS)	P	Algorithm used with DRSP with DSM-V criteria	–	Reliable, valid protocol companion to DRSP	Availability as a worksheet	https://ajp.psychiatryonline.org/doi/10.1176/appi.ajp.2016.15121510?url_ver=Z39.88-2003&rfr_id=ori:rid:crossref.org&rfr_dat=cr_pub%20%200pubmed or https://www.ncbi.nlm.nih.gov/pmc/articles/PMC5205545/ Worksheet available in the supplementary material of article

(DSM: Diagnostic and Statistical Manual of Mental Disorders; P: prospective; R: retrospective) within the last 4 weeks. The total score, which ranges from 0 to 48, is obtained by summing the scores of each individual item scored from 0 to 4.

- *Sexual Function Questionnaire (SFQ):*[60] The SFQ, a screening instrument for FSD, comprises 31 validated items. It assesses seven domains, namely pleasure, orgasm, pain, partner relationship, physical arousal-sensation, and lubrication. The SFQ28, a 28-item scale, has been recently developed through SFQ's refinement HSDD (hypoactive sexual desire disorder) and validated for female sexual arousal disorder (FSAD) and HSDD. It has demonstrated good internal consistency and reliability, except for pain. Moreover, it has shown satisfactory test–retest reliability, recognized group validity, and strong convergent validity with the FSDS and SQOL-F (sexual quality of life-female). Notably, a cutoff score of 14 on the SFQ has been validated among Indian women, indicating the presence of sexual dysfunction.[61]
- *Female Sexual Well-being (FSWB) Scale:*[62] The present instrument is a reliable, self-rated assessment tool that has undergone validation for the purpose of evaluating the sexual health of women across all age groups. Multiple domains, including cognitive–emotional, interpersonal, physical arousal, and orgasm satisfaction, are assessed. The initial psychometric validation studies have demonstrated good internal consistency, test–retest reliability over a 2-week interval, and construct validity.
- *Sexual Quotient—Female Version:*[63] The female version of the sexual quotient is a rating scale consisting of ten items which aim to evaluate various aspects of sexual function, including but not limited to desire, foreplay, sexual arousal, harmony with a partner, and comfort during sexual intercourse. Additionally, this scale accounts for sexual pleasure and the attainment of orgasm. Scores on this scale range from 0 to 100, with a score of <62 indicating inadequate sexual functioning.

The details of scales used for female sexual functioning such as type of scale, factors/domains, number of items, psychometric properties, and resources has been summarized in **Table 3**.

- *Perinatal Mental Health:* The period of pregnancy and postpartum is considered a time of heightened vulnerability for the development or exacerbation of mental illnesses in women. Within this peripartum period, mental illnesses can manifest as either peripartum common mental disorders (PCMDs) or peripartum severe mental disorders (PSMDs). The former encompasses a range of nonpsychotic mental health conditions, such as anxiety spectrum disorders, nonpsychotic depression, and somatoform disorders, among others. The latter includes affective

TABLE 3: Scales on female sexual functioning.

S. No.	Name of scale	Type of scale	Factors/domains assessed	No. of items Cutoff (if any)	Psychometric properties	Remarks	Resource
1.	Female sexual functioning index (FSFI)	Self-report	Six: Arousal, sexual desire, lubrication, orgasm, satisfaction, and pain	19 Cutoff: 26	Established discriminant validity	Urdu version available	https://cdn-links.lww.com/permalink/aog/a/aog_124_2_2014_06_02_reed_14-218_sdc1.pdf
2.	Arizona sexual experience scale (ASEX)	Self and clinician administered	Five: drive, arousal, penile erection/vaginal lubrication, capacity for orgasm, and orgasmic satisfaction	5 Likert scale (1–6)	High measures of reliability, validity, and sensitivity	Available for both men and women Hindi version available	https://www.mirecc.va.gov/visn22/Arizona_Sexual_Experiences_Scale.pdf
3.	Female sexual distress scale—revised	Self-administered	Female sexual distress for past four weeks	12 Scored 0–4 (maximum score 48)	Well-validated	Short scale, easy to administer	Copyrighted

Contd...

Contd...

S. No.	Name of scale	Type of scale	Factors/domains assessed	No. of items Cutoff (if any)	Psychometric properties	Remarks	Resource
4.	Sexual function questionnaire (SFQ)	Clinician administered screening tool	*Seven:* Pleasure, orgasm, pain, partner relationship, and physical arousal–sensation and lubrication	Initial 31 items Now refined to 28 items (SFQ28) Cutoff: 14	Established convergent and group validity, internal consistency, test-retest reliability for SFQ28 Validated on Indian women	Screening for both FSAD and HSDD validated	Copyrighted
5.	Female sexual well-being (FSWB) scale	Self-rated	*Four:* Interpersonal, cognitive–emotional, physical arousal and orgasm satisfaction	17	Construct validity, internal consistency and test-retest validity established	Sexual health can be assessed for women of all ages	Copyrighted
6.	Sexual quotient—female version	Self-rated	• Sexual function, desire, foreplay, sexual arousal, harmony with a partner, and comfort during sexual intercourse • Sexual pleasure and orgasm	• 10 items Score 0–100 • Below 62 indicative of inadequate sexual functioning	• Established internal consistency in a sample of 30 • Validity tested by comparing to control group	Covers a wide range of aspects of sexual functioning.	https://www.researchgate.net/figure/Female-Sexual-Quotient-Questionnaire-FSQ_fig1_321431952

psychosis, schizophrenia, as well as nonpsychotic and psychotic bipolar disorder presentations. These conditions may emerge or worsen during the peripartum period, and it has been observed that the prevalence of both PCMDs and PSMDs is high in LMICs. Antenatal and postnatal anxiety disorders have been estimated at 15-20% and 10%, respectively.[64] Antenatal depression has been observed in over 20% of pregnant women in LMICs, while postpartum depression has been noted in 22% of women in an Indian study.[65,66] Estimates of postpartum psychosis are around 1-2 per 1000 postpartum women.[67]

- *Pregnancy:* The methodical assessment of anxiety scales utilized during pregnancy has revealed a deficiency in research on the psychometric characteristics of these scales. While anxiety scales with strong psychometric properties used in the general population may not be appropriate for pregnant women, as they tend to focus on somatic concerns that are a natural part of the physiological changes in pregnancy. It has been argued that assuming that anxiety scales designed for the general population are suitable for use during pregnancy is incorrect, given the overemphasis on physical symptoms and a lack of established cut-off scores and standards for pregnant populations.[68] Moreover, studies have suggested that pregnancy-specific anxiety may exist as a distinct phenomenological entity.[69]
  - *Cambridge Worry Scale:*[70] This scale is composed of 16 distinct items, which encompass a variety of concerns specific to pregnancy, such as potential complications with the fetus and the possibility of miscarriage as well as more general concerns surrounding finances and interpersonal relationships. Respondents are asked to indicate the degree to which they are worried about each item, ranging from minimal to substantial levels of concern. Analysis of this scale has identified four distinct elements related to social and medical concerns following childbirth, financial difficulties, the mother's and infant's health, and various relationship issues. These factors have demonstrated a consistent level of stability across multiple studies.[71-73] Furthermore, there is empirical support for the notion that several items on this scale exhibit strong psychometric properties when used during pregnancy.[68]
  - *Wijma Delivery Expectancy/Experience Questionnaire (W-DEQ-Version A and Version B):*[74] The W-DEQ is a self-administered tool utilized to evaluate the fear of childbirth. The questionnaire comes in two variants, namely A and B, which are designed to assess fear of delivery during pregnancy and postpartum individually. Both versions of the W-DEQ have a total of 33 items, with responses ranging from "not at all" to "extremely". This measurement

scale is unique to the areas of "unfavorable emotions toward childbirth" and the "anxiety of labor and delivery". Studies reveal that this instrument possesses robust psychometric properties in gauging one aspect of anxiety during pregnancy, specifically the apprehension toward labor and delivery and the absence of positive anticipation, in multiple cultures.[75,76] Moreover, the Hindi version of WDEQ version B has undergone validation in India.[77]

- *Pregnancy-related Anxiety Questionnaire-Revised (PRAQ-R) and PRAQ-R2:*[78] The PRAQ-R is a comprehensive 10-item scale utilized to assess anxiety related to current pregnancy. Each item is rated on a 5-point scale, ranging from "never" to "very often". The scale evaluates three pregnancy-specific anxiety domains, namely, "fear of giving birth", "fear of bearing a physically or mentally handicapped child", and "concern about one's appearance". The PRAQ-R2 was developed to determine pregnancy-specific anxiety in both nulliparous and parous mothers. To ensure that the scale is applicable for all pregnant women, regardless of parity, three components were replaced with the more generalized statement, "I am anxious about the delivery", while maintaining the 10-item scale (PRAQ-R2).

- *Postpartum:* The postpartum period is a time where a woman is vulnerable to the onset and exacerbations of psychiatric disorders. The notable clinical entities during the postpartum period are those of postpartum psychosis, which is an umbrella term for psychosis, mania, and psychotic depression in the postpartum period, the spectrum of postpartum depressive symptomatology, including postpartum blues and postpartum depression, anxiety disorders and OCD, and mother–infant bonding disorders.[79] Tools for assessment of bonding are given as a separate section. Given below are scales for the assessment of anxiety and depression. The disorders coming under postpartum psychosis are assessed using scales for the disorder in question, i.e., BPRS/PANSS (Brief Psychiatric Rating Scale/Positive and Negative Syndrome Scale) for psychosis/schizophrenia, Young Mania Rating Scale (YMRS) for mania, etc.[79] The scale for obsessive–compulsive symptoms is given in the section on perinatal scales.

  - *Edinburgh Postnatal Depression Scale (EPDS):* The existing array of scales for depression, though vast, are seemingly constrained for the postpartum period due to their emphasis on somatic symptoms of depression, which could have been attributable to the physiological changes that emerge during the puerperium. In 1987, John Cox and his team developed the EPDS following pilot interviews with mothers who had young babies. This involved an examination of extant depression scales, with items suited for the postpartum period being selected based on thorough interviews with mothers who had newborns. The items' level of acceptance, especially with regard to language, were duly assessed.[80]

The research that was carried out to validate the scale for usage demonstrated good levels of validity and split-half reliability. Additionally, it was found to possess sensitivity to changes in intensity throughout the follow-up period. The female participants found the scale to be acceptable, and it was administered with ease, with completion times averaging 5 minutes. The research was conducted inside the participants' homes, thereby eliminating any possible selection bias. Furthermore, it was noted that sensitivity and specificity may be improved if the test is taken by the mother alone, without any presence of family members.[80]

The scale has been translated into 60 languages, including various Indian languages and has been implemented for screening purposes in clinics. It is recommended to authenticate the scale first in the language of the population as there may be variations in metaphors, semantics, and concepts when a different language is used for screening. Furthermore, it is important to acknowledge that the EPDS is not an instrument for diagnosis. An elevated score only indicates the existence of symptoms and does not affirm the presence of a disorder.[81]

- *Psychometric Properties:* By utilizing the scientific diagnostic criteria that were available during the time of assessment, a cutoff score of 12 out of 13 (with a range of 0–30) demonstrated a sensitivity of 86% and a specificity of 78% for detecting instances of both "major" and "minor" depression. Moreover, the positive predictive value was determined to be 73%. In certain studies that scrutinized the validity of this scale as a screening tool, a lower cutoff score of 9 or 10 was deemed appropriate in select cases; nevertheless, utilizing the score of 12/13 resulted in enhanced accuracy.[82] In the initial trial study, the split-half reliability was calculated to be 0.88, and the standardized coefficient was 0.87. False negatives were reported when family members were present, and it was observed that women may either overstate or understate their symptoms in the presence of family. The acceptability of the scale was increased due to its concise nature and ease of scoring.[80]
  - *Edinburgh Postnatal Depression Scale (EPDS):* Anxiety subscale or the EDS-3A:[83,84] Studies have indicated that the EPDS scale, which was originally designed for depression screening, includes a subscale that targets anxiety. The results of factor analyses

conducted across different studies demonstrate that three specific items in the EPDS align with a solitary factor and more accurately gauge affective and cognitive symptoms of anxiety.[83] These items include: "I had blamed myself unnecessarily when things went wrong", "I have been anxious or worried for no reason", and "I have felt scared or panicky for no very good reason". According to a specific study, it has been suggested that the EDS-3A scale, consisting of the 3 items mentioned, may exhibit better performance in comparison to other scales, such as the Hospital Anxiety and Depression Scale (HADS-A) and PRAQ-R.[85]

- *Perinatal Period:* These scales are not specific to any particular phase of the perinatal period and can be used both in the antepartum and postpartum periods.
  - *The Stafford Interview:*[86] A clinical interview based probing and rating of women's mental health was developed by Ian Brockington along with his team members from India, Italy, New Zealand, Egypt, Spain, and Taiwan in 1992 and subsequently several revisions are made. The "Stafford Interview" is extensively covers the women's mental health from prepregnancy to 1 year after child birth such as social, psychological, and obstetric background to pregnancy, response to conception, prepartum relationship with husband (partner) or father of baby, changes in lifestyle during pregnancy, wellbeing of unborn child, prepartum psychiatric disorders, parturition, social, psychological, and obstetric background to puerperium, postpartum relationship with husband (partner) or father of baby, postpartum psychiatric disorders, and the mother–infant relationship. Considering the fact that "Stafford Interview" developed by perinatal psychiatrists from different nations, the sociocultural factors were considered to frame each of the questions. Though time-consuming, it can be used both in community and clinical settings.
  - *Perinatal Obsessive–Compulsive Scale (POCS):*[87] Studies have revealed that the prevalence of symptoms of obsessive–compulsive disorder (OSD) during the postnatal phase could be as much as 4%–9%, in comparison to a general lifetime risk of 2%. During the perinatal period, certain obsessions may pertain to the baby's health and overall well-being, which may hamper the bonding between the mother and the child. Additionally, aggressive obsessions and the fear of unintentionally or intentionally causing harm to the infant are also common.

The POCS is a self-administered questionnaire that requires women to report the presence or absence of undesired thoughts and actions.

The prenatal version comprises seven pregnancy and infant-related thoughts and nine behaviors, while the postpartum version has 14 behaviors and 19 thoughts. The questionnaire assesses concerns regarding being judged, contamination of the baby, unintentional harm to the baby, and the baby being afflicted, among other factors. The POCS also evaluates the severity and interference caused by these thoughts and behaviors, with 12 questions on the severity scale and scores ranging from 0 to 4 indicating the severity level, resulting in a total score of 0–48. The scale includes postpartum behaviors such as constant cleaning of the baby's surroundings, monitoring of the newborn, and seeking reassurance repeatedly, among others.

It was seen during an initial validation study that the POCS recorded a greater number of clinically relevant symptoms than the Y-BOCS (Yale-Brown Obsessive Compulsive Scale). On the POCS checklist, pregnant women with OCD reported around 25% more symptoms, and postpartum mothers reported about 8% more symptoms. On the POCS severity and interference scales, women with OCD performed better than they did on the YBOCS severity scale. This is due to the fact that most women gave themselves higher ratings on the subscales for distress.

- *Reliability and Validity:* Internal consistency has been demonstrated to be high, with Crohnbach's alpha values of 0.95 in general, 0.94 and 0.95 in pregnant and postpartum women respectively. Test–retest reliability research is ongoing.

  The pilot study has demonstrated that the scale has excellent psychometric characteristics, with representative items, high consistency, good concurrent validity, and determinative capability, thus affirming its good construct validity. Ongoing detailed validation research is currently underway. Although the use of the POCS scale has minimal supporting evidence, it holds considerable potential as a valuable tool for detecting obsessions throughout the pregnancy and postpartum periods.

  - *Perinatal Anxiety Screening Scale (PASS):*[88] The PASS is a self-report assessment tool that examines anxiety symptoms among women during the perinatal period. The test consists of 31 items and evaluates anxiety symptoms experienced in the previous month. Responses are measured on a Likert 0–3 scale, and the final score is calculated by summing the individual ratings. Higher scores indicate greater levels of anxiety, with a maximum score of 93. It classifies symptoms into three categories: minimal anxiety (0–20), mild–moderate anxiety (21–41), and severe anxiety (42–93).[89] The clinical anxiety cutoff is 26. Principal component analyses (PCA) have identified a four-factor structure consisting of symptoms related to acute anxiety and adjustment (8 items), general and specific worries (10 items), perfectionism, control, and trauma (8 items), and social anxiety (5 items). Research on the PASS has shown acceptable test–retest reliability (rho = 0.74), with a sensitivity of 70% and specificity of 30% at the cutoff. The scale is also available in Hindi.[90]

- Scales frequently used but not specific to the perinatal period: There are some scales, as described below, that were not developed for the perinatal population, yet have been used frequently as screening tools for anxiety and depression in the perinatal period because of their ease of use and ability to correctly screen symptoms in this population.
  - *Patient Health Questionnaire-9 (PHQ-9):* The PHQ-9 is a self-rated questionnaire that measures the nine DSM-IV criteria of depression on a Likert scale of 0 (not at all) to 3 (nearly every day). It has been validated as a reliable and valid measure to screen for depression. The cutoff score is 10. It has also been validated as a measure of severity in the same study. The scores of 5, 10, 15, and 20 have been seen to be representing mild, moderate, moderately severe, and severe depression, respectively.[91] The PHQ-9 has been well-validated for use in the perinatal population. A systematic review and meta-analysis explored the psychometric properties of PHQ-9 on perinatal depression. In the study, a total of 35 articles met the eligibility criteria for either criterion or convergent validity. Through a meta-analysis of the studies evaluating criterion validity, utilizing the standard PHQ-9 cut point ≥10, a pooled sensitivity, specificity, and area under the curve (AUC) of 0.84, 0.81, and 0.89, respectively, were observed. In head-to-head comparison studies, it was observed that the operating characteristics of the PHQ-9 and EPDS were almost identical. The median correlation between the PHQ-9 and EPDS was determined to be 0.59, with moderate categorical agreement being demonstrated.[92]
  - *Generalized Anxiety Disorder Scale-7 (GAD-7):* The GAD-7 is a self-rated scale comprising seven items that was developed to function as a screening tool and severity indicator for GAD. Its scoring is facile, and it was primarily designed to enhance the recognition of GAD in primary care settings. The cutoff score maximizing sensitivity and specificity is set at 10. The original validation of the GAD-7 in a sizable primary care sample evinces its commendable reliability, as well as its satisfactory criterion, factorial, and procedural validity.[93] In a validation study on perinatal Greek Cypriot women, it was demonstrated to have good internal consistency (Cronbach's alpha 0.907) and good model fit. However, the study's design lacked

the establishment of a discernible cutoff point to optimize both sensitivity and specificity.[94] Nevertheless, GAD-7 is a widely used screening measure for perinatal anxiety.

- *Mother–fetus–infant Bonding:* It has been observed that mothers experiencing the onset or exacerbation of mental illness during the perinatal period encounter impediments in developing a bond with their infants. Despite the existence of a multitude of instruments for evaluating parenting behavior, only a limited number have been utilized specifically for mothers with mental illness. We present a discussion of commonly employed scales for evaluating bonding in mothers with mental illness during the postpartum phase.
  - *Postpartum Bonding Questionnaire (PBQ):*[95] The PBQ, a self-administered questionnaire, is utilized to assess maternal–infant bonding from the perspective of the mother. This tool features a scale consisting of 25 statements, each accompanied by one of six response options, ranging from "always" to "never". Positive responses are scored from 0 (indicating "always") to 5 (indicating "never"), while negative responses are scored from 5 (indicating "always") to 0 (indicating "never"). The mother is instructed to evaluate each statement according to their current and most extreme symptoms. The cumulative score of the 25 items is classified into four factors, and a high score denotes the presence of pathology. The factors are delineated below in **Table 4**.

    The preliminary validation research conducted by the authors uncovered that the general factor displayed a sensitivity of 0.82 for all forms of mother–infant relationship disorders. In contrast, the sensitivity of newborn rejection stood at 0.88, whereas that of intense rage was a mere 0.67. The performance of infant-focused anxiety, unfortunately, proved to be unsatisfactory. While the prevalence of aggressiveness towards the infant (incipient abuse) was limited to a few women, it was instrumental in identifying individuals with the highest probability of child abuse. The refinement of the cutoff points can enhance sensitivity, especially in the case of anger and rejection, where a threshold of 12 = normal and 13 = high can more effectively

TABLE 4: Factors and items of Postpartum Bonding Questionnaire (PBQ).

No.	Factor	Items	Cutoff
F1	General factor (Positive/negative affective response to baby)	12	11
F2	Anger and rejection	7	16
F3	Confidence and anxiety	4	9
F4	Aggression to the baby	2	2

recognize mothers at risk of threatened rejection. Nevertheless, the validation of these adjusted cutoff values would require a distinct data set.[95] This screening tool possesses the capability of identifying mothers who are at risk of impaired bonding and is commonly employed in scientific research.[96]

The PBQ has undergone translation and validation in the Tamil language resulting in the PBQ-T. Composed of 19 items, the PBQ-T's five factors [General Bonding (F1A), Frustration (F1B), Anxiety (F2), Feeling Trapped (F3A), and Aggression/Rejection Dimensions (F3B)] were identified through component analysis and subsequently loaded into three subscales. These subscales, with cutoffs at 2/3 for subscales 1 and 2 and 0/1 for subscale 3, proved useful in detecting moderate disorders of bonding as well as infant-focused anxiety and anger/rejection. For the detection of any disorder of bonding, a cutoff of 5/6 for the total score is most effective.[97]

- *Bethlem Mother–Infant Interaction Scale (BMIS):*[98] The BMIS scale has been devised to evaluate maternal behavior toward their infants. The BMIS instrument gauges the appropriateness of the mother's caregiving behavior by means of direct observation carried out by a trained nurse. The scale assesses seven elements of mother–infant adjustment, namely eye contact, physical touch, voice contact, maternal mood, routine in general, risk to the baby, and the baby's participation in interaction. The minimum score of zero indicates suitable or sufficient care, whereas the maximum score (four) represents a severely disturbed and chaotic contact pattern. Indicators of the mother's involvement in the conversation with the child are reflected in scores on synchronous and sensitive mood towards the infant, physical touch, vocal contact, and visual contact. The subscale measuring general routine ratings encompasses the scores on the mother's overall proficiency in handling the daily routine, as well as her ability to take care of the baby's physical needs. On the subscale pertaining to physical danger to the neonate, the evaluation of any potential hazards to the infant from the mother, regardless of their intent, is appraised. The contribution of the infant to the quality of interaction is assessed on a distinct subscale, as with the other subscales. The cumulative BMIS score is the summation of the scores for the initial four subscales in addition to the ratings for the general routine and the danger to the neonate. A total BMIS score ranging from 0 to 5 is deemed within the normal range. The BMIS instrument is ideally suited to well-resourced settings that have specialized mother–baby units (MBUs) with highly trained nurses and a favorable nurse-to-patient ratio. The process of scoring the items in BMIS necessitates specialized training, expert knowledge, and considerable time investment.

The present scale has undergone standardization with a commendable degree of interrater reliability and was subject to validation against a standard measure of mother-infant interaction as conducted by Ainsworth et al. in 1971.

- *NIMHANS Maternal Behavior Scale (NIMBUS):*[99] The NIMBUS instrument was formulated to evaluate the interactions between mothers with SMI and their infants via direct observation. Specifically, the NIMBUS comprises five distinct domains: infant care provision, expressions of affection towards the infant, significant occurrences, overall assessment of safety, and maternal response to separation from the infant, in addition to an extra component that examines infant separation from the mother during inpatient care. These domains were developed through a thorough literature review and a retrospective clinical examination of 100 mother–infant dyads admitted to the MBU to gain insight into maternal behavior. For individuals with postpartum psychosis, the NIMBUS demonstrates high internal consistency and inter-rater reliability. Furthermore, external validity has been confirmed via BMIS.
- *Formal Initial Risk Assessment for Mothers and Babies (FIRST-MB):*[100] This is a tool developed in NIMHANS (National Institute of Mental Health and Neurosciences) for risk assessment in a MBU. It assesses risk in the domains of risk to self, risk to the infant, risk to others and other risks, and infant health. It is used in perinatal patients to assess suitability for admission and to assess risk thereafter as well. It has been used to measure risk in studies from the NIMHANS MBU.[100,101]

■ *Perimenopause and Menopause:* The process of menopause, according to the Stages of Reproductive Aging Workshop (STRAW), is characterized by the time period between the initial significant changes in the duration of the menstrual cycle up until 1 year after the final menstrual cycle, with a typical duration ranging from 4 to 5 years.[102] This transitional phase is accompanied by numerous biological and psychosocial changes, such as alterations in endocrine function including changes in sex hormones as well as psychosocial factors, such as increased stressful life events, distress related to changes in role, physical changes associated with reproductive aging, and other health conditions.[103] Notably, an Indian study found that a significant proportion of perimenopausal women experienced psychiatric illness, with the most common mental illness being depression (31%), followed by anxiety.[104]

- *Women's Health Questionnaire (WHQ):*[105] The WHQ is a comprehensive questionnaire consisting of 36 items that assess nine domains of physical and emotional health. The questionnaire utilizes a 4-point scale to rate the various domains of symptom experience, which includes vasomotor symptoms relevant to menopause, as well as psychosocial factors, general health, aging, sleep, sexual problems, and cognitive difficulties. The versatility of the WHQ is demonstrated through its application in various settings, such as evaluating the quality of life for middle-aged women, assessing hormone treatments for menopause-related problems, and conducting epidemiological studies with healthy women populations. The questionnaire has established test–retest reliability and concurrent validity. The external validity has been established with the Mental Health SF36 scale and Vitality scale. Internal consistency is established for seven domains (Cronbach's alpha 0.7–0.84); however, the domains of menstrual problems and sexual problems have alpha values of 0.64 and 0.59, respectively. The scale is provided in the referenced article.

- *Meno-D:*[106] The Meno-D questionnaire serves as a valuable tool for evaluating the severity of perimenopausal depression symptoms through self-report or clinician evaluation. Its comprehensive assessment includes a total of 12 symptoms, such as anxiety, physical discomfort, irritability, self-esteem, vitality, focus, loneliness, sleep patterns, weight changes, libido, memory loss, and suspicion. The scoring system ranges from 0 to 4 for each symptom, yielding a total score from 0 to 48. The research focused on the validity and reliability of the Meno-D, which involved a sample of 93 perimenopausal women. Confirmatory factor analysis demonstrated that the Meno-D questionnaire possesses excellent internal consistency and reliable and valid assessments of the five factors: self, somatic, cognitive, sleep, and libido. All these factors achieved alpha above the 0.70 threshold, indicating that they possess strong internal consistency.

- *Menopause Rating Scale (MRS):*[107] The establishment of the MRS was prompted by the paucity of standardized measurement tools for evaluating the severity of aging-related symptoms and their impact on health-related quality of life (HRQoL) during the early 1990s. In its initial iteration, the MRS was administered by a physician; however, a self-administered version was subsequently developed. The MRS comprises 11 items that encompass both physical and psychological symptoms. The severity of symptoms experienced by the respondent determines the score assigned to each item, ranging from 0 (no symptoms) to 4 (severe symptoms). A large-scale multinational survey utilizing the MRS was carried out in nine countries, including Germany, Spain, France, Sweden, the United States, Mexico, Argentina, Brazil, and Indonesia, which demonstrated robust reliability and validity of the scale across these nations.

- *Scales for Neurodevelopmental Disorders:* It is being recognized that the gender difference in the prevalence of attention-deficit hyperactivity disorder (ADHD) and autism may be due to delay and lack of identification of both the disorders in girls.[108,109] This may stem from the assumption that it presents the same way in both sexes. Though there is marked difference in the prevalence between the sexes in childhood ADHD, the differences are not very apparent when adult ADHD rates are compared. The diminished rates of identification and referral may have far reaching consequences in the life of these girls.[108] Given below are scales developed for identification of these disorders in girls.
  - *ADHD:* There are two checklists that have been developed for assessing ADHD in girls, the ADHD self-rating scale for girls,[110] and the ADHD self-assessment symptom inventory (SASI).[111] The former measures 14 domains on a 0–3 Likert scale and the latter has two parts assessing childhood and adulthood ADHD symptoms on a variety of domains including clinical, learning problems, social and problem behaviors.
  - *Autism:* The Girls Questionnaire for Autism Spectrum Condition (GQ-ASC) is a parent-rated questionnaire for girls 13 years and older. It assesses symptoms of autism in four sections: play, friendships and social situations, abilities and interests, and sensory profile and medical history. A version of this scale has been modified as an autism screening measure in adult women.[109]
- *Resilience:* Resilience is a multi-dimensional construct describing a process of using positive adaptive skills in the face of traumatic adversity.[112] The Connor-Davidson Resilience Scale (CD-RISC) is a 25-item scale validated to assess resilience covering domains including "personal competence, high standards, and tenacity," "trust in one's instincts, tolerance of negative affect, and strengthening effects of stress," "positive acceptance of change and secure relationships".[113] A Kannada version of this scale has been validated among adolescent girls in India.[114]
- *Ecological Momentary Assessments (EMA):* EMA is a measure which comprises repeated sampling of a person's actions in their natural habitat. Usually, a phone application or electronic journal is used to gather these data. Participants are instructed to record answers anytime they experience a specific emotion or at preestablished intervals.[115] In women's health, it has been explored for assessing domains of PMDD. Variation in mood and cognitive states that are cycle related have been picked up by EMA. Ruminations influencing mood have also been seen in the late luteal phase. These measurements have the advantage of nullifying retrospective memory biases and prospective real-time measurements can be made.[116] EMA is also being explored in a pilot study as a means of early detection of postpartum depression.[117]

CONCLUSION

There are a variety of scales available to assess various biological and psychosocial factors causing distress throughout their lifespan and their effect on mental health. The assessment of these conditions is necessary, as knowing of their existence or severity via appropriate objective measures will enable the formulation of a comprehensive plan of intervention. Separate scales for various mental health problems in the perinatal and perimenopausal periods are important, as the symptom profile is unique to women in that phase due to various biological mechanisms.

Most of these scales have established reliability and validity in the target populations. However, due to cultural and language differences in the expression of various phenomena, scales developed in one part of the world may be difficult to apply in another. Thus, more vernacular language translations are warranted to adapt these scales to the context of the various cultures and languages in India.

> **KEY POINTS**
> - There are various assessment measures available for psychiatric illnesses and psychosocial issues encountered by women throughout their lives.
> - The selection of the measure may be based on the target population's characteristics and needs.
> - There is a dearth of availability of vernacular language translations of scales, which is a problem more prominent in India due to the variety of languages spoken throughout the country.

REFERENCES

1. Seedat S, Scott KM, Angermeyer MC, Berglund P, Bromet EJ, Brugha TS, et al. Cross-National Associations Between Gender and Mental Disorders in the World Health Organization World Mental Health Surveys. Arch Gen Psychiatry. 2009;66(7):785-95.
2. World Health Organization. (2000). Women's Mental Health: An Evidence Based Review. [online] Available from https://iris.who.int/bitstream/handle/10665/66539/WHO_MSD_MDP_00.1.pdf?sequence=1 [Last accessed December, 2023].
3. Malhotra S, Shah R. Women and mental health in India: An overview. Indian J Psychiatry. 2015;57(6):205.
4. Ministry of Health and Family Welfare. (2021). National Family Health Survey (NFHS-5). [online] Available from https://main.mohfw.gov.in/sites/default/files/NFHS-5_Phase-II_0.pdf [Last accessed December, 2023].
5. Matud MP. Gender differences in stress and coping styles. Pers Individ Dif. 2004;37(7):1401-15.
6. Toribio Caballero S, Cardenal Hernáez V, Ávila Espada A, Ovejero Bruna MM. Gender roles and women's mental health: their influence on the demand for psychological care. Anales de Psicologia. 2022;38(1):7-16.

7. World Health Organization (2021). Violence against women prevalence estimates, 2018: global, regional and national prevalence estimates for intimate partner violence against women and global and regional prevalence estimates for non-partner sexual violence against women. [online] Available from https://apps.who.int/iris/handle/10665/341337 [Last accessed December, 2023].
8. Hegarty K, Fracgp null, Bush R, Sheehan M. The composite abuse scale: further development and assessment of reliability and validity of a multidimensional partner abuse measure in clinical settings. Violence Vict. 2005;20(5):529-47.
9. Ford-Gilboe M, Wathen CN, Varcoe C, MacMillan HL, Scott-Storey K, Mantler T, et al. Development of a brief measure of intimate partner violence experiences: the Composite Abuse Scale (Revised)—Short Form (CAS R-SF). BMJ Open. 2016;6(12):e012824.
10. Straus MA, Hamby SL, BONEY-McCOY S, Sugarman DB. The Revised Conflict Tactics Scales (CTS2): Development and Preliminary Psychometric Data. J Fam Issues. 1996;17(3):283-316.
11. García-Moreno C, Jansen H, Ellsberg M, Heise L, Watts C. WHO Multi-country Study on Women's Health and Domestic Violence Against Women. Initial Results on Prevalence, Health Outcomes and Women's Responses, volume 204. Geneva: World Health Organization; 2005.
12. Indian Council of Medical Research. Health consequences of domestic violence with special reference to reproductive health. 2011. (https://main.icmr.nic.in/sites/default/files/annual_repoorts/Annual-Report_2005-2006_ICMR_Headquarters-Delhi-English.pdf)
13. Oram S, Fisher HL, Minnis H, Seedat S, Walby S, Hegarty K, et al. The Lancet Psychiatry Commission on intimate partner violence and mental health: advancing mental health services, research, and policy. Lancet Psychiatry. 2022;9(6):487-524.
14. Government of India. (2005). Protection of Women from Domestic Violence Act. 2005. [online] Available from https://www.indiacode.nic.in/bitstream/123456789/15436/1/protection_of_women_from_domestic_violence_act%2C_2005.pdf [Last accessed December, 2023].
15. Kalokhe AS, Stephenson R, Kelley ME, Dunkle KL, Paranjape A, Solas V, et al. The Development and Validation of the Indian Family Violence and Control Scale. PLoS One. 2016;11(1):e0148120.
16. Indu P, Remadevi S, Vidhukumar K, Anilkumar T, Subha N. Development and validation of the domestic violence questionnaire in married women aged 18-55 years. Indian J Psychiatry. 2011;53(3):218.
17. Krug EG, Dahlberg LL, Mercy JA, Zwi AB, Lozano R. World Report on Violence and Health. Geneva: World Health Organization; 2002.
18. National Crime Records Bureau. (2021). Crime in India 2021. [online] Available from http://www.indiaenvironmentportal.org.in/files/file/crime%20in%20india%202021.pdf [Last accessed December, 2023].
19. Rai R, Rai AK. Sexual violence and poor mental health of women: An exploratory study of Uttar Pradesh, India. Clin Epidemiol Glob Health. 2020;8(1):194-8.
20. Koss MP, Gidycz CA. Sexual Experiences Survey: Reliability and validity. J Consult Clin Psychol. 1985;53(3):422-3.
21. Karabatsos G. The Sexual Experiences Survey: interpretation and validity. J Outcome Meas. 1997;1(4):305-28.

22. Johnson SM, Murphy MJ, Gidycz CA. Reliability and Validity of the Sexual Experiences Survey–Short Forms Victimization and Perpetration. Violence Vict. 2017;32(1):78-92.
23. Perrin N, Marsh M, Clough A, Desgroppes A, Yope Phanuel C, Abdi A, et al. Social norms and beliefs about gender based violence scale: a measure for use with gender based violence prevention programs in low-resource and humanitarian settings. Confl Health. 201913(1):6.
24. Marshall LL. Development of the severity of violence against women scales. J Fam Viol. 1992;7(2):103-21.
25. Brand B. Trauma and women. Psychiatric Clinics of North America. 2003;26(3):759-79.
26. Bernstein DP, Fink L, Handelsman L, Lovejoy M, Wenzel K, Sapareto E, et al. Initial reliability and validity of a new retrospective measure of child abuse and neglect. Am J Psychiatry. 1994;151(8):1132-6.
27. Liebschutz JM, Buchanan-Howland K, Chen CA, Frank DA, Richardson MA, Heeren TC, et al. Childhood Trauma Questionnaire (CTQ) correlations with prospective violence assessment in a longitudinal cohort. Psychol Assess. 2018;30(6):841-5.
28. Patil DM, Bajaj A, Supraja TA, Chandra P, Satyanarayana VA. Lifetime traumatic experiences and postpartum depressive symptoms in a cohort of women in South India. Arch Womens Ment Health. 2021;24(4):687-92.
29. Gupta M, Madabushi JS, Gupta N. Critical Overview of Patriarchy, Its Interferences With Psychological Development, and Risks for Mental Health. Cureus. Cureus 15(6): e40216.
30. Singh A, Chokhandre P, Singh AK, Barker KM, Kumar K, McDougal L, et al. Development of the India Patriarchy Index: Validation and Testing of Temporal and Spatial Patterning. Soc Indic Res. 2022;159(1):351-77.
31. Yoon E, Adams K, Hogge I, Bruner JP, Surya S, Bryant FB. Development and validation of the Patriarchal Beliefs Scale. J Couns Psychol [Internet]. 2015;62(2):264-79.
32. Gillespie BL, Eisler RM. Development of the Feminine Gender Role Stress Scale. Behav Modif. 1992;16(3):426-38.
33. García-Cueto E, Rodríguez-Díaz FJ, Bringas-Molleda C, López-Cepero J, Paíno-Quesada S, Rodríguez-Franco L. Development of the Gender Role Attitudes Scale (GRAS) amongst young Spanish people. International Journal of Clinical and Health Psychology. 2015;15(1):61-8.
34. Blumberg RL. Gender, Family, and Economy: The Triple Overlap.. California: Thousand Oaks; 2023.
35. Chandra PS, Satyanarayana VA. Gender disadvantage and common mental disorders in women. Int Rev Psychiatry. 2010;22(5):513-24.
36. Stepanikova I, Acharya S, Abdalla S, Baker E, Klanova J, Darmstadt GL. Gender discrimination and depressive symptoms among child-bearing women: ELSPAC-CZ cohort study. EClinicalMedicine. 2020;20:100297.
37. de la Torre-Pérez L, Oliver-Parra A, Torres X, Bertran MJ. How do we measure gender discrimination? Proposing a construct of gender discrimination through a systematic scoping review. Int J Equity Health. 2022;21(1):1.

38. Satyanarayana VA, Chandra PS, Sharma MK, Sowmya HR, Kandavel T. Three sides of a triangle: gender disadvantage, resilience and psychological distress in a sample of adolescent girls from India. Int J Cult Ment Health. 2016;9(4):364-72.
39. Klonoff EA, Landrine H. The Schedule Of Sexist Events: A Measure of Lifetime and Recent Sexist Discrimination in Women's Lives. Psychol Women Q. 1995;19(4):439-72.
40. Zaman S, Naqvi I. Development and Validation of a Perceived Gender Discrimination Scale (PGDS) for Pakistani Women. FUJP. 2022;6(1):1-7.
41. Steiner M. Hormones and mood: from menarche to menopause and beyond. J Affect Disord. 2003;74(1):67-83.
42. Frank RT. The Hormonal Causes of Premenstrual Tension. Arch NeurPsych. 1931;26(5):1053.
43. American Psychiatric Association. Diagnostic and Statistical Manual of Mental Disorders. DSM-5-TR. Washington, DC: American Psychiatric Association Publishing; 2022.
44. Moos RH. The Development of a Menstrual Distress Questionnaire. Psychosom Med. 1968;30(6):853-67.
45. Hawes E, Oei TPS. The menstrual distress questionnaire: Are the critics right? Curr Psychol. 1992;11(3):264-81.
46. Clare A WR. The construction of a modified version of the Menstrual Distress Questionnaire for use in general practice populations. In: Carenza L, Zichella L (Eds). Emotions and Reproduction, volume 20A. London: Academic Press. 1979. pp. 177-84.
47. Haywood A, Slade P, King H. Assessing the assessment measures for menstrual cycle symptoms. J Psychosom Res. 2002;52(4):223-37.
48. Halbreich U, Endicott J, Schacht S, Nee J. The diversity of premenstrual changes as reflected in the Premenstrual Assessment Form. Acta Psychiatr Scand. 1982;65(1):46-65.
49. Allen SS, McBride CM, Pirie PL. The shortened premenstrual assessment form. J Reprod Med. 1991;36(11):769-72.
50. Steiner M, Macdougall M, Brown E. The premenstrual symptoms screening tool (PSST) for clinicians. Arch Womens Ment Health. 200;6(3):203-9.
51. Raval C, Panchal B, Tiwari D, Vala A, Bhatt R. Prevalence of premenstrual syndrome and premenstrual dysphoric disorder among college students of Bhavnagar, Gujarat. Indian J Psychiatry. 2016;58(2):164.
52. Endicott J, Nee J, Cohen J, Halbreich U. Premenstrual changes: Patterns and correlates of daily ratings. J Affect Disord. 1986;10(2):127-35.
53. Mortola JF, Girton L, Beck L, Yen SS. Diagnosis of premenstrual syndrome by a simple, prospective, and reliable instrument: the calendar of premenstrual experiences. Obstet Gynecol. 1990;76(2):302-7.
54. Endicott J, Nee J, Harrison W. Daily Record of Severity of Problems (DRSP): reliability and validity. Arch Womens Ment Health. 2006;9(1):41-9.
55. Eisenlohr-Moul TA, Girdler SS, Schmalenberger KM, Dawson DN, Surana P, Johnson JL, et al. Toward the Reliable Diagnosis of DSM-5 Premenstrual Dysphoric Disorder: The Carolina Premenstrual Assessment Scoring System (C-PASS). Am J Psychiatry. 2017;174(1):51-9.

56. McCool-Myers M, Theurich M, Zuelke A, Knuettel H, Apfelbacher C. Predictors of female sexual dysfunction: a systematic review and qualitative analysis through gender inequality paradigms. BMC Womens Health. 2018;18(1):108.
57. Wiegel M, Meston C, Rosen R. The Female Sexual Function Index (FSFI): Cross-Validation and Development of Clinical Cutoff Scores. J Sex Marital Ther. 2005;31(1):1-20.
58. A. McGahuey Alan J. Gelenberg CC. The Arizona Sexual Experience Scale (ASEX): Reliability and Validity. J Sex Marital Ther. 2000;26(1):25-40.
59. Derogatis LR, Rosen R, Leiblum S, Burnett A, Heiman J. The Female Sexual Distress Scale (FSDS): Initial Validation of a Standardized Scale for Assessment of Sexually Related Personal Distress in Women. J Sex Marital Ther. 2002;28(4):317-30.
60. Symonds T, Abraham L, Bushmakin AG, Williams K, Martin M, Cappelleri JC. Sexual Function Questionnaire: Further Refinement and Validation. J Sex Med. 2012;9(10):2609-16.
61. Krishna K, Avasthi A, Grover S. Validation of Sexual Functioning Questionnaire in Indian Patients. Indian J Psychol Med. 2014;36(4):404-7.
62. Rosen RC, Bachmann GA, Reese JB, Gentner L, Leiblum S, Wajszczuk C, et al. Female Sexual Well-Being ScaleTM (FSWB ScaleTM): Development and Psychometric Validation in Sexually Functional Women. J Sex Med. 2009;6(5):1297-305.
63. da Costa CKL, Spyrides MHC, de Sousa MBC. Consistency of three different questionnaires for evaluating sexual function in healthy young women. BMC Womens Health. 2018;18(1):204.
64. Howard LM, Khalifeh H. Perinatal mental health: a review of progress and challenges. World Psychiatry. 2020;19(3):313-27.
65. Biaggi A, Conroy S, Pawlby S, Pariante CM. Identifying the women at risk of antenatal anxiety and depression: A systematic review. J Affect Disord. 2016;191:62-77.
66. Upadhyay RP, Chowdhury R, Aslyeh Salehi, Sarkar K, Singh SK, Sinha B, et al. Postpartum depression in India: a systematic review and meta-analysis. Bull World Health Organ. 2017;95(10):706-717C.
67. Sit D, Rothschild AJ, Wisner KL. A Review of Postpartum Psychosis. J Womens Health. 2006;15(4):352-68.
68. Sinesi A, Maxwell M, O'Carroll R, Cheyne H. Anxiety scales used in pregnancy: systematic review. BJPsych Open. 2019;5(1):e5.
69. Huizink AC, Mulder EJH, de Medina PG, Visser GHA, Buitelaar JK. Is pregnancy anxiety a distinctive syndrome? Early Hum Dev. 2004;79(2):81-91.
70. Green JM, Kafetsios K, Statham HE, Snowdon CM. Factor Structure, Validity and Reliability of the Cambridge Worry Scale in a Pregnant Population. J Health Psychol. 2003;8(6):753-64.
71. Carmona Monge FJ, Peñacoba-Puente C, Marín Morales D, Carretero Abellán I. Factor structure, validity and reliability of the Spanish version of the Cambridge Worry Scale. Midwifery. 2012;28(1):112-9.
72. Petersen JJ, Paulitsch MA, Guethlin C, Gensichen J, Jahn A. A survey on worries of pregnant women - testing the German version of the Cambridge Worry Scale. BMC Public Health. 2009;9(1):490.

73. Gourounti K, Lykeridou K, Taskou C, Kafetsios K, Sandall J. A survey of worries of pregnant women: Reliability and validity of the Greek version of the Cambridge Worry Scale. Midwifery. 2012;28(6):746-53.
74. Wijma K, Wijma B, Zar M. Psychometric aspects of the W-DEQ; a new questionnaire for the measurement of fear of childbirth. J Psychosom Obstet Gynecol. 1998;19(2):84-97.
75. Han L, Wu J, Wu H, Liu J, Liu Y, Zou Z, et al. Validating the use of the Wijma Delivery Expectancy/Experience Questionnaire in Mainland China: a descriptive, cross-sectional study. BMC Pregnancy Childbirth. 2022;22(1):931.
76. Khwepeya M, Huang HC, Lee GT, Kuo SY. Validation of the Wijma delivery expectancy/experience questionnaire for pregnant women in Malawi: a descriptive, cross-sectional study. BMC Pregnancy Childbirth. 2020;20(1):455.
77. Jha P, Larsson M, Christensson K, Svanberg AS. Fear of childbirth and depressive symptoms among postnatal women: A cross-sectional survey from Chhattisgarh, India. Women Birth. 2018;31(2):e122-33.
78. Huizink AC, Delforterie MJ, Scheinin NM, Tolvanen M, Karlsson L, Karlsson H. Adaption of pregnancy anxiety questionnaire–revised for all pregnant women regardless of parity: PRAQ-R2. Arch Womens Ment Health. 2016;19(1):125-32.
79. Bharadwaj B, Endumathi R, Parial S, Chandra P. Management of psychiatric disorders during the perinatal period. Indian J Psychiatry. 2022;64(8):414.
80. Cox JL, Holden JM, Sagovsky R. Detection of Postnatal Depression: Development of the 10-item Edinburgh Postnatal Depression Scale. Br J Psychiatry. 1987;150(6):782-6.
81. Cox J. Thirty years with the Edinburgh Postnatal Depression Scale: voices from the past and recommendations for the future. Br J Psychiatry. 2019;214(3):127-9.
82. Gibson J, McKenzie-McHarg K, Shakespeare J, Price J, Gray R. A systematic review of studies validating the Edinburgh Postnatal Depression Scale in antepartum and postpartum women. Acta Psychiatr Scand. 2009;119(5):350-64.
83. Brouwers EPM, van Baar AL, Pop VJM. Does the Edinburgh Postnatal Depression Scale measure anxiety? J Psychosom Res. 2001 Nov;51(5):659-63.
84. Tuohy Alan, McVey Cynthia. Subscales measuring symptoms of non-specific depression, anhedonia, and anxiety in the Edinburgh Postnatal Depression Scale. Br J Clin Psychol. 2008;47(2):153-69.
85. Matthey S, Valenti B, Souter K, Ross-Hamid C. Comparison of four self-report measures and a generic mood question to screen for anxiety during pregnancy in English-speaking women. J Affect Disord. 2013;148(2-3):347-51.
86. Brockington I, Chandra P, Bramante A, Dubow H, Fakher W, Garcia-Esteve Ll, et al. The Stafford Interview. Arch Womens Ment Health. 2017;20(1):107-12.
87. Lord C, Rieder A, Hall GBC, Soares CN, Steiner M. Piloting the Perinatal Obsessive-Compulsive Scale (POCS): Development and validation. J Anxiety Disord. 201;25(8):1079-84.
88. Somerville S, Dedman K, Hagan R, Oxnam E, Wettinger M, Byrne S, et al. The Perinatal Anxiety Screening Scale: development and preliminary validation. Arch Womens Ment Health. 2014;17(5):443-54.
89. Somerville S, Byrne SL, Dedman K, Hagan R, Coo S, Oxnam E, et al. Detecting the severity of perinatal anxiety with the Perinatal Anxiety Screening Scale (PASS). J Affect Disord. 2015;186:18-25.

90. Dwivedi A, Sandhu N, Datta S, Gumber A, Shukla L, Yadav U, et al. Association of antenatal anxiety with adverse pregnancy outcomes: A prospective hospital-based study. Indian J Psychiatry. 2023;65(3):368.
91. Kroenke K, Spitzer RL, Williams JBW. The PHQ-9: Validity of a brief depression severity measure. J Gen Intern Med. 200;16(9):606-13.
92. Wang L, Kroenke K, Stump TE, Monahan PO. Screening for perinatal depression with the Patient Health Questionnaire depression scale (PHQ-9): A systematic review and meta-analysis. Gen Hosp Psychiatry. 2021;68:74-82.
93. Spitzer RL, Kroenke K, Williams JBW, Löwe B. A Brief Measure for Assessing Generalized Anxiety Disorder. Arch Intern Med. 2006;166(10):1092.
94. Vogazianos P, Motrico E, Domínguez-Salas S, Christoforou A, Hadjigeorgiou E. Validation of the generalized anxiety disorder screener (GAD-7) in Cypriot pregnant and postpartum women. BMC Pregnancy Childbirth. 2022;22(1):841.
95. Brockington IF, Fraser C, Wilson D. The Postpartum Bonding Questionnaire: a validation. Arch Womens Ment Health. 2006;9(5):233-42.
96. Wittkowski A, Vatter S, Muhinyi A, Garrett C, Henderson M. Measuring bonding or attachment in the parent-infant-relationship: A systematic review of parent-report assessment measures, their psychometric properties and clinical utility. Clin Psychol Rev. 2020;82:101906.
97. Vengadavaradan A, Bharadwaj B, Sathynarayanan G, Durairaj J, Rajaa S. Translation, validation and factor structure of the Tamil version of the Postpartum Bonding Questionnaire (PBQ-T). Asian J Psychiatr. 2019;40:62-7.
98. Kumar R, Hipwell AE. Development of a Clinical Rating Scale to Assess Mother-Infant Interaction in a Psychiatric Mother and Baby Unit. Br J Psychiatry. 1996;169(1):18-26.
99. Ganjekar S, Prakash A, Thippeswamy H, Desai G, Chandra PS. The NIMHANS (National Institute of Mental Health and Neuro Sciences) Maternal Behaviour Scale (NIMBUS): Development and validation of a scale for assessment of maternal behaviour among mothers with postpartum severe mental illness in low resource settings. Asian J Psychiatr. 2020;47:101872.
100. Chandra P, Saraf G, Desai G, Harish T, Reddy D, Gandi S. Detecting and managing risk to mother and infant in a mother-baby unit in India using a tool--The FIRST MB (Formal Initial Risk Assessment for Mothers and Babies. Arch Womens Ment Health. 2015;18:371-2.
101. Chandra P, Desai G, Reddy D, Thippeswamy H, Saraf G. The establishment of a mother-baby inpatient psychiatry unit in India: Adaptation of a Western model to meet local cultural and resource needs. Indian J Psychiatry. 2015;57(3):290.
102. Soules MR, Sherman S, Parrott E, Rebar R, Santoro N, Utian W, et al. Executive summary: Stages of Reproductive Aging Workshop (STRAW) Park City, Utah, July, 2001: Menopause. 2001;8(6):402-7.
103. Maki PM, Kornstein SG, Joffe H, Bromberger JT, Freeman EW, Athappilly G, et al. Guidelines for the Evaluation and Treatment of Perimenopausal Depression: Summary and Recommendations. J Womens Health. 2019;28(2):117-34.
104. Jagtap B, Prasad BS V, Chaudhury S. Psychiatric morbidity in perimenopausal women. Ind Psychiatry J. 2016;25(1):86.
105. Hunter M. The women's health questionnaire: A measure of mid-aged women's perceptions of their emotional and physical health. Psychol Health. 1992;7(1):45-54.

106. Kulkarni J, Gavrilidis E, Hudaib AR, Bleeker C, Worsley R, Gurvich C. Development and validation of a new rating scale for perimenopausal depression—the Meno-D. Transl Psychiatry. 2018;8(1):123.
107. Heinemann K, Ruebig A, Potthoff P, Schneider HPG, Strelow F, Heinemann LAJ, et al. The Menopause Rating Scale (MRS) scale: A methodological review. Health Qual Life Outcomes. 2004;2(1):45.
108. Young S, Adamo N, Ásgeirsdóttir BB, Branney P, Beckett M, Colley W, et al. Females with ADHD: An expert consensus statement taking a lifespan approach providing guidance for the identification and treatment of attention-deficit/hyperactivity disorder in girls and women. BMC Psychiatry. 2020;20(1):404.
109. Brown CM, Attwood T, Garnett M, Stokes MA. Am I Autistic? Utility of the Girls Questionnaire for Autism Spectrum Condition as an Autism Assessment in Adult Women. Autism Adulthood. 2020;2(3):216-26.
110. Nadeau K, Littman E, Quinn P. AD/HD Self-rating Scale for Girls. United States: Advantage Books, LLC; 2015.
111. Nadeau KG, Quinn PO. AD/HD Self-assessment symptom inventory (SASI). In: Nadeau KG, Quinn PO (Eds). Understanding Women with AD/HD. Silver Spring: Advantage Books; 2002. p. 465, vii, 465-vii.
112. Haddadi P, Besharat MA. Resilience, vulnerability and mental health. Procedia Soc Behav Sci. 2010;5:639-42.
113. Connor KM, Davidson JRT. Development of a new resilience scale: The Connor-Davidson Resilience Scale (CD-RISC). Depress Anxiety. 2003;18(2):76-82.
114. Sidheek KPF, Satyanarayana VA, Sowmya HR, Chandra PS. Using the Kannada version of the Connor Davidson Resilience Scale to assess resilience and its relationship with psychological distress among adolescent girls in Bangalore, India. Asian J Psychiatr. 2017;30:169-72.
115. Shiffman S, Stone AA, Hufford MR. Ecological Momentary Assessment. Annu Rev Clin Psychol. 2008;4(1):1-32.
116. Beddig T, Reinhard I, Ebner-Priemer U, Kuehner C. Reciprocal effects between cognitive and affective states in women with Premenstrual Dysphoric Disorder: An Ecological Momentary Assessment study. Behaviour Research and Therapy. 2020;131:103613.
117. Krohn H, Guintivano J, Frische R, Steed J, Rackers H, Meltzer-Brody S. App-Based Ecological Momentary Assessment to Enhance Clinical Care for Postpartum Depression: Pilot Acceptability Study. JMIR Form Res. 2022;6(3):e28081.

CHAPTER 21

Neuromodulation in Women

Nishant Goyal, Shobit Garg

ABSTRACT

Neuromodulation is defined as "the alteration of nerve activity through targeted delivery of a stimulus, such as electrical stimulation or chemical agents, to specific neurological sites in the body." This chapter describes varied neuromodulation techniques and their classification as per invasiveness. Techniques such as electroconvulsive therapy (ECT), transcranial magnetic stimulation (TMS), magnetic seizure therapy (MST), transcranial electric stimulation (tES), vagus nerve stimulation (VNS), and deep brain stimulation (DBS) system and their approved indications across all psychiatric disorders are described in this chapter in context with their usage in women across various age groups. Neuromodulation techniques, their efficacy, safety, applicability, and feasibility are reviewed in the context of women's mental health. Specific situations such as pregnancy and postpartum phase and operator safety are specifically detailed. There is a need to study the online paradigms utilizing the aforementioned neuromodulation techniques keeping in mind the differential gender-based cortical reactivity of the human cortices. We would further need to replicate or devise protocols in the native context.

Keywords: Noninvasive neuromodulation, women, pregnancy, mental health

CASE VIGNETTE

A patient named Mrs SG, 42-year-old married female, known case of hypertension (HTN), type II diabetes mellitus (DM), and hypothyroidism, with well-balanced management plan, with a past history symptomatic of a depressive episode 10 years back (treatment details not known) that precipitated post demise of her father [due to stroke], came to psychiatry outpatient department (OPD) with complaints of 2 years' duration with abrupt onset, continuous illness and deteriorating course of increased need for sleep, low mood, reduced energy and pleasure in activities, and suicidal attempts precipitated by financial loss. On physical examination, the patient had a body mass index (BMI) of 44 kg/m^2. On mental status examination (MSE), the patient showed reduced eye contact, established rapport with difficulty, increased reaction time, had a depressed and communicable affect, a retarded thought stream, ideas of guilt and hopelessness, impaired judgment, and insight grade 3 **(Fig. 1)**.

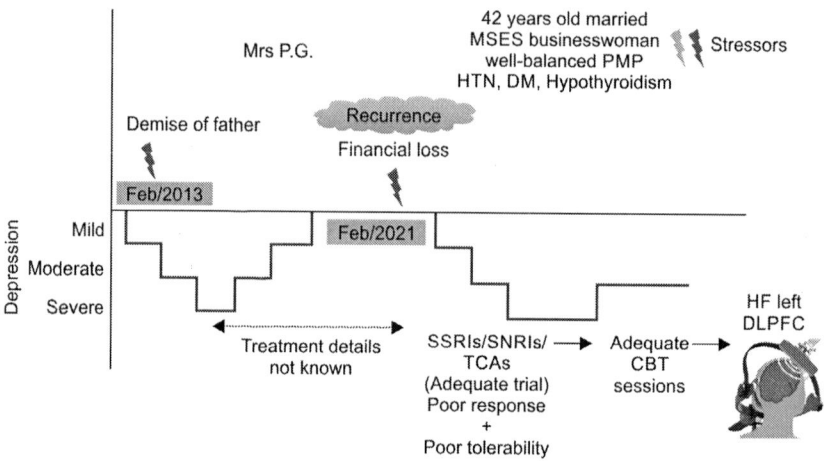

Fig. 1: Illness graph. (DM: diabetes mellitus; HTN: hypertension; MSES: mini-mental state examination; PMP: patient management plan; SNRIs: serotonin and norepinephrine reuptake inhibitors; SSRIs: selective serotonin reuptake inhibitors; TCAs: tricyclic antidepressants)

The patient was diagnosed with the recurrent depressive disorder, a current episode of severe depression (second episode) without psychotic symptoms with morbid obesity, HTN, type II DM, and hypothyroidism.

On investigation, her complete blood count (CBC), liver function test (LFT), kidney function test (KFT), lipid profile, and sugar fasting/postprandial (F/PP) were within normal limits (WNL). Thyroid function test (TFT) was normal. Her recent MADRS (Montgomery-Åsberg Depression Rating Scale) score was 40. The patient did not show adequate response to the trial of antidepressants [both selective serotonin reuptake inhibitors (SSRIs) and serotonin and norepinephrine reuptake inhibitors (SNRIs)] in the past with significant tolerability issues (e.g., weight gain). Subsequent cognitive behavioral therapy (CBT) sessions were not beneficial. So, she was psychoeducated about repetitive transcranial magnetic stimulation (rTMS) and started on 20 sessions (five per week) of high frequency (10 Hz) rTMS targeting the left dorsolateral prefrontal cortex (DLPFC). The stimulus parameters details of each session were 3,000 pulses per session, 5% seconds per train with intertrain interval (ITI) of 26 seconds, at 100% motor threshold (MT).

INTRODUCTION

Neuromodulation is defined as "the alteration of nerve activity through targeted delivery of a stimulus, such as electrical stimulation or chemical agents, to specific neurological sites in the body" as per the International Neuromodulation Society.[1] This expanding family of treatments, which has

Flowchart 1: Various neuromodulation techniques.

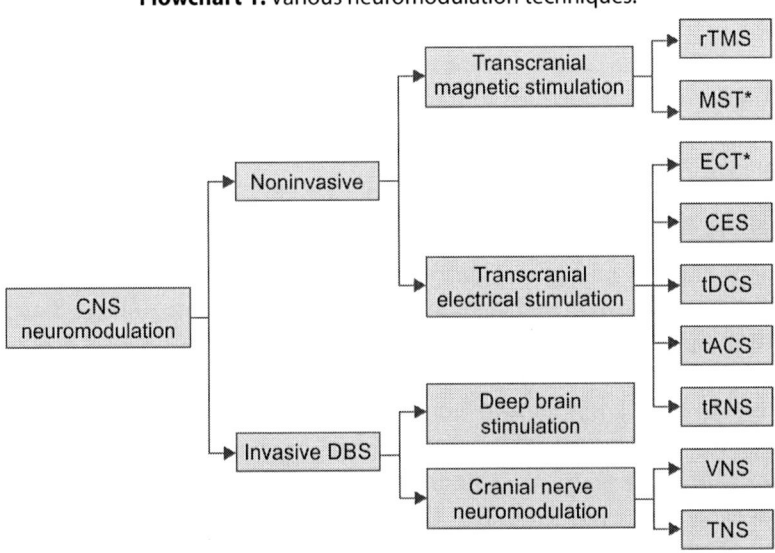

(CES: cranial electrotherapy stimulation; CNS: central nervous system; DBS: deep brain stimulation; ECT: electroconvulsive therapy; MST: magnetic seizure therapy; rTMS: repetitive transcranial magnetic stimulation; tACS: transcranial alternating current stimulation; tDCS: transcranial direct current stimulation; TNS: trigeminal nerve stimulation; tRNS: transcranial random noise stimulation; VNS: vagus nerve stimulation. *ECT and MST induce seizures to induce therapeutic benefits)

been in use since the 1980s, can help restore function or reduce symptoms with a neurobiological basis in psychiatry. Neuromodulation techniques range from noninvasive ones such as transcranial magnetic stimulation (TMS)[2] to implanted ones such as a deep brain stimulation (DBS) system (**Flowchart 1**).[3] Different neuromodulation techniques utilize either electrical impulses, magnetic forces, or both to modulate the faulty neural pathway behavior brought on by the disease process.[1] Modalities such as electroconvulsive therapy (ECT)[4] and magnetic seizure therapy (MST)[5] work via induction of seizure in their specific indications (**Flowchart 1**).

Brain is not sexually dimorphic, but it is known that there are sex and gender differences in brain structure and cognitive processes. For example, females have larger hippocampal size and better reading, writing, perceptual, and fine motor coordination skills when compared to males. Due to the influence of sex hormones and reduced hypothalamic–pituitary–adrenocortical (HPA) axis stress responses, women have been found to be more susceptible to psychosocial environmental stressors, which increases the prevalence of mental disorders. Thereby, women have a substantially higher chronic prevalence of anxiety, depression, and bipolar illnesses than men.[6] Interestingly, different levels of estrogen, testosterone, and progesterone are associated with differential cortical excitability and have varied psychopathological and treatment implications in the context of neuromodulation. Intricacies are invited in physiological states such as pregnancy and applications to treat psychopathology via neuromodulation. In this chapter, we will discuss the role of neuromodulation in the context of women's mental health and its disorders.

INDICATIONS

Perhaps the most important feature of neurostimulation that sets it apart from medications is its "targeted fashion" approach. Neurostimulation techniques have far superior spatial resolution bringing therapeutic effects and negligible or no effects "below the neck." For example, DBS has the highest (roughly 1 mm) and transcranial direct current stimulation (tDCS)[7] has the lowest (in centimeters) spatial resolution. With the exception of ECT and MST, the majority of other neurostimulation techniques have spatial resolutions that fall between these two extremes **(Table 1)**.

Various modalities have received the Food and Drug Administration (FDA) approvals such as ECT, TMS, vagus nerve stimulation (VNS),[8] and DBS for varied clinical phenotypes. Details of the equipment (machines) and specific conditions are mentioned in **Table 2**.

PERINATAL PERIOD AND NEUROMODULATION

The perinatal period lasts from pregnancy till 1 year postpartum. A woman's life undergoes substantial physical, biochemical, emotional, and psychosocial changes throughout the perinatal period. This puts her at risk for acute psychiatric problems.[9] Psychiatric illnesses during the perinatal phase are very difficult to manage. Psychotherapies are, in fact, quite difficult to access, specifically in our native context, and there is reluctance to employ psychotropics due to concerns about their safety, particularly about their possible effects on prenatal development or potential toxicity to the nursing infant. In fact, most of the psychotropics used during pregnancy are category C.[10] Due to this, brain stimulation modalities as an alternative to medication during pregnancy are gaining popularity. Intriguingly, patients' lack of awareness regarding the safety and effectiveness of neuromodulation techniques in peripartum psychiatric disorders defines their acceptability.[11] We shall discuss each neuromodulation modality and its efficacy, safety, and acceptability.

ELECTROCONVULSIVE THERAPY

For unipolar depression, bipolar disorder, schizophrenia, and other psychiatric disorders that are life-threatening or treatment resistant, ECT is a very effective and secure treatment option **(see Table 2)**. With only

TABLE 1: Characteristics of neuromodulation approaches.

Modality	Medium	Convulsive	Invasive	Spatial resolution	Depth of penetration	Applied strength	FDA approval*
ECT	Electrical	Yes	No	NA	NA	800 mA	Yes
MST	Magnetic	Yes	No	NA	NA	2 Tesla	No
TMS	Magnetic	No	No	~1 cm	1–3 cm[†]	2 Tesla	Yes
tDCS[‡]	Electrical	No	No	in cms	Varying	1–2 mA	No[§]
VNS	Electrical	No	Yes	NA	NA	0.1–6 mA	Yes
DBS	Electrical	No	Yes	~1 mm	Varying	2.4–4.4 V	Yes

(DBS: deep brain stimulation; ECT: electroconvulsive therapy; FDA: Food and Drug Administration; MST: magnetic seizure therapy; tDCS: transcranial direct current stimulation; TMS: transcranial magnetic stimulation, VNS: vagus nerve stimulation)
*See Table 2 for details.
[†]H coils: 0.7 cm more depth of penetration than figure of eight.
[‡]Transcranial electrical stimulation.
[§]Investigational.

TABLE 2: The United States Food and Drug Administration (FDA) approval for neuromodulation modalities.

Equipment	Disorder
rTMS	
Neuronetics (Neurostar®) ± TBS/Deep TMS (BrainSway)/Rapid[2] (Magstim)/ Tonica Elektronik (MagVenture) ± TBS/ navigated brain therapy (NBT) system (Nexstim)/Apollo TMS (MAG & More)/ CloudTMS (Soterix Medical)	MDD
Deep TMS (BrainSway)/Tonica Elektronik (MagVenture)	OCD
eNeura	Migraine
Deep TMS (BrainSway)	Smoking cessation
Deep TMS (BrainSway)	Anxiety comorbid with MDD
tDCS	
For medical use is considered "investigational use only" (FDA). European Union (EU): 1 × 1 tDCS™ Therapy System (Soterix Medical, Inc.) approved for MDD (2015)	
VNS	
NCP M100-106, SenTiva® M1000	• Refractory partial-onset epilepsy (>4 years of age) • Difficult to treat depression
ECT	
Devices—Class II (moderate risk)	Catatonia or a severe MDE associated with MDD or bipolar disorder in patients aged 13 years and older who are treatment resistant or who require a rapid response treatment due to the severity of their psychiatric or medical condition
Devices—Class III (high risk)	Class III (premarket approval) for the following intended uses: Schizophrenia, bipolar manic states, schizoaffective disorder, schizophreniform disorder, and catatonia or a severe MDE associated with MDD or BPD in: • Patients under 13 years • Or patients aged 13 years and older who are not treatment resistant or who do not require a rapid response due to the severity of their psychiatric or medical condition

Contd...

Contd...

Equipment	Disorder
Deep brain stimulation (DBS)	
Medtronic's device Vercise™ PC, Vercise Gevia™, and Vercise Genus™ DBS systems	• The ventral intermediate nucleus of the thalamus (1996), STN or GPi (2001) DBS for essential tremor and severe tremor in PD. Humanitarian device exemption (HDE) for dystonia (2002) • Refractory OCD as a HDE (H050003) (2009)
MST	
Since MST has not yet received FDA approval and is currently in the experimental stages, there are no clinical algorithms available at this time.	

(BPD: borderline personality disorder; ECT: electroconvulsive therapy; GPi: globus pallidus internus; HDE: humanitarian device exemption; OCD: obsessive-compulsive disorder; MDD: Major depressive disorder; MDE: major depressive episode; MST: magnetic seizure therapy; PD: Parkinson's disease; rTMS: repetitive transcranial magnetic stimulation; STN: subthalamic nucleus; TBS: theta burst stimulation; tDCS; transcranial direct current stimulation; TMS: transcranial magnetic stimulation; VNS: vagus nerve stimulation)

2 deaths per 10,000 procedures, ECT has one of the lowest fatality rates of any procedure carried out under general anesthesia. It is also well known that the underutilization of ECT in pregnancy is a result of stigma, patient access issues, and provider discomfort when referring patients for ECT evaluation.[12]

The *first ECT* to be administered in peripartum depression in pregnancy was in a lady in her second trimester who underwent unilateral ECT to the nondominant hemisphere for eight sessions.[13] There are no randomized controlled studies on the effectiveness of ECT during pregnancy. The majority of the safety information is inferred from case studies of ECT therapy during pregnancy and ECT usage in nonpregnant patients. Fortunately, the negative effects of ECT on pregnant and nonpregnant individuals are comparable.[12] Most of the ECTs were delivered in the second and third trimesters, and seizure duration lasted from 17 to 186 seconds.[14] According to the official joint statement from the American Psychological Association and the American College of Obstetricians and Gynecologists, ECT should be regarded as a secure and efficient therapy option for pregnant women who are suffering from refractory or life-threatening depression.[15] Despite the safe outcomes, there are risks of ECT-induced seizure causing a decrease in the uteroplacental unit's perfusion and risks of aspiration.

There are several modifications that can be made to increase the safety in pregnancy, as follows:[12]

- Pregnancy should not affect the required number of ECT treatments.
- It is important to record the presence of fetal doptones in the previous period both before and after treatment.

- Aspiration risks can be decreased by taking sodium citrate, histamine-2 receptor antagonists (H2 blockers), prokinetic drugs, or proton-pump inhibitors prior to the procedure.
- Routine intubation needs to be avoided because of the pregnancy-related increase in vascularity and airway edema.
- Preoxygenation, left lateral tilt positioning using a wedge, and intravenous fluid prehydration can all improve uteroplacental perfusion and fetal oxygenation.
- Prior to the anesthesia, it is best to prevent hyperventilation because it is linked to decreased placental blood flow and can cause fetal acidosis and hypoxia through vasoconstriction, decreased venous return, and a left shift in the maternal oxygenation curve.
- After 23 weeks, preprocedure and postprocedure nonstress testing or continuous fetal monitoring should be carried out, and the procedure should be carried out in a facility that can handle an emergency delivery if necessary.
- Pregnancy necessitates changes to some drugs used in the delivery of ECT; for instance, glycopyrrolate should be used if an anticholinergic substance is required. Propofol may reduce fetal heart rate abnormalities linked to prolonged seizure duration and is associated with shorter seizures without losing effectiveness.
- Patients should undergo reassuring antenatal testing and be monitored until they are alert and comfortable. An early postpartum visit (within 2 weeks following delivery) would certainly be beneficial citing the risk of postpartum exacerbations of mood disorders.

Safety Evidence

The most frequent side effects of ECT reported are temporary and self-limited fetal heart rate fluctuations and contractions, which rarely would progress to labor. Importantly, it does not seem that individuals who got ECT during pregnancy have a higher incidence of vaginal bleeding/placental abruption, prolonged fetal heart rate anomalies, preterm delivery, or stillbirth. Reported congenital abnormalities in children of women who received ECTs were possibly unrelated to the intervention as ECTs were applied in the second or third trimester.[16] It is interesting to note that, for ECT in the postpartum, just one study found transitory memory loss.

Importantly, there is a higher prevalence of reporting bias regarding adverse or unusual outcomes following ECT in pregnancy. As we know, none of the routine cases of ECT in pregnancy at their institution are reported in the general literature because there have been no adverse events.[12]

Acceptability

Treatment interruption was reported in pregnant women due to adverse effects such as contractions and the risk of preterm labor, cognitive decline, transportation difficulties, etc. The estimated acceptability of ECT during pregnancy is 83.2%. All the postpartum patients reported to have finished their treatment, indicating a 100% acceptance.[14]

■ REPETITIVE TRANSCRANIAL MAGNETIC STIMULATION

Another type of neuromodulation is TMS, which depolarizes neural networks by applying intense, focused magnetic pulses to specific brain areas (**see Table 1**). Unlike ECT, no pharmaceutical agent is required for its delivery during pregnancy.

Evidence in Peripartum Depression

The first case report on a pregnant woman was published in 1999.[17] With no prior psychiatric history, the 36-year-old gravida 1 para 0 female declined antidepressants and showed no response to psychotherapy. At 22 weeks of gestation, TMS treatment for major depressive disorder (MDD) with pronounced anxiety was started on the dorsolateral prefrontal cortex (DLPFC) [14 left-sided sessions at 100% motor threshold (MT), high-frequency protocol]. She made quick progress and gave birth to a healthy full-term baby. Almost a decade later, two more cases of antenatal depression were reported with healthy outcomes.[17] Subsequently, open-label trials and controlled trials in peripartum depression were conducted which are discussed in the following section.

Efficacy

There are three meta-analyses (**Table 3**) till date reporting the effect of TMS over peripartum depression comprising mixed partum and postpartum depression (till 6 months) data.[18-20] Majority of the randomized controlled trials (RCTs) were from postpartum phase, except one reporting pregnancy data.[21] Remission rates reported by Kim et al. in peripartum depression were 27.27% in the active group and 18.18% in the sham group.

Majority of studies employed high-frequency left DLPFC stimulation than low-frequency right DLPFC. Interestingly, majority of studies were from Southeast Asia (China). The effect sizes reported by the three meta-analyses range from 0.65 to 1.394. In a subgroup analysis, a larger sample size and longer duration of intervention (>2 months) were found to have a better effect size than otherwise. Interestingly, cognition scores showed significant improvement with TMS.

TABLE 3: Description of meta-analysis of TMS in peripartum depression.

Article	Total number of studies	Age group	Disorder	rTMS type	Reduction in severity	Response	Remission
Lee et al. 2021[18]	5	Any	Peripartum depression	Any rTMS	SMD 1.394 (0.944–1.843)	NA	NA
Liu et al. 2020[19]	10	Any	Peripartum depression	Any rTMS	SMD 0.65 (0.31–0.98)	OR 1.47 (0.99–2.17) Not significant	OR 1.83 (1.05–3.18)
Peng et al. 2020[20]	14	Any	Postpartum depression	Any rTMS	SMD 1.02 (0.66–1.37) SMD of 2.47 (3.03 –1.91) (Longer duration of intervention) MMSE: MD = 3.64, CI (0.19– 7.09)	NA	NA

(CI: confidence interval; MD: mean differences; MMSE: mini-mental state examination; rTMS: repetitive transcranial magnetic stimulation; SMD: sensory modulation disorder; TMS: transcranial magnetic stimulation)

Acceptability

The acceptability of ECT was computed using the total number of withdrawals. 84.6% of the women in the rTMS RCT during pregnancy finished the protocol, according to Kim et al.[21] In the single-arm studies and case reports, every woman finished the course of treatment.

Regarding the postpartum rTMS investigations, acceptance rates varied from 76% to 100% among the women who were included in the single arm and RCTs reflecting the higher rates of acceptability.[14]

Safety

The documented adverse events in the published cases were brief, mild, and typically limited to headache, scalp pain, and dry mouth. None of the side effects reported were grave and were equally distributed between active and sham conditions. Difficulty concentrating and anxiety have been recorded as isolated events that resolved on their own. Supine hypotension syndrome or inferior vena cava compression syndrome are reported in a couple of cases during TMS. Supine hypotension syndrome is indicated by pallor, dizziness, low blood pressure (BP), sweating, nausea, and increased heart rate. Symptoms usually occur within 3–10 minutes after lying down. Supine hypotension syndrome is diagnosed with a decrease in systolic BP of at least 15–30 mm Hg. In severe cases, loss of consciousness is also reported. Since symptoms are less likely to manifest with at least a 30° left pelvic tilt, it shall be feasible that any woman who is over 24 weeks pregnant should be positioned on her left side while using a wedge cushion.[22]

Is transcranial magnetic stimulation a fetal risk factor?
The physics of typical clinical rTMS seems compatible with pregnancy, notwithstanding the lack of trials particularly designed to verify TMS safety in pregnancy. According to a finite element model, when the distance between the coil and the uterus was 60 cm, the TMS-induced E-field produced by a figure-of-eight coil next to DLPFC was around 100 mV/m.[23] The International Commission on Nonionizing Radiation Protection guidelines state that 800 mV/m is the safety threshold for stimulating myelinated central and peripheral neurons, and this number is much lower. The magnetic field produced by single-pulse TMS drops from 0.9 T at 1 cm away from the coil surface to 11×10^{-6} T at the distance the uterus may travel at full term. Citing safe and minimal exposure of the fetus to magnetic forces, minimal adverse effects are expected.[23]

Pridmore et al.,[24] in a recent review, located 10 studies including 67 births followed up to a peripartum period of 62 months. Most of them were offsprings of depressed mothers who received TMS in all the trimesters. Stimulation included either high or low frequency and theta burst stimulation (TBS).

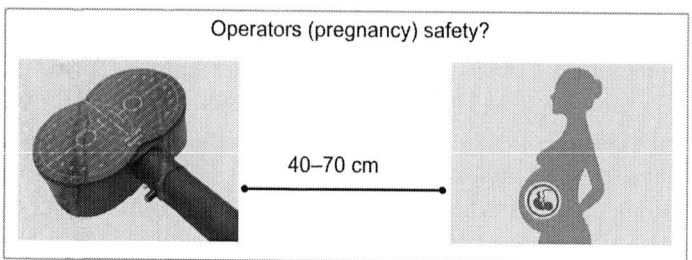

Fig. 2: Safety parameters (distance between the coil and self) for operators.

Interestingly, no serious event was observed. Only one baby developed irritability which resolved within a week. Three preterm births were reported but were explained by associated medical conditions. Moreover, no neurodevelopmental issues were screened positive.

Safety Parameters for Operators

Transcranial magnetic stimulation delivery with precision is very paramount and ought to be given by a "TMS operator." In addition to having received training in identifying and appropriately handling seizures, a "TMS operator" shall be able to "recognize potentially the serious changes in a patient's mental status and know when to alert an attending physician." Therefore, any nonmedical staff member might be the "TMS operator."[2]

It is important to note that no specific reports of TMS adverse events in operators exist. Even though operators are exposed to magnetic fields for several hours everyday, sometimes even for years, safety concerns are rarely addressed for them. Studies have explored the distance needed from the coil to avoid magnetic field exposure exceeding these limit values—40–70 cm (Fig. 2).[23] But these findings call for more investigation to determine the limiting distance to the coil based on the following factors: exposure duration, stimulation frequency and intensity, and TMS machine type and coil configuration.

Status of Theta Burst in Peripartum Depression

Theta burst stimulation is one of the recently developed patterned TMS which has more robust neuroplastic effects, is more efficient, and takes lesser stimulation time when compared to conventional rTMS. TBS has been recently studied in antenatal depression, but the data is at large anecdotal (case reports and case series).[25,26] TBS in suprathreshold protocol was applied in left DLPFC in cases either in second or third trimester. A maximum of 21 sessions were given to one of the cases. All patients responded with three achieving remission. All pregnancies were full term, and all the infants had an

APGAR (appearance, pulse, grimace, activity and respiration) score of 10 (10 minutes). This establishes the need for a controlled trial to establish efficacy and safety.

Evidence in Other Psychiatric Disorders

The use of rTMS in the perinatal phase is studied barely in psychiatric conditions apart from depression. Single case reports of rTMS and its effects are reported in three psychiatric conditions: (1) Bipolar depression (2) chronic akathisia, and (3) tokophobia and psychogenic nonepileptic seizures (PNES) during pregnancy including two reports from India.[27-30]

A 32-year-old G2P1 woman with bipolar II depression presented at 20 weeks' gestation and responded to bilateral DLPFC with 41 sessions.[27] There is a case report of tokophobia (fear of pregnancy and childbirth) being treated with TMS. The patient received intermittent TBS over the left DLPFC and continuous TBS(at 90% of resting MT) over the right DLPFC. She needed 20 sessions until 28 weeks of gestation and tolerated them well.[29]

There is a report of managing chronic akathisia (worsening with fluoxetine) in a pregnant lady with MDD with a single session of 1 Hz rTMS on the right M1, at 90% of resting motor threshold (RMT) using a figure-of-eight coil in her 20 weeks of gestation. She achieved remission after a 6-week course of rTMS.[28]

Furthermore, there is a single case report of pregnant women with PNES who had been treated with TBS.[30] Three cases were successfully treated with single-pulse TMS in the second trimester for treatment-refractory migraine.[31]

■ TRANSCRANIAL ELECTRIC STIMULATION

Transcranial electric stimulation (tES) is a noninvasive brain stimulation technique that modifies brain activity by applying a brief, low-intensity electric current through two electrodes applied to the scalp: (1) The cathode, which decreases spontaneous neuronal activity, and (2) the anode, which increases it.[32] tES comes in a variety of forms: tDCS uses a weak direct continuous electric current, transcranial alternating current stimulation (tACS) employs a sinusoidal alternating electric current, and transcranial random noise stimulation (tRNS) uses a weak alternating current.[32]

Of late, these tES techniques are increasingly being used for the treatment of several psychiatric disorders such as depression and schizophrenia. It is important to know that tDCS is the most popular tES technique. Major reasons are that it is simple to use (no anesthesia required), its safety profile (no major side effects), and acceptability (dropout rates < 10%).[33] tES studies reviewed largely consist of case reports employing tDCS and are conducted in the pregnancy phase of peripartum.[32]

Efficacy

Transcranial electric stimulation efficacy data is available across psychiatric conditions such as unipolar depression (four case reports, two open-label trials, and one RCT), bipolar depression (one case report), schizophrenia (two case reports), and post-traumatic stress disorder (PTSD) (one case report) **(Table 4)**. All the available studies have employed tDCS therapeutic modality, except in two case studies which have used tACS and trigeminal nerve stimulation (TNS), albeit both for unipolar depression[25,34] **(Table 4)**.

Two case reports studying the effects of tDCS and tACS in MDD (F3 anode; F4 cathode) have respectively reported short-term improvements (47% and 72%). But two open-label trials of tDCS in MDD have reported mixed short-term outcomes. Vigod et al.[35] evaluated the effectiveness of tDCS versus placebo in 20 pregnant women in a RCT design. The efficacy of tDCS over placebo in depression was not established. However, the rate of remission in the postpartum period was higher in the tDCS group. Interestingly, sustained improvement (till 6 months) has been reported in a single case of bipolar II depression with tDCS (F3 anode; F4 cathode). Two case reports studying the role of tDCS (F3 anode; TP3 cathode) in schizophrenia have reported >90% reduction in auditory hallucinations over 1 month. Interestingly, one study reported the effect of sham tDCS in PTSD adjuvant to pharmacotherapy has reported remission till delivery. Laurin et al.[32] reported the effect of tDCS in postpartum depression in a lactating female with modest short-term improvement and a relapse subsequently.

Safety

In terms of safety, different authors suggested different methods for monitoring obstetrical and fetal parameters, but the information that is now available indicates that there are no impacts on pregnancy or delivery, and all studies show that tES is well tolerated, with modest and temporary side effects (burning, tingling, itching at electrode site, and phosphenes) for tDCS being well known **(see Table 4)**. It would be extremely improbable that tES therapies would have any negative consequences on a pregnant woman, embryo, or fetus, despite the fact that there is currently available data that is anecdotal regarding its use during pregnancy.

Acceptability

Vigod et al.[35] discovered an 88% retention rate of tDCS which is comparable to the rate observed in the general population. Also, reported satisfaction rates with tDCS were good, estimated at 87.5%. This means that tES is a successful treatment with low dropout rates, even for expectant mothers. tES therapies could be a feasible option in nursing mothers who would refuse medications.

TABLE 4: Description of studies of tES modalities in peripartum psychiatric disorders.

Article	tES	N	Trimester	Sessions	Reduction in severity	Electrode	Stimulus parameters	Safety
Major depressive disorder								
Sreeraj et al., 2016[36]	tDCS	One case report	First	10	• 1 month after the end of treatment, HAM-D reduced from 18 to 5 and HAM-A reduced from 32 to 6 • The patient was in remission	Anode: F3 Cathode: F4	2 mA, 20 s fade-in/fade-out, 30 min/day over 10 days	Transient, mild burning sensations, and fleeting experience of phosphenes Fetal or obstetrical data not stated
Palm et al., 2017[43]	tDCS	Three open-label trial	Second and third	30	• Mean HAMD-21 score reduced from 24.7 (SD 10.7) to 15.7 (SD 3.7) after 2 weeks, then 7.0 (SD 7.1) after 4 weeks • One patient achieved remission	Anode: F3 Cathode: F4	2 mA Two sessions over 30 min/day, over 10 days	• No adverse effect • Fetal or obstetrical data not stated

Contd...

Contd...

Article	tES	N	Trimester	Sessions	Reduction in severity	Electrode	Stimulus parameters	Safety
Vigod et al., 2019[35]	tDCS	20 (10/10) RCT	Second to third	15	Remission rate (MADRS score < 10) in the active and sham groups was 37.5% and 22% at posttreatment phase After 4 and 12 weeks postpartum, remission rates increased to 75% in active group and 22% at 4 and 25% at 12 weeks respectively in sham group	Anode: F3 Cathode: F4	2 mA (or sham), 30 min/day, 15 days over 3 weeks	• Buzzing/tinging at the electrode site • Retention rate and satisfaction rates are 88% and 87.5%, respectively • No abnormalities noted on continuous fetal monitoring (>24 weeks) • One infant in each group had an APGAR score < 8 (5 min) with no known sequelae

Contd...

Contd...

Article	tES	N	Trimester	Sessions	Reduction in severity	Electrode	Stimulus parameters	Safety
Kurzeck et al., 2021[37]	tDCS	Six open-label trials	First to third	20	• Mean HAMD-21 total score decreased by 39% after 2 weeks • Two patients were responders defined by a 50% reduction in the HAMD-21 total score	*Anode:* F3 *Cathode:* F4	2 mA, 15 s fade-in/fade-out, Two sessions 30 min/day, 10 days	• Mild headache, phosphenes, and feeling of itching • No antenatal or neonatal complications
Laurin et al., 2022[32]	tDCS	One case report	Lactation period	19	Reduction of MADRS score from 36/60 to 25/60 (−30%) after tDCS treatment with a relapse of depression at 1 month	*Anode:* F3 *Cathode:* F4	2 mA, 15 s fade-in/fade-out, 30 min/day session, 5 days/week, over 3 consecutives weeks, then 4 weekly maintenance tDCS sessions	Mild fatigue, scalp paresthesia, and low-intensity headache

Contd...

Contd...

Article	tES	N	Trimester	Sessions	Reduction in severity	Electrode	Stimulus parameters	Safety
Wilkening et al., 2019[34]	Gamma-tACS	One case report	First	9	• The scores at baseline after nine stimulations and then at 2 weeks follow-up were respectively 19–11 and then 10 for HAMD-21 • After 3 months, the patient was in remission	Anode: F3 Cathode: F4	• 2 mA, 20 min, 40 Hz, 48,000 cycles • Offset at 1 mA without ramp-in/ramp-out	• Mild Phosphenes was reported • No complication was reported till 27 weeks of gestation
Trevizol et al., 2015[25]	TNS	One case report	Second to third	10	• Baseline HAMD-21 score was 27 • After 10 sessions remission was achieved (HAMD-21 <7) • Improvement sustained for 4 months	Supraorbital trigeminal branches (V1) bilaterally	120 Hz with a pulse wave duration of 250 ms for 30 min/day	• No adverse effect • Elective cesarean delivery • No neonatal complications

Contd...

Contd...

Article	tES	N	Trimester	Sessions	Reduction in severity	Electrode	Stimulus parameters	Safety
Bipolar depression II								
Laurin et al., 2022[32]	tDCS	One case report	First	15	Reduction in MADRS scores from 32/60 to 15/60 (−53%) 4 days after the end of treatment, then 18/60 (−43%) and 13/60 (−59%) at 2 and 6 months, respectively	*Anode:* F3 *Cathode:* F4	−2 mA, 15 s fade-in/fade-out, 1 × 30 min/day	• Scalp paresthesia and asthenia reported • Induced labor at 40 weeks • No neonatal complications
Schizophrenia								
Shenoy et al., 2015[38]	tDCS	One case report	Second	10	Progressive reduction in AHRS score from 29/42 to 22/42 (−24%) after treatment and then 2/42 (−93%) after 1 month follow-up	*Anode:* F3-FP1 *Cathode:* T3-P3	2 mA, 2 × 20 min/day, 3 hours between two daily sessions	• No adverse effect • USG normal

Contd...

Contd...

Article	tES	N	Trimester	Sessions	Reduction in severity	Electrode	Stimulus parameters	Safety
Strube et al., 2016[39]	tDCS	One case report	Third	20	Changes in clinical scale scores at baseline, 2 weeks, and 5 weeks follow-up were, respectively, 18/49, 12/49, and 10/49 for PANSS positive; 22/49, 23/49, and 24/49, for PANSS negative; 39/112, 27/112, and 33/112 for PANSS general; 27/42, 0/42, and 0/42 for AHRS	Anode: F3 Cathode: TP3	2 mA, 20 min/day, 3 hours between two daily sessions	• No adverse effect • USG normal • Spontaneous delivery • No neonatal complications

Contd...

Contd...

PTSD

Article	tES	N	Trimester	Sessions	Reduction in severity	Electrode	Stimulus parameters	Safety
Laurin et al., 2022[32]	tDCS	One case report	First	10	Sham (placebo) tDCS during the reading of a traumatic script 1 month after tDCS treatment, reduction in CAPS-5 scores from 23/80 to 17/80, PCL-5 from 50/80 to 35/80, and BDI-13 from 12/39 to 8/39 PTSD in remission at delivery	Anode: F3 Cathode: FP2	Sham stimulation, 30 seconds fade-in/fade-out, two sessions/day, over 5 consecutive days, 30 minutes between two daily sessions	• Minor effects reported such as tingling, fatigue, scalp pain, and itching • Elective cesarean at 39 weeks APGAR score 10/10 (5 min) • No neonatal complications

(AHRS: attitude and heading reference system; BDI: Beck depression inventory; CAPS-5: clinician-administered PTSD scale; HAM-A: Hamilton Rating Scale for Anxiety; HAM-D: Hamilton Rating Scale for Depression; MADRS: Montgomery–Åsberg Depression Rating Scale; PANSS: positive and negative syndrome scale; PCL: post-traumatic stress disorder checklist; PTSD: post-traumatic stress disorder; SD: standard deviation; tACS: transcranial alternating current stimulation; tDCS: transcranial direct current stimulation; tES: transcranial electric stimulation; USG: ultrasonography)

DEEP BRAIN STIMULATION

In DBS, electrodes are inserted into the brain that are calibrated by an implanted pulse generator, sometimes known as a "brain pacemaker." To alter neuronal activity, electrical impulses are produced and sent via the electrodes to particular brain areas. Currently, DBS is not FDA-approved for treating depression, but approved for Parkinson's disease, dystonia, and obsessive-compulsive disorder (OCD).[17]

King et al.[40] recently reviewed 27 subjects with DBS leads and 29 pregnancies. All the subjects became pregnant after the placement of DBS leads. Except for one subject who was suffering from OCD, all other females were prescribed DBS for Tourette's syndrome ($n = 2$), Parkinson's ($n = 3$), epilepsy ($n = 4$), and dystonia ($n = 17$). The most common adverse effect reported was discomfort from the DBS battery (i.e., impulse generator) ($n = 3$) at the placement site. There was one preterm birth reported at 35 weeks. Though heterogeneously reported, there were no adverse neurodevelopmental outcomes as few babies were followed up till 108 months.

Interestingly, DBS shall preferably be installed before becoming pregnant because it would need to be inserted under anesthesia.

VAGUS NERVE STIMULATION

Another method that necessitates surgical intervention is VNS. To activate the left vagus nerve, VNS implants a tiny pulse generator in the left thoracic area. The FDA approved VNS for treating refractory epilepsy and refractory depression.[41] As per a recent review by Ding et al.,[41] around 42 subjects had 48 pregnancies with VNS systems. Except for one, all other cases have had one or more pregnancies after VNS implantation. Interestingly, amongst all the subjects, only one woman was implanted with VNS for depression as an indication. Two of the pregnancies resulted in miscarriages, while two pregnancies resulted in congenital abnormalities, which could be attributed to antiepileptic medication polytherapy. Interestingly, a patient receiving VNS therapy for severe depression (nonresponse to six antidepressants) experienced sustained remission during pregnancy while receiving citalopram 80 mg/day and bupropion 400 mg/day combination and an uneventful perinatal phase.[41,42]

A summary of the various neuromodulation modalities and their role in antepartum and postpartum phases is given in **Table 5**.

CONCLUSION

Neuromodulation is a potential treatment modality in psychiatric morbidities which have a poor response to available therapeutic options or develop poor tolerance for the same. Available evidence suggests a definite role of ECT

TABLE 5: Clinical utility of neuromodulation techniques in the perinatal phase.

Modality	Indication	Best evidence		Efficacy	Safety	Acceptability	Feasibility
		Antenatal	Postpartum				
ECT	Depression	Case reports	Case reports	+	+	+	±
TMS	Depression	RCT	Meta-analysis/RCT	+	+	+	–
tDCS	Depression	One RCT	Case report	±	+	+	+
VNS*	Depression	Case reports	Case reports	±	±	+	–
DBS*	OCD	Case report	Case report	±	±	+	–
MST	NA	NA	NA	NA	NA	NA	NA

(DBS: deep brain stimulation; ECT: electroconvulsive therapy; MST: magnetic seizure therapy; OCD: obsessive-compulsive disorder; RCT: randomized controlled trial; tDCS: transcranial direct current stimulation; TMS: transcranial magnetic stimulation; VNS: vagus nerve stimulation)
+ Adequate; ± Modest; – Poor
*VNS and DBS were implanted before the pregnancy.

and rTMS in peripartum psychiatric conditions, specifically depression. The role of other neuromodulation modalities such as tDCS, VNS, and DBS needs to be elucidated further in controlled conditions. We also need to study the online paradigms utilizing the aforementioned neuromodulation techniques, keeping in mind the differential gender-based cortical reactivity of the human cortices. We would further need to replicate or devise protocols in the native context.

> **KEY POINTS**
> - Neuromodulation holds promise in the management of psychiatric disorders especially in women.
> - Non-invasive brain stimulation techniques including rTMS, tDCS etc. have shown sizable efficacy in women as well.
> - These techniques are safe and well tolerated during pregnancy and postpartum.

REFERENCES

1. Wang J, Chen Z. Neuromodulation for Pain Management. Adv Exp Med Biol. 2019;1101:207-23.
2. Tikka SK, Siddiqui MA, Garg S, Pattojoshi A, Gautam M. Clinical Practice Guidelines for the Therapeutic Use of Repetitive Transcranial Magnetic Stimulation in Neuropsychiatric Disorders. Indian J Psychiatry. 2023;65(2):270-88.
3. Dougherty DD. Deep Brain Stimulation: Clinical Applications. Psychiatr Clin North Am. 2018;41(3):385-94.
4. McDonald WM, Weiner RD, Fochtmann LJ, McCall WV. The FDA and ECT. J ECT. 2016;32(2):75-7.
5. Singh R, Sharma R, Prakash J, Chatterjee K. Magnetic seizure therapy. Ind Psychiatry J. 2021;30(Suppl 1):S320-1.
6. Zelco A, Wapeesittipan P, Joshi A. Insights into Sex and Gender Differences in Brain and Psychopathologies Using Big Data. Life (Basel). 2023;13(8):1676.
7. Fregni F, Nitsche MA, Loo CK, Brunoni AR, Marangolo P, Leite J, et al. Regulatory Considerations for the Clinical and Research Use of Transcranial Direct Current Stimulation (tDCS): review and recommendations from an expert panel. Clin Res Regul Aff. 2015;32(1):22-35
8. Johnson RL, Wilson CG. A review of vagus nerve stimulation as a therapeutic intervention. J Inflamm Res. 2018;11:203-13.
9. Munk-Olsen T, Maegbaek ML, Johannsen BM, Liu X, Howard LM, di Florio A, et al. Perinatal psychiatric episodes: a population-based study on treatment incidence and prevalence. Transl Psychiatry. 2016;6(10):e919.
10. Payne JL. Psychiatric Medication Use in Pregnancy and Breastfeeding. Obstet Gynecol Clin North Am. 2021;48(1):131-49.
11. Kim DR, Sockol L, Barber JP, Moseley M, Lamprou L, Rickels K, et al. A survey of patient acceptability of repetitive transcranial magnetic stimulation (TMS) during pregnancy. J Affect Disord. 2011;129(1-3):385-90.
12. Rose S, Dotters-Katz SK, Kuller JA. Electroconvulsive Therapy in Pregnancy: Safety, Best Practices, and Barriers to Care. Obstet Gynecol Surv. 2020;75(3):199-203.

13. Wise MG, Ward SC, Townsend-Parchman W, Gilstrap LC 3rd, Hauth JC. Case report of ECT during high-risk pregnancy. Am J Psychiatry. 1984;141(1):99-101.
14. Pacheco F, Guiomar R, Brunoni AR, Buhagiar R, Evagorou O, Roca-Lecumberri A, et al. Efficacy of non-invasive brain stimulation in decreasing depression symptoms during the peripartum period: A systematic review. J Psychiatr Res. 2021;140:443-60.
15. Yonkers KA, Wisner KL, Stewart DE, Oberlander TF, Dell DL, Stotland N, et al. The management of depression during pregnancy: a report from the American Psychiatric Association and the American College of Obstetricians and Gynecologists. Gen Hosp Psychiatry. 2009;31(5):403-13.
16. Leiknes KA, Cooke MJ, Jarosch-von Schweder L, Harboe I, Høie B. Electroconvulsive therapy during pregnancy: a systematic review of case studies. Arch Womens Ment Health. 2015;18(1):1-39.
17. Kim DR, Snell JL, Ewing GC, O'Reardon J. Neuromodulation and antenatal depression: a review. Neuropsychiatr Dis Treat. 2015;11:975-82.
18. Lee HJ, Kim SM, Kwon JY. Repetitive transcranial magnetic stimulation treatment for peripartum depression: systematic review & meta-analysis. BMC Pregnancy Childbirth. 2021;21(1):118.
19. Liu C, Pan W, Jia L, Li L, Zhang X, Ren Y, et al. Efficacy and safety of repetitive transcranial magnetic stimulation for peripartum depression: A meta-analysis of randomized controlled trials. Psychiatry Res. 2020;294:113543.
20. Peng L, Fu C, Xiong F, Zhang Q, Liang Z, Chen L, et al. Effects of repetitive transcranial magnetic stimulation on depression symptoms and cognitive function in treating patients with postpartum depression: A systematic review and meta-analysis of randomized controlled trials. Psychiatry Res. 2020;290:113124.
21. Kim DR, Wang E, McGeehan B, Snell J, Ewing G, Iannelli C, et al. Randomized controlled trial of transcranial magnetic stimulation in pregnant women with major depressive disorder. Brain Stimul. 2019;12(1):96-102.
22. Kim DR, Wang E. Prevention of supine hypotensive syndrome in pregnant women treated with transcranial magnetic stimulation. Psychiatry Res. 2014;218(1-2):247-8.
23. Rossi S, Antal A, Bestmann S, Bikson M, Brewer C, Brockmöller J, et al. Safety and recommendations for TMS use in healthy subjects and patient populations, with updates on training, ethical and regulatory issues: Expert Guidelines. Clin Neurophysiol. 2021;132(1):269-306.
24. Pridmore S, Turnier-Shea Y, Rybak M, Pridmore W. Transcranial Magnetic Stimulation (TMS) during pregnancy: a fetal risk factor. Australas Psychiatry. 2021;29(2):226-9.
25. Trevizol AP, Vigod SN, Daskalakis ZJ, Vila-Rodriguez F, Downar J, Blumberger DM. Intermittent theta burst stimulation for major depression during pregnancy. Brain Stimul. 2019;12(3):772-4.
26. Sylvén SM, Gingnell M, Ramirez A, Bodén R. Transcranial magnetic intermittent theta-burst stimulation for depression in pregnancy - A case series. Brain Stimul. 2020;13(6):1665-7.
27. Xiong W, Lopez R, Cristancho P. Transcranial magnetic stimulation in the treatment of peripartum bipolar depression: a case report. Braz J Psychiatry. 2018;40(3):344-5.

28. Guerrero Solano JL, Molina Pacheco E. Low-Frequency rTMS Ameliorates Akathisia During Pregnancy. J Neuropsychiatry Clin Neurosci. 2017;29(4):409-10.
29. Nanjundaswamy MH, Varshney P, Thanki MV, Arunya B, Rai V, Mehta UM, et al. Theta burst stimulation for tokophobia during pregnancy. Brain Stimul. 2019;12(5):1322-24.
30. Agarwal R, Garg S, Tikka SK, Khatri S, Goel D. Successful use of theta burst stimulation (TBS) for treating psychogenic non epileptic seizures (PNES) in a pregnant woman. Asian J Psychiatr. 2019;43:121-2.
31. Bhola R, Kinsella E, Giffin N, Lipscombe S, Ahmed F, Weatherall M, et al. Single-pulse transcranial magnetic stimulation (sTMS) for the acute treatment of migraine: evaluation of outcome data for the UK post market pilot program. J Headache Pain. 2015;16:535.
32. Laurin A, Nard N, Dalmont M, Bulteau S, Bénard C, Bonnot O, et al. Efficacy and Safety of Transcranial Electric Stimulation during the Perinatal Period: A Systematic Literature Review and Three Case Reports. J Clin Med. 2022;11(14):4048.
33. Woods AJ, Antal A, Bikson M, Boggio PS, Brunoni AR, Celnik P, et al. A technical guide to tDCS, and related non-invasive brain stimulation tools. Clin Neurophysiol. 2016;127(2):1031-48.
34. Wilkening A, Kurzeck A, Dechantsreiter E, Padberg F, Palm U. Transcranial alternating current stimulation for the treatment of major depression during pregnancy. Psychiatry Res. 2019;279:399-400.
35. Vigod SN, Murphy KE, Dennis CL, Oberlander TF, Ray JG, Daskalakis ZJ, et al. Transcranial direct current stimulation (tDCS) for depression in pregnancy: A pilot randomized controlled trial. Brain Stimul. 2019;12(6):1475-83.
36. Sreeraj VS, Bose A, Shanbhag V, Narayanaswamy JC, Venkatasubramanian G, Benegal V. Monotherapy With tDCS for Treatment of Depressive Episode During Pregnancy: A Case Report. Brain Stimul. 2016;9(3):457-8.
37. Kurzeck AK, Dechantsreiter E, Wilkening A, Kumpf U, Nenov-Matt T, Padberg F, et al. Transcranial Direct Current Stimulation (tDCS) for Depression during Pregnancy: Results from an Open-Label Pilot Study. Brain Sci. 2021;11(7):947.
38. Shenoy S, Bose A, Chhabra H, Dinakaran D, Agarwal SM, Shivakumar V, et al. Transcranial direct current stimulation (tDCS) for auditory verbal hallucinations in schizophrenia during pregnancy: a case report. Brain Stimul. 2015;8(1):163-4.
39. Strube W, Kirsch B, Padberg F, Hasan A, Palm U. Transcranial Direct Current Stimulation as Monotherapy for the Treatment of Auditory Hallucinations During Pregnancy: A Case Report. J Clin Psychopharmacol. 2016;36(5):534-5.
40. King C, Parker TM, Roussos-Ross K, Ramirez-Zamora A, Smulian JC, Okun MS, et al. Safety of deep brain stimulation in pregnancy: A comprehensive review. Front Hum Neurosci. 2022;16:997552.
41. Ding J, Wang L, Wang C, Gao C, Wang F, Sun T. Is vagal-nerve stimulation safe during pregnancy? A mini review. Epilepsy Res. 2021;174:106671.
42. Husain MM, Stegman D, Trevino K. Pregnancy and delivery while receiving vagus nerve stimulation for the treatment of major depression: a case report. Ann Gen Psychiatry. 2005;4:16.
43. Palm U, Leitne rB, Kirsch B, et al. Prefrontal tDCS and sertraline in obsessive compulsive disorder: a case report and review of the literature. Neurocase. 2017;23(2):173-177. doi:10.1080/13554794.2017.1319492

CHAPTER 22

General Principles of Psychopharmacology in Women

Vikas Menon, Chandrima Naskar

ABSTRACT

Sex is an important source of variability in the pharmacokinetics and pharmacodynamics of psychotropics. Yet, this factor is systematically underexplored, underreported, and undervalued in day-to-day practice. A clear example of its consequence is the commonplace practice of prescribing the same psychotropic doses to men and women; illustrative examples show that this practice may be neglectful and even harmful. Despite regulatory changes, such data have been hard to come by, limiting comprehensive guidance for tailored psychotropic prescribing. Key sex differences in pharmacokinetics include altered drug absorption, distribution, metabolism, and excretion. These differences contribute to varying drug availability and clearance rates, leading to differences in plasma levels and potential adverse effects. The efficacy and tolerability of psychotropics vary based on sex, hormonal levels, and age. Women are more prone to adverse effects with psychotropic medications due to differences in receptor binding, neurotransmitter regulation, and hormone-mediated modulation. Hormonal fluctuations during menstrual cycles, pregnancy, and postmenopausal years, further influence drug pharmacokinetics, necessitating adjustments in dosing to optimize therapeutic outcomes and minimize adverse effects. Addressing sex and gender disparities in research will result in safer and, potentially more effective prescribing for all; the Sex and Gender Equity in Research (SAGER) guidelines represent an important step in this direction. It is hoped that this chapter will spotlight the issues of sex differences in psychopharmacologic prescribing, highlight key knowledge gaps, and provide inputs for further research.

Keywords: Sex, gender, drugs, psychotropics, pharmacokinetics, pharmacodynamics

INTRODUCTION

Before 1993, women were systematically excluded from clinical bioequivalence trials. The two main reasons were associated risks to those with childbearing potential and the belief that including women would lead to greater interindividual variability, necessitating larger samples. This situation was sought to be remedied with the US National Institute of Health (NIH) Revitalization Act of 1993 which mandated the inclusion of women in federally funded clinical trials. Though there was a perceptible improvement in the enrolment of women following this act, few studies reported sex-specific differences in outcomes or included sex as a covariate.

Consequently, little data is available to guide sex-specific prescribing of psychotropics. This issue assumes greater significance when juxtaposed with empirical evidence showing that women are more likely to use (and abuse) psychotropics and, thus, be more prone to adverse effects. In a classic example, it took years of postmarketing surveillance and reports of cognitive adverse effects of zolpidem, approved by the United States Food and Drug Administration (FDA) before the Revitalization Act, to frame sex-specific dosing recommendations for the drug. Zolpidem quickly became the "poster" drug for advocacy surrounding the study of women's health, in general, and biological sex differences, in particular.

Psychotropic pharmacokinetics may differ in women due to their lower body weight, greater body fat, reduced gastric elimination, decreased gastric pH, increased intestinal transit time, and slower glomerular filtration rate. Likewise, the best examples of pharmacodynamic differences are differences in rates and extent of pharmacological response and adverse effects. A well-documented example here is the increased propensity of women to experience adverse effects, such as lithium-induced hypothyroidism. Another example is the recent evidence suggesting that women may preferentially respond to selective serotonin reuptake inhibitors (SSRIs) while males prefer tricyclic antidepressants (TCAs).

Accordingly, in this chapter, we discuss the principles of sex-specific psychotropic prescribing by examining sex differences in pharmacokinetics, pharmacodynamics, safety, and tolerability. Subsequently, we discuss these differences in the context of reproductive cycles and events. Gaps in the data are highlighted, and specific recommendations for more research in this area are offered. Finally, we discuss the Sex and Gender Equity in Research (SAGER) guidelines and their implications for research and advocacy in women's health. The chapter will summarize what is known about sex differences in psychotropic pharmacokinetics and pharmacodynamics and also provide useful inputs for further research in this area.

■ SEX DIFFERENCES IN PHARMACOKINETICS

Differences in Absorption

Several factors determine the extent of drug absorption in the gastrointestinal (GI) tract. These can be broadly divided into drug-related factors, such as the formulation, route of administration, and lipophilic nature of the drug in question and its degree of ionization, and local GI factors, such as the prevalent acid-base balance, presence of bile and mucus, and nature of epithelial membranes.

Women have slower gastric emptying times and faster intestinal transit; both serve to reduce plasma drug levels because less drug reaches/stays in the small intestine, where there is a larger surface area available for absorption. Further, the gastric pH is lower in women; this means that base compounds such as tricyclics and benzodiazepines are absorbed more rapidly, enabling higher plasma concentrations. Though less well quantified, the activity of certain gastric enzymes is lowered among women; since enzymes denature proteins, this may also contribute to variations in drug absorption. Further, sex differences have also been noted in bile acid composition, a determinant of drug solubility. For instance, men have higher levels of cholic acid, while levels of chenodeoxycholic acid are higher among women.

In a given patient, it is difficult to delineate the influence of each of these variables on the absorption equation. One can only speculate about general possibilities. For instance, decreased gastric emptying means increased exposure to denaturing gastric enzymes and reduced drug availability in the small intestine for absorption. However, if intestinal transit time is prolonged in a patient, it may counterbalance this effect. Similarly, an acidic environment favors the absorption of weak acids by establishing a nonionic state, while it disfavors the absorption of weak bases by promoting ionization. Ultimately, gender-related differences in bioavailability must be established by studying every compound separately.

Differences in Distribution

Factors influencing the distribution of a drug can be divided into drug-related and individual factors. Drug-related factors include its physical and chemical properties, such as its pH, lipophilic nature, and protein-binding affinity. Individual constitutional factors include body weight, percentage of body fat, and blood perfusion. Additionally, a greater relative proportion of adipose tissue mass, compared to lean body mass, can influence drug disposition.

Women tend to have a lower ratio of lean body mass to adipose tissue mass. In the case of highly lipophilic drugs, such as diazepam, this implies a greater volume of distribution for the drug initially. The result is lower plasma levels at initial administration. However, over time, the potential for the drug to sequester in the adipose tissue is higher. This may lead to increased serum levels and longer half-life for those with lower lean body mass and greater adipose tissue, such as older women, increasing their exposure to adverse effects. There is a striking paucity of information on the sex-specific effects of these variables on individual psychotropic drug disposition.

After absorption, the extent of protein binding determines the passage of a drug into the central nervous system. Only the unbound fraction is free to pass through the blood–brain barrier. The plasma protein binding capacity is generally lower among women than men. This fact has two important implications. First, for highly protein-bound drugs such as benzodiazepines,

SSRIs, and TCAs, there is a higher free fraction for the same dose among women than men. This suggests a greater probability of adverse effects. Second, coprescribing two highly protein-bound drugs may lead to displacing one of them, again increasing the chances of adverse effects, for example, coadministration of benzodiazepine (BZD) and TCA may lead to increased TCA levels; even small increases in TCA levels may be clinically relevant due to their narrow therapeutic index.

Differences in Metabolism and Excretion

Most psychotropic drugs undergo varying degrees of hepatic metabolism. Both phase 1 reactions (such as oxidation, reduction, and hydrolysis) and phase 2 reactions (such as glucuronidation) are slower in women than men leading to greater plasma drug concentrations. Further, renal drug elimination is also lower among women owing to reduced glomerular filtration rate. Thus, drug metabolism and excretion are slower in women resulting in lower elimination and higher plasma levels; this increases exposure to adverse effects.

The cytochrome P450 enzymatic system, comprising >30 different isozymes, is an important regulator of hepatic metabolism. Sex differences have been noted in the activity of certain, but not all, isozymes. For instance, women appear to have increased activity of cytochrome P450 2C19 (CYP2C19). Drugs that are CYP2C19 substrates, such as diazepam, and antidepressants, such as clomipramine and imipramine, would therefore be expected to have a faster metabolism and lower plasma concentrations among women than men for the same dose. Another important isozyme that has been shown to have slower activity in women is cytochrome P450 family 1 subfamily A polypeptide 2 (CYP1A2). Important CYP1A2 substrates among psychotropic drugs include clozapine, olanzapine, and, to a lesser extent, tricyclics, and fluvoxamine. One must remember this when prescribing these drugs to women as they are at greater risk of adverse effects at the same dose than men.

Sex and age-dependent differences in action also exist in CYP3A4, the most abundant isozyme subfamily in the liver. Specifically, young women in the reproductive age group exhibit greater activity of this isozyme than men and postmenopausal women. Young women, therefore, could be expected to have lower therapeutic activity of benzodiazepines; such as alprazolam, and antidepressants; such as amitriptyline, imipramine, fluoxetine, escitalopram, and antipsychotics; such as quetiapine and ziprasidone, all of which are metabolized predominantly through the cytochrome P450 3A4 (CYP3A4) pathway. On a related note, older women should be prescribed lower doses of alprazolam compared to young women or older men due to declining CYP3A4 activity with age and lower lean body mass to adipose tissue mass ratio.

Sex differences have also been noted for renal functions such as glomerular filtration rate, tubular reabsorption, and tubular secretion. All of these functions are slower in women, decreasing the renal clearance of drugs. Since the kidney is the main organ of drug excretion for both the parent compound and its active metabolites, these differences can affect the disposition of virtually every psychotropic drug. However, empirical studies examining sex differences in renal clearance of specific psychotropic agents are lacking. **Table 1** summarizes key sex differences in psychotropic pharmacokinetics and their implications.

TABLE 1: Sex differences in pharmacokinetics and implications.

Pharmacokinetic aspect	Sex differences	Implications
Absorption	• Slower gastric emptying and faster intestinal transit in women • Lower gastric pH and altered enzyme activity • Women may experience altered drug availability in the small intestine	Drug absorption rates and bioavailability may differ between sexes, affecting therapeutic levels and dosing requirements
Distribution	• Higher adipose tissue to lean body mass ratio in women • Greater volume of distribution initially for lipophilic drugs • Higher plasma levels initially followed by potential accumulation in adipose tissue	Women may experience altered drug distribution and prolonged exposure to lipophilic drugs, potentially leading to increased side effects over time
Metabolism	• Slower hepatic metabolism in women due to slower phase 1 and phase 2 reactions • Variability in cytochrome P450 enzymatic activity, particularly CYP2C19 and CYP1A2	Women may have slower drug metabolism and elimination, resulting in higher plasma drug concentrations and increased risk of adverse effects
Excretion	Slower renal clearance in women due to reduced glomerular filtration rate and altered tubular functions	Differences in renal clearance can impact the elimination of drugs and their metabolites, potentially affecting drug efficacy and toxicity

(CYP1A2: cytochrome P450 family 1 subfamily A polypeptide 2; CYP2C19: cytochrome P450 2C19)

■ SEX DIFFERENCES IN PHARMACODYNAMICS

Pharmacodynamics is the study of a drug's effect on the body, which includes both the intended therapeutic effects and the unintended adverse reactions. The pharmacodynamics of psychotropics is affected by various individual factors, such as sex, age, hormonal levels, frailty, and genetic factors. These factors may determine variations in the degree of therapeutic and adverse effects in individuals when administered the same dose of specific psychotropics. For instance, antidepressant medications have a higher incidence and severity of side effects in women, and the risk of developing tardive dyskinesia with antipsychotics is significantly higher in older women than in men.[1-3]

Because women use psychotropics more frequently than men,[3-5] it is important for clinicians to be aware of sex differences in the pharmacodynamics of psychotropics. This will aid decision-making on the choice and dosage of medications. Notwithstanding similar mechanisms of action for drug classes such as antipsychotics and antidepressants, the clinical response and adverse effects can be moderated by sex, age, hormonal influences, or genetic factors. Various studies have shown that women experience more frequent and severe side effects with psychotropic medications.[6,7] An Indian study also noted that females experienced significantly higher adverse psychotropic drug reactions as compared to men.[8] One of the reasons for these differences is the impact of female sex on the pharmacokinetics and pharmacodynamics of psychotropics. Hence, a knowledge of pharmacodynamic patterns of psychotropics in men and women is necessary to guide clinical practice and research.

Antipsychotics

Conventional antipsychotic medications exert their action primarily by blocking dopamine type 2 (D2) receptors. For optimal control of symptoms, without significant extrapyramidal side effects, approximately 60% of D2-receptor blockade is necessary.[9,10] Various lines of evidence testify to the role of sex in moderating the extent of the D2 blockade. For instance, women have higher D2-receptor binding potential than men, particularly in the left and right anterior cingulate cortex.[11] Next, in preclinical studies, male rats had higher upregulation of D2-receptors after 12 weeks of treatment with haloperidol or clozapine.[12] A study assessing the degree of receptor blockade by positron emission tomography (PET) imaging found that women need a lesser dose of antipsychotics to achieve the same level of receptor occupancy. This finding was subsequently replicated in another study where women needed half the daily doses of olanzapine than men to achieve the same occupancy level.[9,13]

While dopamine receptors are the primary targets of conventional antipsychotics, certain antipsychotics like clozapine have been shown to affect multiple other receptors such as alpha 1, alpha 2, muscarinic, and 5-hydroxytryptamine (serotonin) receptor 1A (5HT1A) receptors. In certain brain areas, the density and distribution of 5HT1A and muscarinic receptors are higher in women than in men. These differences can lead to variations in therapeutic effects and side effects of clozapine in female patients.[14] An important confounder here is the higher cerebral blood flow in women compared to men, the role of which is yet to be fully delineated.[15]

The antipsychotic side effects that have shown a female preponderance are tardive dyskinesia, metabolic derangements, agranulocytosis, hyperprolactinemia, and cardiac arrhythmias.[16] The possible confounding factors for tardive dyskinesia might be the higher age of women included in the studies, as old age is an independent risk factor. Still, as per the pharmacodynamic hypothesis of women needing a lower than the usual daily dose for receptor occupancy, the higher risk of tardive dyskinesia in women can be because of the long-term supratherapeutic dosage. For agranulocytosis, while small studies with small female samples have shown a higher risk in women, a large-scale meta-analysis failed to report any significant difference in the risk between the two sexes.[17] The higher risk of cardiac arrhythmias might be because of the longer baseline QTc interval in adult women, which increases further during pregnancy.[18]

The interactions between psychotic illness, antipsychotic use, and metabolic disorders (obesity, type 2 diabetes, dyslipidemia, etc.) are multifactorial, with genetics, variations in metabolizing enzymes, drug transporters, and receptors playing important roles. Yet, females have been found to have a higher tendency to gain weight, develop metabolic side effects, and experience cardiovascular mortality compared to males.[19] The long-term higher levels of antipsychotic exposure and pharmacokinetic differences in drug metabolism have been considered to be the risk factors for the same.[16] It has also been seen that hyperprolactinemia and its consequences such as hirsutism, acne, osteoporosis, and even breast cancer, are higher in women. Due to multiple confounding factors, whether this is a direct consequence of the pharmacokinetic and pharmacodynamic differences in the antipsychotic action or a multifactorial effect of other risk factors related to genetics and endocrine status remains unanswered.[20]

Antidepressants

Estrogen has been shown to affect the production of serotonin, the binding of serotonin to transporters, and the expression of transporter receptors in the synapse. This can explain why women of reproductive age respond better to SSRIs (due to their higher-circulating estrogen levels) while men respond more favorably to pronoradrenergic medications.[6] Further, younger women respond better to SSRIs than older women (>50 years of age); hormone replacement therapy, however, eliminates this difference.[6] No intraclass variation in pharmacodynamics has been noted. For other antidepressants, such as bupropion and venlafaxine, no consistent sex-specific differences in response have been found.

Women have almost twice the prevalence of depression as men, and they also experience an earlier age of onset for depression, more atypical symptoms, longer duration, greater severity, and higher incidence of comorbid anxiety. Pharmacologically, they experience an overall tendency to have higher side effects.[21] Most trials do not report gender-based differences in the side effect profile of antidepressants. The available data shows that with SSRIs, complaints of sexual problems and distress regarding weight gain might be more common in women. However, more large-scale well-structured studies are needed to identify if these differences are true.[22]

In a recent study from the Netherlands that assessed how sex affected the incidence of adverse drug reactions of common groups of medications, SSRIs had significantly higher side effects in women with a high odds ratio of 6.2.[23] Numerous studies have reported that females experience significantly more frequent and severe side effects such as sedation, constipation, dry mouth, sweating, and tremors with TCAs like imipramine than men. This leads to a higher dropout rate in women prescribed TCAs than in men receiving the same dose of TCAs. A possible explanation for this is the higher plasma level of TCA achieved in females due to the sex-based difference in pharmacokinetics.[22]

Mood Stabilizers

A recent systematic review on sex differences in lithium efficacy and side effects showed no robust sex-based difference in the efficacy of lithium in symptom reduction irrespective of bipolar disorder subtype, including the rapid cycling variant. However, it did note that women might be at a higher risk of gaining weight and developing hypothyroidism after long-term lithium treatment. In comparison, men have a higher risk of developing tremors.[24,25] A South Indian study on 57 patients suffering from early onset bipolar disorder associated female gender with lithium nonresponse.[26]

Not many studies have explored the effect of sex on anticonvulsant pharmacodynamics, and findings from available studies are inconsistent. Interestingly, whereas the natural cyclic changes in female sex hormone levels during the menstrual cycle do not affect anticonvulsant serum levels, oral contraceptive pills (OCPs) significantly reduce the serum concentrations of lamotrigine and valproic acid.[27]

On the other hand, anticonvulsants such as carbamazepine and lamotrigine are known to reduce the efficacy of all hormonal methods of contraception through hepatic enzyme induction.[28] The use of valproic acid in reproductive age group women is discouraged as it produces various gender-specific side effects, such as increasing the risk of polycystic ovary syndrome, hyperinsulinism, hyperandrogenism, hyperprolactinemia, hypothalamic amenorrhea, and teratogenic effects on the fetus.[29] Further, one study found that females with bipolar disorder respond poorly to anticonvulsant mood stabilizers relative to males.[30]

Other Agents

Females have higher sublingual absorption, systemic exposure, and overall lower clearance rate of hypnotic benzodiazepine receptor agonists (HBRA) such as zolpidem, and experience more adverse effects due to the same. The FDA has suggested halving the dosage of HBRAs for women; however, this has not been implemented in most of the countries.[31] Similarly, for pregabalin, the concentration–dose ratio achieved in women may be up to 42% higher than in men. For a given dose, this means that women may experience significantly higher rates of side effects, such as weight gain and sedation.[31] **Table 2** summarizes the differences in pharmacodynamics between the sexes for various classes of psychotropics. **Table 3** summarizes the major

TABLE 2: Sex differences in the pharmacodynamic profile of psychotropics.

Antidepressants	*Antipsychotics*	*Mood stabilizers*
• Estrogen affects the production and binding of serotonin and the expression of serotonin receptors • Women of reproductive age respond better to SSRIs due to their higher circulating estrogen levels, while men respond more favorably to pronoradrenergic medications	• Women have been found to have higher D2-receptor binding potentials than men, more so in the left and right anterior cingulate cortex • In certain brain areas, the density and distribution of 5HT1A and muscarinic receptors are higher in women than in men • Possibility of higher dopaminergic as well as nondopaminergic side effects in women	• Valproate is contraindicated in females of reproductive age • Overall, the response to anticonvulsant mood stabilizers is better in males than females • Lithium causes a higher incidence of tremors in men but higher weight gain and hypothyroidism in women

(D2-receptor: dopamine receptor type 2; SSRI: selective serotonin reuptake inhibitor; 5HT1A: 5-hydroxytryptamine receptor 1A)

TABLE 3: Sex differences in side effect profile of psychotropics in females versus males.

Antidepressants	Antipsychotics
With tricyclic antidepressants, females tend to experience significantly more: • Sedation • Constipation • Dryness of mouth • Sweating and tremor	Antipsychotic side effects that have shown a female preponderance are: • Tardive dyskinesia • Metabolic derangements • Agranulocytosis and hyperprolactinemia • Cardiac arrhythmias

differences in adverse drug reactions to antidepressants and antipsychotics between the two sexes.

PHARMACODYNAMICS AND PHARMACOKINETICS IN THE CONTEXT OF REPRODUCTIVE CYCLES AND EVENTS

While the basic pharmacokinetic differences in drug absorption, metabolism, distribution, and elimination exist between men and women, the pharmacokinetic parameters in women show further cyclic changes based on the menstrual cycle, and it shows significant alterations in the periods of pregnancy and postmenopausal years. While each of these has been dealt with in detail in this book's respective chapters, a summary is provided in this chapter. Sex steroid hormones such as androgens, estrogens, and progestins influence pharmacokinetic parameters and receptor-binding properties of drugs in the heart, bone, muscle, vasculature, immune system, and brain.

Fluctuations of these hormones during the menstrual cycle, pregnancy, and postmenopausal period can alter drug clearance rates and volume of distribution leading to changes in serum levels and differential occurrence of adverse effects. Not only the natural hormonal fluctuations but also hormonal therapies for in vitro fertilization, hormone replacement therapy for gender transition, endocrine therapies for certain malignancies, and commonly used medications such as oral contraceptive medications can all contribute to changes in pharmacokinetic and pharmacodynamic parameters of psychotropics.[32]

Antipsychotics

D2-receptor availability has been noted to change with fluctuations in the level of plasma sex steroid hormones across the menstrual cycle. These changes can alter drug dosages required for antipsychotic efficacy and the occurrence of adverse effects like hyperprolactinemia.[33]

Antidepressants

The effect of pregnancy on antidepressant serum concentrations is variable. Decreased dose-adjusted levels of fluvoxamine and nortriptyline, especially between the 6-9 months of pregnancy, have been found. Likewise, clomipramine, imipramine, and paroxetine showed a small reduction in dose-adjusted concentrations in the third trimester. On the other hand, escitalopram, venlafaxine, and fluoxetine concentrations were not significantly altered in pregnancy, while plasma sertraline levels tended to increase.[34]

Mood Stabilizers

Some studies have shown that women tend to clear lithium less efficiently than men, and clearance varies with the menstrual cycle phases.[35] Lithium clearance decreases significantly during pregnancy and is inversely related to changes in serum lithium concentration; these changes revert to baseline at 4-9 weeks postdelivery. Thus, repeated lithium serum level monitoring and dose adjustment are essential in the peripartum period to prevent toxicity and relapse of symptoms.[36] However, the teratogenicity of lithium is much lesser than what was assumed earlier, and it is considered a safe and effective mood stabilizer in women of reproductive age.[37]

Other Agents

Progesterone-containing OCPs have been found to increase the receptor binding of benzodiazepines. Oxidized benzodiazepines like triazolam and alprazolam have been found to have reduced receptor binding in women taking OCPs, while for conjugated benzodiazepines such as lorazepam and temazepam, the receptor binding is accelerated.[31]

LIMITATIONS TO DATA ON SEX DIFFERENCES AND RECOMMENDATIONS

Often, females are systematically excluded from animal and human research because of the general assumption that their hormonal complexity might affect the results. When pharmacological research includes female participants, a larger sample size may be necessary to account for participant variability based on their hormonal status. This principle also extends to research on drug development and drug trials for safety and efficacy. Even in studies and trials where women are adequately represented, sex-related differences in outcome measures are often not reported.

There is little recent cross-cultural data on sex differences in drug pharmacokinetics and pharmacodynamics; most such available studies are from the late 1990s and early 2000s. For clinicians, a good understanding of the general variations in the effect of psychopharmacology in various populations is essential to minimize adverse drug reactions and improve treatment outcomes. To gain this understanding, drug trials at every stage of drug development need sufficient representation from both sexes to establish significant differences. Further, reporting of sex-specific differences in outcomes should be mandated.[6]

SEX AND GENDER EQUITY IN RESEARCH GUIDELINES AND THEIR IMPLICATIONS

Sex and gender have important biopsychosocial implications for health-related scenarios. Whereas sex is a biological variable determined by anatomy, physiology, genetics, and hormones and traditionally used to differentiate males from females, gender refers to a person's self-representation (identity) based on a socially constructed set of norms, behaviors, roles, and power for women and men. Both sex and gender impact social factors, such as differences in occupational risks, the prevalence of certain diseases, differences in healthcare-seeking behavior, and healthcare utilization. Sex and gender-related differences exist in psychological domains affecting health outcomes, such as level of risk-taking behavior and perceived experience with healthcare, to name a few. Biologically, as elaborated earlier, sex affects the pharmacokinetics and pharmacodynamics of various psychotropics leading to differences in treatment outcomes as well as the nature and extent of adverse effects. Therefore, focusing on how sex and gender impact health-related behavior and its management may be important in determining health outcomes.

Multiple large-scale assessments have clarified that female under-representation commonly exists in biomedical research.[38,39] This has been labeled the "gender gap" in research. To reduce this gap and promote sex and gender equity in research, a panel of 13 international experts deliberated during a two-day workshop in 2016; the group's work led to the SAGER guidelines. This guideline has been designed to guide researchers and journal editors in reporting sex and gender-related information in manuscripts.[39,40] Recently, the European Journal of Science Editing (EASE) has developed an easily usable checklist for gender-sensitive reporting of all kinds of research[41] based on the original guideline by Heidari et al. and the work by Van Epps et al. for better implementation of SAGER guidelines.[42] The guideline has two separate checklists: (1) For research involving human participants and (2) for studies with a biological or applied science approach. A summary of the guidelines for studies with human participants is enumerated in **Box 1**.

> **BOX 1:** Summary of SAGER guidelines for research with human participants.
> - Appropriate use of the terms—sex/gender
> - Title to specify the sex/gender of participants if only one category is included
> - Abstract to specify the sex/gender of participants if only one category is included and the population is to be described with sex/gender breakdown
> - Introduction to include the relevance of sex/gender in the context of the topic from previous literature and the current study
> - Methods to clearly mention the definition of sex/gender considered in the study and how the authors have ensured adequate representation of participants from both male and female sexes
> - Results to include the gender/sex breakdown for each of the categories reported, including sex differences for all outcomes and adverse effects
> - Discussion should report the implications of sex/gender on the findings and whether findings can be generalized to all sexes/genders in the population
>
> The guideline also necessitates the authors to provide a rationale if sex/gender reporting has not been done in the methods, results, and discussion section.

CONCLUSION

This chapter summarizes the intricate realm of sex-specific psychotropic prescribing, focusing on the multifaceted interplay between sex-related factors, pharmacokinetics, and pharmacodynamics. The complex relationships between sex-related factors and drug absorption, distribution, metabolism, excretion, and drug-receptor interactions underscore the need for sex-specific prescribing practices that are yet to be adopted widely. There is a striking paucity of data on sex-specific desirable and undesirable psychotropic outcomes, though this is an important area. For drugs such as lithium with a narrow therapeutic index, there are well-documented changes in drug pharmacokinetics in the context of reproductive cycles and events; this knowledge is essential to facilitate safe prescribing practices. Additionally, the emergence of the SAGER guidelines highlights the significance of acknowledging and addressing gender disparities in scientific investigation, paving the way for equitable advancements in psychopharmacology. We hope the present chapter provides useful insights for practice and research in this field.

> **KEY POINTS**
> - Women exhibit distinct psychotropic pharmacokinetics. Key considerations here include (1) slower gastric emptying and faster intestinal transit which may reduce plasma levels, (2) greater volume of distribution for lipophilic drugs due to greater adipose tissue mass, and (3) differences in hepatic metabolism such as increased activity of CYP2C19 and reduced activity of CYP1A2.
> - Sex differences in pharmacodynamics are less robustly established. These stem from differences in receptor density, distribution, and binding affinity. There are well-documented examples of sex differences in adverse effects, such as a higher incidence of lithium-induced hypothyroidism in women and preliminary evidence of differences in therapeutic effects, notably a greater response of women to SSRIs.

- Practitioners need to be aware of subtle pharmacokinetic changes in the context of reproductive cycles and events to prescribe safely, for example, the renal clearance of lithium is increased in the third trimester of pregnancy and returns to normal 4–9 weeks postpartum. This may necessitate an increased frequency of serum lithium monitoring in this period which must form the basis of individualized dose adjustments.
- In recognition of the important implications of sex and gender-related factors on health-related outcomes, the SAGER guidelines (2016) mandate reporting of sex and gender information in research design, data analysis, study findings, and their interpretation.

REFERENCES

1. Yonkers KA, Kando JC, Cole JO, Blumenthal S. Gender differences in pharmacokinetics and pharmacodynamics of psychotropic medication. Am J Psychiatry 1992;149(5):587-95.
2. Yassa R, Jeste DV. Gender differences in tardive dyskinesia: a critical review of the literature. Schizophr Bull. 1992;18(4):701-15.
3. Boyd A, Van de Velde S, Pivette M, Ten Have M, Florescu S, O'Neill S, et al. Gender differences in psychotropic use across Europe: Results from a large cross-sectional, population-based study. Eur Psychiatry 2015;30(6):778-88.
4. Estancial Fernandes CS, de Azevedo RCS, Goldbaum M, Barros MBA. Psychotropic use patterns: Are there differences between men and women? PLoS One. 2018;13(11):e0207921.
5. Maestre-Miquel C, López-de-Andrés A, Ji Z, de Miguel-Diez J, Brocate A, Sanz-Rojo S, et al. Gender Differences in the Prevalence of Mental Health, Psychological Distress and Psychotropic Medication Consumption in Spain: A Nationwide Population-Based Study. Int J Environ Res Public Health 2021;18(12):6350.
6. Romanescu M, Buda V, Lombrea A, Andor M, Ledeti I, Suciu M, et al. Sex-Related Differences in Pharmacological Response to CNS Drugs: A Narrative Review. J Pers Med. 2022;12(6):907.
7. Iversen TSJ, Steen NE, Dieset I, Hope S, Mørch R, Gardsjord ES, et al. Side effect burden of antipsychotic drugs in real life - Impact of gender and polypharmacy. Prog Neuropsychopharmacol Biol Psychiatry. 2018;82:263-71.
8. Lucca J, Ramesh M, Ram D. Gender differences in the occurrences and pattern of adverse drug reactions in psychiatric patients: A prospective observational study. Trop J Med Res. 2017;20(1):84.
9. Seeman MV. Gender differences in the prescribing of antipsychotic drugs. Am J Psychiatry. 2004;161(8):1324-33.
10. Kapur S, Zipursky R, Jones C, Remington G, Houle S. Relationship between dopamine D(2) occupancy, clinical response, and side effects: a double-blind PET study of first-episode schizophrenia. Am J Psychiatry. 2000;157(4):514-20.
11. Kaasinen V, Någren K, Hietala J, Farde L, Rinne JO. Sex differences in extrastriatal dopamine d(2)-like receptors in the human brain. Am J Psychiatry 2001;158(2):308-11.
12. Bouvier M, Fehsel K, Schmitt A, Meisenzahl-Lechner E, Gaebel W, von Wilmsdorff M. Sex-dependent alterations of dopamine receptor and glucose

transporter density in rat hypothalamus under long-term clozapine and haloperidol medication. Brain Behav. 2020;10(8):e01694.
13. Lako IM, van den Heuvel ER, Knegtering H, Bruggeman R, Taxis K. Estimating dopamine D_2 receptor occupancy for doses of 8 antipsychotics: a meta-analysis. J Clin Psychopharmacol 2013;33(5):675-81.
14. Cosgrove KP, Mazure CM, Staley JK. Evolving Knowledge of Sex Differences in Brain Structure, Function and Chemistry. Biol Psychiatry. 2007;62(8):847-55.
15. Aanerud J, Borghammer P, Rodell A, Jónsdottir KY, Gjedde A. Sex differences of human cortical blood flow and energy metabolism. J Cereb Blood Flow Metab. 2017;37(7):2433-40.
16. Seeman MV. The Pharmacodynamics of Antipsychotic Drugs in Women and Men. Front Psychiatry. 2021;12:650904.
17. Li XH, Zhong XM, Lu L, Zheng W, Wang SB, Rao WW, et al. The prevalence of agranulocytosis and related death in clozapine-treated patients: a comprehensive meta-analysis of observational studies. Psychol Med. 2020;50(4):583-94.
18. Bett GCL. Hormones and sex differences: changes in cardiac electrophysiology with pregnancy. Clin Sci (Lond). 2016;130(10):747-59.
19. Castellani LN, Costa-Dookhan KA, McIntyre WB, Wright DC, Flowers SA, Hahn MK, et al. Preclinical and Clinical Sex Differences in Antipsychotic-Induced Metabolic Disturbances: A Narrative Review of Adiposity and Glucose Metabolism. J Psychiatr Brain Sci. 2019;4:e190013.
20. Sørup FKH, Eriksson R, Westergaard D, Hallas J, Brunak S, Andersen SE. Sex differences in text-mined possible adverse drug events associated with drugs for psychosis. J Psychopharmacol 2020;34(5):532-9.
21. LeGates TA, Kvarta MD, Thompson SM. Sex differences in antidepressant efficacy. Neuropsychopharmacology. 2019;44(1):140-54.
22. Sramek JJ, Murphy MF, Cutler NR. Sex differences in the psychopharmacological treatment of depression. Dialogues Clin Neurosci. 2016;18(4):447-57.
23. de Vries ST, Denig P, Ekhart C, Burgers JS, Kleefstra N, Mol PGM, et al. Sex differences in adverse drug reactions reported to the National Pharmacovigilance Centre in the Netherlands: An explorative observational study. Br J Clin Pharmacol. 2019;85(7):1507-15.
24. Henry C. Lithium side-effects and predictors of hypothyroidism in patients with bipolar disorder: sex differences. J Psychiatry Neurosci. 2002;27(2):104-7.
25. Viguera AC, Tondo L, Baldessarini RJ. Sex Differences in Response to Lithium Treatment. Am J Psychiatry. 2000;157(9):1509-11.
26. Selvarajan S, Srinivasan A, Sakkarabani P, Verma A, Rajendran P, Kandasamy P. Genetic polymorphisms influencing response to lithium in early-onset Bipolar disorder from south India. Asian J Psychiatr. 2022;70:103018.
27. Herzog AG, Blum AS, Farina EL, Maestri XE, Newman J, Garcia E, et al. Valproate and lamotrigine level variation with menstrual cycle phase and oral contraceptive use. Neurology. 2009;72(10):911-4.
28. Patsalos PN. Drug interactions with the newer antiepileptic drugs (AEDs)--Part 2: pharmacokinetic and pharmacodynamic interactions between AEDs and drugs used to treat non-epilepsy disorders. Clin Pharmacokinet. 2013;52(12):1045-61.
29. Bauer J, Isojärvi JIT, Herzog AG, Reuber M, Polson D, Taubøll E, et al. Reproductive dysfunction in women with epilepsy: recommendations for evaluation and management. J Neurol Neurosurg Psychiatry. 2002;73(2):121-5.

30. Menculini G, Steardo L, Sciarma T, D'Angelo M, Lanza L, Cinesi G, et al. Sex Differences in Bipolar Disorders: Impact on Psychopathological Features and Treatment Response. Frontiers Psychiatry. 2022;13:926594.
31. Farkouh A, Riedl T, Gottardi R, Czejka M, Kautzky-Willer A. Sex-Related Differences in Pharmacokinetics and Pharmacodynamics of Frequently Prescribed Drugs: A Review of the Literature. Adv Ther. 2020;37(2):644-55.
32. Bartkowiak-Wieczorek J, Wolski H, Bogacz A, Kujawski R, Ożarowski M, Majchrzycki M, et al. Gender-specific implications for pharmacology in childbearing age and in postmenopausal women. Ginekol Pol. 2015;86(2):143-9.
33. Arakawa R, Okumura M, Ito H, Takano A, Takahashi H, Takano H, et al. Positron emission tomography measurement of dopamine D_2 receptor occupancy in the pituitary and cerebral cortex: relation to antipsychotic-induced hyperprolactinemia. J Clin Psychiatry. 2010;71(9):1131-7.
34. Schoretsanitis G, Spigset O, Stingl JC, Deligiannidis KM, Paulzen M, Westin AA. The impact of pregnancy on the pharmacokinetics of antidepressants: a systematic critical review and meta-analysis. Expert Opin Drug Metab Toxicol. 2020;16(5):431-40.
35. Dawkins K, Potter WZ. Gender differences in pharmacokinetics and pharmacodynamics of psychotropics: focus on women. Psychopharmacol Bull. 1991;27(4):417-26.
36. Clark CT, Newmark RL, Wisner KL, Stika C, Avram MJ. Lithium Pharmacokinetics in the Perinatal Patient With Bipolar Disorder. J Clin Pharmacol. 2022;62(11):1385-92.
37. Yonkers KA, Little BB, March D. Lithium during pregnancy: Drug effects and their therapeutic implications. CNS Drugs. 1998;9(4):261-9.
38. Johnson JL, Greaves L, Repta R. Better science with sex and gender: Facilitating the use of a sex and gender-based analysis in health research. Int J Equity Health. 2009;8(1):14.
39. Heidari S, Babor TF, De Castro P, Tort S, Curno M. Sex and Gender Equity in Research: rationale for the SAGER guidelines and recommended use. Res Integr Peer Rev. 2016;1(1):2.
40. Peters SAE, Babor TF, Norton RN, Clayton JA, Ovseiko PV, Tannenbaum C, et al. Fifth anniversary of the Sex And Gender Equity in Research (SAGER) guidelines: taking stock and looking ahead. BMJ Glob Health. 2021;6(11):e007853.
41. EASE. The SAGER Guidelines. [online] Available from https://ease.org.uk/communities/gender-policy-committee/the-sager-guidelines/ [Last accessed December, 2023].
42. Epps HV, Astudillo O, Martin YDP, Marsh J. The Sex and Gender Equity in Research (SAGER) guidelines: Implementation and checklist development. Eur Sc Ed. 2022;48:e86910.

Index

Page numbers followed by *b* refer to box, *f* refer to figure, *fc* refer to flowchart, and *t* refer to table

A

Absorption 470, 473
Abuse 129
Acetylcholine 255
Acne 254
Acquired immunodeficiency syndrome 137, 353, 393
Acute agitation, management of 235, 236*b*
Adenosine triphosphate 167
Adjustment disorder 215, 257
Adrenarche 271
Adult separation anxiety, self-report measure of 44
Aggression 36, 430
Agoraphobia 41, 42, 44
Agranulocytosis 8, 188, 475, 478
Akathisia, chronic 455
Albumin-bound drugs 188
Alcohol 131, 132, 140, 240
　anonymity 135
　dependence 136
　effects of 126
　metabolism of 125, 126, 126*t*
　scale, clinical institute withdrawal assessment for 190
　use 131
　　disorder identification test 131, 132
Allopregnanolone 242
Alpha-2 norepinephrine agonist 139
Alprazolam 222, 472, 479
Amalgamation 205
Amenorrhea
　drug-induced 228
　hypothalamic 477
American College of Obstetrics and Gynecology 243
American Psychiatric Association 151
Amitriptyline 472
Amnesia, dissociative 83, 84
Amphetamine 139, 240
Amygdala 36
　volumes 81
Anal penetration 349
Androgens 38, 478
Anergia 183
Anger 430
Anode 455
Anorexia nervosa 64
Anorgasmia 186
Antenatal depression 414
　prevalence of 299
Anterior cingulate cortex 54, 82
Anthropometry 282
Anticonvulsant
　mood stabilizers 477
　serum levels 476
Antidepressants 40, 49, 185, 186, 204, 221, 225, 228, 231, 233, 472, 475, 477-479
　effects of 48
　medications 48
　resistance 183
　response 36
　serum concentrations 479
　use of 47
Antiepileptics 186
　medication polytherapy 464
Antihistamine 236
Antihistaminics 185
Antihypertensives 185, 186
Antiobsessive medication 221
Antiparkinsonian drugs 185
Antipsychotics 204, 226, 228, 230, 233, 243, 474, 475, 477, 478
　drugs 8, 11
　efficacy 478
　first-generation 230, 236, 242, 243
　medication, high dose of 11
　second-generation 191, 230, 236, 243
Antisocial personality disorder 127
Anxiety 45, 125, 131, 132, 177, 180, 190, 244, 250, 254, 257, 285, 294, 295, 298, 306, 333, 390, 430, 431
　biopsychosocial model of 43
　disorders 33, 36, 41, 45-47, 77, 112, 219, 257, 260, 271, 272, 276, 335
　　assessment of 44
　　epidemiology 41
　　selective 41
　　separation 42, 44
　　social 41, 61, 83
　higher chronic prevalence of 445
　higher risk of 299

mild-moderate 428
minimal 428
mixed 257
severe 428
subscale 426
Anxiolytic 233
Apathy 183
Apomorphine 170
Aripiprazole 54, 223
Arizona sexual experience scale 162, 417, 422
Arthralgia 338
Atomoxetine 139
Attention-deficit hyperactivity disorder 123, 124, 132, 299
    prevalence of 434
    treatment of 139
Attitude and heading reference system 463
Augmentation agents 54
Autism 434
    spectrum condition 434
Autoimmune disorders 186
Autonomy, lack of 199
Awareness, lack of 297, 380

B

Basal ganglia 176
Beck's depression inventory 39, 190, 416, 463
Beck's suicidal intent scale 190
Behavioral disturbances 203
Below poverty line status 8
Benzodiazepines 186, 191, 222, 225, 233, 237, 240, 243, 471
    activity of 472
    clinical institute withdrawal assessment for 190
    coadministration of 472
    dependence 138
    oxidized 479
    receptor binding of 479
    withdrawal 138
Beta-blockers 185
Bethlem mother-infant interaction scale 431
Binge eating disorder 64
Biopsychosocial paradigms 405
Bio-socio-occupational dysfunction 94
Bipolar affective disorder 390
Bipolar disease, late-onset 184

Bipolar disorders 39, 46, 183, 184, 284, 390
    early-onset 184
    neurobiology of 284
Bipolar illness 284, 445
Birth
    defects 225, 226
    premature 11
    weight, low 11
Bisexual 335, 336
Bleeding 188
Blood alcohol
    concentration 126, 127
    level 126
Blood-brain barrier 275, 471
Blunted cortisol response 334
Bodily distress disorder 78
Body
    dissatisfaction, levels of 67
    mass index 6, 189, 443
    temperature rhythm, blunted amplitude of 281
Body dysmorphic disorder 52, 57, 61, 62, 112
    epidemiology 57
    etiology 60
    evaluation 61
    examination 61
    treatment 61
Body focused repetitive behaviors
    clinical features 63
    disorders 52, 62
    epidemiology 62
    etiology 63
    treatment 64
Borderline personality disorder 87, 196-198, 203, 205, 297, 449
    diagnostic criteria for 198*b*
Brain 78
    derived neurotrophic factor 284
Breast
    cancer 49
    milk production, abnormal 11
Breastfeeding, benefits of 48
Breathing 305
Bremelanotide 170*t*, 171
Brexanolone 242
Brief psychiatric rating scale 425
Bulimia nervosa 64
Bupropion 137, 154, 170, 191
Burning 456
Burst stimulation 454
Buspirone 222

Index 487

C

Cambridge worry scale 424
Canadian Network for Mood and Anxiety Treatments guidelines 283
Cancer
  gynecological 249, 259
  nature of 259
Candidiasis 158
Cannabis 132, 138, 140
  abuse screening test 132
  use 138
Cannabis use disorder identification test 132
  revised 132
Capsaicin 169
Carbamazepine 224, 242
Cardiac arrhythmias 475, 478
Cardiovascular diseases 132
Cardiovascular disorders 186, 254
Cardiovascular malformations, risk of 139
Carolina premenstrual assessment scale 417
  scoring system 420
Catamenial psychosis 276
Catastrophization 159
Catatonia 191
  management of 237
  stuporous conditions of 237
Cathode 455
Central nervous system 33, 86, 445, 471
  dysregulation, stress induced 159
  multiple 280
Cervical cancer 259
  screened for 336
Chemical
  agents 443
  properties 471
Chemotherapy 186
Child Welfare Committee 324
Childhood trauma 125
  questionnaire 411
Chlordiazepoxide 222
Chlorpromazine 223
Chorionic gonadotropin 217
Circadian rhythms 281
Cirrhosis 132
Clinical opioid withdrawal scale 190
Clitoris 155
Clomipramine 221
Clonazepam 222
Clonidine 139, 472

Clozapine 8, 188, 223, 474, 475
  side effects of 475
Cocaine 240
Coerced sex 350
Coercion, type of 350
Cognitive behavioral therapy 8, 18, 45, 47, 54, 59, 61, 135, 156, 165, 256, 293, 308, 356, 444
Cognitive impairment 126
Coital alignment techniques 164
Columbia-suicide severity rating scale 190
Commercial sex workers 133
Communication 19, 151
Complete blood count 444
Complex human behaviors 119
Complex posttraumatic stress disorder, prevalence of 296
Composite abuse scale 407
Computer-based data collection 410
Conduct disorder 299
Confusion assessment scale 190
Connor-Dresilience scale 434
Consciousness 190
Consequences 134
Constipation 188, 478
Contraceptive
  alternatives 243
  bidirectional impact of 242b
  combined oral 252
  effects of 242
  interaction, oral 243t
  pills
    combined hormonal 46
    oral 55, 476
  planning 214, 242
Conversion disorder 77
  cause of 373
Convulsions, dissociative 89
Copper intrauterine devices 46
Cortico-limbic disconnection model 82
Cortico-striato-thalamo-cortical circuits 54
Couples therapy 135
COVID-19 pandemic 60, 285
Cranial electrotherapy stimulation 445
Crisis 203
  humanitarian 321
  major disruptive 179
  management 196
  plan 202b
Cronbach's alpha 407, 429, 433
Crying spells 272

Cultural formulation interview 365, 367, 368
  domains of 369*fc*
Culture-bound syndromes 371
Curiosity 130
Cyclic adenosine monophosphate 167
Cyclic guanosine monophosphate 167
Cytochrome P450 enzymatic system 472
Cytokines, proinflammatory 37, 38, 255

D

Daily living scale, Lawton instrumental activities of 190
Daily rating form 416, 419
Danazol 252
Death 34
Deep brain stimulation 55, 445, 447, 464, 465
  system 443, 445
Dehydroepiandrosterone 169
Delirium 190
  higher risk for 191
  rating scale 190
Delivery 225, 226
Delusions 182
Dementia 176, 177, 180, 181
  behavioral symptoms of 181
  psychological symptoms of 181
  rating scale 190
  risk factors for 180
  type of 181
Depersonalization disorder 83, 86
Depletion syndrome 183
Depression 34, 35*t*, 36, 37, 40, 47, 48, 125, 131, 132, 160, 177, 180, 182, 183, 187, 190, 244, 250, 254, 255, 257, 258, 260, 271, 272, 277, 282, 294, 295, 298, 299, 333, 335, 342, 370, 374, 380, 381, 390, 445
  antenatal 414
  bipolar 455
  development of 255
  diagnosis of 38
  disorder 257
  exacerbation of 285
  genesis of 272
  late-onset 182, 183
  low rate of 36
  management of 40, 283
  mild-to-moderate 40, 48
  neurobiology of 37
  neurotic 177

perimenopausal 39, 48, 49
perinatal 33
peripartum 39, 451, 452*t*, 454
postmenopausal 33
postnatal 299
postpartum 46, 414
preoperative history of 253
psychotic 425
risk 282
severe 444
somatic veil of 374
trigger 255
unipolar 184, 456
vascular 183
Depressive
  disorder 33, 34, 219
  mood 34
  symptoms 255
    development of 182
Derealization disorder 86
Derogatory auditory hallucinations 182
Diabetes mellitus 132, 443, 444*f*
  gestational 230
Dialectical behavior therapy 205
Diazepam 222
Dietary calcium 180
Disability 77, 190
  adjusted life 177
  higher rates of 78
Discharge per vagina 249
Discrimination 332, 343
Disruptive disorder 269
Dissociation 77, 78, 370
  disorders 77, 78, 82, 88, 96
Dissociative disorders 77, 82, 84, 84*t*, 85-87, 380
  assessment of 83
  course of 83
  outcome of 83
  section speaks of 83
  treatment of 87
Dissociative experiences scale 87, 351
Dissociative identity disorder, symptoms of 83
Distress
  idiom of 381
  psychological 18, 349
  tolerance 205
District Level Services Authority 326
District Mental Health Programme 392
Domestic abuse 293
Domestic violence 117, 373, 378, 389, 409
  questionnaire 409

Dopamine 38, 55, 56, 255, 474
   agonist 170
   receptors 477
      sensitivity of 284
   release 56
Dopaminergic agonists 166
Dorsolateral prefrontal cortex 36, 451
Dowry system, abolition of 117
Drospirenone 46
Drug 125, 469
   adverse effects 8
   interaction 243
   pharmacokinetics 479
Dual sex therapy 163
Dysbiosis 38
Dyschezia 250
Dyslipidemia 178
Dysmenorrhea 281
Dysmorphic disorder 52
Dyspareunia 186, 250
Dysphoria 338
   premenstrual 257
Dysthymia 272
Dystonia 236, 464

E

Early pubertal maturation 268
   effects of 271
Eating disorders 46, 52, 53, 64-67, 112, 125, 132, 271, 273, 294
   epidemiology 65
   etiology 65
Eating disturbance, type of 273
E-cigarettes 137
Edinburgh postnatal depression scale 425, 426
Electrical stimulation 443
Electroconvulsive therapy 40, 191, 236, 237, 238b, 443, 445-447, 449, 465
   indications of 40
Electrode 455-463
Electroencephalogram 86
Emotional
   abuse 179, 407
   distress 26, 413
   intimacy 151
   lability 128, 188
   regulation 88, 205, 334
   violence 294
Emotions 83, 365
   self-regulation of 205

Endocrine therapies 478
Endometriosis 249-251, 253
   peritoneal 250
   treatment for 251
Endometriotic ovarian cysts 250
Endometrium tissue 250
Epidemiological studies depression scale, center for 282
Epigenetics 81
   modification 37
Epochal menstrual psychosis 276
Escitalopram 221, 306, 472
Estradiol 55, 169
Estrogen 38, 56, 168, 184, 275, 284, 475, 477, 478
   fluctuations 38
   inhibits monoamino oxidase-A 55
   levels 180, 186, 445
   modulates dopamine 274
   protective role of 181
   receptors for 38
Euthymia 284
Exacerbation
   potential triggers for 233
   premenstrual 46
Excessive stimulation 373
Excretion 472
Exposure response prevention 54, 59
Exposure therapy 308
Externalizing disorders 271
Extrapyramidal side effects 285
Eye movement desensitization 308, 356
Eysenck inventory questionnaire 201

F

Fallopian tube 259
Family accommodation scale 54
Family-centric rehabilitation 26
Fantasy 155
Fat, loss of 186
Fear disorders 41
Feasibility 465
Female dhat syndrome 90
Female orgasmic disorders 155, 156, 170
   etiology of 157f
Female sexual arousal disorder 151-153, 167, 170, 421
   etiology of 155f
Female sexual distress scale revised 417, 422
Female sexual dysfunction 150, 161t, 162t, 169t, 170, 417

classification, evolution of 152*t*, 153*t*
comprehensive management of 161
concept of 150
treatment of 168*t*, 171*t*
type of 150
Female sexual functioning index 417, 422, 422*t*
Female sexual interest 151-153
   etiology of 155*f*
Female sexual pain disorders, prevalence of 158
Female sexual well-being scale 421, 423
Female suicidal behavior 112
Feminine
   gender role stress scale 412
   norms inventory 412
Feminist intervention principles 301
Fetal acidosis 450
Fetal heart rate 238
   monitoring of 235
Firearms 110
   suicide 110
First information report 354
Fistulas 259
Flibanserin 166
Fluctuations, hormonal 271*f*, 469
Fluoxetine 221, 308, 455, 472
Fluvoxamine 221
Folic acid, high-dose of 227, 230
Follicle-stimulating hormone 270
   tests 262
Follicular phase 270
Folstein mini-mental status examination 190
Forensic psychiatry 396
Frailty index 190
Free-floating anxiety 41
Frustration 130, 431
   tolerance, low 129

G

Gabapentin 306
Gamma-aminobutyric acid 36, 255
Gastric enzymes 471
Gastric pH 471
Gastrointestinal diseases 132
Gastrointestinal disorders 91
Gay 335
Gay-straight alliances 334
Gender
   based violence 130, 291, 374, 381, 406
   disadvantage 413
   discrimination 406, 413
   inequality 389
   minority 333
   responsive care 395
   role
      attitudes scale 412
      expectations 378
   sensitive
      mental health services 387
      training 327
      treatment facilities 325
   violence, lifetime spiral of 388
Generalized anxiety disorder scale 190, 429
Genetic 37, 125
   vulnerabilities 94, 125
Genital
   blood flow 166
   herpes 158
   injury 353
Genito-pelvic
   examination 158
   pain 156, 157*t*, 158, 159*t*, 169
Geriatric
   depression scale 190
   psychiatry 176
   syndrome 180
Gestalt therapy 206
Gestrinone 252
Glasgow coma scale 190
Global adult tobacco survey 124
Globus pallidus internus 449
Glomerular filtration rate 472
Glutamate 55
   levels 255
Glycogen, epithelial 186
Gonadal hormones 34
Gonadarche 271
Gonadotropin-releasing hormone agonists 46, 252
Good enough sex 164
Grounding techniques 305, 306*b*
Group psychotherapy 308
Guanfacine 139
Guilt 34, 36
   feelings of 12
   ideas of 272
Gums 137
Gut
   microbiome 38
   microbiota 38
Gynecological disorder 249, 250

H

Habit reversal therapy 64
Haloperidol 54, 223, 474
Hamilton anxiety rating scale 463
Hamilton depression rating scale 39, 190, 463
Hanging 110
Harassment 407
Hatzenbuehler's framework 332
Headache 338
Health
    disparities 342
    problems 293
Heart
    defects, congenital 140
    diseases, chronic 178
Helplessness 183
    feelings of 180
Hepatitis
    B 353
    C virus 132
Hirsutism 254
Histamine-2 receptor antagonists 450
Homelessness 27, 34, 36, 183
Homophobia, internalized 332, 333, 340
Homosexuality, depathologizing 332
Hormonal disorders 186
Hormone 166, 478
    influence of 55
    mediated modulation 469
    replacement therapy 178, 285, 478
Hospital anxiety and depression scale 427
Human immunodeficiency virus 27, 132, 137, 353, 393
    heightened risk of 298
    infection 10, 393
    transmission of 130
Human rights and mental illness 317
Human sexual response cycle 150
Hydroxytryptamine receptor 477
Hygiene 323
Hyperactive-impulse symptoms, symptom severity for 128
Hyperactivity disorder 128
Hyperandrogenism 255, 477
Hyperchromocysteinemia 180
Hyperinsulinism 477
Hyperprolactinemia 475, 477, 478
Hypersomnia disorders 185
Hypertension 139, 186, 443, 444f
Hypervigilance 159
Hypnotics 231
    benzodiazepine receptor agonists 477
Hypoactive sexual desire disorder 151, 152, 167, 169t, 170, 170t, 421
Hypoestrogenism 262
Hypogonadism 262
Hyponatremia 188
Hypospadias 140
Hypotension, orthostatic 180, 236
Hypothalamic-pituitary-adrenal axis 38, 255, 334
    systems 89
Hypothalamus 56
Hypothesis, inflammatory 33
Hypothyroidism 186, 443, 444
Hypoxia 450
Hysterectomy 249, 252, 253
    small proportion of 253
Hysteria 79, 80, 370
    cause of 372, 372t, 373

I

Illness
    explanatory model of 376
    stage of 44
Imipramine 472
Imperforate hymen 158
Impulsive-aggressive personality traits 37
In vitro fertilization 478
India patriarchy index 411
Indian Council of Medical Research 399
    Task Force Study on Domestic and Partner Violence 408
Indian Disability Evaluation and Assessment Scale 190
Indian Family Violence and Control Scale 409
Indian Interpersonal Trauma Interview 411
Infanticide 213
    risk assessment 235, 235t
Infections 158
    perinatal 139
    vaginal 132
Infectious diseases 17, 27
Infertility 249, 251, 254-257, 375
    cause of 257
    diagnosis of 257
Inflammation 33, 37, 38
Inflammatory response systems 160
Influence immune cell population 38
Insensitive reactions 353
Insomnia 185, 233
Insulin resistance 255

International Classification of Diseases 34, 35, 41, 42, 79t, 153, 156, 157
International Classification of Mental And Behavioral Disorders 214
International Personality Disorder Examination 201
International Society for Traumatic Stress Studies 356
Interpersonal therapy 67
Intimate partner violence 293, 296f, 298, 300-302, 389, 406
  assessment of 303
  impact of 299
  mental health impact of 294, 299
  perpetrators of 300
  screening tool 131
  signs of 304
  type of 348
Intimate personal violence 374
Intrauterine growth restriction 136
Irritation 165
Ischemia 139
Isolation 12
Isozyme 472
Itching 456

K

Katz index 190
Kegel exercises 163
Kidney
  diseases, chronic 178
  function test 444

L

Labia majora 186
Labiaplasty 62
Lactation 25, 48, 213, 225, 226, 233t, 392
  advice 233
  Hales category for 221-224
  labeling rule 220
Lamotrigine 54, 224, 231
Language
  barriers 381
  sensitive use of 389
Large-scale epidemiologic catchment area study 182
Late luteal phase dysphoric disorder 414
Lesbian 335, 336
Levator ani, hypertonicity of 186
Levodopa 185
Lewy body dementia 185
Limbic system 176

Lipid profile 444
Lipophilic nature 470
Lipopolysaccharide 38
Lithium 224, 225, 228, 231, 232, 479
  efficacy 476
  teratogenicity of 479
Liver
  disease 132, 178
  function test 444
  injury 126
Lives model 356b
Loneliness 333, 334
Lorazepam 222, 237
Lozenges 137
Lubricants 261
Lung diseases, chronic 178
Luteal phase 270
Luteinizing hormone 262, 270

M

Magnetic seizure therapy 443, 445, 447, 449, 465
Mahatma Gandhi National Rural Employment Guarantee Act 20
Major depressive disorder 36, 187, 390, 449
  treatment for 451
Major depressive episode 449
Major psychiatric disorders 37
Malformation, congenital 140
Malignancy 478
Manchester scale 190
Mania 231, 425
Marijuana screening inventory 132
Marital therapy 252
Masculine norms inventory 412
Massage, form of 235
Masturbation 164
Maternal infant attachment disorders 214, 234, 234t
Mayhem personality disorder 196
Medroxyprogesterone acetate 252
Melancholic depressive episodes 35
Melanocortin 4 receptor 170
Memantine 54
Membranes, premature rupture of 299
Memory 83
  long-term 139
  pain related 93
Menarche 268, 271, 405, 414
Menopause 158, 162, 178, 268, 282-284, 405, 414, 432
  process of 432
  rating scale 433

Menstrual abnormality 228
Menstrual bleeding 250, 282
Menstrual cycle 11, 66, 268-270, 274, 469, 478
    effects of 280
    phases of 270, 271
Menstrual distress questionnaire 415, 418
Menstrual hygiene 22
Menstrual irregularities 254
Menstrual psychosis 275
    type of 276, 276*t*
Menstruation 414
Mental disorders 177, 200, 228, 229*fc*, 230, 233, 243, 244, 244*t*, 405
    diagnostic and statistical manual of 78, 79*t*, 151, 152*t*, 153, 156, 157, 199, 279, 420
    management of 220, 227, 230
    prevalence of 445
    several 366
    severe 25, 298
    stigma of 379
Mental health 80, 249, 253, 261, 268, 280, 282, 293, 302, 331, 365-367, 380, 382, 387, 443
    assessments 341
    concerns 338
    condition 215, 216
    consequences 348, 351
    disorders 114, 269, 295, 297
        assessment of 341
    establishments 322
    issues 214, 294, 298, 331, 333
    outcomes 348
    practitioner 257, 367
    problems 293, 298, 300, 381
    professionals 349
        shortage of 26
    Review Board 322
    services 137
Mental Healthcare Act 244*f*, 316, 321, 327, 396
Mental illness 10, 11, 27, 116, 131, 155, 177, 219*b*, 242, 316-320, 323, 323*t*, 324, 326, 351, 366, 370, 370*t*, 378, 391
    experience of 387
    impact of 218
    individual's experience of 366
    maternal 219
    nature of 390
    severe 3, 16, 318, 405

Mental scars 348
Mental status
    assessment 189
    examination 443
Metabolic derangements 475, 478
Metabolic syndrome 186
Metabolism 126, 472
Methylphenidate 139
Meyer's minority stress model explores 332
Michigan alcoholism screening test 132
Migration 375, 381
Millon clinical multiaxial inventory 201
Mind-body interventions 308
Mindfulness 88, 165, 205
    based stress reduction 165
    interventions, type of 165
    techniques 164
Minilaparotomy 253
Mini-mental state examination 444*f*, 452
Minnesota multiphasic personality inventory 201
Minority stress 338, 343
    impacts 334
    influence cognitive processes 334
Mirtazapine 191, 221
Modafinil 139
Modulate intracellular signaling pathways 284
Mons pubis 186
Montgomery-Åsberg depression rating scale 39, 190, 463
    score 444
Montreal cognitive assessment 190
Mood
    constellation of 45
    disorders 33, 45, 77, 176, 177
    dysfunction, predictive of 178
    elevation 284
    stabilizers 204, 224, 226, 228, 231, 233, 242, 243, 476, 477, 479
    state assessments, profile of 416
    swings 46, 196
    symptoms 45
Mother-infant attachment disorders 57, 214, 227
Mouth, dryness of 478
Movement disorders 183
Multi-episode psychoses 6
Multiple large-scale assessments 480
Multiple somatic symptoms 80

Muscle
    dysmorphia 60
    relaxation 305
    tone 158
Myalgia 338
Myocardial infarction 139

N

Narcolepsy 185
Narrative exposure therapy 308, 356
National AIDS Control Organization 393
National Commission for Women 319
National Epidemiologic Survey on Alcohol and Related Conditions analysis 337
National Family Health Survey 349, 408
National Health and Social Life Survey 186
National Human Rights Commission 317
National Institute of Medicine 336
National Institute of Mental Health and Neurosciences 319
National Institute on Drug Abuse quick screen 131
National Mental Health Study 34, 282
Neonatal withdrawal syndrome 231
Neural dysregulation 125
Neuroactive steroids, formation of 46
Neurodegenerative disorders, manifestations of 185
Neurodevelopmental disorders 434
Neuroendocrine responses 391
Neurological disorders 177
Neuromodulation 213, 443, 444, 446, 464
    noninvasive 443
    techniques 443, 445fc, 465t
    therapies 214
Neuroplasticity 217
Neuropsychiatric inventory 190
Neurostimulation, feature of 446
Neurotransmitter
    imbalance of 255
    mechanisms 277
    regulation 469
Nicotine
    dependence
        smokeless tobacco, Fagerstrom test for 131
        test for 131
    replacement therapy 137
NIMHANS maternal behavior scale 432
Nitric oxide 167
    synthase 167

N-methyl-D-aspartate 38
Norepinephrine reuptake inhibitor 45, 139, 252, 444, 444f
Nucleus
    accumbens 56
    subthalamic 449
Nutritional deficiencies 39

O

Obesity 255
    morbid 444
Obsessive-compulsion disorder 46, 52, 53, 55, 56, 59, 83, 236, 449, 464, 465
    prevalence of 57
    symptoms of 425, 427
Obstructive sleep apnea syndrome 185
Olanzapine 191, 223, 230, 236, 472
Opiates 186
Opioid 134, 138, 140, 241
Oppositional defiant disorder 129
Orbitofrontal cortex 54
Organ damage 126
Orgasm
    dysfunction, form of 251
    satisfaction 421
Orgasmic disorder 155, 156t, 162
Orofacial clefts 140
Osteoarthritis 186
Osteoporosis 180
Ovarian failure 186
Ovarian hormones fluctuate 43
Ovarian insufficiency, primary 249
Ovulation 270
    induction, cycles of 257
Oxcarbazepine 242
Oxidative stress pathways 82
Oxytocin 60, 89, 171
    response 391

P

Pain 186, 233
    focused hypothesis 251
    mapping 158
    processing 81
Panic disorder 41, 42, 44, 83
    severity scale 44
Parkinson's disease 449, 464
Paroxetine 47, 221, 228, 308
Patriarchal beliefs scale 412
Patriarchy 411

Pelvic
  floor
    muscles 158
    tone 159
  inflammatory disease 353
  muscle physiotherapy 164
  pain 338, 353
Penetration
  depth of 447
  disorders 156, 157t, 158, 159t, 169
Perceived gender discrimination scale 414
Perimenopaus disorders 414
Perinatal anxiety
  disorder 215
  screening scale 428
Perinatal depressive disorder 215
Perinatal mental disorders 214, 217, 242, 243, 405
  intrapartum management of 231
  magnitude of 214
  management of 229
  nosological status of 214, 214b
  postnatal management of 232
Perinatal mental health 214, 421
  conditions
    course of 215t
    spectrum of 214
  team 231
Perinatal obsessive-compulsion
    disorder 216
  assessment of 58t
  management of 57
  treatment of 58t
Perinatal obsessive-compulsion scale 427
Perinatal period 62, 118, 218, 299, 427, 446
Perinatal post-traumatic stress
    disorder 216
Perinatal psychiatric disorders
    management 237
Perineal membrane 186
Peripartum period 218, 479
Peripartum psychiatric disorders 457t
Peripheral vascular disease 186
Personality assessment
  inventory 201
  schedule 201
Personality disorder 197, 199b, 200, 201, 203, 204, 207, 208b, 294, 297, 300
  development pathway of 197
  evidence-based treatment for 205
  interview 201
  pathology of 203
  specific 204

Personality traits 36, 37, 197
Pesticide ingestion 110
Pharmacodynamics 469, 474, 479
Pharmacokinetics 169, 170, 469, 470, 473
Pharmacotherapy 45
Phenomenology 54, 59, 62
Phobia, specific 41, 42, 44
Phosphenes 456
Phosphodiesterase 5 inhibitors 167
Physical abuse 407
Physical scars 348
Placental corticotropin-releasing
    hormone 217
Plasma sertraline levels 479
Poisoning 110
Polycystic ovarian syndrome 55, 249, 254-256
  risk of 477
Polysomnography 280
Poor mental health, roots of 368
Positive and negative syndrome
    scale 190, 425
Positron emission tomography 474
Postassault safety, lower
    perceptions of 349
Post-hysterectomy syndrome 253
Postmenopausal obsessive compulsion
    disorder 57
Postpartum bonding questionnaire 234, 430, 430t
Postpartum disorders 383
Postpartum period 25, 36, 62, 116, 299, 425
Post-traumatic stress disorder 82, 86, 125, 132, 137, 180, 205, 294, 296, 338, 348, 350, 375, 391, 456, 463
Pregnancy 11, 25, 47, 48, 135, 139, 213, 217, 219, 225-227, 229, 375, 392, 405, 414, 424, 455, 469, 478
  effect of 479
  high-risk 229
  medical termination of 399
  related anxiety questionnaire-revised 425
  stages of 225t
  unwanted 353
Premature ovarian insufficiency 262
  mental health implications of 262
Premenstrual assessment form 415, 418
Premenstrual dysphoric disorder 33, 45, 46, 268, 277, 279, 281, 414
Premenstrual experiences, calendar of 416, 419

Premenstrual period 36
Premenstrual symptom 277
    screening tool 39, 416, 419
Premenstrual syndrome 277, 281, 414, 418*t*
Prenatal fetal attachment scale 234
Prenatal substance abuse screen 132
Progesterone 38, 56, 217, 284, 479
    increasing amount of 270
    receptors for 38
    role of 56
Progestins 478
Prokinetic drugs 450
Promethazine 236
Prostaglandins
    E1 167
    inhibitors 167
Protein binding determines 471
Proton pump inhibitors 450
Pseudo-seizures 89
Psoriasis 186
Psychiatric
    assessment, components of 189*b*
    comorbidities 132, 134
    conditions 455
    disorders 116, 176-178, 257, 269, 278, 279, 366, 370, 414, 455
        assessment of 187, 200, 339
        impact of 176, 177
        postpartum 376
        pre-existing 257
        pregnancy related 382
        risk factors for 178
        specific 180
    homes, review of 327
    illness 81, 112, 159, 368
        severe 3, 16
    label 89
    morbidity 118, 274
    screening 94
    services 387
Psychiatry
    health 80
    perinatal 213, 214
    reproductive 211
Psychoeducation 18, 59, 163
Psychological aggression 389
Psychological disturbances 249, 257, 259, 260
Psychological health 177, 304
Psychological intervention 140, 348, 355
Psychological therapies, use of 381

Psychological violence 294
Psychometric properties 418-420, 422, 423, 426
Psychomotor
    agitation 34
    retardation 183, 272
Psychoneuroimmunology pathway 258
Psychopathology stressors 119
Psychopharmacological agents, usage of 214
Psychopharmacology, general principles of 469
Psychosexual dysfunctions 152
Psychosis 61, 160, 231, 274, 275, 284, 294, 391, 425
    increasing risk for 339
    mid cycle 276
    paramenstrual 276
    postpartum 213, 216, 414
    premenstrual 276
Psychosocial dimension 7
Psychosocial factors 35, 35*t*, 43, 176, 262, 338
    influence of 269
Psychosocial groups 24
Psychosocial interventions 18, 150
    cognitive interventions for 19
Psychosocial screening programs 118
Psychosomatic disorders 80
Psychostimulants 185
Psychotherapy 40, 45, 48, 49, 88, 205
    psychodynamic 88
    supportive 206
Psychotic disorders 176, 181, 191, 238, 335, 339
Psychotic symptoms 444
    frequencies of 366
Psychotropics 213, 242, 469
    class 233
    decrease metabolism of 242
    drugs 218
    increase metabolism of 242
    pharmacodynamics of 469, 474, 477*t*
    safety data, interpretation of 220
    tolerability of 366
    use of 33
Pubarche 271
Puberty 36, 43, 65, 269, 274
    early 273
    marker of 271
    onset of 199
Pubic hair, reduction of 186

Index 497

Q
Quetiapine 223, 230

R
Raloxifene 285
Randomized controlled trial 169, 465
Rape 350
Rapid eye movement 185, 280
Receptor blockade, degree of 474
Recurrent depressive disorder 444
Rehabilitation 13, 16, 21, 22
    centers 326
    programs 18
    psychosocial 16, 17
Repetitive transcranial magnetic stimulation 55, 444, 445, 449, 451, 452
Reproductive
    disorders 268
    health 336
    hormones
        influence of 33
        role of 36
    life span 36
Resilience 306, 434
Restless leg syndrome 185
Restrictive food intake disorder 64
Rhinoplasty 62
Risperidone 54, 191, 223
Ritz point 394
Rugae, loss of 162
Rumination disorder 64

S
Sad person scale 190
Sanitary napkins 320
    disposal facilities for 323
Schema-focused therapy 206
Schizophrenia 4, 9, 11, 17, 25, 26, 46, 181, 190, 219, 231, 275, 285, 391, 425
    challenges of 7
    early-onset 182
    late-onset 181, 182
    research foundation 20
    spectrum disorders 11, 284
Sclerosis, multiple 186
Sedation 188, 478
Sedative 231, 233
Seizures, psychogenic nonepileptic 455
Selective mutism 42, 44
    Frankfurt scale of 44
Selective norepinephrine reuptake inhibitor 45
Selective serotonin reuptake inhibitors 45, 167, 204, 231, 233, 243, 252, 444, 444*f*, 470, 477
    treatment 154
Self-assessment symptom inventory 434
Self-harm 108, 110, 119, 297, 333, 380, 391
    elevated risk of 297
    episodes 109
    largest proportion of 108
Self-help groups 21, 26
Self-immolation 110, 112
Self-report questionnaire 24
Self-stigma 393
Sensorimotor stimulation, adequate 235
Sensory modulation disorder 452
Serious mental illnesses 16
    diagnosis of 16
Serotonin 38, 255
    neurons 55
    reuptake inhibitor 45, 61, 444, 444*f*
        high-dose of 54
    transporter 55
Sertraline 47, 221, 308
Severe mental illness 3, 16, 318, 405
    symptoms of 231, 232*fc*
Sex
    chromosomes 38
    differences 36, 470, 473, 474, 476, 479
    hormones 445
        role of 269
    specific differences 476
        reporting of 480
    steroids 38
        hormones 478
Sexist events, schedule of 413
Sexual abuse 17
    childhood 93, 318, 351
    victimization 351
Sexual act 349
Sexual arousal 154
    low 154
Sexual assault, long-term impact of 353
Sexual coercion 318
Sexual contact, type of 349
Sexual cycle 176
Sexual difficulties 261
Sexual disorders 176, 336
Sexual dysfunction 152, 154, 160, 161, 186, 228, 251, 253, 254, 256, 258, 260, 298
    concept of 150

genesis of 161
posthysterectomy 254
presence of 421
prevalence rates of 186
Sexual education 261
Sexual experiences survey 410
Sexual fantasy, frequencies of 186
Sexual function questionnaire 421, 423
Sexual functioning 259, 414, 417
Sexual harassment 348, 413
Sexual health 336
Sexual identity disclosure 339
Sexual interest, low 154
Sexual intimate partner violence 350
Sexual maturation 271
Sexual minority
    community 340
    groups 343
    populations 337
Sexual orientation 366
    concealment of 332
Sexual problems 150, 159, 160, 162, 186, 190
Sexual quality 421
Sexual quotient 421, 423
Sexual stigma 342
Sexual victimization 11
Sexual violence 294, 298, 348, 349, 351, 358, 409
    characteristics of 349
    context of 399
    disclosure of 353
    medicolegal care for victims of 355
    prevalence of 348
    risk of 352f
    survivors of 351, 356
    victimization 351
Sexuality 10, 258
Sexually transmitted
    diseases 137, 318
    infections 131, 306, 336, 351, 353
        risk of 11
Shiny vaginal secretions, lack of 162
Shock, cultural 368
Shorter rapid eye movement latency 184
Sildenafil 167
Single-photon emission computed tomography 60
Skill-based therapy 205
Skin picking disorder 61, 62
Sleep 176, 280, 281
    behavioral disorders 185
    deprivation 56
    disorders 184, 336
    disturbances 91, 280, 281, 306
    duration 281
    efficiency 280
    hygiene education 261
    problem 185, 190
    quality 280
Social impairment 134
Social phobia 44
    inventory 44
Social support 352
    role of 352
Sodium citrate 450
Somatic symptoms 45, 80, 91, 94, 370
    scale 91
Somatization 77, 78, 80, 338, 374, 381
    disorders 77, 78, 82, 83, 90-92, 96, 337, 366
        assessment of 93
        clinical delineation of 91
        treatment of 94, 96f
    prevalence of 92
Somatoform expression 380
Somatostatin, reduced expression of 36
Somatothymic symptoms 80
South Asian Women's Social Isolation 374
Spinal injuries 186
Spousal sexual violence 350
Stafford interview 427
Steroids 38, 185
Stigma 10-12, 116, 255, 301, 333, 343, 373, 380, 381
    fear of 381
    intersectional 12
Stimulus parameters 457-463
Stress 33, 37, 81, 89, 125, 130, 178, 214, 340, 391
    interpersonal 373
    reduction exercises 305
    response 334
    sources of 177
    stigma related 332
Stressors 116, 254
    occupational 373
    psychosocial 119
Substance abuse 160, 190, 204, 294
    and mental health services administration 357, 382, 392
Substance misuse 295
Substance use 123, 135, 177, 273, 296, 390
    disorders 36, 113, 123, 133f, 135, 137t, 160, 161, 239, 276, 377, 382
        developing severe forms of 377

diagnosis of 131
epidemiology of 124
management of 135, 140t, 213, 239
therapies 214
patterns 129, 134t
perinatal 136
prevalence of 123, 124t
risk profile-pregnancy scale 132
Suffocation 110
Suicidal behavior 111, 112, 118, 119, 348
context of 119
methods of 110
spectrum of 119
Suicidal ideation 36
Suicidal prevention, interventions for 118f
Suicidal thoughts 294, 297
Suicidality 115b, 116b, 179, 333, 342
general theory of 114
Suicide 9, 34, 36, 108, 109, 119, 176, 187, 190, 213, 235, 235t, 280, 337, 378, 391
contemplate 299
deaths 109
elevated risk of 297
media reporting of 116
prevention
gender specific interventions for 116
interventions 115
strategies 115, 116
risk
assessment 235
factors of 36
Swartz somatization index 91
Sweating 478
Sympathetic nervous system 160
Systemic lupus 186

T

Tadalafil 167
Tardive dyskinesia 191, 474, 475, 478
Telepsychiatry program 24
Temazepam 306
Teratogenic effect 219, 477
Teratogenicity 136
Testosterone 168, 169, 445
intranasal gel 171
Thalamus 176
Thelarche 271
Thematic apperception test 201
Theta burst
stimulation 449
status of 454

Thyroid function test 444
Tissue lesions 158
Tobacco 132, 140
use 239
risk factors for 125
Tokophobia 455
Topiramate 242, 308
Toxicity 479
Transcranial alternating current
stimulation 445, 455, 463
Transcranial direct current stimulation 55, 445-447, 449, 463, 465
Transcranial electric
stimulation 443, 455, 463
Transcranial magnetic stimulation 443, 445, 447, 449, 452, 465
fetal risk factor 453
Transcranial random noise
stimulation 445, 455
Transference focused
psychotherapy 206
therapy 196
Transgender group 335
Trauma 125, 129, 293, 353, 395
effects of 306
focused cognitive behavioral
therapy 308
informed care 307, 388
interpersonal 411
multiple 388
Traumatic memory recovery 87
Tremor 478
Triazolam 479
Trichotillomania 61, 62
Tricyclic antidepressants 47, 243, 444f, 470
Trigeminal nerve stimulation 445, 456
Trustworthiness 357
Tuberculosis 186

U

Ultrasonography 463
Urinary tract infection 299
recurrent 353
Uterine 259
bleeding, abnormal 253
prolapse 253
Uterus 79, 80

V

Vagina 155
penetration of 157
Vaginal agenesis 158
Vaginal atrophy 162

Vaginal bleeding 299
Vaginal dilators 164, 261
Vaginal discharge 91
Vaginal dryness 166
Vaginal epithelium 186
Vaginal estrogen cream 261
Vaginal lubricants 169
Vaginal microbial environment 186
Vaginal moisturizer 169
Vaginal penetration, type of 158
Vaginal pH measurement 158
Vaginal secretions 186
Vaginal stenosis 259
Vaginal wall, elasticity of 186
Vague dissatisfaction 183
Vagus nerve stimulation 443, 445-447, 449, 464, 465
Validation techniques 205, 304
Valproate 224, 228, 231
Vasoactive intestinal peptide 167
Vasorelaxant 166
    effects 166
    type of 167*t*
Venlafaxine 191, 221, 308
Vernacular language translations 435
Vigilance 333
Violence 93, 318, 389
    against women scales, severity of 410
    physical 294
    risk of 336
Violent victimization, risk of 9
Visual analog scale 7
Vitamin 180
Vulvovaginal pain syndrome 166

W

Weight gain 444
    excessive 230
White discharge per vagina 249, 261
Women's health questionnaire 432
Women's mental health 316, 327, 366
Women's Refugee Commission 321
World Mental Health Report 368
Worsening 455
Worthlessness, feelings of 34

X

X chromosome 38

Y

Yale midlife study 186
Yale-brown obsessive compulsive scale 54, 428
Young mania rating scale 425

Z

Ziprasidone 236
Zolpidem 222, 470, 477